Clare Stapley.

Core Topics in Cardiothoracic Critical Care

Core Topics in Cardiothoracic Critical Care

Edited by

ANDREW KLEIN
Consultant in anaesthesia and intensive care

ALAIN VUYLSTEKE
Consultant in anaesthesia and intensive care

SAMER A.M. NASHEF
Consultant in cardiothoracic surgery

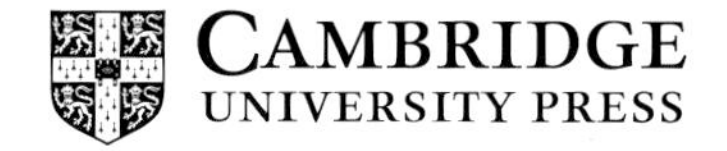

CAMBRIDGE UNIVERSITY PRESS
Cambridge, New York, Melbourne, Madrid, Cape Town, Singapore, São Paulo, Delhi

Cambridge University Press
The Edinburgh Building, Cambridge CB2 8RU, UK

www.cambridge.org
Information on this title: www.cambridge.org/9780521872836

First published 2008
Reprinted 2008

Printed in the United Kingdom at the University Press, Cambridge

A catalogue record for this publication is available from the British Library.

ISBN 978-0-521-87283-6 hardback

Contents

3.8 NEUROLOGICAL SYSTEM IN CARDIOTHORACIC CRITICAL CARE

SECTION 4 Procedure-Specific Care in Cardiothoracic Critical Care

SECTION 5 Discharge and Follow-up From Cardiothoracic Critical Care

SECTION 6 Structure and Organization in Cardiothoracic Critical Care

SECTION 7 Ethics, Legal Issues and Research in Cardiothoracic Critical Care

Contributors

S.J. Allen, MD, FCARCSI
Consultant, Cardiothoracic Anaesthesia and Intensive Care
Royal Victoria Hospital, Belfast, UK

J.E. Arrowsmith, MD, FRCP, FRCA
Consultant, Cardiothoracic Anaesthesia and Intensive Care
Papworth Hospital, Cambridge, UK

C.C. Arvieux, MD
Professor, Head of Department Anaesthesiology and Intensive Care
University Hospital of Brest, France

C.R. Bailey, FRCA
Consultant Cardiothoracic Anaesthesia
Guys and St. Thomas' Hospitals, London, UK

A.P. Barker, BMSc, MBChB, MRCS
Specialist Registrar, Cardiothoracic Surgery
Papworth Hospital, Cambridge, UK

L. Barrow, BPharm (TAS), BSc (Deakin), MRPharmS
Pharmacist, Critical Care
Papworth Hospital, Cambridge, UK

R.J. Bosman, MD
Consultant, Critical Care
Institution Onze Lieve Vrouwe Gasthuis
Amsterdam, the Netherlands

D.E.P. Bramley, MBBS, FANZCA
Staff Specialist, Anaesthesia
Western Health Melbourne, Australia

N. Breitenfeldt, PhD, MRCS
Department of Surgery
Royal Devon & Exeter Hospital, Devon, UK

S.J. Brett, MD, FRCA
Consultant and Honorary Senior Lecturer in Intensive Care
Hammersmith Hospital, London,
Imperial College, London, UK

A. Brice, BSc, MCSP
Senior Physiotherapist
Royal Brompton and Harefield NHS Trust
London, UK

C.J. Broomhead, BSc, MBBS, FRCA
Consultant, Anaesthesia
Barts and the London NHS Trust, London, UK

W.F. Buhre, MD
Consultant, Anaesthesia
University Medical Centre, Utrecht, The Netherlands

J.M. Bygott, BMedSci, MB, BS, MPHTM, FRACGP, MRCPath
Specialist Registrar
Microbiology, Addenbrooke's Hospital,
Cambridge, UK

E. Cameron, MD, MA, MB, BChir, MRCP
Consultant, Gastroenterology
Addenbrooke's Hospital, Cambridge, UK

L. Chapman, MRCP
Consultant, Palliative Medicine
Marie Curie Palliative Care Institute, Liverpool, UK

M.L. Cheatham, MD, FACS, FCCM
Director, Surgical Intensive Care Units
Orlando Regional Medical Center, Orlando, Florida, USA

D. Cheng, MD, MSc, FRCPC, FCAHS
Professor & Chair/Chief, Anesthesia & Perioperative Medicine
University of Western Ontario, Ontario, Canada

D.V. Collins, MRCP, FCARCSI, FJFICM
Consultant, Anaesthesia and Critical Care
St. Vincent's University Hospital, Dublin, Ireland

J. Cordingley, MB, ChB, FRCA, MD
Consultant, Anaesthesia & Critical Care
Royal Brompton Hospital, London, UK

A.N.G. Curry, MA, MBBChir, FRCA
SPR Anaesthetics & Intensive Care
Southampton General Hospital, UK

B.H. Cuthbertson, MBChB, FRCA, MD
Senior Lecturer, Health Service Unit
University of Aberdeen, UK

A.J. Dawson, MBChB, FANZCA
Specialist Anaesthetist
Auckland City Hospital, Auckland, New Zealand

M. De Kock
Professor, Anaesthesia and Critical Care
Cliniques Universitaires St Luc, Brussels, Belgium

B. Delvaux, MD
Fellow, Anaesthesia and Critical Care
Cliniques Universitaires St Luc, Brussels, Belgium

K. Dhital, BSc, BM BCh, FRCS-CT, PhD
Consultant, Cardiothoracic Surgery
Papworth Hospital, Cambridge, UK

N.E. Drury, BM(Hons), MRCS
Cardiothoracic Surgery
Papworth Hospital, Cambridge, UK

M. Durand, MD
Anesthesiologist and Head of Cardiovascular Intensive Care Unit
University Hospital of Grenoble, Grenoble, France

D. Dykes, BSc (Hons), MCSP
Clinical Specialist in Cardiorespiratory Physiotherapy
St. Richards Hospital, Chichester, UK

J. Eddleston, FRCA
Consultant, Critical Care
Manchester Royal Infirmary, Manchester, UK

F. Falter, MD
Consultant, Anaesthesia and Intensive Care
Papworth Hospital, Cambridge, UK

R. Feneck, MD
Consultant, Anaesthesia
St. Thomas' Hospital, London, UK

J.E. Foweraker, MA, MB, BChir, PhD, FRCPath
Consultant, Microbiology
Papworth Hospital, Cambridge, UK

M. Furlanut, MD
Professor, Director of the Institute of Clinical Pharmacology & Toxicology
Department of Experimental and Clinical Pathology and Medicine, University of Udine, Italy

S.P. Fynn, MD
Consultant, Cardiology
Papworth Hospital, Cambridge, UK

H.F. Galley, PhD
Senior Lecturer in Anaesthesia & Intensive Care
School of Medicine, University of Aberdeen, UK

M. Georgieva
Resident, Dept. of Anesthesia and Critical Care Medicine
Hadassah Hebrew University Medical School, Jerusalem, Israel

H. Gerlach
Consultant, Anesthesiology and Intensive Care Medicine
Virchow Clinic, Humboldt University, Berlin, Germany

S. Ghosh, BSc, MBBS, FFARCS
Consultant, Anaesthesia
Papworth Hospital, Cambridge, UK

F.M. Gibson, MD, FRCA, FFARCS(I)
Consultant, Anaesthesia and Critical Care
Royal Victoria Hospital, Belfast, UK

R.S. Gill, FRCA
Consultant, Anaesthesia and Intensive Care
Southampton General Hospital, Southampton, UK

C. Gillbe, FRCA, MBChB
Consultant, Critical Care & Anaesthesia
Royal Brompton Hospital, London, UK

C.D. Gomersall, MD
Consultant, Anaesthesia and Intensive Care
The Chinese University of Hong Kong, Sha Tin, Hong Kong

J. Gooi, MBBS, FRACS
Consultant, Cardiothoracic Surgery
Alfred Hospital, Melbourne, Australia

J.A. Griffiths, DICM, FRCA, MRCP, MA, MBBS
Honorary Research Associate, Nuffield Department of Anaesthetics
John Radcliffe Hospital, Oxford, UK

R. Hall, FRCA
Consultant, Anaesthesia and Intensive Care
Papworth Hospital, Cambridge, UK

D.K. Hamilton, BArch, MS
Associate Professor of Architecture
Texas A&M University, College Station, Texas, USA

S.J. Harper, MD, FRCA
Consultant, Intensive Care
Royal Liverpool University Hospital, Liverpool, UK

A. Harvey, BSc Hons, MSc, MCSP
Lecturer Practitioner Physiotherapist
Royal Brompton Hospital/Brunel University, London, UK

P.C. Hébert, MD, MHSc
Professor of Medicine, Surgery, Anesthesiology and Epidemiology
University of Ottawa
Critical Care Physician
The Ottawa Hospital
Senior Scientist
Ottawa Health Research Institute (OHRI), Ottowa, Ontario, Canada

M. Hiesmayr, MD
Professor, Cardiothoracic Anaesthesia & Intensive Care
Medical University Vienna, Austria

C.W. Hogue, MD
Staff, Anesthesiology and Critical Care
The John Hopkins University Hospital, Baltimore, Maryland, USA

P. Holder, MB, ChB, FRCA
Specialist Registrar, Critical Care
Aberdeen Royal Infirmary, Aberdeen, UK

S.P. Hoole, BM, BCh, MA, MRCP
Specialist Registrar, Cardiology
Papworth Hospital, Cambridge, UK

L.S.G.E. Howard, MA, MB, BChir, DPhil, MRCP
Consultant, Pulmonary Medicine
Hammersmith Hospital, London, UK

A.M. Ingle, RGN, RNT, BSc
Assistant Director of Nursing
Papworth Hospital, Cambridge, UK

D.P. Jenkins, BSc, MS (Lond), FRCS (Eng), FRCS (CTh)
Consultant, Cardiothoracic Surgery
Papworth Hospital, Cambridge, UK

G.M. Joynt, MD
Professor, Anaesthesia and Intensive Care
The Chinese University of Hong Kong, Sha Tin, Hong Kong

S. Kaul, BSc, MB, ChB, MRCP, AFRCS
Specialist Registrar, Respiratory and Intensive Care Medicine
London Deanery, London, UK

P. Kesteven, MB, BS, FRACP, FRCP, FRCPath, PhD
Consultant, Haematology
Freeman Hospital, Newcastle, UK

A.A. Klein, MBBS, FRCA
Consultant, Anaesthesia and Intensive Care
Papworth Hospital, Cambridge, UK

A. Koster, MD
Vice Chair, Department of Anesthesia
German Heart Centre, Berlin, Germany

P.F. Laterre, MD
Consultant, Critical Care
Cliniques Universitaires St. Luc, Brussels, Belgium

M. Leemans, FRCA
Specialist Registrar, Anaesthesia
Guys and St. Thomas' Hospital, London, UK

C. Leonard, FRCP
Consultant, Respiratory and Transplant Medicine
Wythenshawe Hospital, Manchester, UK

E. Lin, MBBS, BMed Sci, FANZCA
Consultant, Cardiothoracic Anaesthesia
The Alfred Hospital, Melbourne, Australia

J.H. Mackay, MRCP, FRCA
Consultant, Cardiothoracic Anaesthesia
Papworth Hospital, Cambridge, UK

M.L.N.G. Malbrain, MD, PhD
Director, Critical Care
Ziekenhuis Netwerk Antwerpen, Stuivenberg Hospital, Antwerp, Belgium

W.T. McBride, BSc, MD, FRCA, FFARCS(I)
Consultant, Cardiac Anaesthesia
Royal Victoria Hospital, Belfast, UK

S. McCorkell, FRCA
Consultant, Anaesthesia
Guy's and St. Thomas' Hospital, London, UK

B. McGrattan, FRCA
Clinical Fellow, Cardiothoracic Anaesthesia
Royal Victoria Hospital, Belfast, UK

A.F. Merry, MBChB, FANZCA, FFPMANZCA, FRCA
Professor and Head of Department of Anaesthesiology
University of Auckland, Auckland City Hospital, New Zealand

J. Moore, FRCA, MRCP
Specialist Registrar, Critical Care
Manchester Royal Infirmary, Manchester, UK

S. Mordzynski, MD
Resident, Department of Anesthesia and Critical Care Medicine
Hadassah Hebrew University Medical School, Jerusalem, Israel

C. Moro, MD
Consultant, Anaesthesia
Centre Hospitalier Louis Pasteur, Bagnols sur Cèze, France

S.A.M. Nashef, MB, ChB, FRCS
Consultant, Cardiothoracic Surgery
Papworth Hospital, Cambridge, UK

J. Osgathorp, RN, BSc Hons
Senior Nurse, Critical Care
Papworth Hospital, Cambridge, UK

J. Parameshwar, MD, FRCP
Consultant, Transplant Cardiology
Papworth Hospital, Cambridge, UK

F. Pea, MD
Institute of Clinical Pharmacology & Toxicology
Department of Experimental and Clinical Pathology and Medicine, University of Udine, Udine, Italy

A. Pearce, FRCA
Consultant, Anaesthesia
Guy's and St Thomas' Hospital, London, UK

G.J. Peek, FRCS, CTh
Consultant, Cardiothoracic Surgery & ECMO
Glenfield Hospital, Leicester, UK

H. Powell, MB, BS, FRCA
Consultant, Cardiothoracic Anaesthesia and Critical Care
Freeman Hospital, Newcastle, UK

S. Rex, MD
Utrecht, The Netherlands

Z. Ricci, MD
Staff Cardiothoracic and Paediatric Anesthesiology
Bambino Gesù Hospital, Rome, Italy

L.S. Ring, MBBS, MRCP
Specialist Registrar, Cardiology
Papworth Hospital, Cambridge, UK

P.J. Roberts, MD, FRCP
Consultant/Clinical Director, Gastroenterology
Hinchingbrooke Hospital, Huntingdon, UK

C. Ronco MD
Head, Department of Nephrology, Dialysis and Transplantation
S. Bortolo Hospital, Vicenza, Italy

A. Roscoe, FRCA
Consultant, Cardiothoracic Anaesthesia & Intensive Care
Wythenshawe Hospital, Manchester, UK

S.T. Runnels, MD
Assistant Professor, Anesthesia
University of Utah Medical Center,
Salt Lake City, Utah, USA

T. Ryan, MRCP, FFARCSI
Consultant, Anaesthesia & Intensive Care
Dublin, Ireland

R.A. Sayeed, MA PhD MRCP FRCS (C-Th)
Consultant, Cardiothoracic Surgery
John Radcliffe Hospital, Oxford, UK

D. Schmidlin, MD, MBA
Director, ICU
Klinik am Park, Hirslanden Group, Zürich,
Switzerland

P.M. Schofield, MD, FRCP
Consultant, Cardiology
Papworth Hospital, Cambridge, UK

W.E. Scott, MB, ChB, FRCA, DRCOG
Consultant, Anaesthesia
Derby Hospitals NHS Foundation Trust, Derby, UK

M. Screaton, RGN, MSc
Senior Nurse Practice Development, Critical Care
Papworth Hospital, Cambridge, UK

N.J. Screaton, BM, BCh, MRCP, FRCR
Consultant, Cardiothoracic Radiology
Papworth Hospital, Cambridge, UK

P.J. Shirley, MBChB, FRCA, FIMC, RCSEd, EDIC
Consultant, Intensive Care Medicine and Anaesthesia
Royal London Hospital, London, UK

D.A. Sidebotham, MBChB, FANZCA
Consultant, Anaesthesia and Intensive Care
Auckland City Hospital, Auckland, New Zealand

E.P. Smith, BSc, MBChB, MRCP, FRCR
Consultant, Radiology
University Hospital of South Manchester,
Wythenshawe, Manchester, UK

L. Spencer, MRCP
Specialist Registrar, Thoracic Medicine and Transplantation
Wythenshawe Hospital, Manchester, UK

J.D. Stearns, MD
Department of Anesthesiology and Critical Care
The Johns Hopkins University Hospital, Baltimore,
Maryland, USA

T. Strang, FRCA
Consultant, Cardiothoracic Anaesthesia
Wythenshawe Hospital, Manchester, UK

M. Thavasothy, FRCA, MD
Consultant, Anaesthesia
Royal London and St Bartholomew's Hospitals,
London, UK

B. Thomson, MD
Consultant, Cardiothoracic Surgery
Prince Charles Hospital, Brisbane, Australia

A.A. Tinmouth, MD
University of Ottawa Center for
Transfusion Research and Clinical
Epidemiology Program of the Ottawa
Health Research Institute, Ottawa,
Ontario, Canada

R. Tiruvoipati, FRCS
CESAR Trial Fellow, Cardiothoracic Surgery
University of Leicester, Leicester, UK

S. Toussaint, MD
Consultant Anesthesiology and Intensive Care Medicine
Virchow Clinic, Humboldt University,
Berlin, Germany

S.S.L. Tsui, MBBCh, MA, MD, FRCS(C-Th)
Consultant, Cardiothoracic Surgery,
Director of Transplantation
Papworth Hospital, Cambridge, UK

A.F. Turgeon, MD, FRCPC
Staff, Anaesthesiology and Critical Care Medicine
Ottawa Health Research Institute,
Ottawa Hospital, Ottawa, Canada

R.S. Ulrich, PhD
Professor, Architecture
Texas A&M University, College Station, Texas, USA

K. Valchanov, MD, FRCA
Consultant, Anaesthesia and Intensive Care
Papworth Hospital, Cambridge, UK

J. Varley, MD, FRCA
Specialist Registrar, Anaesthesia
East Anglican Deanery, UK

A. Vuylsteke, MD, FRCA
Consultant, Cardiothoracic Anaesthesia and Intensive Care
Lead Consultant Critical Care, Papworth Hospital, Cambridge, UK

T.K. Waddell MD, MSc, PhD, FRCSC, FACS
Associate Professor, Division of Thoracic Surgery
University of Toronto, Toronto General Hospital, Toronto, Ontario, Canada

S.T. Webb, MB, BCh, BAO, FRCA
Specialist Registrar, Anaesthesia & Intensive Care Medicine
Royal Victoria Hospital, Belfast, UK

C.R. Weinert, MD, MPH
Associate Professor of Medicine, Division of Pulmonary, Allergy and Critical Care
University of Minnesota Medical School, Minneapolis, Minnesota, USA

Y.G. Weiss, MD, FCCM
Senior Lecturer in Anesthesia and Critical Care Medicine
Hadassah Hebrew University Medical School, Jerusalem, Israel,
Adjunct Assistant Professor in Anesthesia and Critical Care Medicine
University of Pennsylvania Medical School, Philadelphia, Pennsylvania, USA

P.A. White, MSc, PhD, DIC, MIPEM
Consultant, Clinical Scientist,
Head of Clinical Engineering
Addenbrooke's Hospital, Cambridge, UK

J.M. Williams, FRCA
Consultant, Cardiothoracic Anaesthesia & Intensive Care
Glenfield Hospital, Leicester, UK

C.H.A. Willmott, MBChB, FANZCA
Fellow, Anaesthesia and Critical Care
Princess Alexandra Hospital, Brisbane, Australia

N. Yonan, MD, FRCS(CTh)
Consultant, Cardiothoracic Surgery, Honorary Senior Lecturer
Wythenshawe Hospital, Manchester University, Manchester, UK

R. Zarychanski, MD, FRCPC
Staff, Haematology and Critical Care
Ottawa Health Research Institute, Ottawa Hospital, Ottawa, Ontario, Canada

Preface

In the corner, a patient is recovering well after a heart operation. Even so, the lights of five infusion pumps are blinking regularly, the ventilator is sighing, the electrocardiograph, several pressures, temperature and oxygen saturation are continuously displayed and massive amounts of data are being generated and recorded, and this is when things are going well!

Elsewhere, another patient may be on an intra-aortic balloon pump, a third may be on haemofiltration, a fourth may be on a ventricular assist device and occasionally, behind drawn curtains, a mad-eyed surgeon may be performing open heart surgery on the unit due to unexpected complications.

The cardiothoracic critical care area can be a frightening place indeed.

Don't panic!

Managing the critically ill cardiothoracic patient is no different from any other patient. The principles of good clinical practice apply here as they do elsewhere. Knowing the history helps. Clinical examination, as in every field of medicine, yields valuable information.

However, critical care provides additional, hard clinical data like no other area of medical practice. Continuous and regular monitoring of physiological and haematological parameters makes most diagnoses easy to make. If there is still doubt about the status of the patient, further information is easy to obtain, whether by pulmonary artery flotation catheter, transoesophageal echocardiography or computed tomography. This is one area where most decisions are made on the basis of sound evidence rather than on a clinical hunch. All that is required is some basic knowledge, a degree of thoroughness and sound judgment.

This book aims to guide caregivers from all disciplines in the management of cardiothoracic patients during their time in the critical care environment. The work is not exhaustive nor, we hope, exhausting. It is written by experts in their fields and its primary aims are to explain and demystify the approach to various areas of cardiothoracic critical care.

We truly believe the topic of cardiothoracic critical care can be accessible and easy to learn. We hope, with this book, to have made it more so.

Thanks also to Graham Hilton for photographs, including the cover.

Andrew Klein
Alain Vuylsteke
Samer Nashef
Editors

Foreword

Cardiac intensive care is a peculiarity in the United Kingdom. In many hospitals, it is the only single specialty critical care area. We should not be too surprised at this; cardiac disease is common and its frequency has spawned many new and innovative treatments. Changes in the organization of our hospitals may mean more patients with cardiac disease are treated in specialist centres and even fewer seen in general intensive care units, thus reducing the skill base and so comfort of many intensivists in managing these patients. Patients do not just present with heart disease, they also require surgery for other problems and familiarity with cardiac support is essential for all who work in general units.

This is not an in-depth tome, but rather a practical text full of the kind of tricks of the trade that make a skilled cardiac intensivist. One potential problem of a single specialty unit is a tendency to "forget" about the other systems; these are all addressed herein, along with other essential elements such as ethics and the running of a successful unit.

This is a welcome text targeting a multidisciplinary audience. It will be useful for those approaching an attachment to a cardiac unit as well as for those of us outside who want to update ourselves on the latest treatments available.

Anna M. Batchelor,
MB,ChB, FRCA
Consultant, Anaesthesia and Intensive Care
Royal Victoria Infirmary Newcastle
President of the Intensive Care Society

Abbreviations

A	
A-	Angiotensin
ABG	Arterial blood gas
ACE	Angiotensin-converting enzyme
ACEI	Angiotensin-converting enzyme inhibitor
ACLS	Advanced cardiac life support
ACS	Abdominal compartment syndrome
ACT	Activated coagulation time
ACTA	Association of Cardiothoracic Anaesthetists
ACTH	Adrenocorticotrophic hormone
ACV	Assist-control ventilation
ADL	Activity of daily living
ADP	Adenosine diphosphate
AED	Automatic external defibrillator
AEP	Auditory evoked potential
AF	Atrial fibrillation
AIDS	Acquired immunodeficiency syndrome
ALI	Acute lung injury
ALS	Advanced life support
ANH	Acute normovolaemic haemodilution
AP	Anteroposterior
APACHE	Acute Physiology and Chronic Health Evaluation
APC	Activated protein C
aPTT	Activated partial thromboplastin time
ARDS	Acute respiratory distress syndrome
ARF	Acute renal failure
ASV	Adaptive support ventilation
A_{sys}	Area under the systolic fraction
AT	Antithrombin
ATG	Antithymocyte globulin
ATN	Acute tubular necrosis
AUC	Area under the curve
AV	Atrioventricular
B	
BAEP	Brainstem auditory evoked potentials
BiPAP	Bi-level positive airway pressure, bi-level pressure assist
BIS	Bispectral (index)
BiVAD	Biventricular assist device
BLS	Basic life support
BMI	Body mass index
BMR	Basal metabolic rate
BPF	Bronchopleural fistula
bpm	Beats per minute
BUN	Blood urea nitrogen

C

CABG Coronary artery bypass graft
CAM-ICU Confusion assessment method for the intensive care unit
cAMP Cyclic adenosine monophosphate
CBF Cerebral blood flow
CCO Continuous measurements of cardiac output
CCP Critical care practitioner
CCT Certificate of completion of training
CDC Centers for Disease Control and Prevention (USA)
CF Cystic fibrosis
CI Cardiac index
Confidence interval
CIS Clinical information system
CML Chronic myelomonocytic leukaemia
$CMRO_2$ Cerebral metabolic rate (for oxygen)
CMV Controlled mechanical ventilation
Cytomegalovirus
CNS Central nervous system
CO Cardiac output
CoA Coarctation of the aorta
CoBaTriCE Competency based training for intensive care medicine
COPD Chronic obstructive pulmonary disease
COX Cyclo-oxygenase
CPAP Continuous positive airway pressure
CPB Cardiopulmonary bypass
CPOE Computer-aided physician order entry
CPP Cerebral perfusion pressure
CPR Cardiopulmonary resuscitation
CR Computed radiography
CRBSI Catheter-related bloodstream infection
CSF Cerebrospinal fluid
CT Computed tomogram/tomography
CTEPH Chronic thromboembolic pulmonary hypertension
CVA Cerebrovascular accident
CVP Central venous pressure
CVVH Continuous venovenous haemofiltration
CVVHD Continuous venovenous haemodialysis
CVVHDF Continuous venovenous haemodiafiltration
Cx Circumflex artery (coronary artery)
CYP3A4 Cytochrome microsomal system isoform 3A4

D

DC Direct current
DDAVP Desmopressin (1-desamino-8-D-arginine vasopressin)
DHCA Deep hypothermic circulatory arrest
DIC Disseminated intravascular coagulation
DL_{CO} Transfer coefficient for carbon monoxide
DNAR Do not attempt resuscitation
DR Direct radiography
DST Down slope time
DVT Deep venous thrombosis

E

EAA Excitatory amino acid
EBM Evidence-based medicine
ECG Electrocardiograph
ECMO Extracorporeal membrane oxygenation
ECT Ecarin clotting time
EDIC European Diploma in Intensive Care
EDTA Ethylenediamine tetra-acetic acid
EDV End-diastolic volume
EEG Electroencephalograph
EF Ejection fraction
EHR Electronic health record
EJV External jugular vein
EMR Electronic medical record
EPAP Expiratory positive airway pressure
EPO Erythropoietin

EQ-5D EuroQoL five-dimension
ESR Erythrocyte sedimentation rate
ETco_2 End-tidal CO_2
EVLW Extravascular lung water
EWS Early warning scores

F

FEV_1 Forced expiratory volume in 1 second
FFD Film to focus distance
FFP Fresh-frozen plasma
FG Filtration gradient
Fio_2 Fraction of inspired oxygen
FRC Functional residual capacity

G

GABA γ-Aminobutyric acid
GCS Glasgow Coma Scale
G-CSF Granulocytes colony stimulating factor
GEDV Global end-diastolic volume
GFR Glomerular filtration rate
GI Gastrointestinal
GTN Glyceryl trinitrate

H

HADS Hospital anxiety and depression scale
Hb Haemoglobin
HBOC Haemoglobin-based oxygen carriers
Hb-S Haemoglobin S
HCSW Health care support worker
HDU High-dependency unit
HF Haemofiltration
HFFI High frequency flow interruption
HFJV High frequency jet ventilation
HFOV High frequency oscillatory ventilation
HFPV High frequency percussive ventilation
HFPPV High frequency positive-pressure ventilation
HFV High frequency ventilation
HIT Heparin-induced thrombocytopenia
HLA Human leukocyte antibody
HMT Heparin management test
HP Haemoperfusion
HPA Human platelet antigen
HR Heart rate
HRQOL Health-related quality of life

I

IABP Intra-aortic balloon pump
IAH Intra-abdominal hypertension
IAP Intra-abdominal pressure
IBTICM Intercollegiate Board for Training in Intensive Care Medicine
ICA Internal carotid artery
ICAM Intercellular adhesion molecule
ICD Implantable cardiac defibrillator
ICP Intracranial pressure
ICU Intensive care unit
IE Infective endocarditis
IFN Interferon
Ig Immunoglobulin
IHD Intermittent haemodialysis
IJV Internal jugular vein
IL Interleukin
IMV Intermittent mandatory ventilation
INR International Normalized Ratio
IPAP Inspiratory positive airway pressure
IPD Intermittent peritoneal dialysis
IPF Idiopathic pulmonary fibrosis
IPPV Intermittent positive-pressure ventilation
IRV Inverse ratio ventilation
ISHLT International Society of Heart and Lung Transplantation
ISI International Sensitivity Index
IT Information technology
ITBV Intrathoracic blood volume
ITP Idiopathic thrombocytopenic purpura
ITTV Intrathoracic thermal volume

ITU	Intensive therapy unit
IV	Intravenous
IVC	Inferior vena cava
K	
K	Clearance
K_m	Membrane coefficient
KPS	Karnofsky performance status
L	
LAD	Left anterior descending (coronary artery)
LAP	Left atrial pressure
LCP	Liverpool Care Pathway for Dying Patients
LDH	Lactate dehydrogenase
LIMA	Left internal mammary artery
LMS	Left main stem (coronary artery)
LMWH	Low-molecular-weight heparin
LOS	Length of stay
LPS	Lipopolysaccharide
LSV	Long saphenous vein
LV	Left ventricle/ventricular
LVAD	Left ventricular assist device
LVEDP	Left ventricular end-diastolic pressure
LVEDV	Left ventricular end-diastolic volume
LVRS	Lung volume reduction surgery
M	
MAP	Mean arterial pressure
MCA	Middle cerebral artery
MCAEP	Midcortical auditory evoked potentials
MCP	Monocyte chemotactic protein
MDD	Major depressive disorder
MDE	Major depressive episode
MDT	Multidisciplinary team
MEP	Motor evoked potential
MET	Medical emergency team
MEWS	Modified early warning scores
MHC	Major histocompatibility complex
MI	Myocardial infarction
MIDCAB	Minimally invasive direct coronary artery bypass
MMV	Mandatory minute ventilation
MOD	Multiorgan dysfunction
MOF	Multiorgan (system) failure
MPAP	Mean pulmonary artery pressure
MRI	Magnetic resonance imaging
MRSA	Methicillin-resistant *Staphylococcus aureus*
MTT	Mean transit time
MU	Million units
N	
NEEP	Negative end-expiratory pressure
NF-κB	Transcription factor nuclear factor κB
NHP	Nottingham Health Profile
NIRS	Near-infrared spectroscopy
NIV	Noninvasive ventilation
NK	Natural killer (cells)
NMDA	*N*-methyl-D-aspartate
NSAID	Nonsteroidal anti-inflammatory drug
NSE	Neuron-specific enolase
NYHA	New York Heart Association
P	
PA	Pulmonary artery
PAC	Pulmonary artery catheter
$Paco_2$	Carbon dioxide alveolar pressure
PACS	Picture archiving and communication system
PADP	Pulmonary arterial diastolic pressure
PAF	Platelet activating factor
PAH	Pulmonary arterial hypertension
PAMP	Pathogen-associated molecular patterns
Pao_2	Oxygen alveolar pressure
PAP	Pulmonary artery pressure
PC	Personal computer
	Pericardial collection
	Protein C

PCA	Patient-controlled analgesia
PCI	Percutaneous coronary intervention
PCP	*Pneumocystis carinii*
PCR	Polymerase chain reaction
PCV	Pressure-controlled ventilation
PCWP	Pulmonary artery wedge pressure
PD	Peritoneal dialysis
PDE	Phosphodiesterase
PDMS	Patient data management system
PE	Pulmonary embolus/embolism
PEA	Pulmonary endarterectomy
PEEP	Positive end-expiratory pressure
PEG	Percutaneous endoscopic gastroscopy
PHT	Pulmonary hypertension
PICC	Peripherally inserted central catheter
PMN	Polymorphonuclear neutrophils
Po_2	partial pressure of oxygen
POC	Point of care
PPE	Personal protective equipment
PPH	Primary pulmonary hypertension
PPV	Pulse pressure variation
PRBC	Packed red blood cells
PRVC	Pressure-regulated volume-controlled ventilation
PSV	Pressure-support ventilation
PT	Prothrombin time
PTP	Proximal tubular pressure
PTT	Partial thromboplastin time
PTSD	Post-traumatic stress disorder
PTV	Pulmonary thermal volume
PVAD	Paracorporeal ventricular assist device
$Pvco_2$	Pulmonary venous CO_2
PVR	Pulmonary vascular resistance

Q

Q_b	Blood flow
Q_d	Dialysis flow
Q_f	Filtration flow
QOL	Quality of life

R

RA	Right atrium/atrial
RATG	Rabbit antithymocyte globulin
RBC	Red blood cell
RCA	Right coronary artery
RFID	Radiofrequency identification
RIJ	Right internal jugular
RRT	Renal replacement therapy
RSTP	Risk score for transport patient
RV	Right ventricle/ventricular
RVAD	Right ventricular assist device

S

SAH	Subarachnoid haemorrhage
SAM	Systolic anterior motion (of the anterior mitral leaflet)
Sao_2	Arterial oxygen saturation
SBT	Spontaneous breathing trial
s/c	Subcutaneous
SC	Membrane sieving coefficient
$Scvo_2$	Central venous oxygen saturation
SCUF	Slow continuous ultrafiltration
SDD	Selective decontamination of digestive tract
SF-36	Short Form Health Survey
SI	Système Internationale
SIMV	Synchronized intermittent mandatory ventilation
SIRS	Systemic inflammatory response syndrome
$S_{JV}o_2$	Jugular venous oxygen saturation
SNP	Sodium nitroprusside
SOFA	Sequential Organ Failure Assessment
SPV	Systolic pressure variation
SSEP	Somatosensory evoked potential
SSRIs	Selective serotonin reuptake inhibitors
STS	Society of Thoracic Surgeons (risk scoring)
SV	Stroke volume
SVC	Superior vena cava
Svo_2	Mixed venous oxygen saturation

SVR Systemic vascular resistance
SVT Supraventricular tachycardia
SWG Standard Wire Gauge

T
TAH Total artificial heart
TAT Thrombin–antithrombin complex
Tc Lymphocytes T cytotoxic
TCD Transcranial Doppler
TEG Thromboelastogram/thromboelastography
TFPI Tissue factor pathway inhibitor
Th Lymphocytes T helpers
TLR Toll-like receptor
TMP Transmembrane pressure
TNF Tumor necrosis factor
TOE Transoesophageal echocardiography
TPN Total parenteral nutrition
TRALI Transfusion-related acute lung injury
TREM-1 Triggering receptor expressed on myeloid cells
TRIM Transfusion-related immunomodulation
TRS Toronto Risk Score
TSH Thyroid-stimulating hormone
TTE Transthoracic echocardiography
UF Ultrafiltration
UTI Urinary tract infection

V
VAD Ventricular assist device
VALI Ventilator-associated lung injury
VAS Visual analog scale
VATS Video-assisted thoracoscopic surgery
V_{CO_2} Total volume of CO_2 exhaled over a defined period
VF Ventricular fibrillation
VILI Ventilator-induced lung injury
V_{O_2} Oxygen consumption
V/Q Ventilation–perfusion
VT Ventricular tachycardia
vWF von Willebrand factor

W
WCC White cell count

SECTION 1 Admission to Critical Care

Chapter 1

Who needs cardiothoracic critical care?

M. HIESMAYR AND D. SCHMIDLIN

What is critical care?

Critical Care Units (or intensive care units [ICU]) can be defined as "specialized sections of a hospital containing the equipment, medical and nursing staff and monitoring devices necessary to provide continuous and closely monitored health care to critically ill patients." Such patients may be at high risk of acquiring a life-threatening condition or require a high level of nursing and medical care to maintain physiologic equilibrium. Critical care is a complex and diverse network that interacts with all areas of the hospital.

Level of care

Critical care areas have traditionally been divided into Intensive Therapy Units, where the highest level of care is given to the sickest patients, and high-dependency units or step-down units, where an intermediate level of care between the ICU and the ward is provided. Another classification divides patients according to the level of care required.

The nurse at the bedside is the primary critical care provider. The complexity of the care and monitoring of most critical care patients and the machinery required to treat them means that the majority require one nurse per patient, and this is the standard in level 3 care in some countries such as the United Kingdom. Patients who require less intensive monitoring and treatment may require less nursing time, and level 2 care may be provided by one nurse for two or more patients.

Regardless of the level of care, specialized doctors provide medical supervision. These physicians are usually intensivists who work together with surgeons, physicians, microbiologists and other medical disciplines. The multidisciplinary team includes physiotherapists, pharmacists, dieticians and other support staff as well.

Cardiothoracic critical care provision

All patients are admitted to a critical care environment after cardiac surgery whether cardiopulmonary bypass was used or not. Many recover quickly if the postoperative period is uncomplicated. This rapid change in status (from highest level of intensive care to low-dependency cardiac monitoring over a few hours) has moulded the current cardiothoracic critical care environment. This allows patients to progress from level 3 to level 1 care ready for discharge to the ward in less than 24 hours.

Some patients need critical care longer. This may be because of the complexity of surgery, because comorbidities dictate a more prolonged recovery, or because of the development of postoperative complications. Transplantation and other invasive treatment for severe heart failure often requires prolonged critical care. Medical patients with unstable cardiac conditions and all patients with respiratory or renal disease may also need a prolonged stay. The number of such patients varies, making critical care planning difficult, but up to 10% of patients

Table 1.1 Classification of critical care

Level	Care required
0	Care can be provided on a normal ward within an acute hospital.
1	Patients whose condition is at risk of deteriorating or who are recovering from a serious illness, whose care may be provided on an acute ward with additional support.
2	Patients who require detailed observation or intervention, including support for a single failing organ system or postoperative care, including those "stepping down" from higher levels of care.
3	Patients requiring advanced respiratory support or support of at least two organ systems.

Adapted from Comprehensive Critical Care, London, Department of Health.

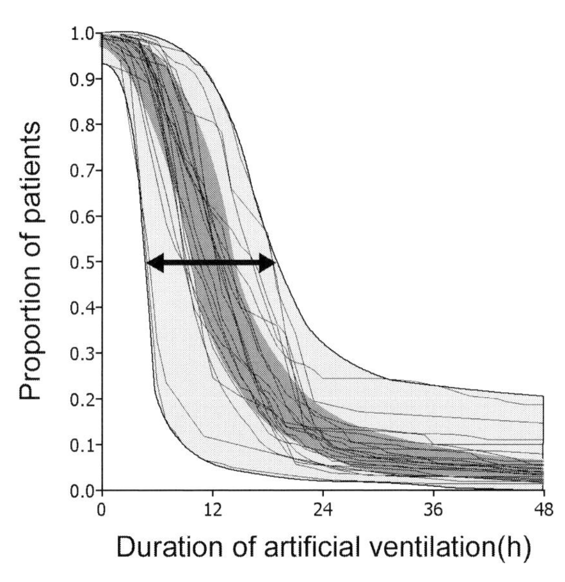

Figure 1.1 Proportion of extubated patients after cardiac surgery. (The proportion of intubated and surviving patients is displayed versus duration since admission in critical care. Each line represents one individual critical care unit. The light grey area indicates the total variability and the dark grey area the main stream behaviour. The arrow indicates the range of time until 50% of patients have been extubated. (From Lassnigg *et al. Intensive Care Medicine* 2002.)

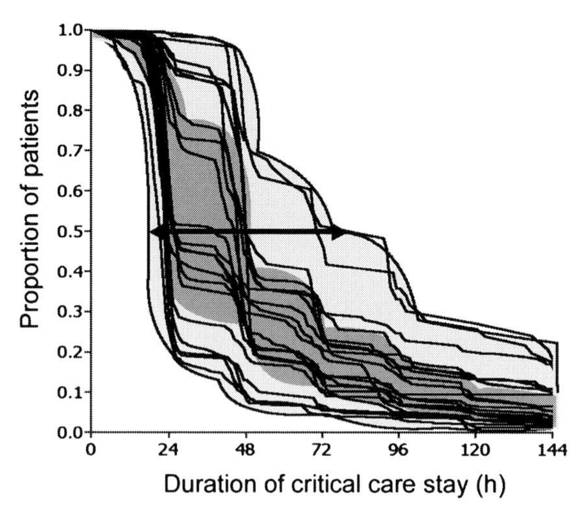

Figure 1.2 Proportion of patients staying in critical care after cardiac surgery. The proportion of surviving patients in critical care is displayed versus duration since admission in critical care. Each line represents one individual critical care unit. The light grey area indicates the total variability and the dark grey area the mainstream behaviour. The arrow indicates the duration range until 50% of patients have been discharged from critical care. (From Lassnigg *et al. Intensive Care Medicine* 2002.)

undergoing cardiac surgery are admitted for longer than 7 days. The service should be flexible; a prolonged stay is not always expected.

Managers and intensivists often struggle to determine the number of critical beds needed in an institution, taking into account elective admissions from theatre and emergency admissions from within the hospital and from other institutions. In an ideal world, there would always be reasonable spare capacity, but in reality few spare beds can be provided, and bed occupancy is often more than 90%. This allows for rapid turnover, but places strain on the critical care staff and environment.

Critical care provision is expensive, and typically consumes 15–25% of the total budget of a tertiary care centre. Use and availability is therefore subject to control owing to financial restrictions, which often dictate the number of available beds and staff.

Discharge

The decision that intensive care is no longer required and reduced monitoring is safe, is straightforward after uncomplicated recovery from surgery. However, readiness for discharge after complex surgery or prolonged critical care is more difficult to determine, and careful consideration by the multidisciplinary team is necessary. Adequate planning and support is required, and follow-up by critical care staff may be beneficial. Some patients may experience long-term complications or psychological effects, and follow-up should allow assessment and treatment of such sequelae.

Shortage of beds due to unexpected emergency admissions or pressure of elective operating work may necessitate early discharge of some patients. This is associated with increased readmission rates and possibly morbidity and mortality. In such circumstances, careful discharge planning and follow-up care arrangements may help to reduce these risks.

Intensive care without walls

Sick patients are not always located in critical care areas. This may be because of an unexpected deterioration in their condition, a postoperative complication, or after premature discharge to the ward when close monitoring is still required. Lower staffing levels on wards and lack of experience managing very sick patients has led to the development of critical care outreach services. These usually consist of nursing and medical staff from the ICU, who may advise, assist and above all educate ward staff. The effect of such services on morbidity, mortality, readmission to critical care and incidence of cardiac arrest is currently the subject of intense scrutiny.

When does a patient receive cardiothoracic intensive care?

After cardiac surgery

All cardiac surgery patients need a period of intensive postoperative care because of the nature of their surgery and the relatively high incidence of complications such as bleeding and respiratory failure. Immediately after surgery, many patients have a relatively unstable phase during which a number of interventions may be indicated without delay to prevent further deterioration and a poor outcome. The risk of such complications is related to the patient's premorbid condition and the success of the surgical procedure.

After thoracic surgery

The majority of thoracic surgical patients are looked after in the postsurgical recovery unit for a short period before discharge to the ward. After more extensive surgery such as pneumonectomy or as a result of complications of surgery or their premorbid condition, patients may require critical care. This may occasionally be prolonged or unexpected.

Nonsurgical cardiothoracic admissions

CARDIAC FAILURE

Medical and surgical management of cardiac failure is rapidly evolving, and recent data suggests that mortality is reducing as a result. Patients in severe heart failure need monitoring and treatment in a critical care environment, and some may require transfer to a specialized unit where mechanical support or transplantation can be offered. Admissions for intensive management of heart failure can be expected to increase in the future.

UNSTABLE CARDIAC CONDITIONS

The medical management of patients with unstable angina or after myocardial infarction may also require intensive monitoring and support. Admission may be prolonged, and surgical treatment may be indicated after a period of treatment and further investigation. Depending on the provision of services, transfer to surgical units may be necessary.

RESPIRATORY FAILURE

Intensive management of respiratory failure is a common indication for critical care. Intervention may range from noninvasive support to tracheal intubation and invasive ventilation; prolonged care is often needed. Some patients may require more specialized intervention such as extracorporeal oxygenation in dedicated units. Long-term ventilatory support may also be necessary in some instances, and this is usually offered in regional centres.

SPECIALIZED WORK

Some units (usually regional or national referral centres) admit patients for highly specialized critical care. This can be for the treatment of complex medical conditions such as cystic fibrosis or pulmonary hypertension, or after super-specialist surgery (e.g. heart and lung transplantation, pulmonary endarterectomy, ventricular assist device implantation).

Readmission

Readmission to critical care after cardiac surgery is needed in 3–4% of patients; the commonest causes are renal, respiratory and cardiac complications. Readmission is associated with greatly increased morbidity and mortality, and because of this, stringent efforts are made to reduce its incidence.

Key points

- There is wide variability in the level of care required after cardiothoracic surgery.
- The number of cardiothoracic critical care beds needed in a hospital is not easily predicted and the service should be flexible to match the elective and emergency workload.
- Readmission is a predictor of poor outcome, and may be reduced by careful discharge planning and critical care outreach.

REFERENCES

1 Lassnigg A, Hiesmeyer MJ, Bauer P, *et al.*, Effect of centre-, patient- and procedure-related factors in intensive care resource utilization after cardiac surgery. *Intensive Care Medicine* 2002;28: 1453–61.

2 *Comprehensive Critical Care: A Review of Critical Care Services*. London: Department of Health; May 2000.

Chapter 2

Scoring systems and prognosis

A.P. BARKER AND S.A.M. NASHEF

Crystal balls

Knowing the likelihood of survival after cardiac surgery is useful. If we know the likely outcome, we can compare it with actual outcome and thus gain some insight into the overall performance of the cardiac surgical unit. Knowledge of who is likely to develop major morbidity also has an impact on the use of valuable resources and may allow for sensible planning of operating lists. In addition, some believe that being able to predict mortality with some certitude may help clinicians to determine when further efforts are futile. Unfortunately, the perfect predictor – a crystal ball to foresee the future – has not yet been fully developed.

Risk models or scoring systems

Scoring systems allow reasonable prediction of outcome after cardiac surgery. Many models have been devised to work out the likelihood of survival, and these and others have also been shown to predict major morbidity, long-term survival and resource use with some accuracy. Models can be broadly divided into two groups:

- *preoperative models*, applied before the operation, with no knowledge of intraoperative events; and
- *postoperative models*, applied immediately after the operation on admission into the critical care unit, taking some account of what the operation did to the patient.

Preoperative models

These are most useful for

- establishing the risk of surgery as an adjunct to surgical decision making (determining the indication to operate on the basis of risk-to-benefit assessment);
- providing the patient with information, which is helpful in obtaining consent;
- helping to measure the performance of the service by comparing actual and predicted outcomes; and
- comparing the performance of different institutions, surgeons and anaesthetists by correcting for risk when outcomes are assessed.

Preoperative models take no account of what happens in the operating theatre and are therefore less useful in predicting which of a number of postoperative patients with complications are likely to emerge intact from the critical care unit.

There are probably more risk models in cardiac surgery than in any other branch of medicine. Most rely on a combination of risk factors, each of which is given a numerical "weight." Weights are added, multiplied or otherwise mathematically processed to come up with a percentage figure to predict mortality or survival. In additive models, the weights given to the risk factors are simply summed to give the predicted risk. They are easy to use and can be calculated mentally or "on the back of an envelope." They are less accurate than more sophisticated systems and have a tendency to overscore slightly in low-risk patients and to underscore considerably in very high-risk patients. Examples of such models are Parsonnet and the additive EuroSCORE for cardiac surgery overall. Other models deal specifically with cardiac surgical subsets, like coronary surgery and valve surgery. Sophisticated models use Bayesian analysis, logistic regression or even computer neural networks. They do not allow easy bedside calculation (unless you are Einstein) and need the help of a computer. They are, however, more stable than additive models across the risk range and slightly more accurate in exact risk prediction. Examples of such models are the Society of Thoracic Surgeons (STS) model and the logistic EuroSCORE for overall cardiac surgery.

Preoperative model risk factors

Not surprisingly, the usual suspects are common to all models (age, gender and left ventricular [LV] function). Other risk factors feature in some models but not in others, such as hypertension and diabetes. Models also differ depending on whether they deal with all cardiac surgeries or a specific subset, such as coronary surgery.

AGE

There is an increased risk above the age of 60 years.

GENDER

Females have a higher operative mortality than males, possibly because of smaller coronary artery size, although the reason for the difference is unknown.

LEFT VENTRICULAR FUNCTION

As estimated by echocardiography or angiography, LV function is a good measure of cardiac status, but determination can be operator dependent. It is difficult to produce an accurate and reproducible percentage ejection fraction. Generally, LV function is classified as “good,” “moderate” or “poor.”

TYPE OF SURGERY

General cardiac risk models take into account patients that undergo different surgeries – the risk for coronary artery bypass graft (CABG) surgery is less than for valve surgery, which in turn is less than that for surgery of the thoracic aorta. Combined procedures like CABG with valve carry a higher risk than single procedures.

EXTENT OF CARDIAC DISEASE

The severity of coronary disease is subjective and therefore not included in risk scores, although left main stem disease may be associated with more risk. Objective measures of cardiac disease include recent myocardial infarction (MI), unstable angina or mechanical complications of MI such as acute rupture of the mitral valve or ventricular septum.

REPEAT OPERATION

Previous cardiac surgery (or previous sternotomy) increases difficulty of access and prolongs operative time. These patients therefore carry an increased risk of bleeding as well as possibly having more advanced disease than those undergoing their first cardiac procedure.

LUNG DISEASE

The presence of chronic pulmonary disease such as chronic obstructive pulmonary disease (COPD) has a large impact on how a patient is managed in anaesthetic and ventilatory terms. After cardiac surgery, patients with concurrent lung disease are more likely to require extended ventilation, develop chest infections or require support such as continuous positive airway pressure (CPAP) ventilation. Lung function is difficult to quantify with a single test and severity is based partly on subjective judgments. However, chronic pulmonary disease is taken into account in the EuroSCORE and STS. Parsonnet includes smoking but not the presence of COPD particularly.

Table 2.1 Preoperative cardiac surgery risk assessment scores

EuroSCORE	Parsonnet	STS
Patient-related factors		
Age (yrs)	Age (yrs)	Age (yrs)
Gender	Gender	Gender
Extracardiac arteriopathy	Obesity	Race
Neurological dysfunction	Hypertension	Body mass index
Chronic pulmonary disease	Smoking	Smoking
Creatinine $>200\ \mu$mol/L	Diabetes	Diabetes
Critical preoperative state	Dyslipidaemia	Dyslipidaemia
Previous cardiac surgery	Dialysis	Creatinine
Active endocarditis	Catastrophic state	Renal failure
	Other rare circumstance (e.g. paraplegia, pacemaker dependency)	Dialysis
		Hypertension
		Cerebrovascular accident
		Endocarditis
		Chronic pulmonary disease
		Immunosuppression
		Extracardiac arteriopathy
		Reoperation
Cardiac-related factors		
Unstable angina	LV function	LV function
Pulmonary hypertension	Preoperative IABP	Recent MI
Recent MI		Congestive cardiac failure
LV function		Previous percutaneous coronary intervention
		New York Heart Association classification
		Preoperative inotropes/ventricular assist device/IABP
Operation-related factors		
Emergency	Emergency	Emergency
Post MI septal rupture	Type of procedure	Type of procedure
Other than isolated CABG	Other than isolated CABG	Surgery on thoracic aorta
Surgery on thoracic aorta		

Abbreviations: CABG, coronary artery bypass grafting; IABP, intra-aortic balloon pump; LV, left ventricular; MI, myocardial infarction; PCI, percutaneous coronary intervention.

RENAL DISEASE

Renal dysfunction, as evidenced by dependence on dialysis, increases mortality by as much as 40%, but the spectrum of renal failure is wide and difficult to quantify. Creatinine levels are easy to measure, but are not always an accurate measure of true kidney function. EuroSCORE uses grossly deranged serum creatinine (>200 μmol/L) as a measure of significant renal impairment. Other scores use dialysis dependence. The best measure is probably creatinine clearance.

OTHER RISK FACTORS

These include peripheral vascular disease, neurological dysfunction, degree of urgency, diabetes, hypertension and degree of pulmonary hypertension. In addition, various scoring systems give weight to the type of operation performed.

Postoperative models

Such models benefit from information that is only available after the completion of the operation, such as the physiological parameters on admission to critical care. Many have been devised for critically ill patients outside the cardiac surgical specialty, but have been used and validated in cardiac surgery. The most well-known models are the Acute Physiology and Chronic Health Evaluation (APACHE) and the Sequential Organ Failure Assessment (SOFA). The APACHE score is used on admission to critical care to assess the risk of in-hospital death, whereas the SOFA was developed to quantify the severity of a patient'sillness using the degree of organ dysfunction at any one time.

Postoperative model risk factors

Postoperative risk scores look at each organ system systematically and score according to derangement of function. Basically, the more organ dysfunction, the poorer the prognosis.

RESPIRATORY

Oxygenation and the requirement of respiratory support (ventilation) are measured to determine respiratory function.

CIRCULATORY

Most scores taken postoperatively use mean arterial pressure as an easily measured and monitored parameter. However, whereas APACHE concentrates on derangement of normal physiology, SOFA concentrates on the need for (and level of) inotropic support.

NEUROLOGICAL

Trends are more useful than a snap-shot at a particular point in time, but the Glasgow Coma Scale is easily measured and provides an easily reproducible measure of neurological status.

RENAL

As in score used preoperatively, the mainstay of renal function is serum creatinine level. Easily measured with a relatively inexpensive test, this variable can be used to monitor changes in renal function and to compare current with preoperative function.

GASTROINTESTINAL/HEPATIC

Both APACHE and SOFA use bilirubin levels as a measure of liver function. APACHE is used more widely in general critical care units and includes many more variables, such as amylase, albumin (as a rough measure of nutritional status) and other liver function tests. The APACHE score also contains variables to measure metabolic function and septic status. These criteria are less relevant in cardiac surgery.

Thoracic surgery

Risk modelling is not as developed in thoracic surgery, although recently some attempts have been made to produce models for predicting mortality

Table 2.2 Preoperative cardiac surgery risk assessment scores

Organ system	SOFA	APACHE
Respiratory	Oxygenation (Pao_2/Fio_2) Respiratory support	Respiratory rate nonventilated Pao_2 with Fio_2 1.0 $Paco_2$
Coagulation/haematological	WCC	WCC Haematocrit Platelet count Prothrombin time
Circulatory	Mean arterial pressure Dopamine dose Adrenaline dose Noradrenaline dose Dobutamine use	Mean arterial pressure Heart rate ventricular response Central Venous Pressure Evidence of acute MI Arrhythmia Serum lactate Arterial pH
Neurological	Glasgow Coma Scale	Glasgow Coma Scale
Renal	Creatinine Urine ouput/24 hr	Creatinine Urine output/24 hr Blood urea nitrogen
Gastrointestinal/hepatic	Bilirubin	Amylase Albumin Bilirubin Alkaline phosphatase Liver enzymes Allergy by skin testing
Septic		Cerebrospinal fluid positive culture Blood culture positive Fungal culture positive Rectal temperature
Metabolic		Calcium level Glucose Sodium Potassium Bicarbonate Serum osmolarity

Abbreviations: APACHE, Acute Physiology and Chronic Health Evaluation; Fio_2, fraction of inspired oxygen; MI, myocardial infarction; $Paco_2$, partial pressure of carbon dioxide in arterial blood; Pao_2, partial pressure of oxygen in arterial blood; SOFA, Sequential Organ Failure Assessment; WCC, white cell count.

after lung resection. The most important risk factors associated with a poor outcome are age (older people do less well) and how much functioning remains long after the resection (the more, the better).

Key points

- Many models help to predict the outcome of cardiac surgery, and these can be applied before or after the operation.
- Preoperative models help in the decision making, consent and assessment of clinical performance.
- Postoperative models can help to plan resource use and provide information to relatives.
- No amount of risk modelling can predict with certainty which patient will live and which will die.
- Models devised specifically for mortality have also been found to be useful in predicting major morbidity, resource use and long-term outcomes.
- Risk models are not perfect and should be used as an adjunct rather than as a replacement for sound clinical judgment.

FURTHER READING

- Arts D, de Keizer NF, Vroom MB, *et al.* Reliability and accuracy of sequential organ failure assessment. *Critical Care Medicine* 2005;33:1988–93.
- Knaus WA, Draper EA, Wagner DP, *et al.* APACHE II: A severity of disease classification system. *Critical Care Medicine* 1985;13: 818–29.
- Nashef SA, Roques F, Michel PR, *et al.* European system for cardiac operative risk evaluation (EuroSCORE). *European Journal of Cardiothoracic Surgery* 1999;16:9–13.
- Parsonnet V, Dean D, and Bernstein AD. A method of uniform stratification of risk for evaluating the results of surgery in acquired adult heart disease. *Circulation* 1989;79: I3–12.

Chapter 3

Admission to critical care: The cardiology patient

S.P. HOOLE AND P.M. SCHOFIELD

Introduction

Critical care admission is sometimes required for cardiology patients. This can be for invasive monitoring, supportive therapy, or both, and may be helpful in patients presenting either electively or urgently to the cardiology department. Cardiopulmonary optimization, if instigated promptly or even sometimes preventatively, reduces the risk of developing multiorgan failure and may prevent mortality and major morbidity. When this is a risk, early referral to the critical care unit is paramount.

Elective admissions

Most planned admissions to critical care of elective cardiology patients are for one of three reasons:

- high-risk percutaneous coronary intervention (PCI) by angioplasty or stenting;
- percutaneous heart valve procedures; or
- catheter laboratory procedures involving the use of contrast media in patients with chronic renal failure.

High-risk PCI

Elective PCI of the left main stem (LMS) coronary artery is sometimes offered to patients who are either unsuitable or unwilling to undergo coronary artery bypass grafting ([CABG]; PCI can be done especially if the disease is limited to the ostium or body of the LMS, but disease at the LMS bifurcation is usually not suitable). Such patients are often frail, with preexisting left ventricular (LV) dysfunction and other comorbidities. Because the territory of myocardium supplied by the LMS is large, PCI may cause important haemodynamic instability. The risk of this is reduced or abolished by intra-aortic balloon pump (IABP) counterpulsation. Therefore, when such a procedure is planned, IABP use should be considered along with critical care admission. In addition to averting major haemodynamic compromise during the procedure, IABP use prevents hypotension in the periprocedural period, maximizes peak coronary blood flow velocity and, at least theoretically, reduces the risk of acute stent occlusion. Although the only evidence of clinical benefit of IABP in the setting of LMS intervention is when there is concomitant cardiogenic shock, such patients are often managed on critical care for up to 24 hours after PCI.

In addition to LMS PCI, there are patterns of coronary disease that may also be perceived as posing a high risk of deterioration during or after PCI, such as when the target vessel is

- diffusely diseased;
- totally occluded;
- excessively tortuous proximally; or
- a diseased vein graft from a previous CABG.

Elective admission may also be advisable for such patients.

Table 3.1 Admission from cardiology

Elective
Preventative insertion of IABP.
Recovery and monitoring following percutaneous valvular procedures.
Preventative haemofiltration in patients with renal impairment.
Emergency
Invasive monitoring to establish diagnosis or titrate inotropic support.
Invasive procedures such as IABP, haemofiltration or mechanical support.
Pulmonary oedema and respiratory failure requiring ventilatory support.
Life-threatening complications from catheter laboratory.

Abbreviation: IABP, intra-aortic balloon pump.

Percutaneous valve procedures

Advances in percutaneous techniques have led to the development of percutaneous aortic valve replacement and mitral valve repair in addition to the established aortic and mitral balloon valvuloplasty. At present, most of these therapies are used almost exclusively to palliate elderly patients who are not candidates for open heart surgery. These patients often have comorbidities and impaired LV function, which justifies recovery and monitoring in the critical care unit. Elective admission is therefore arranged.

Chronic renal failure

Radiology contrast media are nephrotoxic and may precipitate acute-on-chronic renal failure in susceptible patients. Periprocedural haemofiltration in critical care may protect renal function in patients with chronic renal failure. This is arbitrarily defined as a serum creatinine >200 μmol/L. Haemofiltration immediately after contrast administration reduces plasma contrast load, although the clearance is modest (20% of total). The expense and complexity of haemofiltration has prevented widespread elective use, and it is generally reserved for patients who are already receiving long-term renal support.

Emergency admissions

Admission of cardiology patients to the critical care area is more likely to be in an emergent or urgent context. These admissions are predicted to increase as early PCI after acute myocardial infarction (MI) becomes more common. Such patients may need critical care admission because of postinfarct or postprocedural cardiac failure, and are more likely to require invasive monitoring, inotropic and IABP support, and ventilatory or renal support.

Although these are discussed in more specific details in subsequent chapters, broad principles are outlined hereafter.

Invasive monitoring

Many acutely ill cardiac patients need inotropic drugs and other supportive measures. Although inotropes can be administered outside the critical

Table 3.2 Most common causes of emergency admission of patient from cardiology ward

Cardiogenic shock and pulmonary oedema.
Uncontrolled acute myocardial ischaemia/refractory angina/acute coronary syndrome.
Prolonged cardiac arrest.
Arrhythmia storm.
Infective endocarditis.
Coronary artery rupture/perforation.
Contrast-induced nephropathy.
Failed PCI.

Abbreviation: PCI, percutaneous coronary intervention.

care setting, titration of treatment to the therapeutic response is best undertaken in conjunction with invasive haemodynamic monitoring. For this reason, the critical care unit is the optimal environment to care for patients requiring inotropic drugs. Insertion of a pulmonary artery flotation catheter (PAC) may be necessary to help guide the titration of vasoactive drugs and the administration of intravenous fluid. It is particularly helpful in guiding the management of patients with shock of any cause and those with acute heart failure. Pulmonary artery wedge pressure provides a direct measurement of LV filling pressure, and is elevated (>18 cmH_2O) in cardiogenic shock. This, in conjunction with a low cardiac index (CI ≤ 2.0 L $min^{-1}m^{-2}$) and a high systemic vascular resistance (>1200 dynes s cm^{-5}), confirms the diagnosis of acute cardiac failure. It enables the severity of cardiovascular compromise to be assessed along with response to therapy by monitoring trends and changes in cardiac indices. Insertion of a PAC is not without risk and therefore should be performed by experienced physicians in the critical care unit.

Supporting the failing heart

In patients with cardiogenic shock, evidence suggests that adrenaline should be the first choice inotrope, although it can increase the ischaemic burden of the LV. Other inotropic agents and their cardiovascular effects are outlined in Table 3.3.

In patients with refractory LV failure and cardiogenic shock, mechanical circulatory support with an IABP may be beneficial as a bridge to surgery for haemodynamically correctable lesions. Inflation of the IABP in early diastole is thought to augment coronary blood flow (although this theory is controversial). Balloon deflation during isovolaemic contraction in early systole reduces afterload, LV wall stress, LV work and myocardial oxygen demand. It can improve the CI by 20–25% and improve myocardial energy efficiency by 15%. Patients with an IABP should be cared for on the critical care unit by appropriately trained staff familiar with triggering and augmentation settings of the pump console and arterial line care to minimize the risks of this intervention. In severe or refractory heart failure, pharmacological treatment and an IABP may not be sufficient to improve cardiac output and tissue perfusion. Worsening organ function may necessitate consideration of more invasive mechanical support modalities. In such cases, specialist referral to and support from heart failure units should be sought; such patients may benefit from transfer to a critical care area in a unit where there is availability of advanced mechanical support with ventricular assist devices or extracorporeal membrane

Table 3.3 Inotropes for cardiology patients with cardiogenic shock

	Heart rate	Inotrope	Systemic vascular resistance	Blood pressure	Cardiac output
Adrenergic agonists					
Dobutamine	↑↑	↑↑	↓	↑	↑↑
Dopamine	↑	↑	↑↑	↑	↑
Isoprenaline	↑↑	↑	→↓	↓	↑
Adrenaline	↑	↑↑↑	↑↑↑	↑↑	→
Noradrenaline	→	→	↑	↑↑	→
Phosphodiesterase inhibitor					
Enoximone	↑	↑↑	↓	↓↓	↑↑

oxygenation. This type of treatment may be used as a bridge to recovery, transplantation or, on occasion, as a permanent solution.

Noninvasive ventilation

Continuous positive airway pressure or other forms of noninvasive ventilation (NIV) are useful in treating acute pulmonary oedema. It reduces the need for endotracheal intubation and may also reduce mortality.

Invasive ventilation

Some patients do not respond to or are not suitable for NIV and need endotracheal intubation and positive pressure ventilation. This may enable higher ventilatory pressures and FiO_2 to be administered. Sedative drugs are required and detrimental haemodynamic changes often ensue. Vasodilatation is common, leading to reduced mean arterial pressure and tissue perfusion. In addition, the increase in intrathoracic pressure may reduce venous return, further compromising cardiac output. Positive pressure ventilation of patients with interatrial shunts can exacerbate a right-to-left shunt by elevating right atrial pressure, which may lead to further deterioration in arterial oxygenation.

Renal failure therapy

Cardiogenic shock and decompensated acute heart failure are associated with oliguria and acute renal failure. Treatment of such patients is problematic. As well as fluid accumulation, serum hydrogen ion concentration rises. Acidosis is negatively inotropic and failure to correct it rapidly is associated with increased mortality. As fluid accumulates, heart failure worsens, leading to further deterioration in renal function and acidosis – a vicious circle that can be broken by continuous venovenous haemofiltration (CVVH), either alone or with dialysis; CVVH rapidly corrects acidosis without the risk of sodium or fluid overload. It enables controlled plasma volume and solute depletion, without the profound hypotension seen with intermittent haemodialysis and can be safely administered to critically ill patients.

Table 3.4 Beneficial effects of continuous venovenous haemofiltration on left ventricular dysfunction

Reduction of myocardial oedema.
Reduction in left ventricular end-diastolic pressure → optimization of the Starling relationship → increased myocardial performance.
Removal of circulating myocardial depressant factors.

Specific scenarios

The following are examples of some (but by no means all) situations in which cardiology patients are admitted urgently to the critical care unit, with salient aspects of their management.

Catheter laboratory complications

In the context of PCI, the guidewire may cause coronary artery perforation and deploying a balloon or stent may cause coronary artery rupture. These are rare complications of PCI, but both may cause cardiac tamponade, which can be rapidly fatal unless pericardial blood is drained. Management is complicated because heparin and antiplatelet agents are usually given before and during the procedure and the patient may be coagulopathic at the time.

The condition may be treated by further PCI with covered stents and distal embolization to achieve haemostasis and percutaneous pericardial aspiration and drainage to treat tamponade in the majority of cases; however, open surgery is required occasionally. A period of close haemodynamic monitoring to detect the signs of tamponade (high central venous pressure with Kussmaul'ssign, hypotension, pulsus paradoxus and tachycardia) may be necessary because diagnosis is often difficult.

Failure to achieve adequate blood flow after PCI in the absence of any detectable compromise of the vessel integrity is known as the 'no reflow' phenomenon. It is believed to be due to microvascular dysfunction. This may be mediated by microemboli and vasoactive substances released downstream in the target vessel. This phenomenon is associated with cardiogenic shock; circulatory support on critical care may be required. However, it has been demonstrated by Doppler that IABP does not significantly improve the coronary blood flow in the no-reflow artery. Therefore, in the absence of cardiogenic shock, IABP support may not be helpful.

Contrast-induced nephropathy

Contrast-induced nephropathy is a recognized complication of the administration of iodine-based contrast used during coronary angiography, particularly in diabetics and those with preexisting renal failure. Preventative strategies, such as preprocedural hydration, the use of low ionic contrast agents and minimization of the contrast load, have been shown to reduce the incidence of contrast-induced nephropathy. However, in severe cases of contrast-induced nephropathy, renal supportive therapy with CVVH in critical care may be required. Rarely, coadministration of iodinated contrast to a diabetic patient taking a biguanide like metformin can lead to severe lactic acidosis, especially if the patient has chronic renal impairment and is haemodynamically unstable.

Uncontrolled acute myocardial ischaemia

When not relieved by medical therapy, acute myocardial ischaemia can be effectively treated by IABP support. Angina is relieved predominantly by off-loading the heart in early systole during aortic balloon deflation, causing a reduction in myocardial wall stress and oxygen demand. This therapy "buys time" and increases the margin of safety before definitive revascularization. The timing and method of intervention depends on the following factors:

- the patient's general condition;
- the coronary anatomy and its suitability for PCI or CABG;
- the extent of myocardial damage and time since the infarct; and
- the success of IABP support in relieving symptoms and ischaemia.

Close cooperation between medical and surgical teams is required.

Cardiogenic shock and acute pulmonary oedema

Cardiogenic shock is a clinical syndrome characterized by hypotension (arterial blood pressure $\leq$90 mmHg systolic or $\leq$60 mmHg mean for $\geq$30 minutes), oliguria (urine output <0.3 mL/kg per hour for 2 consecutive hours), and poor peripheral perfusion with an underlying cardiac aetiology.

Cardiogenic pulmonary oedema occurs due to Starling's law of fluids: the hydrostatic pressure exceeds the oncotic pressure of the blood, causing fluid to leave the pulmonary capillaries and fill the alveoli. This typically occurs when the pulmonary capillary wedge pressure exceeds 20 cm H_2O.

Treatment of patients with cardiogenic shock with vasopressor and inotropic agents alone in a coronary care setting is associated with an in-hospital mortality of 90% in most large series. Although mechanical circulatory support can provide a favourable clinical and haemodynamic response in the short term, mortality remains high.

Table 3.5 Causes of cardiogenic shock
Ischaemic left ventricular dysfunction.
Papillary muscle rupture (severe mitral regurgitation).
Ventricular septal rupture.
Free wall rupture (tamponade).

Ultimately, death is merely delayed unless definitive surgical or percutaneous treatment is instigated.

In acute MI complicated by cardiogenic shock, expeditious revascularization is important. Complete coronary revascularization is recommended for patients with cardiogenic shock.

Postinfarction ventricular septal rupture

When the ventricular septum ruptures after MI, an immediate left-to-right shunt adds to the woes of the patient trying to recover from the infarct. This causes right ventricular strain, pulmonary hypertension and cardiac failure with pulmonary oedema, and is usually rapidly followed by renal failure and death. Ventricular septal rupture is invariably an indication for immediate admission to critical care for monitoring and IABP counterpulsation, which, by off-loading the left ventricle in systole, reduces the shunt and gives the heart a fighting chance. Thereafter, the majority of patients need early surgery. There is controversy as to the timing of ventricular septal rupture repair after acute MI. Early surgery means operating in the immediate aftermath of an infarct, repairing a septum that is friable and with a real likelihood of further rupture. On the other hand, these patients rarely improve without surgery. Poor surgical outcome is associated with haemodynamic instability, a short interval between time of MI and operative repair, an inferior rupture, impaired right ventricular function, diabetes and renal failure.

Up to two thirds of patients also have multivessel coronary artery disease, but surgeons disagree whether concomitant CABG is indicated. Attitudes vary from: 'This is life-saving surgery – keep it simple, stupid' to 'CABG hardly adds anything to the risk of this procedure and will prevent future problems, so do a proper job.' This is an evidence-free zone. Delaying surgical treatment of the postinfarct septal rupture, to increase the time between MI and surgery, must be balanced against the end-organ effects of prolonged haemodynamic instability and the risk of sepsis from a prolonged ICU stay and mechanical circulatory support.

Acute mitral rupture

Like the ventricular septum, the papillary muscle may rupture after MI and cause acute catastrophic mitral regurgitation, cardiac failure and pulmonary oedema. Again, an IABP and aggressive diuresis may stabilize the patient to allow consideration of treatment, and improves mortality and morbidity. Early surgical mitral repair or replacement is now recommended, but the exact timing is subject to similar arguments as in ventricular septal rupture (see above). Poor outcome is associated with haemodynamic instability, renal failure and the need for mechanical ventilation. Without surgery, papillary muscle rupture is almost universally fatal.

Infective endocarditis

Patients diagnosed with infective endocarditis, on the basis of the Duke criteria, have an in-hospital mortality of 20%. The identification at presentation of high-risk patients should enable early transfer to critical care to improve the outcome of the disease.

The best outcomes are achieved in patients whose sepsis can be controlled, so that the affected valve or valves are sterile and surgery can be performed electively or semi-electively in a sterile field. Unfortunately, in many patients this is not possible because of haemodynamic compromise owing to the valve lesion, uncontrollable sepsis or mobile life- and brain-threatening vegetations. In such patients, early surgery may be the only (unattractive) option. Prosthetic valve endocarditis in such situations remains a real risk. Furthermore, the decision whether to perform acute surgery is particularly difficult in unconscious or sedated patients with an uncertain neurological outcome.

Ventricular tachycardia storm

Occasionally, intractable ventricular tachycardia can occur and result in haemodynamic compromise and morbidity. Ventilatory support combined with sedation on the critical care unit may be necessary to allow rhythm stabilization. Case reports have documented that some anaesthetic agents like propofol may suppress the electrical storm, by blocking the sympathetic nervous system, thought to be a contributory factor in cardiac electrical hyperexcitability.

After cardiac arrest

Unless cardiac arrest is very brief and full recovery rapidly ensues, admission to critical care is necessary. Cardiac arrest in the catheter laboratory is often due to ventricular arrhythmias that occur during the procedure and rapid treatment often allows full recovery and observation after the event in a ward setting. After prolonged resuscitation or when neurological recovery is delayed, invasive monitoring and ventilation are required in critical care, and a search for the cause of the arrest must be followed by treatment to prevent recurrence.

Key points

- Early or preemptive referral to the critical care unit is ideal.
- Mechanical circulatory support by IABP is a useful bridge to definitive treatment.
- Noninvasive ventilation is an effective treatment for patients with acute pulmonary oedema.
- Haemofiltration is useful to treat refractory heart failure complicated by oliguric renal failure.

FURTHER READINGS

Chu VH, Cabell CH, Benjamin DK Jr, *et al.* Early predictors of in-hospital death in infective endocarditis. *Circulation* 2004;109:1745–1749.

Hochman JS, Sleeper LA, Webb JG, *et al.* Early revascularization in acute myocardial infarction complicated by cardiogenic shock. SHOCK Investigators. Should We Emergently Revascularize Occluded Coronaries for Cardiogenic Shock. *N Engl J Med* 1999;341: 625–634.

Nolan JP, Morley PT, Vanden Hoek TL, *et al.* Therapeutic hypothermia after cardiac arrest: an advisory statement by the advanced life support task force of the International Liaison Committee on Resuscitation. *Circulation* 2003;108:118–121.

Peter JV, Moran JL, Phillips-Hughes J, *et al.* Effect of non-invasive positive pressure ventilation (NIPPV) on mortality in patients with acute cardiogenic pulmonary oedema: a meta analysis. *Lancet* 2006;367:1155–1163.

Chapter 4

Admission to critical care: Heart failure

J. PARAMESHWAR

Introduction

The combination of the aging of the population and improved survival after myocardial infarction (MI) has increased the prevalence of chronic heart failure. Most patients are admitted to hospital with advanced heart failure as a result of acute decompensation of their disease, but some patients with new onset heart failure present in extremis. In addition, patients with impaired ventricular function who undergo surgery may present with low output states. Coronary artery disease is the cause of heart failure in 60–70% of patients, but in younger patients (such as the population referred for cardiac transplantation), dilated cardiomyopathy (often of unknown aetiology) is the commonest cause. The true incidence of acute myocarditis in patients with a short history of heart failure is not known because of the difficulty in confirming the diagnosis. Forty-five per cent of patients hospitalized with heart failure will be readmitted at least once (and 15% at least twice) within 1 year.

Prognosis

Patients with advanced heart failure have a very poor prognosis. For example, in patients admitted with acute pulmonary oedema, in-hospital mortality has been reported to be 12% and the 1-year mortality, 40%.

Clinical presentation

Classically, patients admitted to critical care because of heart failure have one of two clinical syndromes:

1. pulmonary oedema (verified by chest radiograph), accompanied by severe respiratory distress and low oxygen saturation before treatment; or
2. cardiogenic shock, which is defined as tissue hypoperfusion induced by heart failure after correction of preload. It is usually characterized by hypotension (systolic BP $\leq$ 90 mmHg), oliguria ($\leq$0.5 mL/kg per hour) and perhaps evidence of organ congestion.

The approach to advanced heart failure can be simplified by consideration of the haemodynamic profile using bedside assessment. It is essential to distinguish between elevated and nonelevated cardiac filling pressures (wet or dry) and adequate or severely impaired tissue perfusion (warm or cold). Elevated filling pressure can be diagnosed clinically by orthopnoea or by elevated jugular venous pressure. Blood pressure is only a guide to perfusion; proportional pulse pressure ([systolic pressure − diastolic pressure]/systolic pressure) of less than 25% has been reported to correlate with a cardiac index less than 2.2 L min^{-1} m^{-2} in younger patients referred for cardiac transplantation. Patients admitted to the critical care unit are likely to have elevated filling pressures and inadequate perfusion.

Table 4.1 Factors affecting patients admitted with heart failure

Characteristics at hospital admission	Patients (%)
Female	52
Ejection fraction ≤0.40	50
History of heart failure	77
Hospitalized in previous 6 months	25
NYHA class III	43
NYHA class IV	32
History of hypertension	71
History of MI	31
History of IHD	58
AF, asthma, or COPD	30
Diabetes	44
Chronic renal insufficiency	28
Stroke or TIA	16
Ventricular arrhythmia	8

Abbreviations: AF, atrial fibrillation; COPD, chronic obstructive pulmonary disease; IHD, ischaemic heart disease; MI, myocardial infarction; NYHA, New York Heart Association; TIA, transient ischaemic attack.
From Graves EJ. Vital Health Statistics 13; 1995, pp. 1–63.

Cardiorenal syndrome

Some patients demonstrate a progressive decline in renal function, although diuresis may still relieve symptoms of congestion. These patients often have chronic volume overload, prior renal dysfunction, right ventricular dysfunction and high baseline diuretic requirements. The term 'cardiorenal syndrome' is now used to describe this condition; the term 'pre-renal' does not adequately describe the pathophysiology. When filling pressures are measured in these patients, they exceed the optimal levels required to maintain cardiac output (CO). A change in cardiopulmonary pressures may induce an alteration in the balance of vasoconstrictor and vasodilator hormones and thus affect the kidneys. A stable clinical state may be maintained in some patients with high serum urea and creatinine levels, but the prognosis is poor. Inotropic infusions may relieve the congestion and improve renal function, but the problem often recurs when inotropes are withdrawn.

Investigations

- Electrocardiogram to determine rhythm and aetiology of heart failure, such as acute coronary syndrome or myocarditis.
- Chest radiograph for heart size, pulmonary congestion, consolidation in the lungs or pleural effusion.
- Computed tomography to diagnose pulmonary embolism and confirm consolidation or cavitation.
- Echocardiography to evaluate and monitor regional and global left and right ventricular function, valve structure and function, pericardial effusion and mechanical complications of MI. The pulmonary artery systolic pressure may also be estimated from the tricuspid regurgitation jet, but this has not been validated against right heart catheterization in patients with acute heart failure.
- Blood tests: full blood count, coagulation screen, C-reactive protein, creatinine and electrolytes, glucose, liver function tests in all patients. Troponin and plasma brain natriuretic peptide are indicated in some patients.
- Coronary angiography is sometimes useful if revascularization is indicated.

Monitoring

- Noninvasive monitoring: temperature, respiratory rate, blood pressure, electrocardiogram monitoring and pulse oximetry to monitor arterial oxygen saturation. Occasionally CO can be monitored with the use of Doppler techniques.

- Arterial line: essential in unstable patients for continuous arterial blood pressure monitoring and frequent analysis of blood gases.
- Central venous line: monitoring right-sided filling pressure is often essential in patients with advanced heart failure and a central venous line is required for the delivery of fluids and drugs. Estimation of superior vena caval or right atrial oxygen saturation is a very useful marker of oxygen transport. Central venous pressure (CVP) may be significantly affected by positive end-expiratory pressure ventilation.
- Pulmonary artery catheter (PAC): in patients with heart failure, right atrial pressure does not correlate well with left-sided filling pressure. In many situations, an estimate of left atrial pressure is invaluable. For patients requiring inotropic or vasoconstrictor drugs, monitoring of CO and estimation of systemic vascular resistance (SVR) facilitates rational therapy based on pathophysiological principles. Mixed venous oxygen saturation can also be monitored with a PAC and is particularly useful in the presence of severe tricuspid regurgitation, when the CO derived by thermodilution may be inaccurate. In patients with a high pulmonary vascular resistance associated with heart failure, a PAC provides information not obtained by other techniques. Complications associated with the use of a PAC increase with duration of use and it should not be left in situ longer than necessary. In advanced heart failure, therapy tailored to haemodynamic goals as guided by PAC has been shown to result in sustained improvement in symptoms, stroke volume and CO.

Treatment

The treatment of chronic heart failure has been the subject of several large, randomised clinical trials and well-established guidelines have been published. Patients with acute heart failure can be critically ill and difficult to subject to randomised trials because they are a heterogeneous group with respect to aetiology, haemodynamic abnormalities, and comorbidities. Treatment should be based on the underlying pathophysiology. The aim of therapy is to reverse the haemodynamic abnormalities detected. If an underlying treatable cause is identified, the aim should be to support the patient and optimize the clinical condition so that definitive treatment can be carried out with the minimum of risk. Immediate therapy should focus on relieving symptoms, and reducing congestion is often the most effective way of achieving this.

Oxygenation

Achieving an adequate level of oxygenation at the cellular level is important to prevent end-organ dysfunction. To this end, the aim should be to achieve arterial oxygen saturation above 95%. Endotracheal intubation is indicated if there is compromise to airway patency or if the patient is too tired to maintain adequate spontaneous ventilation with less invasive measures (see below). Increasing the inspired oxygen concentration is logical in the presence of hypoxaemia; in the absence of hypoxaemia, the use of increased concentrations of oxygen is controversial and may cause harm.

Noninvasive ventilation

Either continuous positive airway pressure or noninvasive ventilation should be used before endotracheal intubation and mechanical ventilation. Use of continuous positive airway pressure and noninvasive ventilation results in pulmonary recruitment and an increase in functional residual capacity. This leads to a decrease in the overall work of breathing.

Table 4.2 Treatment goals in advanced heart failure

Clinical	Elimination of peripheral and pulmonary oedema Systolic blood pressure >85 mmHg Stable or improving renal function Improving or normal liver function and coagulation parameters Adequate oxygenation
Haemodynamic	Central venous/right atrial pressure ≤8 mmHg Pulmonary capillary wedge pressure ≤16 mmHg Cardiac index >2 L min^{-1} m^{-2} Mixed venous oxygen saturation >60% A secondary goal is systemic vascular resistance 800–1,200 dynes s cm^{-5} (helps to guide therapy)

Mechanical ventilation with endotracheal intubation

If noninvasive ventilation does not reverse hypoxaemia, endotracheal intubation is indicated. Respiratory muscle fatigue often results from hypoxaemia and low CO.

Drug therapy

ANTICOAGULATION

The role of anticoagulation is well established in acute coronary syndromes and atrial fibrillation. Patients with a history of an embolic event or evidence of ventricular thrombus on echocardiography should also receive anticoagulation. A large, placebo-controlled trial of daily 40 mg enoxaparin in acutely ill patients, including those with heart failure, showed less venous thrombosis but no difference in overall outcome. Pulmonary emboli are also commonly associated with severe heart failure and it seems reasonable to anticoagulate patients who are confined to bed in the intensive care unit. Care is needed as concomitant liver dysfunction may lead to a prolonged prothrombin time. In patients with a creatinine clearance below 30 mL/min, low-molecular-weight heparin in therapeutic doses should be used cautiously, probably with monitoring of factor Xa level.

LOOP DIURETICS

The reduction of elevated filling pressures is the most effective way to relieve symptoms of heart failure. Patients with acute decompensation of chronic heart failure are likely to be on diuretic therapy when admitted. Data are lacking on the relative efficacy and tolerability of different diuretics. In this setting, a loop diuretic is administered intravenously with dose titration to produce optimal urine output. A loading dose followed by intravenous infusion has been shown to be more effective than bolus dosing alone. A large bolus of diuretic may also lead to reflex vasoconstriction and perhaps a higher risk of ototoxicity. An intravenous infusion of furosemide at 5–10 mg/h is sufficient in most patients once steps have been taken to increase the CO. Fluid restriction (usually to 1.5 L/d) is an important adjunct to diuretic therapy in severely fluid-overloaded patients. Using a 'fluid challenge' in such patients with obvious peripheral oedema is irrational; inadequate urine output in these patients is invariably related to a low CO and treating this often requires inotropic therapy. Once filling pressures have been reduced to normal, the dose of diuretic should be reduced promptly; the dose required to maintain euvolaemia is usually less than that required to achieve it.

THIAZIDES

The combination of a thiazide (metolazone is commonly used) with a loop diuretic can produce dramatic diuresis in patients with chronic heart failure and is of use in the acute setting. Heart failure patients are often hyponatraemic in the intensive care unit and care needs to be taken not to exacerbate this with combination diuretic therapy. Thiazides act on the proximal tubule and deliver more sodium to the loop of Henle, where furosemide and other loop diuretics act.

ALDOSTERONE ANTAGONISTS

Once diuresis is induced, it is important to monitor serum potassium, as hypokalaemia may predispose to arrhythmias. It is common practice to use diluted potassium chloride as an intravenous infusion to maintain K^+ levels. However, intravenous K^+ supplements have been shown to induce aldosterone release from the suprarenal gland. Aldosterone acts on the myocardium inducing remodelling, which is associated with adverse outcomes in chronic heart failure. It seems rational, therefore, to combine loop diuretics with an aldosterone antagonist like spironolactone provided the serum K^+ is $\leq$5 mmol/L and serum creatinine $\leq$200 μmol/L. In patients who have been intolerant of spironolactone in the past (usually owing to gynaecomastia), epleronone (a selective aldosterone antagonist) is a suitable alternative.

VASODILATORS

In the absence of severe hypotension, vasodilators are indicated in most patients with acute heart failure. Decreasing preload relieves congestion and decreasing afterload is usually beneficial; most patients with heart failure are vasoconstricted. When administering vasodilators or positive inotropic drugs, the following equation is useful in manipulating the circulation:

$$\text{MAP} - \text{CVP} = \text{CO} \times \text{SVR},$$

where MAP is the mean arterial pressure.

Table 4.3 Intravenous vasodilators in advanced heart failure

Drug	Dose
Glyceryl trinitrate	Start at 20 μg/min, increase up to 200 μg/min
Isosorbide dinitrate	Start at 1 mg/h, increase up to 20 mg/h
Sodium nitroprusside	0.2–5.0 μg/kg/min
Nesiritide	Bolus 2 μg/kg, infusion 0.01–0.03 μg/kg/min

Nitrates

In low doses, nitrates are venodilators; high doses may also cause arterial dilatation. They are particularly useful in acute coronary syndromes associated with heart failure. Oral nitrates in combination with hydralazine have been shown to be beneficial in chronic heart failure and at least two randomized controlled trials have shown that intravenous nitrates in combination with furosemide are superior to furosemide alone. Tolerance to nitrates can develop within 24 hours of commencing an infusion.

Sodium nitroprusside

A powerful arterial dilator, sodium nitroprusside (SNP) can increase CO by lowering afterload in patients whose heart failure is not associated with hypotension. Prolonged administration of SNP may be toxic due to its metabolites. There are few controlled trials of SNP in heart failure and, because many patients are admitted to the intensive care unit with hypotension, it is rarely used.

Nesiritide

This drug (recombinant brain natriuretic peptide) is licensed in the United States for the treatment of acute heart failure. It relaxes smooth muscle, leading to arterial and venous dilatation. It leads to an increase in CO without direct positive inotropic effect. Compared with nitroglycerin, nesiritide produced faster relief of dyspnoea and a more pronounced decrease in pulmonary capillary wedge pressure, and the benefit was sustained for 24 hours. Although the drug has natriuretic and diuretic effects, up to 50% of patients with advanced heart failure have been reported to be resistant to its natriuretic effects. There is no conclusive evidence that nesiritide improves kidney function and there has been recent concern that it actually may worsen it. Clinical studies have not confirmed better clinical outcomes and at present the role of nesiritide in the management of heart failure remains unclear.

Hydralazine

A combination of hydralazine and nitrates has been shown to be beneficial in patients with chronic heart failure. In patients who cannot tolerate an angiotensin-converting enzyme (ACE) because of hyperkalaemia or worsening renal function, it is reasonable to use this combination.

ANGIOTENSIN-CONVERTING ENZYME INHIBITORS

The first drug class shown to improve outcome in severe chronic heart failure, ACE inhibitors are the cornerstone of outpatient heart failure treatment. They have no role in the early stabilization of unstable heart failure patients, but should be introduced as soon as the patient is haemodynamically stable and has acceptable perfusion and renal function. ACE inhibitors decrease renal vascular resistance, increase renal blood flow and promote sodium and water excretion. However, in patients with a very low CO, they may significantly decrease glomerular filtration rate. If patients with acute decompensation of chronic heart failure are admitted to the critical care unit, it may be necessary to discontinue them temporarily.

β-BLOCKERS

The role of β-blockers in the management of chronic heart failure is well established, based on several large trials involving many thousand patients. In volume-overloaded patients, β-blockers are likely to increase the severity of heart failure and are usually avoided. There is no consensus on the management of a patient receiving β-blockers for chronic heart failure admitted to hospital with acute decompensation. Most require at least a decrease in the dose of the drug but in patients requiring (β-agonist) inotropic therapy, it is logical to discontinue β-blockers altogether.

INOTROPIC AGENTS

Inotropic agents are indicated in the presence of tissue hypoperfusion (often manifested by worsening renal function) or fluid retention (peripheral or pulmonary oedema) refractory to treatment with diuretics and vasodilators. A common clinical scenario is a volume-overloaded patient with hypotension, hyponatraemia and a rising serum urea and creatinine on intravenous diuretic therapy. Continuing such therapy is likely to exacerbate the metabolic abnormalities and unlikely to induce a significant diuresis. It is essential to improve the patient's haemodynamic state with intravenous inotropic therapy until some form of definitive therapy or long-term palliation can be considered. It must be remembered that inotropic agents in heart failure are like whipping an exhausted horse: they give short-term beneficial haemodynamic effects at the expense of accelerating the underlying problem. This may be due to the increase in myocardial oxygen consumption that results from inotropic therapy. There is also a risk of inducing life-threatening arrhythmia. Rational use of inotropic therapy in a critically ill population requires some form of haemodynamic monitoring; at the very least the CVP, arterial blood pressure, and CO need to be assessed while on therapy.

Inotropic therapy

Despite the desensitization of β-receptor pathways in the failing human heart, most patients

Table 4.4 Typical doses of Intravenous inotropic agents used in heart failure

Drug	Bolus	Dose
Dopamine	No	2–10 μg/kg/min
Dobutamine	No	2–20 μg/kg/min
Adrenaline	No	0.05–0.50 μg/kg/min
Noradrenaline	No	0.02–0.20 μg/kg/min
Enoximone	0.25–0.75 mg/kg	1.25–7.5 μg/kg/min
Milrinone	25–75 μg/kg	0.375–0.750 μg/kg/min
Levosimendan	12–24 μg/kg	0.05–0.20 μg/kg/min

with advanced heart failure still show a substantial response to adrenergic agents. The lowest effective dose should be used; patients receiving β-blockers may require higher doses. Very few trials have been conducted in patients with advanced heart failure and there is no evidence of the superiority of one agent over any other.

Dopamine

A very small dose of the drug (≤2 μg/kg/min) is said to act predominantly on peripheral dopaminergic receptors leading to vasodilatation. An increase in renal blood flow may lead to diuresis. Higher doses certainly increase CO; above 5 μg/kg/min dopamine also has α-adrenergic effects, increasing peripheral vascular resistance and blood pressure.

Dobutamine

Dobutamine acts through stimulation of β-1 and β-2 receptors in a 3:1 ratio and is positively inotropic and chronotropic. There may be a secondary decrease in sympathetic tone, decreasing peripheral vascular resistance; at low doses it may also induce mild arterial vasodilatation. High doses of dobutamine (>10 μg/kg/min) cause vasoconstriction, but the exact effect at any given dose varies by patient. Heart rate increases as atrioventricular conduction is facilitated. The commonly used dose range is 2 to 10 μg/kg/min.

Adrenaline

This drug has a high affinity for β-1, β-2 and α-receptors and is generally infused at a rate of 0.05 to 0.50 μg/kg/min. Use of adrenaline usually requires invasive arterial pressure and CO monitoring.

Noradrenaline

This drug is used to increase SVR because of its affinity for α-receptors. The lowest dose required to increase the SVR (and hence the blood pressure), and to maintain perfusion of vital organs should be used. Septic shock is a common indication for its use; the occasional patient after acute MI presents with low SVR owing to cytokine release and benefits from noradrenaline. It is essential to monitor CO and the SVR when using this agent. In the absence of appropriate monitoring, a common error is to use a dose that maintains a "normal" blood pressure at the expense of adequate flow. A rise in the SVR in this situation is usually associated with a drop in the CO. In young patients, MAP of 65 mmHg may be adequate to maintain renal and systemic perfusion.

Type III phosphodiesterase inhibitors

Phosphodiesterase (PDE) inhibitors block the breakdown of cyclic adenosine monophosphate; enoximone and milrinone are the two agents used in clinical practice. They cause marked peripheral vasodilatation and have inotropic effects; therefore, they are useful in patients with advanced heart failure who have an elevated SVR but remain hypotensive because of a very low CO. Because of their powerful vasodilating effect, haemodynamic monitoring is recommended whenever they are used. Both agents have a long elimination half-life and tend to accumulate if the patient is oliguric. Because their site of action is distal to the β-adrenergic receptor, PDE inhibitors maintain their effect in patients who have been treated with β-blocking drugs. In patients with atrial fibrillation, they may increase ventricular rate less than dobutamine.

Levosimendan

This drug has two main mechanisms of action: calcium ion sensitization of the contractile proteins (positive inotropic effect) and smooth muscle potassium ion channel opening (peripheral vasodilating effect). There is also a suggestion that levosimendan has a PDE-inhibiting effect. Intravenous infusions of levosimendan are usually maintained for 24 hours, but the haemodynamic effects persist, probably because of the long half-life of its metabolite. Levosimendan infusions in patients with heart failure have been associated with a dose-dependent increase in stroke volume and CO, a decline in the pulmonary capillary wedge pressure, a decrease in SVR and pulmonary vascular resistance, a slight decrease in blood pressure and a slight increase in heart rate. An improvement in symptoms of dyspnoea and fatigue has been shown in trials comparing levosimendan with dobutamine. The haemodynamic effects were seen even in the presence of β-blocker therapy. Tachycardia and hypotension are side effects associated with the use of levosimendan and it is not recommended in patients with a systolic blood pressure below 85 mmHg.

Ultrafiltration

Patients with gross fluid retention and hyponatraemia present a difficult clinical problem. Diuretics often worsen hyponatraemia and sometimes features of the cardiorenal syndrome become apparent. Inotropic drugs may help in this situation, but if therapy needs to be prolonged, the risk of arrhythmia needs to be considered. Continuous venovenous haemofiltration (CVVH) is effective in removing fluid and the rate of fluid removal can be tailored to the patient's needs; CVVH may also remove cytokines with myocardial depressant properties (e.g. tumour necrosis factor) because macromolecules up to 20,000 D can pass through the ultrafiltration membrane. If necessary, large volumes of fluid can be removed in a relatively short time to ready the patient for a definitive procedure (heart transplantation, mechanical circulatory support).

Although CVVH usually requires large-bore central venous access, there are devices that allow ultrafiltration via cannulae in peripheral arm veins. Although the maximum rate of fluid removal is less than that attainable by central CVVH, an adequate rate is achieved for the most common clinical situations.

Compared with high-dose diuretic therapy, ultrafiltration has been reported to induce less neurohormonal activation and vasoconstriction. It is underutilized in the management of fluid-overloaded patients with advanced heart failure.

Intra-aortic balloon pump

Intra-aortic balloon pump (IABP) use may reduce afterload, thereby decreasing left ventricular stroke work and myocardial oxygen consumption, as well as augmenting diastolic blood flow in the coronary and systemic circulation. Functional mitral regurgitation, a common problem in a patient with a dilated left ventricle, decreases with the use of the IABP. The IABP is extremely useful in critically ill patients with heart failure who can be stabilized until definitive therapy can be carried out. It is underused in patients with advanced heart failure in the intensive care unit. In patients requiring support beyond that provided by IABP, consideration should be given to the use of a ventricular assist device.

Conclusion

Advanced heart failure in patients on critical care units carries a high mortality. Optimal management requires close cooperation between a cardiologist with an interest in heart failure, an intensive care physician and a cardiac surgeon. With appropriate therapy, many critically ill patients can be resuscitated and returned to a productive life. In the United Kingdom, there is often a reluctance to admit these patients to critical care units; this is not in the best interests of the patients concerned.

Key points

- Heart failure, most commonly secondary to coronary artery disease, carries a poor overall prognosis.
- Admission to critical care is usually due to pulmonary oedema or cardiogenic shock.
- Aggressive diuresis is indicated, and renal replacement therapy may be necessary to remove an adequate amount of fluid.
- Inotropes are often started to enhance CO, but may lead to other complications; therapy should be closely monitored.
- An intra-aortic balloon pump may improve the clinical picture greatly.

FURTHER READING

ACC/AHA guidelines for the evaluation and management of chronic heart failure in the adult. *J Am Coll Cardiol* 2005;46:1116–1143. Updates available via www.acc.org.

Binanay C, Califf RM, Hasselblad V, *et al.* Evaluation study of congestive heart failure and pulmonary artery catheterization effectiveness, the ESCAPE trial. *JAMA* 2005;294:1625–1633.

Nohria A, Lewis E, Stevenson LW. Medical management of advanced heart failure. *JAMA* 2002;287:628–640.

Steimle AE, Stevenson LW, Chelimsky-Fallick C, *et al.* Sustained hemodynamic efficacy of therapy tailored to reduce filling pressures in survivors with advanced heart failure. *Circulation* 1997;96: 1165–1172.

The Task Force on Acute Heart Failure of the European Society of Cardiology. Executive summary of the guidelines on the diagnosis and treatment of acute heart failure. *Eur Heart J* 2005;26:384–416.

Chapter 5

Admission to critical care: The respiratory patient

S. KAUL AND L.S.G.E. HOWARD

Introduction

Acute respiratory failure is a common reason for admission to critical care. This chapter focuses on acute respiratory failure as a consequence of primary lung or chest wall disease, examining the assessment and specific medical management of these conditions. Acute conditions, such as asthma and community-acquired pneumonia, have clear criteria for referral to critical care; however, admission of patients limited by chronic respiratory disease may not be straightforward.

Primary respiratory conditions in those with previously normal lungs

Community-acquired pneumonia

Clinical assessment of community-acquired pneumonia involves recognizing treatable coexisting complications and comorbidities, including parapneumonic effusion or empyema, which should be drained. Detailed microbiological investigations should be performed, including blood and sputum/tracheal aspirate for culture and sensitivities (preferably before starting antibiotic treatment) and urine for both pneumococcal and legionella antigen. In addition, sputum should be examined by Gram stain and direct immunofluorescence for viral pathogens. Additional investigations for severe community-acquired pneumonia include paired viral and atypical serology. The incidence of *Staphylococcus aureus* and *Legionella pneumophila* is increased in severe pneumonia, and a history of influenza symptoms and foreign travel should be sought.

Empirical intravenous antibiotic therapy with a broad-spectrum β-lactamase–stable antibiotic (e.g. co-amoxiclav) or a second- or third-generation cephalosporin should be initiated, combined with an intravenous macrolide. Where legionella infection is suspected, rifampicin may be added and where aspiration is thought to have occurred, antibiotic cover should be broadened to cover anaerobic organisms. Oxygen therapy should maintain saturations between 94% and 98%. In refractory hypoxaemia, a trial of continuous positive airway pressure (CPAP) or noninvasive ventilation (NIV) can be considered, but this should be instituted in a critical care environment where the patient can be intubated swiftly in the event of failure.

Nosocomial pneumonia

Nosocomial pneumonia can be classified in terms of severity and managed in the same way as community-acquired pneumonia, although empirical antibiotic therapy should be adjusted to reflect the likely different microbiological aetiology. In severe nosocomial pneumonia, a standard regimen should include treatment of methicillin-resistant *S aureus* (e.g. vancomycin) and gram-negative organisms such as pseudomonas and enterobacter (e.g. ciprofloxacin or ceftazidime).

Underlying comorbidities, such as malnutrition (Chapter 35), diabetes (Chapter 43), or chronic heart disease (Chapter 3), need to be managed concurrently.

Pulmonary infiltrates in the immunocompromised host

The development of pulmonary infiltrates is a frequent, life-threatening complication in immunocompromised patients, requiring early diagnosis and treatment. Infection should always be suspected and treated empirically. The cause is often related to the patient's underlying diagnosis, current immunosuppressive regimen, duration of immunosuppression, and prior therapies. More often than not, the diagnosis is unknown at the time of referral to the intensive care unit.

Achieving a diagnosis is central to the management of these patients. New infiltrates may represent a complication or progression of the underlying lung disease, such as the accelerated phase of idiopathic pulmonary fibrosis. Immunosuppressants themselves may be associated with new infiltrates, for example, sirolimus-induced pulmonary hypersensitivity. Noninfectious aetiologies are diverse and responsible for between 25% and 50% of infiltrates in these patients. The initial clinical appearance is rarely helpful in identifying a specific cause.

Standard chest radiographs should be regarded as a screening test and the early use of computed

Table 5.2 Common causes of noninfectious pulmonary infiltrates

Pulmonary oedema (cardiogenic/noncardiogenic)
Acute lung injury/acute respiratory distress syndrome
Idiopathic interstitial pneumonias Acute interstitial pneumonia Cryptogenic organizing pneumonia Accelerated idiopathic pulmonary fibrosis
Acute eosinophilic pneumonia
Hypersensitivity pneumonitis (drug-induced, EAA)
Diffuse alveolar haemorrhage

Abbreviation: EAA, extrinsic allergic alveolitis.

Table 5.1 Infectious agents in immunosuppressed patients

Type of immunosuppression	Common associated conditions	Infectious agent affecting the lung
Neutrophil-mediated immunity	Neutropenia Chemotherapy and cytotoxic agents Bone marrow transplantation Corticosteroids Diabetes	*Staphylococcus* Gram-negative bacteria Fungal infections
T-cell–mediated immunity	Immunosuppressive agents, e.g. used in heart/lung transplantation (cyclosporine, tacrolimus) HIV Corticosteroids	Mycobacterial species *Nocardia* Viruses (HSV, VZV, CMV, adenovirus, RSV, influenza, parainfluenza) *Pneumocystis jiroveci*
Antibody deficiency	Myeloma, lymphoma, CLL Splenectomy Congenital deficiency	Encapsulated bacteria *Mycoplasma*

Abbreviations: CLL, chronic lymphocytic leukaemia; CMV, cytomegalovirus; HIV, human immunodeficiency virus; HSV, herpes simplex virus; RSV, respiratory syncytial virus; VZV, varicella zoster virus.

Table 5.3 Routine microbiological investigations in the immunosuppressed patient with pulmonary infiltrates

	BALF	Blood
Bacteriology and mycology	Gram stain Auramine stain for AFB Culture and sensitivities (including fungal; mycobacterial; opportunistic organisms [e.g. *Legionella*, *Nocardia*])	Culture and sensitivities
Virology	PCR (HSV, VZV, CMV) IF (influenza, parainfluenza, RSV, adenovirus)	PCR (HSV, VZV, CMV)
Cytology	Grocott stain (for *Pneumocystis jiroveci*) Differential cell count	

Abbreviations: AFB, acid-fast bacilli; BALF, bronchoalveolar lavage fluid; CMV, cytomegalovirus; HSV, herpes simplex virus; IF, immunofluorescence; PCR, polymerase chain reaction; RSV, respiratory syncytial virus; VZV, varicella zoster virus.

tomography (CT) scans is recommended, with some aetiologies having characteristic patterns, for example, angioinvasive aspergillosis and cryptogenic organizing pneumonia. Furthermore, CT may help in planning bronchoscopic lavage or biopsy, whether transbronchial or surgical. Bronchoscopy is often the next investigation of choice. If the patient is highly oxygen dependent, invasive or noninvasive ventilation may be required during or after the procedure. With experience, use of sedation may be minimized. Bronchoscopic lavage is commonly favoured for reasons of simplicity and safety, but transbronchial biopsy may increase the diagnostic yield. However, there may be an increased risk of bleeding owing to coagulopathy, thrombocytopenia or pulmonary hypertension. Once intubated, the risk of pneumothorax with transbronchial biopsy increases to at least 5%.

The differential cell count in bronchoalveolar lavage may help in the diagnosis of noninfectious causes, such as hypersensitivity or eosinophilic pneumonia. Nasopharyngeal aspirate may often yield a virological diagnosis when bronchoscopy cannot be undertaken. Blind empirical therapy usually includes coverage against Gram-negative and Gram-positive organisms. Additional empirical therapy is guided by likely immune deficit. If therapy based on CT imaging and available cultures has failed, then surgical lung biopsy may be considered. Ultimately, intubation in the immunocompromised patient carries a grave prognosis and NIV should be attempted in suitable patients.

Pulmonary infiltrates in the immunocompetent host

New pulmonary infiltrates in the immunocompetent host have a broad differential diagnosis and are similar to those in the immunosuppressed, although opportunistic infection is far less likely. Clinical history taking and examination, coupled with standard imaging and haematological and biochemical analyses identifies most causes, the commonest being infection and cardiogenic pulmonary oedema. Where standard therapy has failed and the patient is deteriorating, CT imaging and bronchoscopy may be required.

Table 5.2 lists some of the more common forms of noninfectious pulmonary infiltrate. Some conditions are extremely steroid responsive (e.g. cryptogenic organizing pneumonia, hypersensitivity pneumonitis). Heavy immunosuppression may be beneficial in certain cases and interventions such as plasma exchange may also be considered. Consequently, early lung biopsy can be helpful in managing these conditions, particularly in cases of partial response to steroids.

Pulmonary embolism

Pulmonary embolism (PE) can be classified as follows:

- massive PE in association with hypotension;
- submassive PE in association with right ventricular hypokinesia on echocardiography; and
- nonmassive PE in the absence of the above features.

Emergency imaging in the form of CT pulmonary angiography or transthoracic echocardiography is advocated when massive PE is suspected. In massive PE, CT pulmonary angiography reliably demonstrates proximal thrombus. Both right ventricular dysfunction on echocardiography and an elevated serum troponin I predict a higher mortality.

Thrombolysis (given peripherally) is the first-line treatment and may be instituted on clinical grounds in the peri-arrest situation. Where thrombolysis is contraindicated or has failed, surgical embolectomy, clot lysis by direct fragmentation or high-pressure jet lysis may be considered. Ideally, thrombolysis should be instituted in a critical care setting. Intubation and ventilation should be avoided because of the increase in pulmonary vascular resistance associated with positive pressure ventilation and the added risk of hypotension produced by induction agents. There is considerable disagreement about the role of thrombolysis in submassive PE. It has been shown to improve the clinical course (by reducing the rate of rescue thrombolysis) when compared with intravenous unfractionated heparin, but no change in mortality has been reported and it carries an increased risk of haemorrhage.

Mechanical respiratory failure

Acute ventilatory failure owing to extrapulmonary causes may result de novo, from conditions such as Guillain-Barré syndrome, or decompensation of preexisting conditions that may or may not have been diagnosed previously.

Identifying a cause is vital; specific treatments vary and may be extremely effective in addition to supportive care. Additional processes that contribute to respiratory decompensation include the following.

UPPER AIRWAY COMPROMISE

Weakness of the facial, oropharyngeal and laryngeal muscles can result in swallowing dysfunction and

Table 5.4 Common or important causes of mechanical respiratory failure

	Acute	Chronic
Neuronal	Guillain-Barré syndrome Diphtheria Tick paralysis Poliomyelitis	Motor neurone disease
Neuromuscular junction	Botulism Myasthenia gravis	Myasthenia gravis Lambert-Eaton syndrome
Muscle	Dermatomyositis/polymyositis	Dermatomyositis/polymyositis Duchenne muscular dystrophy Chest wall disorders (e.g. thoracoplasty, kyphoscoliosis)

interfere with secretion clearance and increase the risk of aspiration pneumonia. Furthermore, weakness of those muscles may result in upper airway obstruction, particularly in the supine position.

INSPIRATORY MUSCLE WEAKNESS

This results in poor lung expansion and atelectasis, leading to ventilation/perfusion mismatch, and consequent hypoxaemia.

EXPIRATORY MUSCLE WEAKNESS

This prevents adequate cough and secretion clearance, again increasing the risk of pneumonia.

Additional pathology includes:

- primary respiratory tract infection;
- pulmonary embolus owing to immobility in chronic disease;
- coexistent asthma; and
- pulmonary oedema owing to cardiomyopathy.

Guillain-Barré syndrome is the commonest neurological cause of respiratory failure requiring mechanical ventilation. It is an acute, autoimmune polyradiculoneuropathy. Most commonly it presents as an ascending paralysis spreading to the upper limbs and the face. Bulbar palsy may also be present. Early recognition, treatment with intravenous immunoglobulin or plasmapheresis within the first 2 weeks of presentation and adequate supportive care results in near full functional recovery in most patients. However, it is associated with an appreciable mortality, mainly owing to pulmonary and autonomic complications. About 30% of patients require ventilatory assistance largely owing to diaphragmatic failure.

Close clinical supervision in combination with bedside respiratory function tests is required. Serial measurements (3 times a day) of vital capacity and maximal inspiratory and expiratory pressures should be performed; arterial blood gases may not demonstrate hypoxaemia and hypercapnia until late in the disease process. During the night, ventilatory function is more dependent on the diaphragm and continuous oxygen saturation should be monitored during sleep; transcutaneous CO_2 monitoring may be useful. It is important to note that endotracheal intubation in these patients can trigger autonomic instability. The consequences of respiratory arrest can therefore be devastating and early intubation and assisted ventilation is preferred. At present, there is no evidence supporting the use of CPAP or NIV in patients with respiratory decompensation due to Guillain-Barré syndrome.

Table 5.5 Criteria for intensive care unit admission for Guillain-Barré syndrome

Clinical features	Physiological features
Bulbar dysfunction	MIP $\leq$ 30 cmH_2O or MEP $\leq$ 40 cmH_2O
Autonomic instability	VC $\leq$ 20 mL/kg
Bilateral facial palsy	Fall of 30% over 24 hours in VC, MIP or MEP
Rapid disease progression	$Pao_2 \leq 9$ kPa or increasing $Paco_2$

Abbreviations: MEP, maximum expiratory pressure; MIP, maximum inspiratory pressure; $Paco_2$, partial pressure of carbon dioxide in arterial blood; Pao_2, partial pressure of oxygen in arterial blood; VC, vital capacity.

Other causes of acute respiratory muscle weakness require mechanical ventilation less frequently than Guillain-Barré syndrome. Specific treatments include plasma exchange and acetylcholinesterase inhibitors in myasthenia gravis or immunosuppression in polymyositis. A detailed diagnostic strategy is therefore warranted, but is beyond the scope of this chapter.

Infection is often the triggering event for the first presentation of respiratory failure in the chronic neuromuscular disorders. Unlike the more rapidly progressive conditions, it is reasonable to consider NIV as an initial form of ventilatory support, and this may be required long term. If invasive ventilation is necessary, then early extubation facilitated by NIV or tracheostomy should be considered.

Respiratory conditions in those with previously abnormal lungs

Asthma

A significant proportion of asthma deaths occur during hospitalization. Exacerbations of asthma are reversible; therefore, ensuring institution of correct treatment, adequate monitoring and appropriate critical care admission is a priority.

Patients meeting the criteria for acute life-threatening or near-fatal asthma should be admitted to intensive care and maximal therapy administered. As part of their assessment, additional reversible causes must be excluded, such as pneumothorax and lobar collapse owing to mucus plugging or pneumonia.

Oxygen, nebulized bronchodilators and steroid therapy are required. Arterial blood gases should be sampled to assess $Paco_2$ and pH. Although high-flow oxygen is associated with higher levels of $Paco_2$ and lower peak expiratory flow in patients with acute asthma, this should not prevent the administration of maximal oxygen therapy in patients who are persistently hypoxaemic. Oxygen delivered via reservoir bag mask is dry and cold, potentially worsening bronchospasm. Ideally, oxygen should be delivered warm and humidified. There is currently no good evidence for use of Heliox in acute asthma.

Nebulized bronchodilators and β-agonists should be driven by oxygen and may be administered continuously. If there is no response, intravenous β-agonists can be considered, although evidence for this is limited. Intravenous magnesium sulphate (1.2–2.0 g) is effective and should be administered over 20 minutes; more rapid infusion can cause flushing, hypotension and flaccid paralysis. If repeat boluses are required, admission to critical care is necessary and continuous infusion may be more appropriate. Intravenous aminophylline is rarely administered owing to its side effect profile and paucity of evidence in its favour.

Table 5.6 British Thoracic Society classification of acute asthma severity

Moderate asthma	Severe asthma
One of more of the following: • No features of acute severe asthma • PEFR >50–75% best or predicted	One of more of the following: • Cannot complete sentences • Pulse $\geq$ 110 beats/min • Respiratory rate $\geq$ 25 breaths/min • PEFR 33–50% predicted or usual best
Life-threatening asthma	**Near-fatal asthma**
One or more of the following: • Silent chest, feeble effort • Cyanosis/ $Spo_2 \leq 92\%$ • Bradycardia, hypotension • Exhaustion, confusion, coma • Normal $Paco_2$ • PEFR $\leq$33% predicted or usual best	One of more of the following: Raised $Paco_2$ and/or requiring mechanical ventilation with increased ventilatory pressures

Abbreviations: $Paco_2$, partial pressure of carbon dioxide in arterial blood; PEFR, peak expiratory flow rate; Spo_2, saturation of peripheral oxygen.

It has a narrow therapeutic range and regular monitoring of theophylline and potassium levels is also required. Other agents such as ketamine and halogenated inhalational anaesthetic agents may be necessary in refractory bronchospasm.

Steroids can usually be given enterally (prednisolone 40–50 mg) and intravenous hydrocortisone (100 mg 4 times a day) is reserved for patients unable to swallow or absorb tablets.

Hypovolaemia is common and fluid resuscitation is required. If intubation and invasive ventilation are necessary, the high pressures required for ventilation coupled with often severe gas trapping and intrinsic positive end-expiratory pressure lead to a marked reduction in preload to the left ventricle; systemic hypotension and loss of cardiac output may occur.

There is no role for NIV in asthma outside of critical care. Low-level CPAP offsets intrinsic positive end-expiratory pressure and may be started after critical care admission.

Antibiotics should only be administered if there is objective evidence of infection, such as consolidation on chest radiographs or high C-reactive protein levels.

'Pseudo-asthma' may occur in acute hyperventilation, vocal cord dysfunction and thoracoabdominal asynchrony. It is often extremely difficult to differentiate these from true asthma in an emergency setting. In this instance, if the patient is intubated, then their airway pressures should be documented immediately after intubation. This can be useful when treating subsequent exacerbations.

Chronic obstructive pulmonary disease

Exacerbations of COPD account for about 10% of all emergency medical admissions and around a quarter present with acidosis. There is a high (7.4%) inpatient mortality. In addition, comorbidities often coexist, including heart disease (40%), diabetes (10%), stroke (6%) and other chest disease (11%). Differential or concomitant diagnoses include the following.

- *Pneumonia*.
- *Pneumothorax*: Often this may be difficult to detect on plain radiographs owing to bullae or anterior or posterior pneumothoraces. CT may be required.
- *Pulmonary embolism*: In uncomplicated exacerbation, the incidence of PE is low; however, up to 50% of patients with COPD have post mortem evidence of pulmonary artery thrombosis.
- *Pulmonary oedema*: The features of oedema on radiograph are often atypical in COPD and old radiographs may be helpful.
- *Lung cancer*.
- *Aspiration*.

Hypoxaemia should be prevented, while minimizing acidosis and hypercapnia. Lung function must be optimized while the precipitating cause of the exacerbation is treated. Many patients have an uncomplicated admission responding to the standard regimen of controlled oxygen therapy, bronchodilators (β-agonists and anticholinergics), steroids (prednisolone 30 mg for 7–14 days) and antibiotic therapy. Antiobiotic therapy should be instituted in the presence of increased production of purulent sputum and can usually be given orally. Targeted therapy may often be guided by present or past sputum culture results.

Many patients at risk of hypercapnic respiratory failure are hypoxaemic between exacerbations and do not require high target saturations during an exacerbation. Oxygen therapy may worsen ventilation–perfusion mismatch, cause absorption atelectasis, decrease haemoglobin buffering of CO_2 by the Haldane effect and reduce the hypoxic ventilatory response. These factors lead to an increase in $Paco_2$ via a decrease in effective alveolar ventilation and CO_2 buffering. If a patient is found not be hypercapnic, then their saturations may be kept above 94%. However, either until $Paco_2$ is known or if they are hypercapnic, their saturations should be kept within the range of 88–92% or even lower on occasion.

Twenty per cent of patients remain acidotic (pH $\leq$ 7.35) despite optimal medical therapy and these patients are potential candidates for NIV. It should be considered before intravenous aminophylline and doxapram. These agents may be used in conjunction with NIV, however, or as a ceiling of therapy if NIV is not tolerated and invasive ventilation is not indicated.

A decision regarding invasive ventilation should be made before commencing NIV. Where possible, decisions should be made in consultation with the patient, relatives, nursing staff, admitting medical team members and critical care team. This should not be based on age or forced expiratory volume in 1 second (FEV_1) alone because it is a poor predictor of physical capacity. Furthermore, it should not be based on a personal assessment of quality of life.

The attitude towards mechanical ventilation and COPD is often nihilistic. However, in-hospital survival is better and duration of ventilation shorter in patients ventilated for an exacerbation of COPD than all causes of acute respiratory failure, with a 1-year survival of 40–60%. Paradoxically, previous mechanical ventilation is associated with an improved survival, perhaps suggesting more variable disease. Factors that may influence the decision regarding ventilation include body mass index, functional status and the presence of other organ failure.

Often patients are 'accepted' for mechanical ventilation if there is deemed to be some reversible pathology such as pneumonia. Although there is a component of logic in this, the higher mortality associated with COPD and pneumonia compared with an exacerbation of COPD alone draws this strategy into question. Furthermore, although COPD itself is not reversible, the physiology of the patient improves after treatment of the exacerbation.

The decision to admit to critical care and/or implement invasive mechanical ventilation needs to consider how intensive therapy can improve the patient, whether they have the functional reserve to withstand therapy and whether further treatment could be given safely on the medical wards. Clear communication of the benefits and risks of critical care management is required. Ideally, this should be done in anticipation of critical care referral before the patient becomes unstable, even in the outpatient clinic, where reasonable.

Interstitial lung disease

Underlying causes of deterioration in a patient with a background of interstitial lung disease should be sought, such as anaemia, PE, pneumothorax or infection. Serial chest radiographs are often helpful in diagnosing new infection; if no change is noted, in particular no clear progression of disease, then CT pulmonary angiography should be performed to exclude PE. Patients with idiopathic pulmonary fibrosis and asbestosis are at much higher risk of developing carcinoma of the bronchus, which may cause acute deterioration due to bronchial occlusion.

Idiopathic pulmonary fibrosis may enter an accelerated phase, with rapidly worsening respiratory failure and increased alveolar opacification. The histological features show diffuse alveolar damage akin to acute interstitial pneumonia. Patchy disease on CT is associated with 50% mortality and diffuse involvement is nearly always fatal. Often these patients have been immunosuppressed and consequently, conventional and opportunistic infection must be excluded, often by bronchoscopy. Lung biopsy is not usually required in deteriorations of well-documented idiopathic pulmonary fibrosis; however, where diagnostic uncertainty exists, the cause of the deterioration should be sought and biopsies obtained because intense immunosuppression may be required.

Key points

- Well-evidenced guidelines for management of many respiratory conditions have been produced by various scientific societies (British Thoracic Society).
- The use of diagnostic tests, in particular CT and bronchoscopy, help to guide therapy in cases where the differential diagnosis is broad.
- Noninvasive ventilation can be used successfully outside the critical care setting in COPD. It may also be used in other conditions, but usually within the critical care unit.
- Empirical antibiotic therapy should always take into consideration the provenance and immunocompetence of the patient.

FURTHER READING

British Thoracic Society Standards of Care Committee. Non-invasive ventilation in acute respiratory failure. *Thorax* 2002;57:192–211.

British Thoracic Society Standards of Care Committee Pulmonary Embolism Guidelines Development Group. British Thoracic Society guidelines for the management of suspected acute pulmonary embolism. *Thorax* 2003;58: 470–483.

British Thoracic Society; Scottish Intercollegiate Guidelines Network. British guideline on the management of asthma. *Thorax* 2003;58(Suppl 1):i1–94.

National Collaborating Centre for Chronic Conditions. Chronic obstructive pulmonary disease. National clinical guideline on management of chronic obstructive pulmonary disease in adults in primary and secondary care. *Thorax* 2004;59(Suppl 1):1–232.

Chapter 6

Resuscitation after cardiac surgery

J.H. MACKAY

Introduction

Defibrillation, ventilation, pacing and resuscitation are essential components of cardiac surgical care. The 2005 European Resuscitation Council Guidelines report the incidence of resuscitation as 0.7% in the first 24 hours, rising to 1.4% within the first 8 days of cardiac surgery. Overall in-hospital cardiac surgical mortality rates (>3.0%), together with the low incidence of do not attempt resuscitation (DNAR) orders and the high proportion of treatable arrests in this population all suggest a higher true incidence of postoperative resuscitation. The most likely explanation for the discrepancy is that many resuscitation interventions are undertaken in house on the cardiac surgical critical care. As patients undergoing cardiac surgery become older and sicker, the quality of postoperative care and resuscitation will continue to increase in importance. Conventional advanced life support (ALS) guidelines provide a useful framework but require modification, particularly in the cardiac surgical critical care setting. This chapter highlights some of the key differences.

Resuscitation guidelines

Adult basic life support

Maintaining the circulation has been promoted ahead of airway management and breathing in adult basic life support (BLS) guidelines. The traditional 'ABC' (airway, breathing, circulation) in the previous BLS algorithm has been replaced by 'CAB' (circulation, airway, breathing). Thirty chest compressions should be given before any attempt to deliver rescue breaths. In situations where BLS is undertaken, the recommended ratio of chest compressions to ventilations is now 30:2 for both one- and two-person cardiopulmonary resuscitation (CPR). More chest compressions and fewer interruptions are achieved with this ratio than with 15:2. In the presence of a patent airway, effective chest compressions are considered more important than ventilation in the first few minutes of resuscitation. It should be borne in mind that coronary perfusion pressure progressively rises during chest compressions and rapidly falls with each pause for ventilation. Rescuers can now be instructed to place their hands over the centre of the chest rather than waste time using the 'rib margin' method. The single BLS algorithm facilitates teaching BLS to lay people and reminds rescuers to consider airway obstruction – but it is also a potential flaw. Future adult guidelines should further increase the emphasis on chest compressions in witnessed unexpected sudden collapse (patients with saturated arterial blood) and reserve initial combined assisted ventilations and chest compressions for unwitnessed arrests or primary respiratory arrest (patients with desaturated arterial blood).

Adult advanced life support

The ALS algorithm for the management of cardiac arrest in adults has shockable and nonshockable limbs. Prompt and effective BLS and early defibrillation for shockable rhythms are the two most important interventions after cardiac arrest. There have been fairly radical changes in defibrillation recommendations for shockable rhythms.

PULSELESS VENTRICULAR TACHYCARDIA/VENTRICULAR FIBRILLATION ARRESTS

Pulseless ventricular tachycardia (VT) and ventricular fibrillation (VF) account for the majority of patients who survive cardiac arrest in a general hospital. For every minute that the arrhythmia persists, the chances of successful defibrillation decline by 7–10%. Specialist cardiothoracic units should be capable of early detection, rapid defibrillation and superior outcomes. A single defibrillatory shock (≥150 J biphasic or ≥360 J monophasic) is recommended instead of three stacked shocks. In the setting of the cardiac critical care, when external cardiac massage may be injurious, immediate defibrillation should be the first-line response for all monitored in-hospital VF arrests. First shock efficacy is greater with biphasic than monophasic waveforms. Duration of CPR between shocks has increased to 2 minutes. Contrary to the new guidelines, there is usually no need to commence chest compressions after a successful shock in invasively monitored cardiac surgical patients.

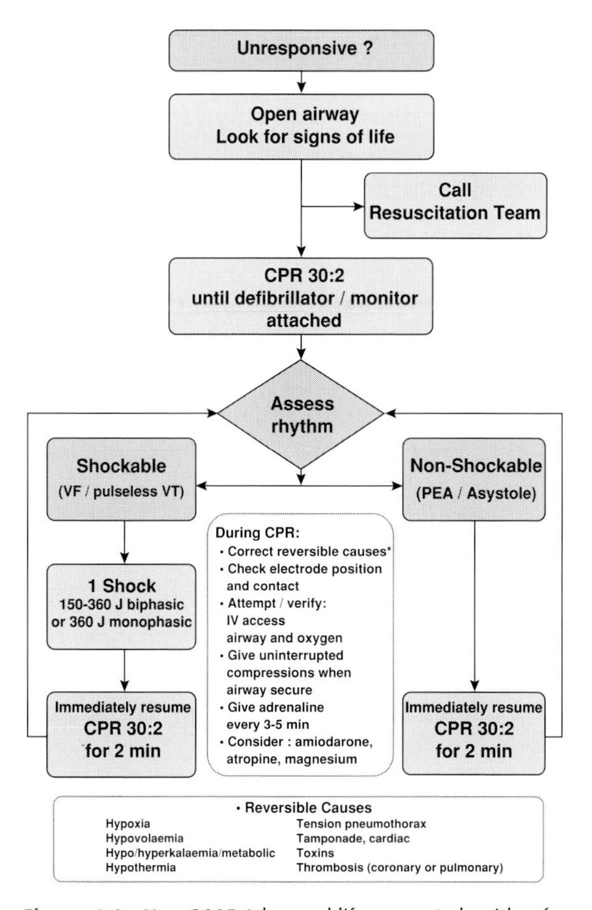

Figure 6.1 New 2005 Advanced life support algorithm for the management of cardiac arrest in adults. (Courtesy of the UK Resuscitation Council and reproduced with permission.)

NON–VENTRICULAR FIBRILLATION/VENTRICULAR TACHYCARDIA ARRESTS

A heterogeneous group of conditions may present as non-VF/VT cardiac arrest. Outcome is generally poor unless a reversible cause can be found and treated effectively. The frequent absence of a readily treatable underlying cause means that this type of arrest has a poor prognosis in general hospitals with only 5–10% patients surviving to discharge. In contrast, in the cardiac surgical critical care – where bleeding, hypovolaemia and tamponade are all readily treatable, and where additional therapeutic options are available – outcomes should be considerably better. Examination of trends in central venous pressure, pulmonary artery wedge pressure and airway pressure all provide useful pointers as to the possible aetiology of arrest. Cessation of drainage from chest drains does not exclude haemorrhage or tamponade because the drains may have become blocked. Although echocardiography is often very useful in the cardiac critical care, transoesophageal echocardiography (TOE) may miss

Table 6.1 An "aide memoire" to the causes of pulseless electrical activity and asystole

The Four *Hs*	The Five *Ts*
Hypoxia	Tension pneumothorax
Hypovolaemia	Tamponade
Hyperkalaemia	Thromboembolic
Hypothermia	Therapeutic substances in overdose
	Toxic substances

localized collections and delay reoperation. Patients with clinical signs suggestive of tamponade should be reopened, even if the TOE is inconclusive.

When faced with an arrest of this type, it is essential to

- confirm that VF is not being missed and that leads or pads are correctly attached;
- treat bradycardias with epicardial pacing if possible;
- exclude underlying VF in the presence of fixed-rate pacing; and
- consider chest reopening if closed chest CPR is unsuccessful.

Symptomatic bradycardia is extremely common in the cardiac surgical critical care unit. The ALS guidelines recommend atropine as first-line treatment. In the cardiac surgical critical care, where tachycardia is equally undesirable, pacing (when possible) is the preferred option. If pacing is not an option (e.g. no wires in situ or failure to capture), isoproterenol or dopamine are often used before atropine is considered. Management of asystole that fails to respond to pacing is an indication for prompt chest reopening.

Drugs in advanced cardiac life support

Although the use of vasopressors at cardiac arrests seems intuitive and has become standard practice, proof of efficacy has been more difficult to achieve. Adrenaline (1 mg) is recommended every 3 minutes to improve coronary and cerebral perfusion. The American Heart Association has suggested that vasopressin may be used as an alternative to epinephrine. Clinical studies, however, have failed to demonstrate that either vasopressin or high-dose epinephrine (5 mg) offer any additional benefit.

On the cardiac surgical critical care, it may be entirely appropriate to modify the recommended pharmacological management of a monitored cardiac arrest. An α-agonist or smaller initial dosages of adrenaline (0.1–0.5 mg) may be administered to minimize the risk of hypertension and tachycardia after successful resuscitation. For patients with VF/VT arrests, it is standard practice to attempt at least two shocks before giving adrenaline. The administration of amiodarone after three unsuccessful shocks increases likelihood of survival to hospital admission, but not survival to discharge. A bolus of 300 mg of amiodarone is recommended for VF/VT arrests that persist after three shocks. A further dose of 150 mg may be given for recurrent or refractory VF/VT, followed by an infusion of 900 mg over 24 hours. Lidocaine can be given for VF/VT if the patient has received amiodarone, but the evidence supporting its efficacy is weak. Consider giving magnesium if there is clinical suspicion of hypomagnesaemia. Administration of bicarbonate should be considered if arterial or mixed venous pH is 7.1 or less.

Chest opening

After surgery via sternotomy, chest reopening is an additional diagnostic and therapeutic option in the cardiac surgical critical care. In addition, chest reopening allows internal cardiac massage, which is considerably more effective than external chest compressions. Bleeding, tamponade, graft occlusion and graft avulsion are conditions likely to be remedied by this approach.

Patients most likely to benefit from chest reopening are those with a surgically remediable lesion, those who arrest within 24 hours of surgery and those in whom the chest is reopened within 10 minutes of arrest. Delayed reopening or the finding of a problem that is not amenable to surgery (e.g. global cardiac dysfunction) is associated with a poor prognosis. Chest reopening should not be used as a 'last-ditch' manoeuvre after a prolonged resuscitation sequence.

Cardiopulmonary bypass

The reinstitution of cardiopulmonary bypass (CPB) after emergency chest reopening may allow the resuscitation of a patient who would otherwise die. Hypothermic CPB restores organ perfusion, decompresses the heart and allows the surgeon to consider all possible options in a more controlled setting. Valve replacement, the repair of bleeding cannulation sites, graft revision and additional grafting may be undertaken with often surprisingly successful clinical outcomes. Whenever possible, the patient should be transferred to the operating theatre before the emergency reinstitution of CPB.

Late resuscitation on critical care

Patients with greater preoperative surgical risk, adverse intraoperative events and poor physiological state at the time of critical care admission are less likely to survive to hospital discharge. Similarly, refractory multisystem organ failure and recurrent nosocomial infection while on the critical care unit have been shown to be important determinants of mortality. For some patients, there comes a point when aggressive resuscitation is inappropriate and cardiopulmonary arrest becomes the terminal event in their illness. It is the duty of a doctor to identify these patients and to ensure that they are spared the indignity of futile interventions.

In the postoperative period, DNAR directives may be instituted if it is believed that death is inevitable and that CPR is unlikely to be successful. Sensible guidelines on implementation of DNAR orders can be found on the UK Resuscitation Council's website.

Resuscitation outside critical care

Ward arrests

The management of a cardiac arrest on a cardiac surgical ward differs little from a cardiac arrest on a general surgical or medical ward. Seemingly trivial symptoms and vague 'early warning' signs should be taken seriously; they may herald a more sinister event. Although some arrests are unheralded, the majority of patients who arrest in the general ward setting display signs of physiological deterioration before the event.

Early intervention seems intuitive and may reduce the incidence of cardiac arrests in the surgical ward setting. Early Warning Scores are used to 'track' the patients' physiological status and 'trigger' a response or intervention. These scoring systems can be adapted for use in cardiothoracic wards.

The use of medical emergency teams (MET) has been shown to reduce both the incidence and mortality from unexpected ward arrests in a general

Table 6.2 Suggested criteria for calling the medical emergency team in a cardiothoracic hospital

Acute change	Physiology
Airway	Threatened
Breathing	All respiratory arrests Respiratory rate ≤5 or >36
Circulation	All cardiac arrests Pulse rate ≤40 or >140
Neurology	Unexplained fall in GCS >2 points
Renal	Urine output ≤0.5 mL/kg/hr for 2 consecutive hours
Oximetry	Spo_2 ≤90% regardless of Fio_2
Other	Patients giving cause for concern who do not meet above criteria

Abbreviations: Fio_2, fraction of inspired oxygen; GCS, Glasgow Coma Scale; Spo_2, saturation of peripheral oxygen.

Table 6.3 Possible Modified Early Warning Scores (MEWS) system for wards in a cardiothoracic hospital

Score	Temp (°C)	AVPU[a]	RR (breaths/min)	SpO_2	HR (if β-blocked; beats/min)	Systolic BP (mmHg)	UO (mL/kg/h)
3		U	≤8	≤85	≤40 (≤35)	≤70	Nil
2	≤35.0	P	9–10	85–89		71–80	≤0.5
1	31.1–36.0	V		90–94	41–50 (35–40)	81–100	
0		A					
1	38.1–38.4	Confused or agitated	20–25		105–120 (100–110)		
2	≥38.5		26–34		121–135 (111–130)	>200	
3			>34		>135 (>130)		

[a]A, alert and orientated; V, responds to voice or confused/agitated; P, response to pain; U, unresponsive.
Abbreviations: BP, blood pressure; HR, heart rate; RR, respiratory rate; SpO_2, peripheral oxygen saturation; UO, urine output.

hospital setting. The effectiveness of the MET concept is significantly hampered by incomplete documentation of patient observations. Given the importance of respiratory rate and urinary output, recording of these values is often poor. Education and redesigning traditional observation charts are often necessary to improve compliance.

The relative success of chest reopening after cardiac arrest on the critical care unit cannot be reproduced when chest reopening is undertaken on the ward. As the time out from surgery increases, the proportion of surgically remediable causes of cardiac arrest decreases exponentially. At this time, thromboembolic phenomena and cardiac failure are far more common than bleeding or tamponade. All patients reopened under such circumstances at the scene of arrest on Papworth wards in the past decade have died in hospital. Surgical reopening trolleys have now been withdrawn from all ward areas and surgical reopening outside theatres and critical care units has been abandoned.

A minority of ward patients who arrest on the wards may benefit from chest reopening. Scooping these patients back to theatre has advantages for the patient, ward staff and arrest team. It also gives the surgeon the option of crashing back onto CPB.

Catheter laboratory arrests

Invariably, VF/VT arrests in the catheter laboratory are iatrogenic, amenable to very early defibrillation and associated with return of spontaneous circulation in more than 90% of cases, as well as a greater than 80% chance of survival to discharge. In hospitals with a cardiac catheterization laboratory, the inclusion of catheter laboratory arrests in overall hospital statistics can significantly skew the overall hospital survival to discharge rate. In cases of coronary dissection or other surgically amenable conditions, early transfer to the operating theatre and emergency CPB should be considered.

Postresuscitation care

Hypothermia

Mild hypothermia improves neurological outcome in comatose patients successfully resuscitated after

Table 6.4 Factors influencing outcome from cardiac arrest and resuscitation on a ward

Geography	The geographical location and layout of cardiac surgical wards are both important.
Monitoring	ECG monitoring is invaluable for detecting asystole and shockable rhythms but less useful at detecting nonshockable rhythms causing PEA.
Prevention	Nowhere is the statement 'Prevention is better than cure' more true than in the field of resuscitation. International studies have shown that many critically ill patients receive suboptimal care on the general wards. Many terminal arrests on general wards are preceded by unrecognized or inadequately treated deterioration in their vital signs. Consideration should be given to the preemptive transfer of a deteriorating patient to the critical care area. The appropriate use of DNAR orders significantly reduces the incidence of unexpected cardiac arrest.
Early detection	Outcomes from witnessed arrests are better than those where the initial arrest is undetected. With early detection, the proportion of primary VF/VT arrests is higher and time to defibrillation reduced.
Equipment	AED are now increasingly being deployed in public sites. They are now so prevalent that BLS training is being extended to include teaching on the use of these straightforward devices. There is a strong argument for putting semi-automated defibrillators on general medical and surgical wards. AED for in-hospital use should include an ECG display and a manual override facility for use by the cardiac arrest team. Accumulating evidence suggests that biphasic defibrillation waveforms may be superior to monophasic waveforms.
Training	Resuscitation training should place greater emphasis on the identification of the at-risk patient and prevention of cardiac arrests. Scenario-based training may be of value.

Abbreviations: AED, automated external defibrillators; BLS, basic life support; DNAR, do not attempt resuscitation; ECG, electrocardiograph; PEA, pulseless electrical activity; VF, ventricular fibrillation; VT, ventricular tachycardia.

out-of-hospital cardiac arrest owing to VF. Mechanisms of action of therapeutic hypothermia include reduced destructive enzyme actions, suppression of free radical actions and inhibition of release and uptake of excitatory transmitters. Cerebral metabolic rate decreases by approximately 7% for every 1°C reduction in temperature.

Therapeutic hypothermia is, however, rarely used in the cardiac surgical critical care, mainly owing to concerns about arrhythmias, hypotension, coagulopathy and infection. Interestingly, cardiac surgeons are increasingly using normothermic rather than hypothermic CPB for routine cardiac surgery.

Key points

- The ALS algorithms require modification after cardiac surgery.
- Consider the possibility of underlying VF in 'asystolic' arrests and paced patients with apparent electromechanical dissociation.
- Look for epicardial pacing wires in bradycardic arrests before giving atropine and adrenaline!
- Resuscitation after cardiac surgery is associated with better outcomes than resuscitation in general hospitals.

FURTHER READING

Buist MD, Moore GE, Bernard SA, *et al.* Effects of a medical emergency team on reduction of incidence of and mortality from unexpected cardiac arrests in hospital: preliminary study. *BMJ* 2002;324:387–390.

Goldhill DR, McNarry AF, Mandersloot G, *et al.* A physiologically-based early warning score for ward patients: the association between score and outcome. *Anaesthesia* 2005;60: 547–553.

The Hypothermia after Cardiac Arrest Study Group. Mild therapeutic hypothermia to improve the neurologic outcome after cardiac arrest. *N Engl J Med* 2002;346:549–556.

Resuscitation Council Website. Available from: www.resus.org.uk

Soar J, Deakin CD, Nolan JP, *et al.* European Resuscitation Council guidelines for resuscitation 2005. Section 7. Cardiac arrest in special circumstances. *Resuscitation* 2005;67(Suppl. 1):S135–170.

Chapter 7

Transport of the cardiac critical care patient

P.J. SHIRLEY

Introduction

When critically ill cardiac patients are moved, either within the hospital or between hospitals, the principles of safe transfer should be applied regardless of the distance travelled or the underlying diagnosis. Interhospital transfers in particular require a high level of expertise because further skilled help may not be readily available if problems occur en route. These transfers have significant associated risk and the transfer period has been shown to be one of the most hazardous phases in any episode of critical care. There must be a local strategy in place to manage the process, so that safe and efficient coordination can take place on a 24-hour basis.

Additional invasive monitoring and organ support before transfer may be required. Compact technology to analyse blood gases and electrolytes during transfer is now readily available and should be used, especially during prolonged journeys. Thrombolytic therapy, pacing and defibrillation have been shown to be both effective and safe during transport. Bypass circuits and left ventricular assist devices represent the current extremes of cardiac support during transfer, used only by selected specialist centres with fully trained medical, nursing and technical staff in attendance.

In general, the aim of transfer is to upgrade the level of care or obtain appropriate specialist diagnostic or treatment facilities. Transfer is associated with complications; even the physical movement from a bed to a stretcher or examination table may be hazardous. Complications range in severity from minor to potentially life threatening and may be related to clinical, equipment or organizational problems. The risk of a complication increases with the extent of instrumentation of the patient and the complexity of the machinery. It has been recognized that the frequency of complications during transport is high and international efforts have been made to improve the standards and organization of transport systems for the critically ill.

Current guidelines

There are currently no specific guidelines relating to the transport of the critically ill cardiac patient, but general guidelines are available, including from intensive care societies. Staff involved in the transfer have a responsibility to ensure that they are adequately trained and experienced in the transfer procedure. Careful planning and detailed knowledge of the equipment are vital to minimizing the risks.

The transfer process

Communication and control

These are vital first elements in the transfer process. The decision to move a critically ill patient must be made by a senior critical care doctor, who can adequately assess the balance of risk to benefit and plan the transfer. This may require discussion with other teams in the hospital, the receiving unit and the ambulance service. Early communication is essential between named senior responsible medical and nursing personnel at both units. This can be a frustrating process, especially for smaller hospitals dealing with tertiary care centres. Ideally, there should be a dedicated telephone number that can be used in the organization of the transfer.

Communication during transfer traditionally relies on the ambulance radio but in practice, mobile phones are a particularly useful, quick and effective mode of communication and they should be carried by the transferring team. To avoid electromagnetic interference, both phones and radios should be used at least 2 metres from all monitoring and electrical clinical equipment.

Team members may have varying levels of experience and training in the transfer process and may benefit from a structured briefing before the transfer process starts.

Table 7.1 Items to be included in checklist used before transfer

CHECKLIST
Airway and NG tube
Breathing and end-tidal CO_2
Circulation and invasive monitoring
Disability/cervical collar and head injury care
Exposed, **e**xamined and **e**quipment sorted out and secure
Family informed
Final considerations ***A***sk for notes and x-rays? ***B***ed confirmed? ***C***ontinuity of care assured? ***D***rugs and spares? ***D***ocumentation ***E***verything secure?

Initial assessment

In general, critically ill patients tolerate transportation poorly. Hypoxia and hypotension occur in at least 15% of transfers and may persist for several hours after arrival at the receiving hospital. In cases of inadequate resuscitation, equipment failure, environmental delays or the transport vehicle being involved in an accident itself, transportation can cause serious morbidity and mortality.

There is no risk model for predicting long-term outcome in such patients. There have been attempts at risk scoring for these patients, but none have gained widespread acceptance. Fundamentally, the more deranged the physiology, the higher the risk.

Preparation and packaging for transfer

A checklist to avoid omissions is helpful and can be incorporated into the transfer documentation. Stabilization and meticulous preparation are the keys to a successful transfer. All personnel should familiarize themselves with the patient, their previous medical history and the current condition. The familiar concept of 'optimization' of perfusion and tissue oxygen delivery before any high-risk procedure should be applied to this group of patients.

Full clinical examination with special reference to on-going monitoring should be carried out. All possible sources of continuing blood loss and sepsis should have been located and controlled if at all possible. Hypovolaemia is associated with greater risk of hypotension during moving; therefore, adequate filling and correction of intravascular volume should be ensured. If there is a risk that bleeding may continue despite best efforts or restart during transport, blood should be ordered and packaged for transport according to laboratory instructions; in general, if packed in an insulated box with ice it may be used for up to 4 hours.

Neurological deficits should be noted both pre- and post-transport and any changes clearly documented. Optimal respiratory function is fundamental. If spontaneous ventilation is compromised, intubation and mechanical ventilation must be initiated before transport. Also, if the consciousness level is depressed or fluctuating or if the patient is confused and agitated, elective intubation should be performed to prevent loss of the airway in transit. Facemask continuous positive airway pressure is rarely possible during transport, and patients who require this for adequate oxygenation should also be electively intubated. Optimization of ventilation and adjusting inspired oxygen fraction should be performed before moving the patient, and blood gases checked, along with a chest radiograph.

Adequate venous access must be in place. A urinary catheter and nasogastric tube should be considered. All lines and tubes must be securely fixed, with sutures if necessary. If transport by air is chosen, chest drains need to be on a non-underwater drainage system and be easily accessible during transfer. This may be achieved by securely connecting a nasogastric drainage bag to the chest drain, and ensuring that this is below the level of the bed at all times. If the chest drain is continuously bubbling because of an unresolved air leak, the underwater system should be retained and continuous suction during the transfer (at 5–7 kPa) prevents an enlarging pneumothorax.

The results of recent investigations including chest radiograph, other radiographs, haematology and biochemistry should be checked and carried with the patient. All documentation, including referral letters, investigations, radiology reports, hard copies of radiographs and computed tomography scans, should be gathered and the receiving hospital recontacted before departure to confirm availability of the bed and give an estimated arrival time. This also allows an update of any changes in the patient's condition.

Monitoring

The standard of monitoring should approach that expected within the hospital setting and minimum standards include:

- the continuous presence of appropriately trained staff;
- electrocardiograph (ECG);
- invasive blood pressure;
- arterial oxygen saturation;
- end-tidal carbon dioxide in a ventilated patient; and
- temperature.

A disconnection alarm should be used whenever mechanical ventilators are used. Additionally, for cardiac patients there should be:

- monitor/defibrillator plus paper/recorder;
- defibrillator pads;
- quick-look paddles or hands-free patches; and
- transcutaneous cardiac pacing facility.

Equipment

Equipment must be suited to the environment, namely, durable, lightweight and with sufficient battery life. A monitored oxygen supply with a safety margin of at least 2 hours on the transfer time should be carried. Modern portable ventilators are sophisticated enough to allow relatively complex modes of ventilation. However, a surprising amount of oxygen may be needed to drive the ventilator, and this needs to be taken into account together with the inspired oxygen fraction when calculating the requirements for the journey. There are published nomograms that can assist with these calculations.

For longer transfers, a large margin of safety is required for unforeseen emergencies or delays en route. Portable monitors, with a single power source, combining oxygen saturation, ECG and invasive and noninvasive blood pressure are essential. A dedicated equipment bridge, containing ventilator, monitoring equipment and infusion devices is becoming the method of choice for providing these requirements. This can be manufactured fairly simply locally, but must be robust enough to withstand the rigors of transport, compatible with stretchers and vehicle fittings and may need formal clearance to be fitted in aircraft.

There are sophisticated commercial integrated equipment bridges available, but their complexity and incompatibility with most ambulances make

Table 7.2 How to calculate if the oxygen supply will last the duration of the transfer

Oxygen requirement = 2 × transport time in minutes × (($MV \times FiO_2$) + ventilator driving gas)

Example.
1 hour transfer, minute volume 10 L/min, FiO_2 = 60% or 0.6, ventilator driving gas 1 L/min.

Oxygen required = 2 × 60 × ((10 × 0.6) + 1) = 840 L

Allowing for extra, this would require 2 × E-sized cylinders or 1 × F-sized cylinder.

Cylinder capacity:
- D, 340 L
- CD, 460 L
- LE, 680 L
- F, 1360 L

Abbreviations: FiO_2, fraction of inspired oxygen; MV, minute volume.

them an impractical and expensive luxury. Alarms should be visible as well as audible. Suction and defibrillation should be immediately available. A warming blanket is also a consideration in cold climates. A reasonable range and supply of medications should be carried with pumps to administer them, ensuring that all such devices have charged and spare batteries. (Some syringe drivers will run off standard AA battery power).

Interhospital management

The safety of all those involved in the transfer is of paramount importance. Travelling in vehicles at high speed is hazardous; therefore, the crew's instructions must be followed. The team should ensure that all equipment is adequately secured or stowed before setting off. Before vehicle departure, attendants should ensure that the patient, the ventilator and monitoring and infusion devices are in view and accessible. They should secure themselves, using the seatbelts provided and should remain seated during the transfer if at all possible.

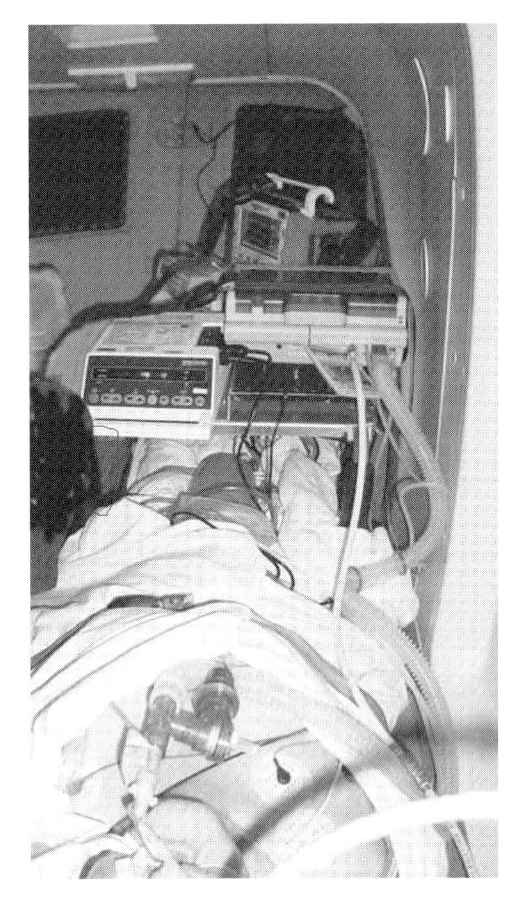

Figure 7.1 Stretcher in an ambulance. The accompanying equipment is not secured and is a risk for both patient and escorting staff.

When staff may be required to move outside the vehicle onto the public highway, high visibility clothing must be worn. This should include a long-sleeved jacket with bands of retro reflective material surrounding the circumference.

Despite meticulous preparation, unexpected clinical events may happen en route. Access for clinical intervention is not easy in a patient who is secured on a transfer stretcher, in a confined space, with monitoring attached and on the move. Stopping the vehicle should always be considered if transport is by road. If an attendant must perform a task while the vehicle is in motion, the ambulance crew must be informed. The attendant then adopts a kneeling

Table 7.3 Troubleshooting during transfer

Common physiological changes
Hypoxia
Cardiac dysrhythmia
Hypotension
Decrease in Glasgow Coma Scale
Hypothermia
Hypoglycaemia
Common equipment problems
Exhaustion of oxygen supply
Ventilator malfunction
Loss of monitoring
Loss of intravenous access
Accidental extubation or tracheal tube blockage

Table 7.4 Handover checklist

HANDOVER
Acute problem
Before admission to intensive care
Current clinical condition
Drugs/infusions and documentation
Examination and any problems during transport
Family

position within the ambulance, using one arm to hold on for stability. After the task has been completed, the attendant should return to a secure seat.

In the past 15 years, technological support on ambulances has improved tremendously. Most critical care facilities can now be packaged into the confines of an ambulance or small aircraft. It should be noted, however, that not all ambulance services possess equipment of the same sophistication.

Air ambulances and helicopters can sometimes appear to be an attractive alternative. However, the lack of familiarity with the environment and the high cost make the use of air transport impractical in many countries. Some regions have integrated land and air ambulance services (fixed-wing and helicopter) for a scattered population. The specifics of air transport are beyond the scope of this chapter; refer to the further reading list for suggestions.

Receiving hospital and hand over

Courtesy is essential when handing over. The patient remains the responsibility of the transferring personnel until safely delivered to a bed in the receiving hospital, with all monitoring in place and a completed hand over. The name and signature of the receiving doctor confirms the continuity of care and provides a point of contact for future queries. All documentation should be completed, including any undocumented transfer events.

Post-transfer analysis

On return to base, all equipment should be accounted for, electrical equipment back on charge and all documentation, including incident and audit forms, completed. Any debriefing required (for training purposes or if there have been problems with the transfer) should take place as soon as practicable.

Special considerations

Power supply

AC power for monitoring can usually be supplied from the vehicle inverter, if fitted. If this power source is interrupted, the internal battery normally takes over. Clearly, the power requirements of all equipment intended for transport use should be checked before the intended transfer and matched with the available power facilities on the available ambulance or aircraft. Some ambulance services have dedicated transfer vehicles with a 240v AC supply delivered through standard plug sockets.

Transport of patients on an intra-aortic balloon pump

Safe air transport of intra-aortic balloon pump (IABP) has been validated mostly in the transfer of patients from peripheral hospitals to tertiary care centres. The most frequent problems encountered are uncoupling of tubing or electronic connections and difficulties with helium cylinders. Experience with such transfers is limited to small numbers of patients, but studies report acceptable transfer outcomes with few adverse incidents.

INTRA-AORTIC BALLOON PUMP EQUIPMENT

- Intra-aortic balloon pump with transport support module.
- Lead cable.
- Skin ECG electrodes.
- Transducer.
- Invasive arterial pressure monitoring (there should be a dedicated separate arterial line in addition to that on the IABP).
- Balloon catheters (8 Fr gauge, 9.5 Fr gauge, with insertion kits).
- Extension tubing.
- Adaptors to enable the connection of various brands of balloon catheters to local equipment.
- Spare helium cylinder.
- Operation manual.
- Stopcocks.
- A 60-mL syringe.

PRETRANSFER CHECKS

Prepare the balloon pump for transport and confirm that the ECG lead cable and transducer are directly connected to the pump and in working order. Check that there is enough battery time available with the IABP for the journey to the receiving hospital or an external power source is available. Arrange intravenous lines, drips, invasive lines and assist in the transfer of the patient from the bed to the stretcher. The transport team should be skilled and experienced in the set-up, operation and troubleshooting of the IABP.

Transport of patients with pacing

Temporary pacemakers (external and/or transvenous) may be in use. External pacing pads should be carried in case of pacemaker failure and the transfer team should be familiar with the pacing function of the defibrillator.

Extracorporeal membrane oxygenation and transfer of extreme high-risk patients

The use of extracorporeal membrane oxygenation (ECMO) during transfer is reasonably well established in certain specialist regional services for both adults and children. Transferring patients on ECMO is clearly complicated and resource dependent. Both venous–arterial and venovenous bypass have been used successfully. Interhospital ECMO has also been reported for patients with cardiogenic shock unresponsive to conventional treatment.

Some ECMO centres have their own dedicated transport team and have transferred patients safely over long distances, despite significant respiratory and cardiovascular compromise. There is no demonstrated excess mortality in this group compared to patients who are not moved.

Recently, pumpless extracorporeal lung assist has been used during transport of high-risk patients with severe adult respiratory distress system to specialist centres. This is an ultracompact extrapulmonary gas exchange system that is perfused by the cardiac output of the patient. It does not need extended technical support and, compared with ECMO, may be easier in terms of personnel and vehicle requirements. Further evaluation is required.

Retrieval models

Centralization of specialist services has led to the development of children's retrieval services in major centres. Unfortunately, the same is not true for adult services despite some evidence that dedicated retrieval teams have reduced morbidity and early mortality. Further prospective investigations may prove the medical efficiency and cost effectiveness of such a system.

Table 7.5 Summary principles for safe critically ill transfers

1. Identify regional hospitals • Local list with telephone numbers • Specialist list with telephone numbers	**2. Identify key staff** • Consultant authorizing transfer • Consultant authorizing reception
3. Identify kit Intrahospital • Ventilator and power lead • Portable monitor and power lead • Syringe drivers and power leads • Spare batteries and extension lead • Transfer bag • Drugs bag • Oxygen and self-inflating bag • Personnel and portering • Notes and radiographs	Interhospital • Ventilator and power lead • Portable monitor and power lead • Syringe drivers • Power inverter/adapter and spare batteries • Transfer bag • Drugs bag • Oxygen and self-inflating bag • Personnel and portering • Notes and radiographs • Documentation/audit form
4. Identify personnel • Core specialty experience • Airway management • Inotropes • Head injuries and trauma • Paediatrics	**5. Familiarity with kit** • Ventilator • Drugs • Syringe drivers • Monitor • Transducers • Defibrillator/external pacer • Specialist equipment (ECMO, IABP)
6. Identify training • Safety training • Everything not included in environment-specific training **Team training** • Incorporating simulated use of kit; safety drills and simulated emergencies. Should include medical, nursing, paramedical and aviation personnel where appropriate. **Vehicle-specific training** • To include escape procedure; use of fire extinguishers, engine cut-off and radio.	**7. Quality control** • Kit check and re-supply • Drug expiry dates • Staff currencies and competencies **Regular audit and feedback** • Supervision of junior staff • Log book review • Critical incident reporting system **On-going equipment improvement and update**

Abbreviations: ECMO, extracorporeal membrane oxygenation; IABP, intra-aortic balloon pump.

Key points

- Planning, training and detailed knowledge of the equipment are vital to minimize the risks of transfer.
- Early communication with the receiving unit is essential.
- Critically ill patients may tolerate transportation poorly and the team should be prepared to intervene en route.
- Stabilization and meticulous preparation are the keys to a successful transfer.

FURTHER READING

Advanced Life Support Group. *Safe transfer and retrieval: The practical approach*. London: BMJ Books; 2002.

Intensive Care Society Standards. 2002 guidelines for the transport of the critically ill adult. Available at: www.ics.ac.uk/icmprof/downloads/icstransport2002mem.pdf.

Lutman D, Petros AJ. How many oxygen cylinders do you need to take on transport? A nomogram for cylinder size and duration. *Emerg Med J* 2006;23:703–704.

Markakis C, Dalezios M, Chatzicostas C, *et al.* Evaluation of a risk score for interhospital transport of critically ill patients. *Emerg Med J* 2006;23:313–317.

Martin T. *Handbook of patient transportation*. London: Greenwich Medical Media; 2001.

SECTION 2 General Considerations in Cardiothoracic Critical Care

Chapter 8

Managing the airway

A. PEARCE AND S. McCORKELL

Introduction

The provision of a patent airway from the external atmosphere to the lower trachea is commonly required to facilitate mechanical ventilation in the critically ill. A cuffed tracheal tube provides the highest degree of airway maintenance and protection and this is the most frequently used device.

Core competencies for airway management in cardiothoracic critical care include relevant physiology and pharmacology, care of the intubated patient, strategies for intubation and extubation, intubation of a patient at risk of aspiration, the management of failed intubation and failed ventilation and specialized techniques for lung isolation.

Physiology

In normal adults breathing air, alveolar minute ventilation is approximately 3.5 L/min. The $Pa{O_2}$ for a given inspired oxygen concentration can be calculated from the alveolar gas equation.

A decrease in alveolar minute ventilation will cause a reduction in $Pa{O_2}$ and elevation in $Pa{CO_2}$. Hypoxaemia secondary only to a reduction in minute ventilation can be treated easily by increasing the inspired oxygen.

The relationship between $Pa{O_2}$ and $Pa{CO_2}$ is more complex and is influenced by venous admixture and cardiac output. With a venous admixture or shunt fraction greater than 20% to 25%, it may prove impossible to raise the $Pa{O_2}$ to normal, even with 100% inspired oxygen.

The procedure of tracheal intubation is often undertaken to permit positive pressure ventilation when spontaneous respiration fails to maintain gaseous homeostasis. Short periods of hypoventilation are inevitable during intubation and major airway interventions in critical care should always be preceded by a period of preoxygenation.

Preoxygenation

Preoxygenation is the term used for the procedure of breathing (or ventilation with) 100% oxygen to replace the nitrogen in the functional residual capacity with oxygen. This oxygen store in the lungs permits a longer time for major airway interventions before the onset of hypoxaemia, and can be life saving. Breathing 100% inspired oxygen for 2 to 3 minutes (3–5 time constants) is sufficient to raise the alveolar (or end-tidal) oxygen to 90% to 91% in normal patients.

During preoxygenation, the mask should fit tightly on the face and the flow of oxygen into the circuit should be high (>10 L/min) to avoid rebreathing of expired gas. The reservoir bag in the circuit should be distended and move with respiration. If the patient is already on continuous positive airway pressure, this should be left in situ and the inspired oxygen increased to 100%.

$$PAO_2 = FIO_2 (P_B - P_{H_2O}) - PACO_2/R$$

Figure 8.1 Alveolar gas equation. *Abbreviations:* PB, barometric pressure (100 kPa at sea level); P_{H_2O}, saturated vapour pressure of water at 37°C (6.3 kPa); R, respiratory quotient (0.8 on mixed diet).

Preoxygenation provides a degree of safety during intubation (and extubation). In critical care patients, oxygen consumption may be high and the functional residual capacity volume small, resulting in much more rapid development of life-threatening hypoxaemia.

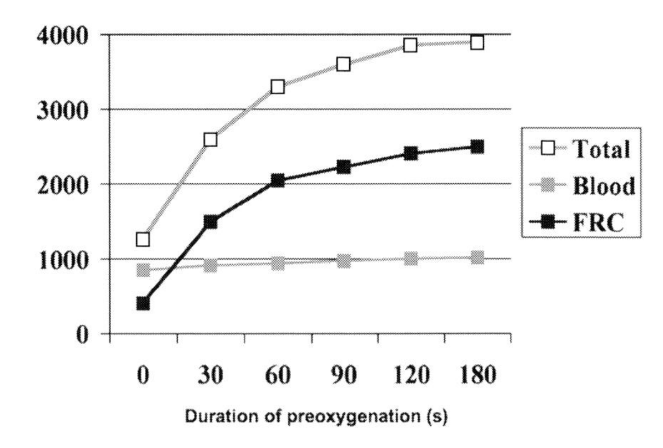

Figure 8.3 Increase in oxygen stores with duration of preoxygenation. Time 0 = air.

Anaesthetic agents

Anaesthetic agents produce unconsciousness. Clinically useful drugs are given intravenously as a bolus over 20 to 30 seconds, act within one arm–brain circulation time and have a dose-dependent effect on length of unconsciousness. The main side effects are hypotension due to reduction in peripheral vascular resistance and myocardial depression.

PROPOFOL

Propofol is the most commonly used induction agent and is also suitable for long-term sedation.

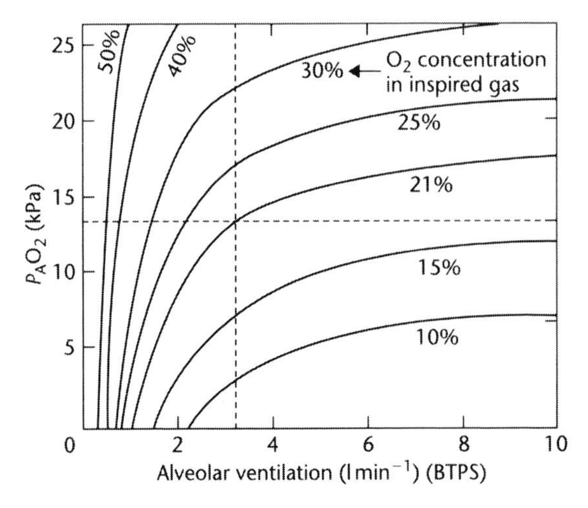

Figure 8.2 Relationship between alveolar minute ventilation and P_{AO_2} for various inspired oxygen concentrations.

It is an isopropylphenol formulated in soybean emulsion; the solution is isotonic with a neutral pH and supports bacterial growth so unused drug should be discarded after 6 hours. The bolus dose for induction is 1 to 2 mg/kg.

ETOMIDATE

Promoted as the induction agent with the least cardiovascular depression, this imidazole derivative is prepared in propylene glycol. The standard induction dose is 0.15 to 0.30 mg/kg. Unfortunately, the drug is a powerful inhibitor of 11-β and 17-α hydroxylation and interferes with synthesis of mineralo- and glucocorticoids. Deaths due to hypoadrenalism have been associated with infusions of the drug, and even single doses have a noticeable biochemical action. Some critical care units do not use the drug at all; some provide steroid cover if it is used, and others allow only a single dose.

OTHER SEDATIVES

Benzodiazepines may be used in the place of anaesthetic agents, particularly when the patient is already hypotensive or is already vasodilated. Agents such as midazolam can be expected to reduce the blood pressure less than propofol or thiopentone, but inadequate anaesthesia is a risk, and increased doses of opioids should be employed.

Opioids

Opioids reduce the cardiovascular response to intubation and prolong the duration of unconsciousness from the induction agent, but cause apnoea and tend to exacerbate hypotension. Clinically useful drugs are fentanyl, 1 to 3 μg/kg, and alfentanil, 10 to 20 μg/kg.

Muscle relaxants

Tracheal intubation is usually possible only if the glottic closure reflex is obtunded. Muscle relaxants are commonly used for this purpose. The drugs are given after the induction agent and appropriate sedation must be continued to avoid the situation of a paralyzed patient who is aware but unable to move.

SUXAMETHONIUM

A rapidly acting depolarizing muscle relaxant, suxamethonium has a duration of action of 3 to 6 minutes, must be stored in the refrigerator and given in a dose of 1.0 to 1.5 mg/kg. Its onset of action, within 45 seconds, is accompanied by visible muscle fasciculation. There are numerous side effects, such as transient hyperkalaemia, particularly severe after major burns or spinal cord injury, and bradycardia. Some physicians believe that the risks outweigh any benefits in the critical care setting.

ATRACURIUM AND CISATRACURIUM

Atracurium and its monoisomeric form cisatracurium are the most commonly used nondepolarizing muscle relaxants in critical care both for intubation and when muscle relaxation must be maintained. Atracurium, a benzylisoquinolinium compound, is not eliminated by renal or hepatic processes, but is broken down in the body by Hofmann degradation, which means that the molecule falls apart under the influence of pH and temperature. There is also nonspecific esterase metabolism. A long shelf life for the drug is produced by storing it in the refrigerator with an acid pH in the ampoule. In clinical use, it is administered in a bolus dose of 0.5 mg/kg and produces adequate muscle relaxation for intubation in 2 to 3 minutes. Larger bolus doses (up to 1 mg/kg) can be used to speed up onset, but these larger doses produce elevated plasma histamine levels, which may produce adverse effects, particularly hypotension, flushing and bronchospasm. Cisatracurium is an isomer that is three times more potent and does not cause histamine release.

VECURONIUM AND ROCURONIUM

Both vecuronium and rocuronium are steroidal, nondepolarizing relaxants. Rocuronium, in a dose of 0.6 to 1.0 mg/kg, is generally acknowledged as the drug with the fastest onset; it produces good conditions for intubation in 60 seconds. Vecuronium does not release histamine, even in high doses of 0.2 mg/kg. Both drugs are mostly metabolized in the liver.

Airway management equipment

Safe management requires immediately available equipment, a knowledgeable/skilled assistant and a back-up plan/protocol for failed intubation. A difficult airway trolley should also be available.

The laryngeal mask may be more reliable as a means of ventilation than the facemask and should always be considered in an unconscious or paralyzed patient in whom facemask ventilation is difficult. It does not protect the airway against aspiration of gastric contents.

Management of the intubated patient

After cardiac surgery, patients often arrive in the critical care unit already intubated and ventilated. The receiving clinician at hand over should acquaint themselves with the following points:

- adequate fixation of the tube;
- size of tracheal tube;
- tube inserted to correct depth;
- any difficulties with intubation;

Table 8.1 Airway equipment required in critical care area

Facemask	Capnography or oesophageal detector device
Oral and nasal airways	Emergency cricothyrotomy kit
Laryngeal mask	Spare laryngoscope batteries/bulbs
Magill forceps	Suction catheters
Catheter mount	Tape or ties for securing tube
Two working laryngoscopes	Syringe for inflating cuff
Introducer (gum elastic bougie)	
Tracheal tubes, sizes 6.0–9.0 mm	

- adequate initial settings for mechanical ventilation;
- back-up ventilation bag with 100% oxygen immediately available;
- equipment required for reintubation; and
- appropriate pharmacological sedation.

The tube should be adequately fixed, usually by a tape encircling the head and tied to the tube, to avoid inadvertent removal or further insertion of the tube. The anaesthetist should specifically hand over any difficulty during intubation, which should trigger special arrangements (staff or equipment) for extubation or reintubation.

The correct depth of insertion of a tracheal tube is when the tip is approximately 2 cm above the carina. Insertion deeper than this risks endobronchial intubation, either continuously or with movements of the head/neck. Clinical examination ought to show symmetrical bilateral chest expansion during inspiration, with equality of breath sounds over all regions of both lungs. If there is any doubt, a chest radiograph should be performed.

Intubated ventilated patients are usually transferred on 100% oxygen with manual ventilation by a simple Waters or Mapleson C circuit. The period of transfer onto mechanical ventilation is a time when critical incidents can occur. The mechanical ventilator should be set according to the protocol of the individual unit and typical settings are as follows.

- Tidal volume of 8 to 10 mL/kg.
- Rate of 10 to 12 breaths/min.
- Inspiratory:expiratory ratio of 1:2.
- 60% inspired oxygen.
- Positive end-expiratory pressure of 3 to 5 cmH_2O.
- Maximum peak inspiratory pressure of 30 cmH_2O.
- Minimum minute volume of 3 L/min.

Another means of ventilation should always be directly available (such as the circuit used for transfer) if there are problems with mechanical ventilation or desaturation.

Thoracic patients are not commonly ventilated electively after surgery and indeed it may be relatively contraindicated. The bronchial stump suture or stapling line would be subjected to positive pressure, the risk of infection is increased and air-leak from cut pulmonary surfaces will be more of a problem.

Intubation

The need to intubate a patient in the cardiothoracic critical care unit commonly indicates deterioration in cardiorespiratory function. It is often a planned intervention, but may be necessary in a crisis situation. Before attempting intubation, an adequately competent clinician should be found (usually an anaesthetist), and equipment, drugs, assistance and suction should be prepared, along with the mechanical ventilator itself.

Indications

The indications for intubation are failure of gaseous homeostasis with spontaneous respiration (pH

Table 8.2 Predictors of difficult direct laryngoscopy in critical care

Limited mouth opening (≤3 cm)
Limited atlanto-occipital extension
Large tongue
Swollen floor of the mouth or neck
Previous head/neck surgery
Oropharyngeal or laryngeal oedema/masses
Stridor or high dysphagia
Oropharyngeal bleeding

≤ 7.2; $Pa{O_2}$ ≤ 7–8 kPa on 60% inspired oxygen), excessive work of breathing or tiredness, cardiovascular instability with hypotension, decreased level of consciousness or other causes of inability to protect or maintain the airway.

Prediction of difficult direct laryngoscopy

Oral intubation by direct laryngoscopy is easy in most patients, but may be very difficult or impossible on occasion. A brief airway evaluation should look for common predictors of difficulty and it is wise then to enlist more senior help.

Oral or nasal intubation?

Oral intubation is common, but a nasotracheal tube may sometimes be better tolerated by the patient and more stable in position. Disadvantages of nasotracheal intubation include nasal haemorrhage, the requirement for a smaller tube, the risk of a transient bacteraemia, the development of paranasal infection and mucosal ulceration.

Tracheal tubes

Tracheal tubes are made from polyvinyl chloride, sized by the internal diameter of the lumen in millimetres and designed for single use. When removed from the packaging, the tubes are uncut and the length can be seen from the markings in centimetres from the tip. Appropriate sizes for use in adult critical care are 8.0 mm for women and 9.0 mm for men. A long tube allows flexibility in depth of insertion and accommodates facial swelling (particularly in burns or oedema associated with anaphylactoid-type reactions), but risks being inserted too far into the airway resulting in endobronchial intubation. For normal-sized adult patients, it is common for the tube to be cut at 24 to 26 cm expecting the depth of insertion (measured in centimetres at the angle of the mouth) to be 20 to 23 cm.

The cuff of the tube is described as 'high volume, low-pressure' to indicate that the seal with the tracheal wall is made by a large surface area of cuff but low intracuff pressure. A high cuff pressure leads to impaired tracheal mucosal blood flow and the cuff pressure should be only slightly more than that required to produce a seal at the inflation pressures used during ventilation. The cuff does not prevent all fluid leaking past it, particularly if there is a column of fluid superior to it.

Technique of direct laryngoscopy

The most common technique of oral intubation is to use the curved Macintosh laryngoscope blade. The laryngoscope blade (usually standard or long length) is held in the left hand, inserted slightly to the right side of the mouth to distract the tongue to the left and slowly advanced in the midline over the base of the tongue until the epiglottis is visualized. The tip of the blade is manoeuvred into the valecula and a vector of force is applied to distract the tongue from the line of sight.

In most patients, correct laryngoscopy technique allows a clear view of the laryngeal inlet and the lubricated tracheal tube can be placed through the glottic aperture under direct vision. In 5% to 8% of the normal population, it is possible to see only the epiglottis and this makes insertion of the tracheal tube more difficult. The first manoeuvre

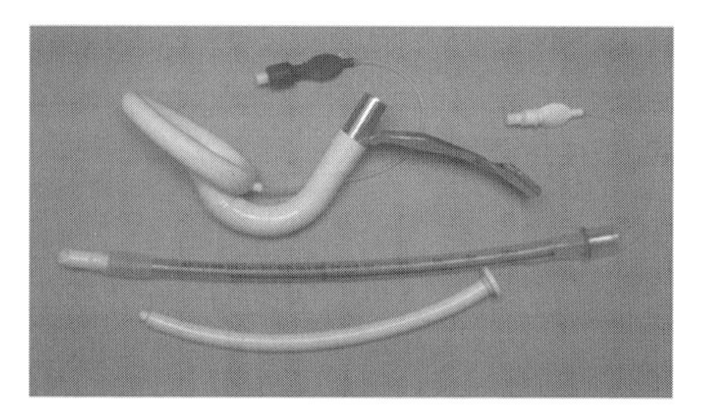

Figure 8.4 Intubating laryngeal mask airway.

used to improve the view is external laryngeal manipulation. The most successful single movement is pressure on the thyroid cartilage to move the larynx *b*ackwards, *u*pwards and to the *r*ight of the *p*atient (*BURP*). If passage of the tube is still difficult, an introducer or gum-elastic bougie should be tried.

Use of the introducer (gum-elastic bougie)

This may be used even if the cords are not well visualized, and the target is estimated using experience and knowledge of anatomy. The introducer should be held at about 25 to 30 cm in the right hand with the tip angled anteriorly. The introducer should be advanced so as to slide the tip along the undersurface of the epiglottis in the midline and continuing to advance without undue force. Keeping the laryngoscope blade in situ, the tracheal tube is advanced over the introducer and if hold-up occurs the tube is withdrawn slightly, rotated 90 degrees anticlockwise and readvanced. The rotation alters the orientation of the tip of the tube, which otherwise commonly impacts on the right vocal cord.

Confirmation of tracheal versus oesophageal intubation

It is essential after intubation to confirm that the tube is within the trachea and not the oesophagus. Occasionally, it is obvious when applying positive pressure ventilation that the chest does not move and a gurgling sound is heard indicating the tube is placed oesophageally. Unfortunately, all the clinical signs of successful tracheal intubation – chest movement, breath sounds, correct 'feel' of the inflating bag, misting of the tube and normal compliance – may occur with oesophageal intubation.

VISUAL CONFIRMATION

The tube is seen on direct laryngoscopy passing between the vocal cords or at least superiorly to the interarytenoid groove.

CAPNOGRAPHY

The best test of tracheal placement is the monitoring of six successive, sustained respiratory carbon dioxide traces on the capnograph. Some carbon dioxide can be detected with oesophageal intubation if facemask ventilation has inflated the stomach with exhaled gas or if a carbonated drink has been recently ingested but the CO_2 is rapidly washed out by ventilation so the end-tidal value declines with each breath. Errors with capnography are always 'fail-safe' – the capnograph will not confirm tracheal intubation when this is not present – but failure to attach the capnograph, a nonfunctioning system or blocked sampling line means that successful tracheal intubation is not accompanied by detectable respiratory gas CO_2. During cardiac arrest, pulmonary blood flow, and hence end-tidal CO_2, are low.

Rapid sequence induction

A rapid sequence induction may be necessary to minimize the risk of aspiration of gastric contents at the time of induction of anaesthesia and intubation. It involves the rapid induction of anaesthesia and muscle relaxation, the application of cricoid force after loss of consciousness, intubation with a cuffed tube and removal of cricoid force only after intubation of the trachea has been verified. It should be considered for all patients in a critical care area who require intubation and may be at increased risk of aspiration. This particularly applies if a full stomach is suspected, such as nasogastric feeding only recently discontinued or the presence of abdominal distention/ileus.

CRICOID PRESSURE

Cricoid pressure is performed by placing two fingers on the cricoid cartilage and applying force posteriorly to move the cricoid ring against the bodies of the cervical vertebrae. The force should be applied to the cricoid cartilage, the most inferior laryngeal structure, and not to the thyroid cartilage, which is the most prominent.

Failed intubation

Intubation by direct laryngoscopy will prove difficult in 2% to 5% of patients. If difficulty is encountered, further attempts at direct laryngoscopy may be attempted only after reoxygenation. However, repeated attempts may lead to airway oedema, and prolonged deoxygenation has deleterious effects on the patient. Therefore, after more than one failed attempt senior assistance should be urgently summoned. The immediate requirement is oxygenation and it is useful to place a laryngeal mask (or return to the facemask) and ventilate with 100% oxygen. This is usually successful, but may fail in the presence of glottic oedema; in this instance, it is necessary to proceed to the failed intubation and failed ventilation protocol, which obviously carries significant risk.

If ventilation by laryngeal mask (or facemask) is possible and oxygenation is satisfactory, intubation is required by another technique. There are four common approaches.

Intubation through the laryngeal mask

Intubation can be undertaken through the classic laryngeal mask. The most successful techniques used are fibreoptic assisted or the employment of the Aintree catheter. A size 6.0 mm tube is suitable for a size 3 laryngeal mask airway (LMA) and a 7.0 mm for size 4 LMA.

Intubating laryngeal mask

The intubating LMA (ILMA) consists of a tightly curved metal stem with a handle, a bowl with an epiglottic elevator bar, dedicated wire spiralled tubes with a novel bevel and a stabilizing rod. The ILMA is the most successful blind method of intubation and can also be used with a fibroscope.

Fibreoptic intubation

The flexible fibroscope may be used to intubate through the nose or mouth, but skill is required and there may not be a suitable fibroscope in the critical care unit. There are a number of oral airways, such as the Berman airway, which may make oral fibreoptic intubation easier, but the skill required may be particularly high in critical care where blood and secretions degrade the view and oedema distorts the anatomy.

Percutaneous tracheostomy

In a patient in whom intubation by a senior clinician has failed in the critical care unit, there is a good case for immediate creation of a percutaneous tracheostomy, maintaining the airway during the procedure by laryngeal mask.

Failed ventilation

The process of tracheal intubation in critical care appears to be more hazardous than during elective anaesthesia. Copious oropharyngeal secretions or blood in the oropharynx, airway oedema, poor or basic equipment, inadequate assistance, imperfect muscle relaxation, poor cardiorespiratory reserve and relatively inexperienced nonanaesthetists may be responsible. At least one serious complication occurs in approximately 25% of patients!

Failed ventilation is the clinical scenario in which it is not possible to maintain oxygen saturations above 90% with 100% oxygen (if the saturations were above this value initially), or reverse signs of inadequate ventilation, by use of the facemask or laryngeal mask.

The situation of 'can't-ventilate-can't-intubate' is managed by introduction of oxygen directly into the trachea either by emergency cricothyrotomy or tracheostomy. Cricothyrotomy is quicker and is undertaken through the cricothyroid membrane, which is superficial, easily located, relatively avascular and inferior to the vocal cords. There are three types of cricothyrotomy: small needle, large-bore cannula (>4 mm diameter) and surgical.

- Needles or cannulae are placed through the cricothyroid membrane and directed caudally into the trachea. Air should be aspirated freely through the inserted cannula to confirm location within the trachea. If a needle or small cannula is used the resistance to gas flow is high and high pressure oxygen (2–4 Bar, 200–400 kPa) is required to allow sufficient ventilation to remove CO_2. Exhalation is through the upper airway, which must be maintained open.
- Large-bore cannulae with an internal diameter greater than 4 mm allow adequate inspiration with a standard breathing system (and pressure-limiting valve shut) and exhalation can occur through the cannula.

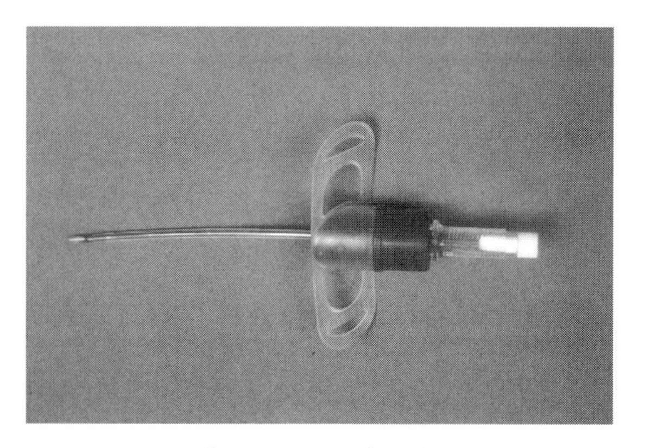

Figure 8.5 Cricothyrotomy cannula with an internal diameter of 2 mm.

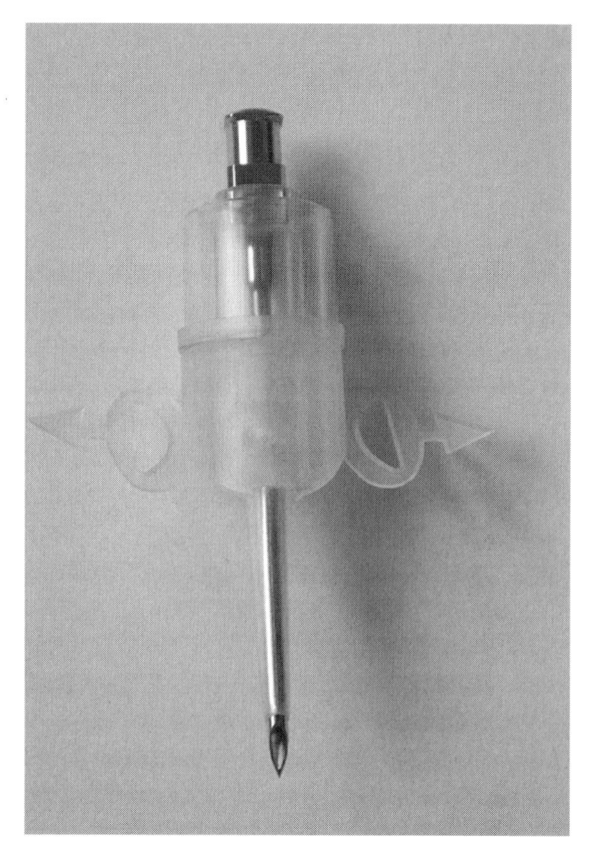

Figure 8.6 Large-bore cricothyrotomy cannula with an internal diameter of less than 4 mm.

- The surgical approach is to make an incision, open the airway by means of a hook on the cricoid cartilage and pass a 5- to 6-mm tube directly into the airway.

Complications of emergency cricothyrotomy include failure of technique, barotrauma with pneumothorax or pneumomediastinum, bleeding or damage to the larynx or surrounding structures.

Changing the tube

Tracheal tubes sometimes need changing, commonly if a leak develops in the cuff. The safest procedure is to assemble the intubation 'kit' and check the new tube, preoxygenate for 3 minutes, suction the oropharynx, ensure abolition of the glottic closure reflex by additional muscle relaxation and undertake direct laryngoscopy.

A tube-exchange catheter is passed through the in situ tube until its tip is near the carina and the defective tube removed. The new tube is passed over the inserted catheter or introducer. Placing an introducer or tube-exchange catheter through the initial tube avoids the problem of taking the defective tube out but being unable to introduce the new one.

Lung separation

In anaesthetic practice during thoracic surgery, it is common to undertake differential lung ventilation, primarily to allow collapse of the lung for surgical access in the appropriate hemithorax. Usually the specialized tubes or blockers are removed or replaced at the end of surgery. However, there are rare indications within the critical care unit for initiating or continuing lung separation, either to protect a 'good' lung from a contralateral disease process or control ventilation to each lung individually. The two most common techniques for providing lung separation are double-lumen tubes and bronchial blockers.

Double-lumen tubes

These tubes contain two separate limbs, one that resides in the bronchus and the other in the trachea. The tubes are known as either 'left' or 'right' to indicate the endobronchial component. The bronchial cuff of a right double-lumen tube must incorporate a slit or orifice to allow ventilation of the upper lobe and the positioning of a right double-lumen tube is more difficult than for a left. The disposable double-lumen tubes are sized in French gauge with 35 or 37 Fr being suitable for women and 39 or 41 Fr for men. The depth of insertion, measured at the teeth, is 29 cm for the average man and 27 cm for a woman.

Bronchial blocker

A bronchial blocker is a long, narrow catheter with a distal cuff. It is designed to be placed under fibreoptic control through a single lumen tube into the bronchus, where inflation of the cuff occludes the bronchus.

Extubation

Extubation is the process of removal of the tracheal tube, after which the patient maintains and protects their airway. Various preconditions exist before extubation can be considered.

- Mechanical ventilation is no longer required.
- There is cardiorespiratory stability.
- The patient is alert enough to maintain their airway.
- There is satisfactory spontaneous ventilation.
- The inspired oxygen is 40% to 60% or lower.
- The work of breathing is satisfactory and can be maintained.

The extubation strategy encompasses the plan for extubation and management for reintubation should extubation fail. Equipment for reintubation should be assembled, the nasogastric tube if present should be suctioned to reduce the likelihood of aspiration and the inspired oxygen increased to 100% for at least 3 minutes. Where copious secretions are present, it is helpful to apply positive pressure and temporarily deflate the cuff to force secretions above the cuff into the oropharynx, where they can be suctioned. At the point of extubation, the fixation tape is untied or cut, positive pressure (approximately 20–30 cmH_2O) is applied, the cuff rapidly deflated and the tube removed. A facemask should be applied attached to the Waters circuit with 100% inspired oxygen and adequacy of spontaneous respiration confirmed before transferring the patient onto a medium oxygen concentration facemask. It is wise to keep nil orally for 1 to 2 hours so that full laryngeal competence can be regained.

Key points

- Induction of anaesthesia and neuromuscular blockade should be used to facilitate tracheal intubation, except in the utmost emergency, such as cardiac arrest.
- When an intubated patient arrives in intensive care unit, adequate handover should include detailed information about the ease of intubation. Careful inspection of the adequacy of the airway is required.
- Intubation in the intensive care unit is potentially difficult and dangerous; suitably trained medical staff are essential and difficult airway equipment and failed intubation protocols must be immediately at hand.
- Exchange of the tracheal tube may lead to significant morbidity and must be undertaken with care.

Chapter 9

Tracheostomy

J. VARLEY AND F. FALTER

Introduction

Despite having existed as a therapeutic intervention since Egyptian times, there remain controversies regarding the timing and method of performing tracheostomy. It is undoubtedly a valuable therapeutic intervention, and is commonly seen on cardiac critical care units.

Indications

The commonest indication is to aid weaning from mechanical ventilation, after either predicted or actual failed removal of the endotracheal tube. The American Society of Thoracic Surgeons has estimated the need for prolonged ventilation (>24 hours) at 5% for first-time coronary artery bypass grafting and more than 10% for other cardiac surgery. If mechanical ventilation is still required after 10 to 14 days, then a tracheostomy is commonly performed. Many clinicians would also consider it necessary after two failed attempts at tracheal extubation. Prolonged ventilation or failed extubation may be due to:

- excessive secretions, persistent chest infection;
- reduced compliance, such as after acute lung injury;
- high oxygen requirements; or
- tracheostomy is also often performed in cases of obtunded neurological state (e.g. after stroke) or reduced airway protection reflexes.

Contraindications

There are no absolute contraindications to tracheostomy. Relative contraindications include:

- previous neck surgery or radiation, because distorted anatomy could lead to damage of associated anatomical structures, including vascular injury;
- impaired coagulation (should be corrected before procedure);
- high oxygen requirements, high positive end-expiratory pressure (PEEP) or airway pressures (may be difficult to ventilate effectively during the procedure).

Timing

There is no consensus about the best timing for tracheostomy. The decision to proceed is based on risk–benefit analysis, but the main determinant is usually the number of days of mechanical ventilation and tracheal intubation that is predicted to be required. The cutoff point may vary, but most commonly is 10 to 14 days. After this time, chronic inflammation and damage to the oropharynx and larynx from the endotracheal tube is likely to cause long-term sequelae.

The advocates of early tracheostomy (within 7 days) have shown that this reduces the duration of mechanical ventilation, and duration of stay in critical care. However, this has not been shown to improve survival or decrease chest infections.

Table 9.1 Benefits of tracheostomy

Facilitation of repeated suctioning of the tracheobronchial tree.
Reduced dead space and airways resistance.
Reduced complications related to translaryngeal intubation: laryngeal oedema, sinusitis, mucosal ulceration, vocal cord dysfunction, subglottic stenosis and tracheomalacia.
Increased patient comfort and better oral hygiene.
May allow speech and swallowing.
Often allows discontinuation of sedation and neurological assessment.

Patients are rarely able to give informed consent for tracheostomy placement, but as a matter of courtesy, relatives should be informed of the reasons for the procedure, and of the advantages and disadvantages. In some countries, specific actions must be taken to comply with current law in relation to consent.

Complications

A tracheostomy is not a benign intervention and can cause patients harm, including death! Complications can be divided into immediate, early and late.

Immediate complications

- Hypoxaemia owing to airway obstruction during the procedure, loss of PEEP and reduced tidal volume.
- Intraoperative bleeding from the thyroid gland and from vessels in the operative field.
- Pneumothorax or pneumomediastinum are the result of direct injury to the pleura or the lung apex, or creation of a false lumen during insertion of the tracheostomy cannula.
- Injury to surrounding structures, including recurrent laryngeal nerve, the great vessels and the oesophagus.
- Tracheal tear.
- Air embolism. This is critical in patients with mechanical assist devices because the device will fail to function.
- Fire; use of diathermy in an oxygen-enriched environment when the trachea is open may lead to flash fire and airway damage.

Early complications

- Obstruction by mucus plug, blood clot or mucosal flap (rare).
- Displacement, leading to loss of the airway. Immediate oral reintubation may be required if the stoma was performed fewer than 7 to 10 days earlier and cannot be recannulated.
- Localized stomal infection (may be less common after percutaneous technique).

Late complications

- Tracheomalacia.
- Tracheal stenosis.
- Tracheoesophageal fistula.
- Granulation tissue (with airway obstruction).
- Scarring.

Technique: percutaneous or surgical

A tracheostomy can be created either surgically or using a percutaneous dilatational technique, and neither has so far proven superior to the other despite passionate arguments by their respective proponents.

Percutaneous dilatational technique is a quicker procedure, usually performed by the critical care team at the bedside; therefore, transfer to theatre is not required. It might be associated with less intraoperative and early complications – certainly less bleeding is seen and lower infection rates have been reported. Torrential haemorrhage during the procedure, although rare, may be catastrophic and necessitates transfer to theatre and involvement of the surgical team. Cosmetic appearance may be better, but studies assessing long-term complications such as

Table 9.2 Conditions unfavourable for percutaneous technique

Abnormal or poorly palpable midline neck anatomy.
Short neck, difficulty palpating cricoid cartilage above the sternum, even with the neck extended.
Need for emergency procedure.
Coagulopathy or thrombocytopenia.
Enlarged thyroid gland.
Obesity (ultrasound guidance to locate anatomical landmarks may be used).

tracheal narrowing owing to overgranulation have been equivocal.

If a percutaneous dilatational technique is carried out, proper training is essential. Use of fibreoptic bronchoscopy to confirm optimal placement is mandatory, and anaesthesia and muscle paralysis are also required; an anaesthetist not undertaking the procedure should perform this.

Without consensus, local preference and resources often determine practice in individual units. Cardiothoracic surgeons may prefer open surgical technique because of perceived lower infection rate of sternotomy wound, although this is not proven.

Choice of tube

A small tube increases air flow resistance, making weaning from the ventilator more difficult. However, the maximum diameter is restricted by the size of the trachea. As a rule the diameter of the tube should be approximately three fourths that of the trachea. The length of the tube is important:

- too short tubes might abut the posterior tracheal wall, which may cause obstruction and ulceration;
- too long tubes might erode the anterior tracheal wall by curving in a forward direction, which can cause erosion and haemorrhage from the innominate artery.

A variety of materials are used to make the tracheostomy cannula. Polyvinyl chloride is thermosensitive and inexpensive, but may retain bacteria. Silicone, although more expensive, is softer and less prone to retain bacteria and secretions. Silver tubes may occasionally be used, when the tracheostomy is required for several months or if the patient is to be discharged home with it in situ.

The tube inserted during the procedure is almost invariably cuffed and consists of a single cannula. Once the tracheostomy tract has healed (7–10 days), the first tube change can be performed. If the tube diameter allows, the new tube should consist of an inner and outer cannula. The inner tube can be cleaned or replaced as necessary, reducing the chance of occlusion with secretions. In the emergency situation of a blocked airway, the inner tube is easily removed; patients are preferably discharged to the ward with such a tube. An inner cannula, however, decreases the inner diameter by up to 1.5 mm, increasing the resistance.

As the patient's recovery progresses, modifications may be made to the tracheostomy to enable phonation and swallowing. The cuff can be deflated, at first temporarily. This allows airflow past the tracheostomy, reducing airway resistance. It may also facilitate swallowing; the inflated cuff can 'anchor' the larynx and occlude the oesophagus. A fenestrated tube is often preferred after the first tube change. This allows greater airflow through the tracheostomy and through the vocal cords, thus allowing the return of phonation. A speaking valve is a one-way valve that caps the tracheostomy tube externally. It allows inspiration through the tracheostomy tube, but closes on expiration, thus directing airflow through the larynx.

Postoperative care

Security of the new tracheostomy is paramount. The original tube is left sutured in place for 5 to 7 days to allow the tract to form. There is commonly a degree of tracheitis after the procedure, and blood-stained secretions may be suctioned for a number of days. Gas exchange may deteriorate immediately after the operation, although this usually recovers in 24 hours.

Humidified gases should be used; the normal warming and moistening mechanisms of the upper airway are bypassed. Motion of the tracheostomy cannula should be minimized in the trachea by effective securing with tapes and a dressing to reduce trauma.

Long-term care

After tracheostomy, sedation is often no longer required; however, confusion or agitation may obviously necessitate pharmacological management. Stopping sedation facilitates weaning from the ventilator and rehabilitation. Patient positioning is usually easier due to increased comfort and reduced pain on movement. More aggressive mobilization and sitting out of bed may be possible. Weaning from mechanical ventilation is easier as the overall work of breathing is reduced – the upper airway is bypassed and dead space is significantly less. Airflow is also more likely to be laminar, with a more homogeneous distribution of inhaled gases. If breathing room air, a Swedish nose device incorporating a heat and moisture exchange filter can be employed.

Because tracheostomy allows use of laryngeal, and later supraglottic, muscles, oedema and atrophy improve, allowing return of function.

Once the patient can tolerate breathing spontaneously without PEEP/continuous positive airway pressure, the cuff can be deflated. This is usually done for short periods at first, as tolerated. As muscle function improves, the cuff can be left deflated for longer periods. Swallowing should be tried, although if this causes coughing, aspiration should be suspected. A food dye or coloured drink can be tried, and the trachea suctioned to ensure none is present, although this does not rule out aspiration. The patient should be as upright as possible whenever swallowing is attempted; conversely, solids and semisolids may be easier to swallow.

Deflation of the cuff may also allow phonation. The proximal end of the tracheostomy tube should be intermittently blocked – the patient may be taught to do this. Air is then forced past the vocal cords and speech may be heard. A speaking valve aids this process, but causes increased work of breathing. In case of difficulties, speech therapist evaluation or videofluoroscopy with or without fibreoptic endoscopic evaluations of swallow may be required. Phonation encourages reestablishment of normal airflow through the vocal cords and may serve to decrease the patient's reliance on the tracheostomy tube.

Decannulation

The decision to remove the cannula is often not straightforward, and requires close cooperation between medical, nursing and physiotherapy staff. Patients are often discharged to the ward with their tracheostomy once they are breathing spontaneously via a tracheostomy mask (humidified

Table 9.3 Criteria for decannulation
Freedom from mechanical ventilation and CPAP – ≥48 hours recommended.
Breathing room air or ≤50% oxygen.
Minimal secretions.
Good cough, spontaneously and in response to tracheal suctioning. Coughing of secretions past tracheostomy into mouth when cuff is deflated preferable.
Adequate protection of airway expected – gag/swallowing reflex present.
Patient cooperative and alert – able to follow commands.
Return of sufficient respiratory muscle tone/strength (difficult to determine).

Abbreviation: CPAP, continuous positive airway pressure.

oxygen) or Swedish nose (air), and the intensive care team may then be asked to advise on timing of decannulation. If the patient is sent to the ward, a fenestrated double tube as described is preferable, because this is safer in an emergency. Whether the tracheostomy is removed on critical care or the ward, all the criteria in Table 9.3 should be observed.

Key points

- Tracheostomy improves patient comfort and facilitates wakening and weaning from mechanical ventilation.
- Early tracheostomy may be associated with faster weaning and shortened critical care stay.
- Percutaneous tracheostomy is an alternative to surgical operation, and may have advantages in terms of long-term complications.
- During period of cuff deflation, swallowing and speech should be encouraged if tolerated.
- Close cooperation between the multidisciplinary team is required for successful management.

FURTHER READING

Freeman BD, Isabella K, Lin N, *et al.* A meta-analysis of prospective trials comparing percutaneous and surgical tracheostomy in critically ill patients. *Chest* 2000;118:1412–1418.

Griffiths J, Barber V, Morgan L, *et al.* Systematic review and meta-analysis of studies of the timing of tracheostomy in adult patients undergoing artificial ventilation. *BMJ* 2005;330:1243–1248.

Heffner JE. The role of tracheotomy in weaning. *Chest* 2001;120(Suppl. 6):477S–481S.

Russel C, Matta B. *Tracheostomy: A multiprofessional handbook*. London: Greenwich Medical Media; 2004.

Chapter 10

Venous access

J.E. ARROWSMITH

Introduction

With very rare exceptions, all patients undergoing critical care will, at some stage during their admission, require an indwelling venous catheter or cannula for fluid and drug administration, invasive monitoring and therapeutic intervention. So ubiquitous is the role of venous access in current medical practice that it is rarely given much consideration in even the most comprehensive textbooks.

This chapter reviews the various sites of venous access, devices in common use, methods of insertion and removal and common complications.

Sites of venous access

Anatomical sites are usually divided into two categories: peripheral and central. Short-term (i.e., 1–3 days) access for infusions of crystalloids, colloids, blood products and nonirritant drugs can be achieved using small to medium sized (e.g. 22- to 14-G) cannulae in a peripheral (i.e., arm and leg) vein. Patients with 'poor' peripheral veins and those requiring long-term (>4 days) venous access, invasive monitoring, inotropic or irritant drugs (e.g. cytotoxic agents), intravenous feeding or therapeutic intervention typically require central venous access with larger (7- to 9-Fr) devices with one or more lumens. Placement of a 'peripherally inserted central catheter' (PICC) allows delivery to a central vein via a long (30- to 55-cm) indwelling catheter.

Peripheral veins

For the purposes of this description, venous access using both the upper and lower limbs is presented.

In the routine perioperative and critical care of the adult, however, it is recommended that only the veins of the arms be considered for peripheral venous access. The application of an elastic tourniquet or similar device proximal to the intended site of cannulation improves the chances of success in most cases.

The small veins of the dorsum of the hand are readily accessible and frequently chosen for short-term access using small (21- to 25-G) cannulae for the administration of sedative, analgesic and anaesthetic drugs. Larger, more proximal veins, such as the cephalic or basilic veins, are more suitable for larger (12- to 18-G) cannulae. A proximally sited cannula is much less prone to inadvertent dislodgement (the radius of rotation is smaller). Whenever possible, veins overlying the wrist and near the elbow should be avoided because movement of the joint may lead to discomfort or extravasation.

In the leg, only the veins overlying the dorsum of the foot and distal part of the long saphenous vein (LSV) are suitable for cannulation. The LSV at the medial malleolus was a favoured site for surgical cannulation ('cut down'). The close proximity of the medial border of the tibia makes percutaneous LSV cannulation rather awkward.

Table 10.1 Indications for venous access

Fluid and drug administration	Crystalloids, colloids, blood products Parenteral drugs Parenteral nutrition
Invasive monitoring	Pressure monitoring Cardiac output measurement Mixed venous O_2 saturation Frequent blood sampling
Therapeutic intervention	Renal replacement therapy Plasmapheresis Extracorporeal oxygenation
Diagnostic intervention	Electrophysiological studies Endocardial biopsy Right heart catheterization studies

Internal jugular veins

The right internal jugular vein (IJV) is the most commonly chosen site for central venous access in patients undergoing general anaesthesia. The route gives near direct access to the right heart via the right innominate (brachiocephalic) vein and superior vena cava, and is well suited to the right-handed operator. In obese, oedematous or tracheostomized patients, however, anatomical landmarks may be obscured. In comparison with subclavian vein cannulation, bleeding complications associated with IJV are generally easier to control.

Table 10.2 Sites of venous access

Peripheral	Dorsal veins of hand Cephalic vein Accessory cephalic vein Median antebrachial vein Basilic vein Median cubital vein
Central	Internal jugular vein External jugular vein Subclavian vein Femoral vein

ANATOMY

The IJV drains blood from the brain, superficial parts of the face and the neck. It begins at the jugular foramen as a continuation of the transverse and sigmoid sinuses, and descends through the neck within the carotid sheath, uniting with the subclavian vein behind the medial end of the clavicle to form the brachiocephalic vein. The left IJV is typically smaller than the right, and each possesses a bicuspid valve located just above the inferior bulb. At its origin the IJV lies on the rectus capitis lateralis – behind the internal carotid artery (ICA) and the glossopharyngeal (cranial nerve IX), vagus (cranial nerve X) and accessory nerves (cranial nerve XI). As it descends through the neck it first lies lateral to the ICA, and then lateral to the common carotid artery. On the right, the vein becomes separated from the common carotid artery in the root of the neck and crosses the first part of the subclavian artery. On the left, the vein usually lies more anterior than lateral to the common carotid artery.

External jugular veins

Cannulation of an external jugular vein (EJV) is occasionally performed in an emergency or when there has been difficulty locating the IJV and the operator is reluctant to move to an alternative anatomical site. Its variable size, superficial location, mobility and tendency to collapse when punctured make the EJV surprisingly difficult to cannulate. In addition, the presence of bicuspid valves at its lower end and its acute passage through deep cervical fascia may impede advancement of a venous catheter.

ANATOMY

The EJV drains blood from the exterior of the cranium and deep parts of the face. It descends obliquely across the sternocleidomastoideus, piercing the deep fascia in the posterior triangle just above the clavicle before draining into the subclavian vein lateral to or in front of scalenus anterior.

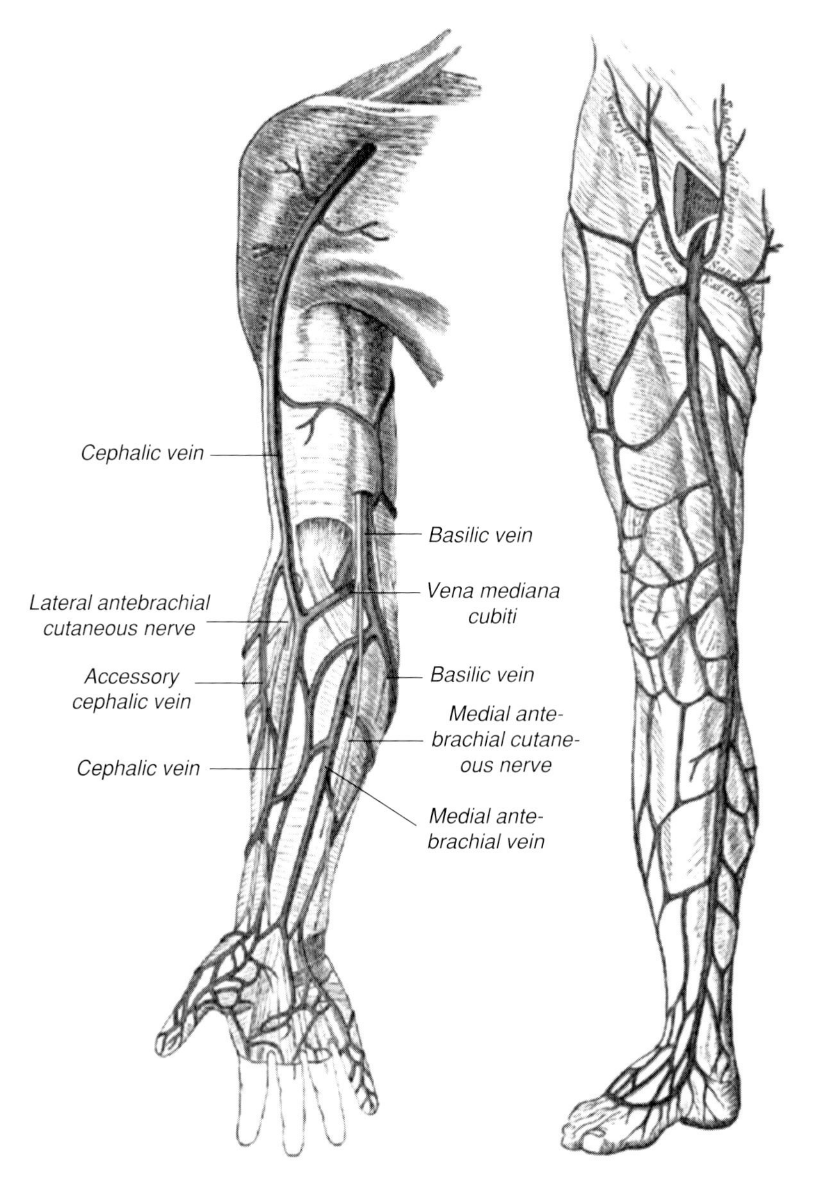

Figure 10.1 The superficial veins of the anterior aspects of the limbs. From Gray's *Anatomy of the Human Body*, with permission.

Subclavian veins

The subclavian veins are arguably the most comfortable site for central venous cannulation and best suited for temporary transvenous pacing and long-term parenteral nutrition. A number of approaches are described: supraclavicular, lateral infraclavicular and medial infraclavicular. Significant local complications are a result of the close proximity of the subclavian artery, brachial plexus, pleura and thoracic duct (on the left). Bleeding complications secondary to arterial puncture or venous laceration are difficult to control by direct pressure alone.

ANATOMY

The subclavian vein is a continuation of the axillary vein. It lies between the outer borders of the first ribs

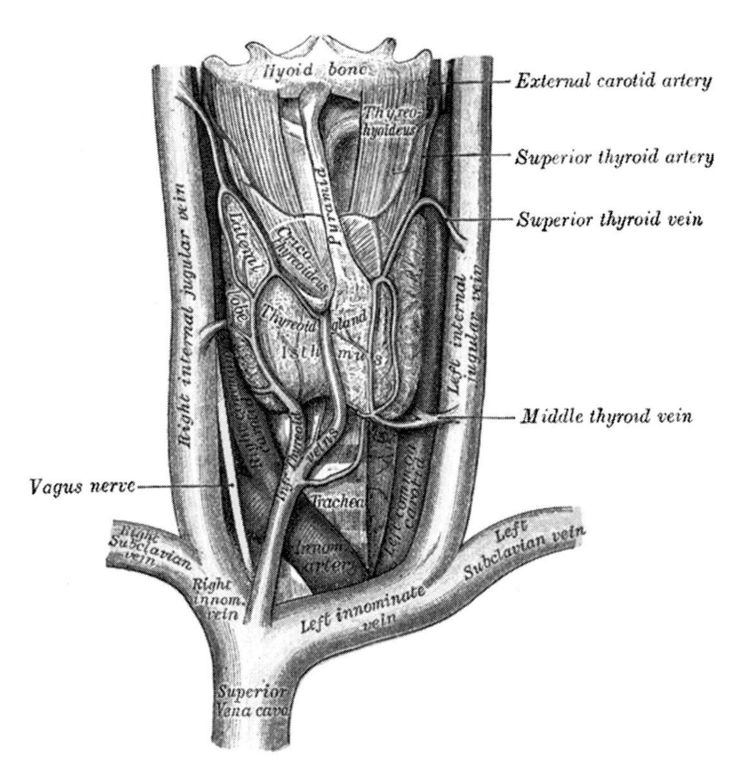

Figure 10.2 The internal jugular veins. From Gray's *Anatomy of the Human Body*, with permission.

and the medial end of the clavicle, where it joins the IJV to form the brachiocephalic vein. It lies posterior to the clavicle and subclavius muscle and superior and anterior to the subclavian artery, from which it is separated medially by the scalenus anterior and the phrenic nerve.

Femoral veins

The variable relationship of the vein to the femoral artery and the high incidence of infective complications means that it is generally used only in an emergency situation and when other sites are unavailable.

ANATOMY

The femoral vein accompanies the femoral artery through the upper two thirds of the thigh. In the lower part of its course it lies lateral to the artery; higher up, it is behind it; and at the inguinal ligament, it lies on its medial side and on the same plane.

Venous access devices

Types of cannulae/catheters

The oldest types of venous cannulae were simply hollow needles – the Butterfly cannula (19, 21, or 23 G) designed by Beck is probably the best-known device of this type. The needle, which has two flexible plastic wings to aid insertion, is attached to an injection port via a length of plastic tubing. The port incorporates the Luer-Lock – an American adaptation of the connection developed by the Luer Company of Paris. The obvious disadvantage of this type of device is the high risk of needle migration, leading to injury to local structures and extravasation.

Plastic (polyvinyl chloride, polyurethane, polytetrafluoroethane) cannulae, inserted over a removable sharpened hollow trocar (stylette), are the most commonly used devices for peripheral venous access. Devices of this type are supplied as a 'plain' catheter or with plastic fixation wings and integrated injection port. Although principally designed

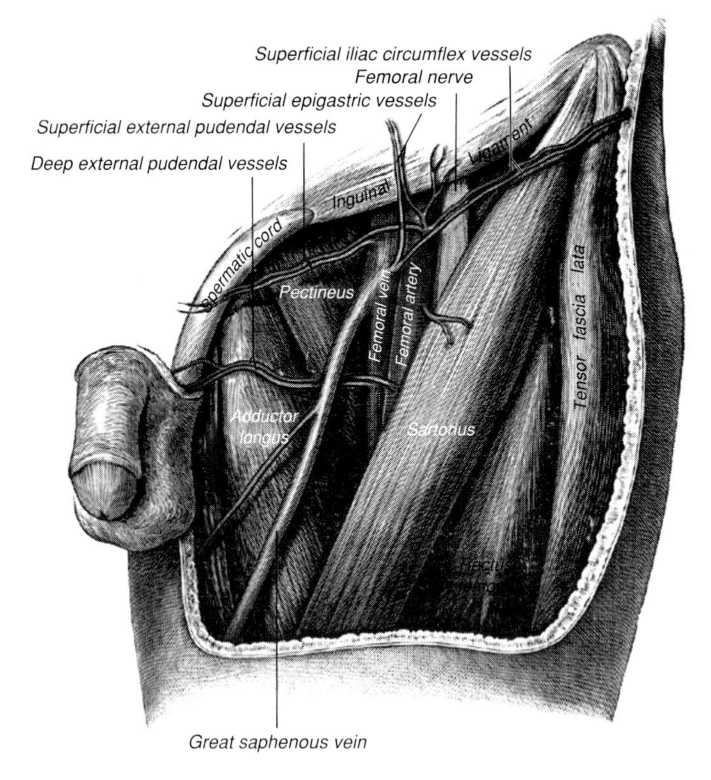

Figure 10.3 The femoral veins. From Gray's *Anatomy of the Human Body*, with permission.

for peripheral venous cannulation, longer versions (15–20 cm) can be used for central venous cannulation using the catheter-over-needle insertion technique (see below).

A wide range of single- and multiple-lumen devices of varying diameters and lengths are available. Thin-walled, large-bore catheters for both peripheral and central venous cannula require stabilization during insertion and are usually supplied with an integral stiffener/dilator and Seldinger-type guidewire. A short (6–8 cm) 7 Fr and 8 Fr rapid infusion catheter is particularly useful for the rapid administration of fluids via a peripheral vein. Longer (15–20 cm) 8 Fr and 9 Fr sheaths suitable for central venous access can be used for either rapid fluid administration or as an access route for pulmonary artery catheterization or transvenous pacing.

Composite devices with two to five separate lumens are particularly useful in perioperative and critical care when there may be a need to administer several types of often-incompatible fluids and monitor pressure continuously.

Long-term (>6 weeks) venous access for parenteral nutrition or chemotherapy is best provided by (1) a PICC, (2) a tunnelled central venous catheter or (3) a totally implanted central venous catheter. Although reduced line-related sepsis is the main reason for choosing this type of device, patient comfort and tolerability are important considerations.

Catheters designed for measuring right heart pressures and cardiac output as well as those used for temporary transvenous endocardial pacing are typically supplied with a small balloon at the distal end to facilitate placement by flotation.

Table 10.3 Sizes of intravenous cannulae

Birmingham/Stubs gauge	French Gauge	Nominal outer diameter (mm)	Nominal internal diameter (mm)
23		0.635	0.318
21		0.813	0.495
	3.0	1.000	—
19		1.067	0.686
18		1.270	0.838
	4.0	1.333	—
17		1.473	1.067
16		1.651	1.194
	5.0	1.667	—
	6.0	2.000	—
14		2.108	1.600
	7.0	2.333	—
	7.5	2.500	—
	8.0	2.667	—
12		2.769	2.159
	9.0	3.000	—

Size matters

The size of many medical tubes and catheters is expressed in French Gauge (Fr), a system of measurement introduced by Joseph-Frederic-Benoit Charriere (1803–1876), a Parisian surgical instrument maker. It is commonly believed that catheter size is the circumference expressed in millimetres (i.e., diameter $\times \pi$), where in fact, it is actually three times the diameter. Thus a 9-Fr (or 9-Ch) catheter has an external diameter of 3 mm.

Somewhat confusingly, needles and simple single-lumen devices for vascular access are sized using a different system – also known as 'gauge' – based on Standard Wire Gauge (SWG). Unlike French Gauge, large cannulae have a smaller gauge number than smaller cannulae. Matters are made more confusing by the fact that there is not one universally accepted and used scale, but several – for example, American or Brown & Sharp; Birmingham or Stubs Gauge; British Imperial Standard SWG; and Washburn & Möen.

When selecting a venous access device for clinical use, it should be kept in mind that the maximal infusion rate is determined by internal diameter, length and fluid viscosity in accordance with the Hagen-Poiseuille law. The selection of a large-diameter device needs to be balanced against the likelihood of successful insertion and patient discomfort.

$$\Phi = \frac{\Delta P \pi R^4}{8 \eta L}$$

Figure 10.4 Poiseuille's law. The relationship between fluid flow rate (Φ) and pressure (ΔP), tube radius (R), fluid viscosity (η) and tube length (L). Described by Gotthilf Heinrich Ludwig Hagen (1797–1884) and Jean Louis Marie Poiseuille (1797–1869).

Methods of insertion

SURGICAL

The vein is exposed by surgical dissection and the catheter placed directly into the vein via a small venotomy. The LSV at the medial malleolus and the femoral vein may be accessed in this way.

DIRECT PUNCTURE

The needle is passed directly through skin into the lumen of the vein.

CATHETER OVER STYLETTE (HOLLOW TROCAR)

The cannula with integral stylette is passed directly through the skin into the lumen of the vein until a 'flashback' of blood is seen in the clear plastic hub of the stylette. The catheter and stylette are advanced a further 1 to 2 mm and then held in a fixed position. The catheter is then advanced over the stylette into the vein. The stylette is removed and discarded.

CATHETER THROUGH INTRODUCER

The catheter (typically a long silicone or plastic tube) is passed though an introducer needle, cannula or sheath and advanced into the vein. This technique is often used for inserting tunnelled lines (e.g. Hickman, Broviac, Leonard, Groshong) and some types of peripheral catheter (e.g. Drum-Cath). Because many of these catheters have fixed Luer hubs that are too large to fit through the introducer sheath, several manufacturers supply a winged introducer sheath that can be 'peeled' apart during removal and then discarded.

CATHETER OVER GUIDEWIRE

Described by Seldinger in 1953, this technique of insertion begins with direct puncture of the vein with a needle of sufficient size to allow the passage of a flexible, metal guidewire into the lumen of the vein. Guidewires are typically composed of a solid wire around which a coil of wire is tightly wound, providing both strength and flexibility. The needle is withdrawn from the vein, pulled back over the guidewire and discarded. The catheter is then threaded over the wire and advanced into the vein – a small skin incision may be required to prevent 'buckling' of the catheter. The guidewire is removed and discarded. Insertion of large-bore and multilumen catheters requires the creation of a subcutaneous track or channel. A tapered, flexible dilator is passed over the guidewire, advanced 1 to 2 cm into the vein and then removed. The incorporation of a removable, intraluminal dilator into the design of large, single-lumen catheters permits creation of a subcutaneous channel and catheter insertion to be achieved in a single manoeuvre.

IMAGING ASSISTED

Real-time two-dimensional (2-D) ultrasound may be used to locate the vein. Video fluoroscopy is particularly useful for ensuring the correct placement of both guidewires and catheters.

ULTRASOUND GUIDANCE

When used to assist IJV cannulation, 2-D ultrasound has been shown to reduce procedure time, catheterization failure, and the number of mechanical complications. Evidence for similar benefits during subclavian or femoral vein cannulation, however, is much less clear. The publication in 2002 of guidelines (United Kingdom) recommending that ultrasound be used to guide IJV cannulation provoked considerable debate. Widespread adoption of these guidelines as the 'routine standard of care' would have significant cost and training implications, and there is concern that 'traditional' techniques that rely on the use of anatomical landmarks would fall into disuse.

The likelihood of successful central venous cannulation can often be improved by the judicious administration of intravenous fluid; attention to optimal patient positioning; ensuring operator comfort; and access to trained assistance.

Contraindications

Other than lack of consent, there are few absolute contraindications to venous cannulation. Relative contraindications include infection at the planned site of insertion, anatomical variations, burns and coagulopathy. The importance of a relative contraindication depends on the experience of the operator and clinical necessity. It is suggested that failure to secure central venous access after three attempts should contraindicate a fourth attempt!

Complications

Complications arise in as many as 1 in 10 central venous cannulations and may, rarely, lead directly to death. Complications may be local or remote and can be classified according to time of onset (immediate, early or late) and their nature (mechanical, infectious or thrombotic).

The likelihood of mechanical complications is increased by (1) the number of cannulation attempts and (2) the frequency of catheter changes. Femoral venous cannulation is much more likely to be accompanied by mechanical complications than either IJV or subclavian vein cannulation.

Table 10.4 Complications of venous cannulation

Mechanical	Guidewire-induced dysrhythmia Embolism: guidewire, catheter, air Misplacement Haematoma, tamponade, venous pseudoaneurysm Arterial puncture (IJV > SCV), arteriovenous fistula, neurological sequelae Pneumothorax (SCV > IJV) Chylothorax (left SCV) Nerve injury – spinal accessory nerve, brachial plexus, sympathetic chain Dural puncture (IJV) Tracheal tube cuff puncture (SCV)
Infectious	Puncture site infection Intraluminal colonization Catheter hub contamination Bacteraemia, septicaemia, endocarditis
Thrombotic	Venous obstruction – superior vena cava syndrome Thromboembolism

Abbreviations: IJV, internal jugular vein; SCV, subclavian vein.

Line-related sepsis

Local and systemic infection is thought to complicate central vein catheterization in 5% to 26% patients. According to the US Centers for Disease Control and Prevention, the median rate of all catheter-related bloodstream infections (CRBSI) in critical care units of all types ranges from 1.8 to 5.2 per 1,000 catheter-days.

The commonest cause of infection is the migration of organisms at the insertion site into the cutaneous catheter tract resulting in colonization of the catheter tip. Contamination of catheter hubs inevitably leads to intraluminal catheter colonization. Occasionally, haematogenous seeding from a remote site of infection may lead to catheter colonization. Infusate-induced catheter colonization is rare.

The diagnosis of CRBSI is based on clinical signs and symptoms, markers of sepsis (leukocyte count, C-reactive protein) and the results of blood cultures. Whereas a negative culture from blood drawn through a catheter makes CRBSI unlikely, a positive result may indicate hub contamination, line colonization or CRBSI. For this reason, it is recommended that blood for cultures be drawn from peripheral sites. Evidence of erythema, induration or frank pus at the insertion site should prompt removal of the catheter and insertion of a new catheter at a new site. A similar approach is recommended in patients with septic shock and no other source of infection.

A considerable body of clinical evidence suggests that a multimodal approach to reducing CRBSI can

Table 10.5 Diagnosis of catheter-related blood stream infections

Presence of a recognized pathogen cultured from ≥1 blood cultures
and
Organism cultured from blood not related to infection at another site
or
Presence of ≥1 of the following: fever (>38°C), chills, hypotension
and
Signs and symptoms and positive results not related to infection at another site
and
Presence of at least one of the following:
- Common skin contaminant (e.g. diphtheroids, bacillus species, propionibacterium species, coagulase-negative staphylococci or micrococci) cultured from ≥2 blood samples drawn on separate occasions.
- Common skin contaminant cultured from ≥1 blood culture in a sample from a patient with an intravascular catheter.
- Positive antigen test on blood (e.g. *Haemophilus influenzae, Streptococcus pneumoniae, Neisseria meningitides*, or group B streptococcus).

result in improved patient care, reduced duration of critical care stay and reduced mortality.

Catheter removal

Little attention is paid to the safe removal of central venous catheters and the task is often delegated to junior or inexperienced staff members. Catheter removal should be undertaken with the same care and attention as catheter insertion. A sterile technique (sterile gloves, field and suture removal kit) should be used. After an explanation of the procedure, the patient should be placed in Trendelenburg

Table 10.6 Methods for reducing incidence of CRBSI

Cannulation site	Preferential use of subclavian route and avoidance of femoral vein
Catheter design	Antimicrobial impregnation Chlorhexidine and silver sulfadiazine; minocycline and rifampicin; platinum and silver impregnation
Insertion	Hand washing
	Full barrier precautions (mask, cap, sterile gown, sterile gloves and large sterile drape) Chlorhexidine skin preparation (in preference to isopropyl alcohol or povidone-iodine) Secure fixation and dressing
Care packages	Health care worker training and education Regular wound surveillance Avoidance of antibiotic ointments – reduces fungal colonization and emergence of resistant organisms Disinfection of catheter hubs Monitoring for signs, symptoms and markers of sepsis Endoluminal brushing Avoidance of 'routine' line change policy – at new site or over guidewire

(reverse Trendelenburg for femoral lines) and any pillows removed. All bandages and dressing should be removed, and all suture material cut and removed. If possible, the patient should be asked to undertake a valsalva manoeuvre while the catheter is swiftly withdrawn. The insertion site should then be covered with occlusive dressing and the catheter tip sent for culture.

Key points

- Venous access is a ubiquitous feature of critical care medicine.
- Central venous access permits a greater degree of monitoring and a wider range of therapeutic interventions, but exposes the patient to greater risk.
- Femoral cannulation should be avoided except in the emergency setting or if no other site can be accessed.
- Weighing benefit against risk, and the adoption of evidence-based practice can reduce the incidence of complications.

FURTHER READING

Hind D, Calvert N, McWilliams R, *et al.* Ultrasonic locating devices for central venous cannulation; meta-analysis. *BMJ* 2003;327:361–364.

National Institute for Clinical Excellence. *Guidance on the use of ultrasound devices for placing central venous catheters.* Technology Appraisal Guidance No 49, 2002. Available at: www.nice.org.uk.

O'Grady NP, Alexander M, Delinger EP, *et al.* Guidelines for the prevention of intravascular catheter-related infections. Centers for Disease Control and Prevention. *MMWR Recomm Rep* 2002;51:1–32. Available at: www.cdc.gov.

Ruesch S, Walder B, Tramer MR. Complications of central venous catheters: internal jugular versus subclavian access – a systematic review. *Crit Care Med* 2002;30:454–460.

Wenzel RP, Edmond MB. Team-based prevention of catheter-related infections. *N Engl J Med* 2006;355:2781–2783.

Chapter 11

Invasive haemodynamic monitoring

P.A. WHITE AND A.A. KLEIN

Introduction

Haemodynamic monitoring is essential in the cardiac critical care unit. Modern monitoring systems provide clinical staff with a plethora of physiological measurements that are used to diagnose and treat patients. Accurate measurements are imperative for patients to obtain the appropriate care. This chapter looks at the general principles involved and applies them to different types of measurement.

Invasive/noninvasive

Haemodynamic monitoring can be generally divided into invasive and noninvasive types. Noninvasive measurements are obtained without breaching the natural body armour (skin or mucosa) and include the electrocardiogram, pulse oximetry, temperature, capnography and blood pressure via a pressure cuff.

Invasive monitoring (obtained after breaching the natural body armour such as when inserting a catheter in an artery) is often preferred because it allows beat-to-beat measurements, greater accuracy of recorded values and the display of a continuous curve.

Pressure

Pressure is the force applied to a unit area of surface in a direction perpendicular to that surface. The internationally approved SI unit for pressure is the Pascal and 1 Pascal is 1 newton per square metre ($1 \text{ Pa} = 1 \text{ N/m}^2$). The standard atmosphere (atm) is an established constant and is approximately equal to typical air pressure at earth mean level and is defined as 1 standard atmosphere = 101,325 Pa. In clinical practice, pressure is still commonly expressed as a depth of a particular fluid, with the most common choices being mercury (Hg) or water. Although no longer measured by reading the displacement of the fluid, pressures are still commonly expressed in manometric units and mmHg is the most common unit. The correlation between the units is as follows: 1 mmHg = 133 Pa = 13.6 mmH_2O.

The transducer

A *transducer* is a device that can change one form of energy into another. A pressure transducer converts the physical measure (pressure) into an electrical signal. Transducers are the first essential component of almost every system of measurement. In most modern patient monitors, this small electrical signal is amplified so that it can be displayed on the monitor.

The most common type of pressure transducer consists of a diaphragm with one side open to the atmosphere and the other connected to the pressure to be measured.

Pressure causes a proportional displacement of the diaphragm. This displacement is converted into an electrical signal by a strain gauge (a silicon crystal). As the resistance of the silicon also changes

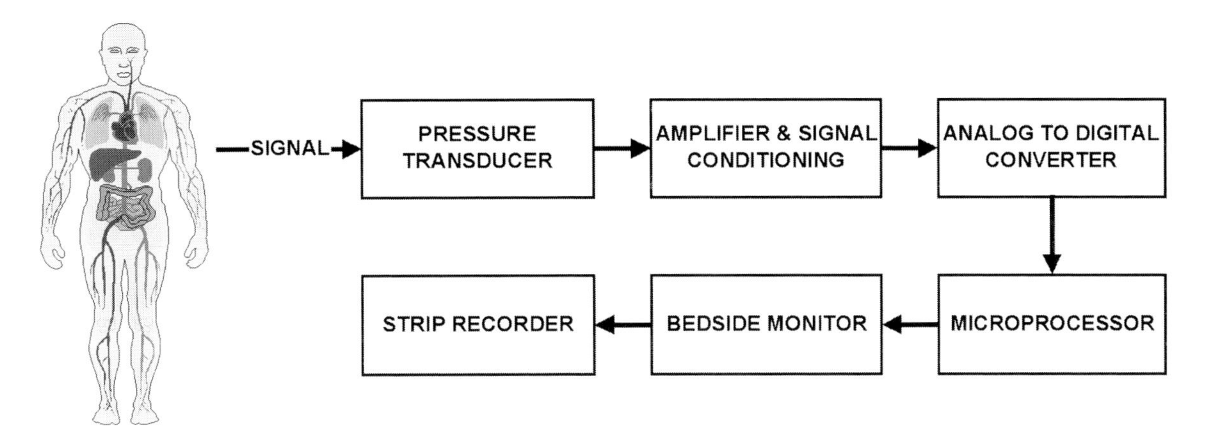

Figure 11.1 Conversion of signal to a number.

with temperature, four further strain gauges are attached to the diaphragm to compensate. These form a resistance bridge, known as a Wheatstone bridge.

The pressure transducer must be zeroed whenever it is connected for the first time and periodically thereafter. This is achieved by exposing both surfaces of the transducer to atmospheric pressure; in practice, the transducer is usually opened to the atmosphere by turning a tab and a button on the monitor is pressed. This is simply to determine the value of the unknown resistance at rest and is referred to as "balancing the bridge."

Transducer characteristics

Sensitivity

For each 100 mmHg pressure applied to the transducer, an output of 5 μV is produced.

Full-range input

The maximum input range of pressure is variable and depends on the model (usually 0–750 mmHg).

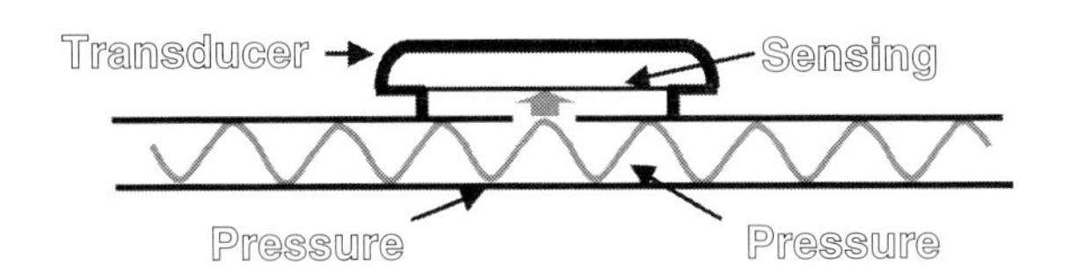

Figure 11.2 Diagram of a pressure transducer.

Elastic stiffness

This is the force needed to produce unit displacement and can be defined as pressure needed to produce unit change of volume within transducer (i.e., 500 mmHg produces a change of volume of 1 mm^3).

Frequency response/response time

The frequency component of a blood pressure waveform is approximately 40 to 50 Hz. The frequency response depends on the volume displacement of the transducer membrane, which in turn is related to the transducer sensitivity. This is affected by

- gas bubbles (as the bubble compresses, more liquid moves than is needed to move the diaphragm);
- compliance of the catheter walls; and
- compressibility of the fluid.

Pressure monitoring

Fluid-filled catheters are generally used in critical care units to measure a variety of physiological parameters, including arterial and venous pressures. A cannula is connected to the pressure transducer through a fluid-filled, noncompliant manometer line incorporating a continuous and intermittent flush device. The transducer is positioned level with the heart, usually at the midaxillary line.

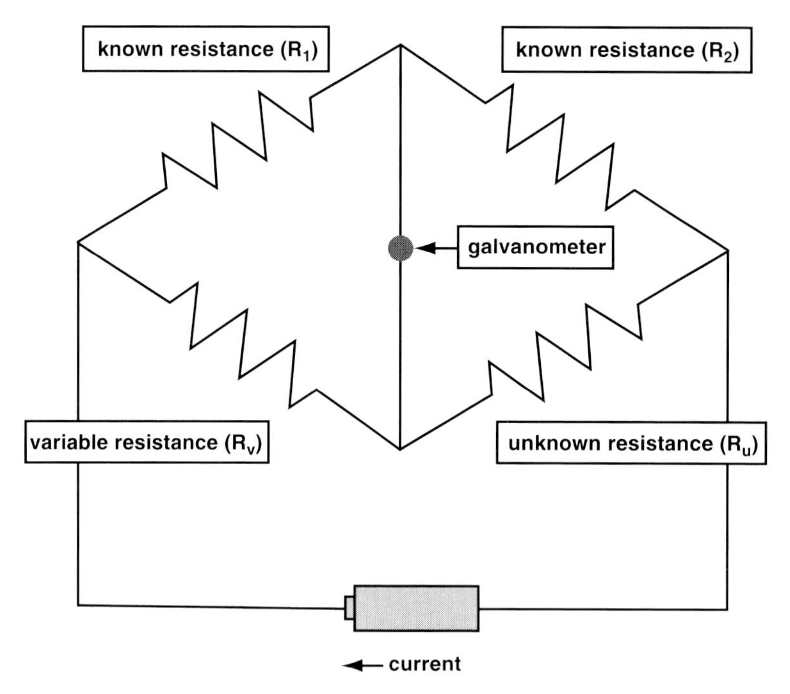

Figure 11.3 Diagram of a Wheatstone bridge.

Components

Intravenous fluid

Most standard intravenous (IV) fluids can be used as transmission fluids in a closed system. In many centres, heparin is added to the fluid bag to prevent clotting in the cannula; however, some studies suggest that the rate of cannula thrombosis and failure is independent of heparin in the flush system. The addition of heparin in the circuit can in itself trigger heparin-induced thrombocytopenia.

Pressure bag

When using an automatic flush, the flush solution is pressurized by using an inflatable pressure cuff. The pressure on the IV bag should be evenly distributed over the entire surface. A pressure of 300 mmHg is usually sufficient to operate the flush system over a long period.

Disposable flush system

To prevent thrombosis and clot at the end of the indwelling catheter and distortion of the pressure waveform, a slow and constant flow of fluid within the circuit is maintained. A typical flow rate of 1 to 3 mL/hr is used. A 'fast flush' exists on the transducer, which can increase the flow to 30 mL/hr.

Pressure line

The interconnecting tubing or "pressure line" that comes with the disposable pressure transducer should be used. This pressure line should have as small a lumen as possible (typically 0.75–1.50 mm) and be made preferably of as stiff (noncompliant) material as possible to minimize errors obtained in the pressure measurements. It is important that the length of the pressure line is as short as possible; it should not exceed 1.5 m.

Dynamic elements of the pressure signal

The blood pressure waveform can be regarded as periodic; it repeats itself in a regular manner with the pulse frequency. A simple periodic signal is a

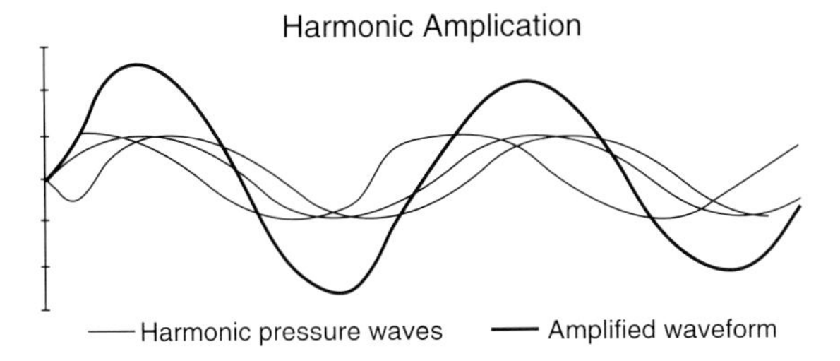

Figure 11.4 Harmonic amplification.

sine wave. A blood pressure waveform constitutes a complex periodical signal that may be built up from a number of sine waves, which when added together reproduce the original complex signal. A complex wave consists of a number of frequencies, namely a fundamental frequency with a series of harmonics.

Damping

Damping is caused by dissipation of stored energy. Removing energy from the pressure system leads to a progressive reduction in the amplitude of oscillations. Increased damping lowers the systolic pressure and elevates the diastolic pressure. Mean arterial pressure is unaltered. Damping can result from air bubbles, blood clots, soft diaphragm or soft tubing.

Resonance

Resonance occurs when the driving force frequency coincides with the resonant frequency of the system. This may occur if the tube or diaphragm is too stiff or noncompliant. The resonant frequency (or natural frequency) is the frequency at which the monitoring system itself resonates and amplifies the signal. It should be at least 10 times the fundamental frequency. If the natural frequency is less than 40 Hz, it falls within the range of the blood pressure and a sine wave is superimposed on the blood pressure wave. The fundamental frequency of this system is the heart rate. This is also known as the *first harmonic*. The first 10 harmonics contribute to the waveform seen.

Arterial pressure

A number of parameters may be derived from the arterial pressure trace.

- Owing to the nonsymmetrical nature, the mean is calculated by dividing the area below the curve with the cycle length. The functional mean can be calculated by adding one third of the difference between the systolic and diastolic pressures to the diastolic pressure.
- The slope of the upstroke of the wave allows estimation of myocardial contractility (dP/dt).

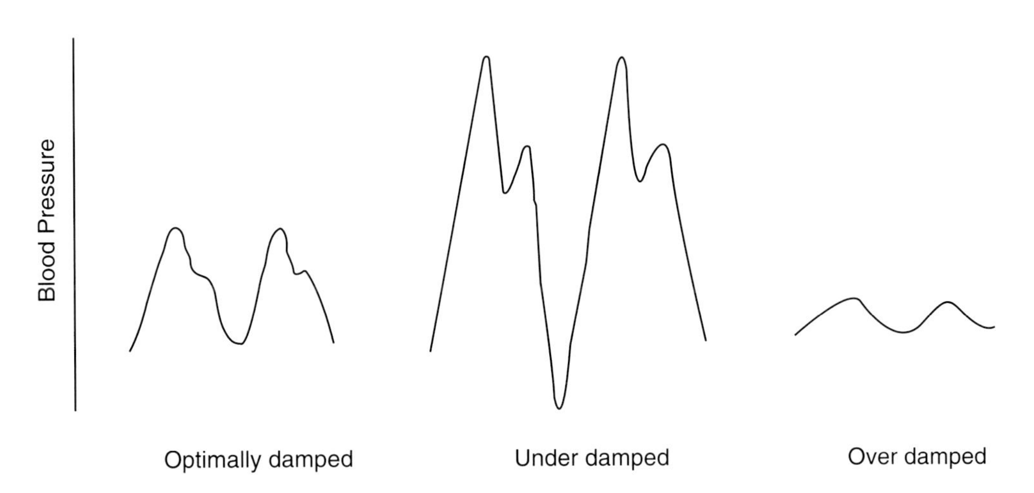

Figure 11.5 Recognition of waveform damping.

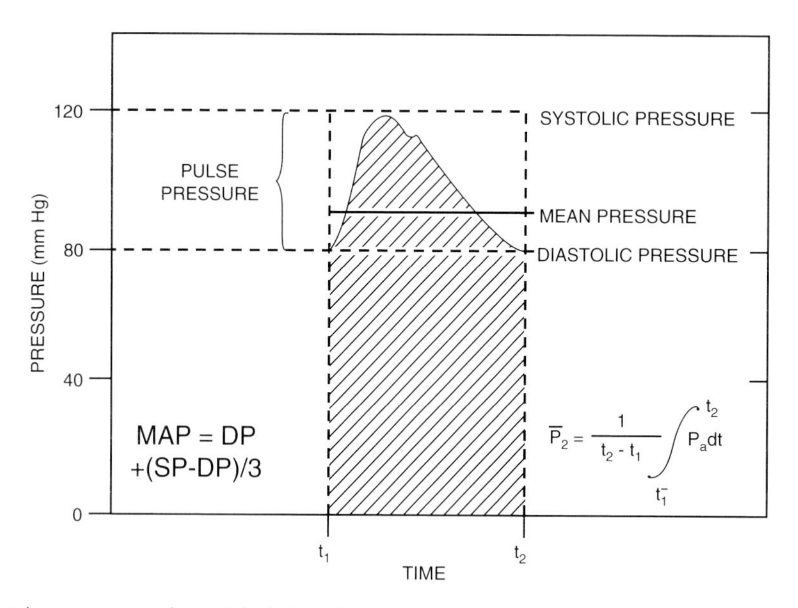

Figure 11.6 Arterial pressure waveform. Calculation of mean pressure.

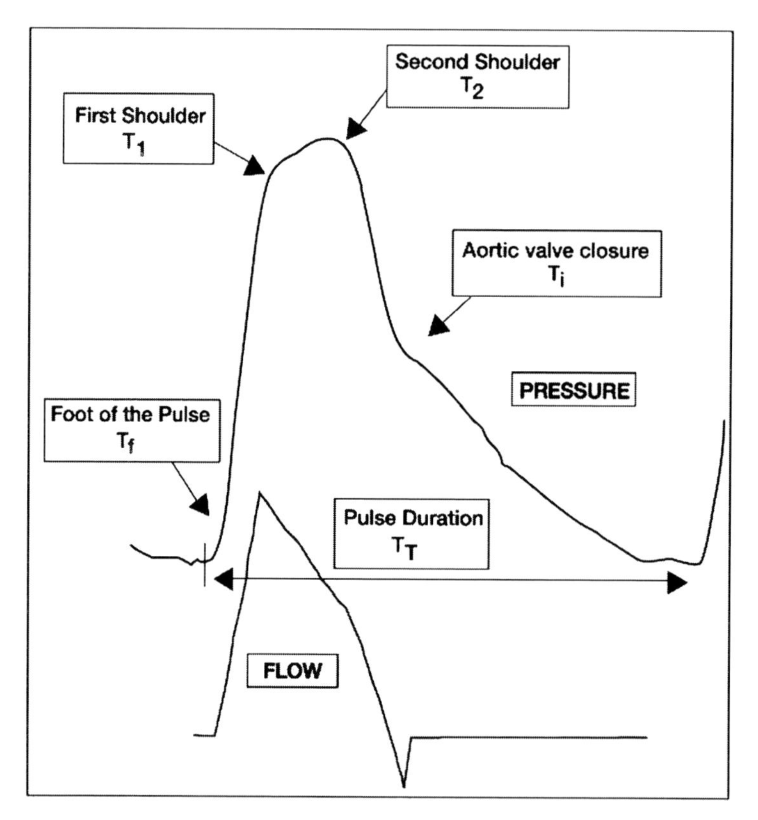

Figure 11.7 Arterial pressure waveform components.

- The stroke volume can be calculated by measuring the area from the beginning of the upstroke to the dicrotic notch. When this is multiplied by the heart rate, cardiac output can be estimated.
- The position of the dicrotic notch on the down stroke. A low dicrotic notch may be associated with underfilling.
- The slope of the diastolic decay indicates resistance to outflow. A slow fall is often seen if vasoconstriction is predominant.

Central venous pressure

- *a Wave*: due to atrial contraction; absent in atrial fibrillation; enlarged in tricuspid stenosis, pulmonary stenosis and pulmonary hypertension.
- *c Wave*: due to bulging of tricuspid valve into the right atrium or possibly transmitted pulsations from the carotid artery.
- *x Descent*: due to atrial relaxation.
- *v Wave*: due to the rise in atrial pressure before the tricuspid valve opens; enlarged in tricuspid regurgitation.

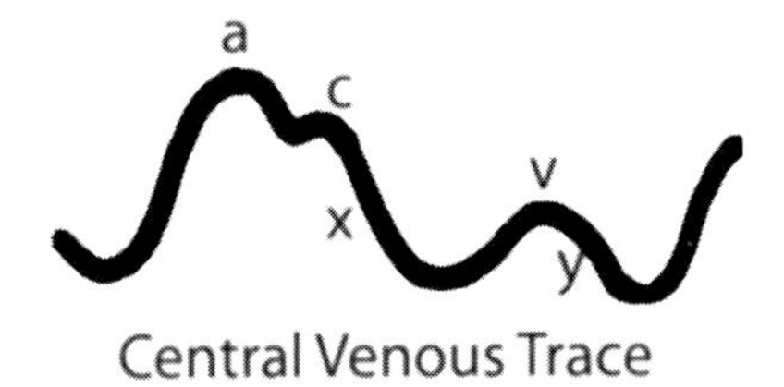

Figure 11.8 Central venous pressure waveform components.

- *y Descent*: due to atrial emptying as blood enters the ventricle.
- *Canon waves*: large waves not corresponding to a, v or c waves; due to complete heart block or junctional arrhythmias.

The central venous pressure trace fluctuates with respiration. Underfilling may be represented be excessive fluctuation in the trace (and the arterial blood pressure trace).

Key points

- Accurate invasive monitoring requires correct set up, including regular zeroing and correct transducer level.
- Overdamping may result from air bubbles or clot within the transducer tubing, and may lead to error (although mean pressure is usually unchanged).
- Inclusion of heparin in the flush solution may not reduce catheter thrombosis or failure, and may be associated with heparin-induced thrombocytopenia.
- Arterial pressure waveform analysis may demonstrate underfilling, poor contractility and excessive vasoconstriction.

FURTHER READING

Oblouc Darovic G. *Hemodynamic monitoring: Invasive and non-invasive clinical application* (3rd edn). Philadelphia: Saunders; 2002.

Chapter 12

Pulmonary artery catheter

S. REX AND W.F. BUHRE

Introduction

Swan, Ganz and colleagues were the first to describe the use of a flow-directed, balloon-tipped catheter for the catheterization of the right heart and the pulmonary artery (PA) in 1970. Since then, the PA catheter (PAC) has become a widespread monitoring tool in the management of critically ill patients. Its use necessitates profound knowledge of cardiovascular (patho) physiology and exhaustive information on current evidence guiding patient selection, particularly in the light of ongoing controversy on its safety and efficacy.

The pulmonary artery catheter

The commonly used PAC has a circumference of 7.0, 7.5 or 8.0 French and is 110 cm long with distances marked at 10-cm intervals. The standard PAC contains four separate internal lumens.

Distal lumen and proximal lumen

These lumen lead to the distal port at the tip of the catheter and to a second port approximately 30 cm proximally to the catheter tip. The distal lumen is used to measure PA pressure (PAP) and sample mixed venous blood, whereas the proximal lumen serves to measure central venous pressure (CVP).

Third lumen

This lumen leads to a balloon just proximal to the catheter tip. Inflating the balloon enables placement of the catheter in the PA and to measure PA occlusion pressure.

Fourth lumen

The fourth lumen contains wires leading to the temperature thermistor located proximally to the balloon. The thermistor enables measurement of blood temperature for the calculation of cardiac output (CO).

Other features

Additional features are available on some catheters and include continuous measurement of CO, mixed venous oxygen saturation (Svo_2) or right ventricular ejection fraction, additional infusion lumens, and pacing leads.

Pulmonary artery catheter insertion

Preparation

Placement of a PAC is not an emergency measure. In life-threatening situations with haemodynamic instability of unknown origin, less invasive procedures like echocardiography are a faster diagnostic tool and should be preferred. Coagulation disorders and electrolyte imbalances should be corrected before insertion. The placement of a PAC can provoke arrhythmias; therefore, continuous electrocardiographic monitoring is mandatory. The availability of a defibrillator is recommended. Separate venous access and drugs for

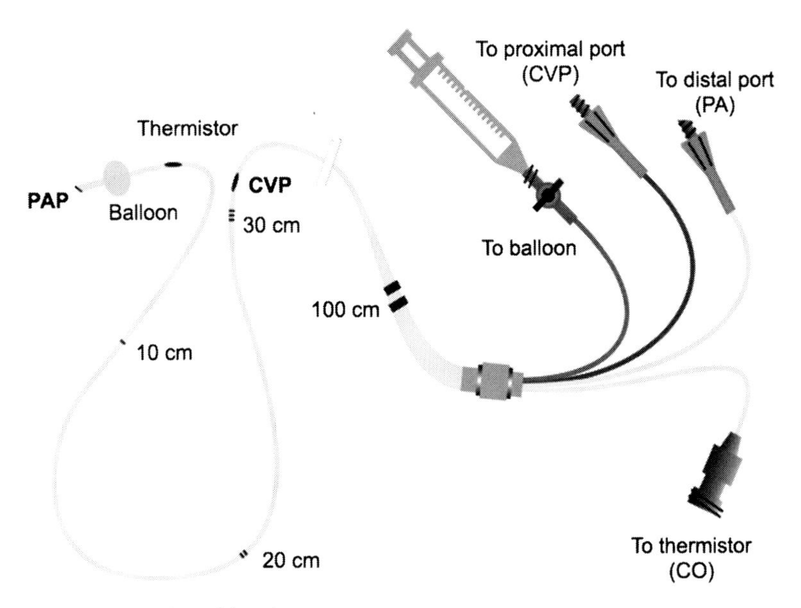

Figure 12.1 Schematic PAC consisting of four lumens.

cardiopulmonary resuscitation must be available. Insertion of the catheter must be performed under sterile conditions.

Access

The PAC is inserted via a large-bore introducer sheath (usually 8.0 to 9.0 Fr in diameter) with a unidirectional valve at its outer end and a sidearm extension for central venous fluid and drug administration. The sheath can be introduced into any central vein. The most direct route to the right heart is provided by the right jugular vein. From other venous insertion sites, the way to the heart is more tortuous, which can result in difficulty or failure of catheterization.

Placement

After flushing the lumens with saline, the PAC is gently inserted through the sleeve that protects the part of the PAC residing outside the patient. The sleeve helps to maintain sterility when manipulating the PAC later in the monitoring period. The balloon is inflated with 1.5 mL of air to ensure that no leak is present and that it inflates without obstructing the distal lumen. The distal port hub is connected to the pressure monitoring device and the integrity of the circuit is checked by gently agitating the catheter and ensuring a trace is visible on the monitor.

The PAC is inserted via the introducer sheath to a depth of 20 cm and the presence of a CVP waveform is identified to confirm correct venous (caval) or intra-atrial position of the PAC tip. The balloon is inflated with 1.0 to 1.5 mL of air and the PAC gently advanced into the right ventricle (RV; using the right internal jugular vein usually at a depth of 30–35 cm), PA (40–45 cm) and finally into the wedge position (45–55 cm). The pressure waves on the monitor are used to ensure adequate position at each of these steps. After obtainment of a wedge curve, the balloon is deflated and the PAP waveform should reappear.

Catheter position should be additionally confirmed with a chest radiograph with the PAC tip within 2 cm of the cardiac silhouette in the anteroposterior projection.

Troubleshooting

Coiling in the right atrium (RA) or RV is a common problem when advancing the PAC. This should be

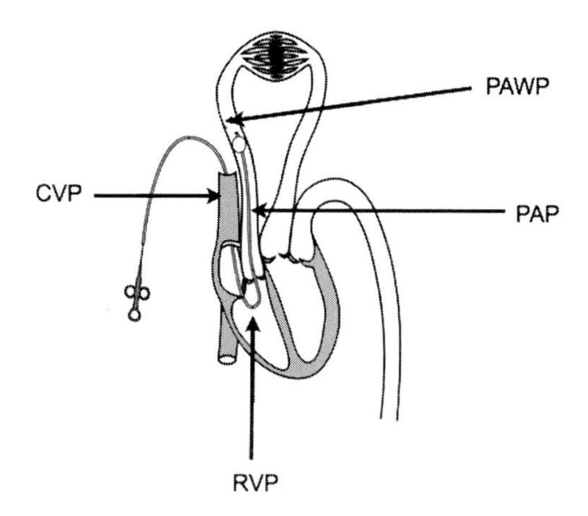

Figure 12.2 Correct position of the PA catheters.

suspected when the expected pressure curve cannot be obtained despite an adequate depth of insertion. After deflating the balloon, the catheter should then be withdrawn to the starting point at 20 cm before repeating the insertion procedure. If it is difficult to reach the RV or PA, simultaneous echocardiography can be helpful in guiding the catheter and visualizing anatomical problems such as a persistent left superior vena cava.

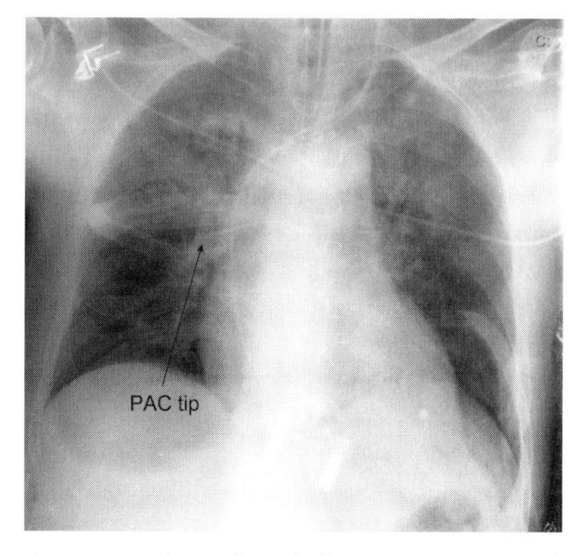

Figure 12.3 Chest radiograph showing correct position of a PAC within the right-sided descending PA.

Occasionally (e.g. in the presence of hypovolemia or tachycardia), it may be difficult to distinguish RV pressure from PAP. Note that RV pressure typically shows a wide pulse pressure with low diastolic pressures. In contrast, the PA can be recognized by the step-up of diastolic pressure. In addition, RV pressure increases during diastole (reflecting venous filling), whereas PAP decreases further during diastole. Radiographic screening may be used in difficult cases. In up to 3% of patients, placement of a PAC is technically impossible.

Pulmonary artery catheter measurements

Cardiac output

The measurement of CO with the PAC is based on the principle of thermodilution. A bolus of saline is injected into the RA and diluted by the blood flow. By analyzing the downstream thermodilution curve in the PA, CO can be computed using the Stewart-Hamilton equation.

For measurement of CO, 0.15 mL/kg (usually 10 mL) of either ice-cooled or room-temperature saline solution is injected as a fast bolus into the proximal CVP port of the PAC. The resulting thermodilution curve should be carefully analyzed to detect artefacts such as unstable blood temperature or recirculation phenomena. Usually, three consecutive measurements are performed, randomly spread over the respiratory cycle and then averaged to account for respiratory variation in RV stroke volumes. For valid and accurate measurements, multiple sources of error must be recognized and avoided.

As an alternative to intermittent bolus thermodilution, PACs are commercially available that allow continuous measurements of CO (CCO). These are equipped with a 10-cm heating filament located 15 to 25 cm from the catheter tip, which normally sits in the RV. The heating filament releases pulses of heat, and CO is calculated using cross-correlation

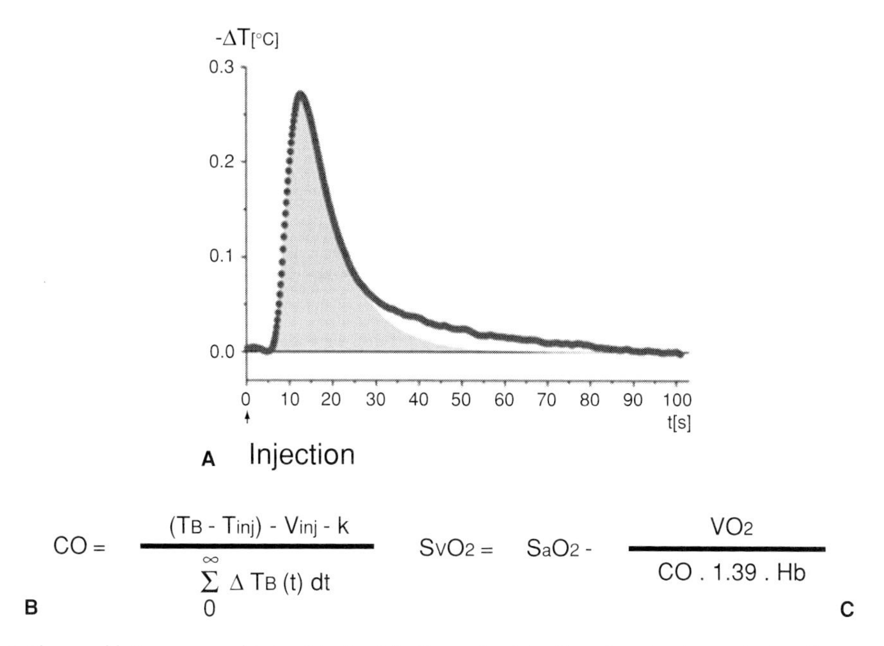

Figure 12.4 *A.* Thermodilution curve obtained in the PA after bolus injection of cold saline solution. The area under the thermodilution curve is obtained by extrapolating the exponential downslope to the temperature baseline. *B.* Stuart Hamilton Equation. k, computation constant (delivered in the PAC package insert, has to be entered manually into the CO computer before measurement of CO); T_B, blood temperature (measured by the thermistor in the PAC tip); T_{inj}, temperature of injectate (measured by an inline temperature sensor at the proximal injection port of the PAC); V_{inj}, volume of injectate; $\sum_0^\infty \Delta T_B(t)dt$, area under the thermodilution curve (integral of temperature change over time). *C.* Equation illustrating the determinants of Svo_2. Hb, haemoglobin concentration; Sao_2, arterial oxygen saturation; Vo_2, oxygen consumption.

of pulmonary arterial blood temperature and the pattern of heating filament activation. Usually, the displayed CO value is updated every 30 to 60 seconds on the CCO computer. It has to be noted that the displayed value represents an average of the CO measured over the last 3 to 6 minutes. Hence, CCO monitors show changes with a delay of up to 15 minutes, reducing their accuracy in detecting acute circulatory alterations. This limits their usefulness in unstable patients. They are also sensitive to thermal noise, such as diathermy. On the other hand, owing to the averaging algorithm, CCO measurements are less susceptible to cyclic changes in CO caused by respiratory variations. Moreover, because CCO systems do not require repeated fluid injections, they may be associated with fewer measurement errors and lower infection rates.

Mixed venous oxygen saturation

The Svo_2 can be measured intermittently by blood sampling from the distal PA port of any PAC. Alternatively, some catheters are commercially available that offer continuous measurements of Svo_2 using reflectance oximetry in the pulmonary arterial blood via implanted fibreoptic bundles. These catheters can be calibrated either in vitro or in vivo and are less prone to wall artifacts since the introduction of reflection intensity algorithms.

The equation above shows the relationship between Svo_2 and CO. Given the assumption that SaO_2, oxygen consumption (Vo_2), and

Table 12.1 Factors that can disturb the accuracy of bolus thermodilution

Source of error	Problem	Solution
Cyclic variations in respiratory pressure	Variations in CO depending on the cycle phase	Averaging multiple measurements randomly spread over the respiratory cycle
Extracorporal temperature losses	Underestimation of CO by 3% for each °C of warming of the injectate	Measuring the temperature of the injectate 'in-line'
Intracorporal temperature losses (central venous injection site within the introducer sheath, or injection of indicator into catheters with a large dead space)	Overestimation of CO	Careful interpretation of thermodilution curve; disregarding the first measurement
Fluctuations of blood temperature (e.g. after CPB owing to redistribution of heat to the periphery, or during rapid intravenous infusions)	Unstable temperature baseline	Measuring only in the presence of a stable temperature baseline; taking ice-cooled saline solution to increase the signal-to-noise ratio
Intra- or extracardiac shunts	Inaccurate CO measurement	No bedside solution
Tricuspid or pulmonary valve insufficiency	Recirculation distorts the decay time of the thermodilution curve usually resulting in an underestimation of CO	None
Wrong constant/wrong volume of injectate	Wrong CO calculation	Verifying the correct constant and volume

Abbreviations: CO, cardiac output; CPB, cardiopulmonary bypass.

haemoglobin remain constant, Svo_2 may be used as surrogate parameter of CO. Therefore, to ensure that a change in Svo_2 truly reflects a change in CO, any changes in one of the other three determinants of Svo_2 have to be excluded.

The Svo_2 reflects the amount of oxygen not taken up by the tissues and gives an indication of the balance between oxygen delivery and oxygen consumption; the lower the Svo_2, the higher the extraction ratio by the tissues, that is, the ratio of oxygen uptake in relation to the amount of oxygen received. A decrease in Svo_2 clearly indicates an inadequacy of oxygen delivery and (in the absence of arterial hypoxaemia and anaemia) of CO. On the other hand, it has to be emphasized that Svo_2 reflects only global oxygen supply-and-demand balance. Hence, patients can have a normal or high value for Svo_2 despite regionally inadequate blood flow.

It is still controversial whether the less invasively determinable central venous oxygen saturation ($Scvo_2$) may also reflect global oxygen balance. Although absolute values of Svo_2 and $Scvo_2$ differ considerably in varying haemodynamic situations, the trend of $Scvo_2$ may be substituted for the trend of Svo_2.

Pulmonary artery pressures

The PAC is currently the only available option for continuous monitoring of PAP. Monitoring PAP can be clinically used for a rough estimation of RV afterload, but the simple interpretation of PAP may be misleading in judging RV outflow impedance; pressures are flow dependent (a failing RV is not able to generate high PAP!). Monitoring of the PAP should be considered in patients with chronic or acute pulmonary hypertension who are at risk of RV failure. It should be used to monitor the efficacy of therapies lowering RV afterload.

Under normal conditions with low pulmonary vascular tone, end-diastolic PAP is in equilibrium with downstream pulmonary venous and left atrial pressure (LAP). In these conditions, PAP monitoring offers the possibility of a continuous estimation of LAP.

Pulmonary artery occlusion wedge pressure

After inflating the balloon, the typical wedge curve appears. Pulmonary artery occlusion wedge pressure (PCWP) is an indirect measurement of pulmonary venous pressure, LAP and left ventricular end-diastolic pressure. For this, a continuous, static blood column has to connect the wedged PAC tip, the left atrium and the left ventricle (LV). This condition is only met if the catheter tip is in lung zone 3, with both pulmonary arterial and pulmonary venous pressure higher than the surrounding alveolar pressure. Position of the PAC in zone I or II should be assumed when respiratory variations of PCWP are markedly increased. Mean PCWP should be measured at end expiration to eliminate confounding effects of cyclic changes in respiratory pressures.

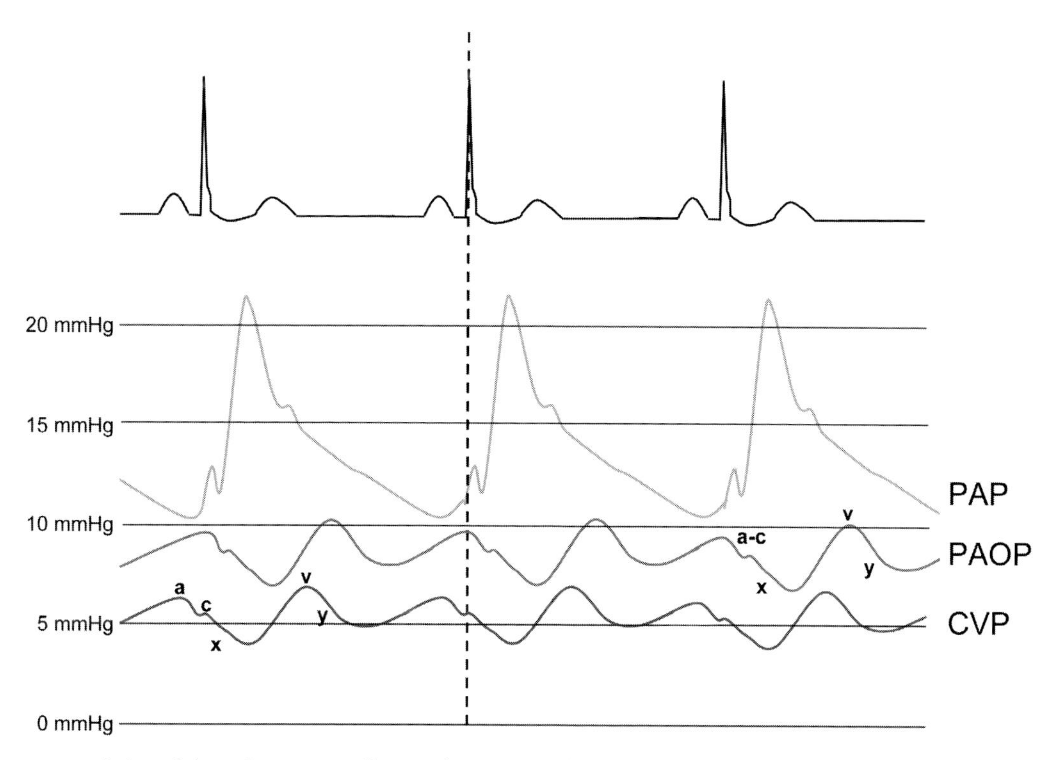

Figure 12.5 Timing of the pulmonary capillary wedge pressure (PCWP) curve in relation to the CVP curve, the PAP curve and the ECG.

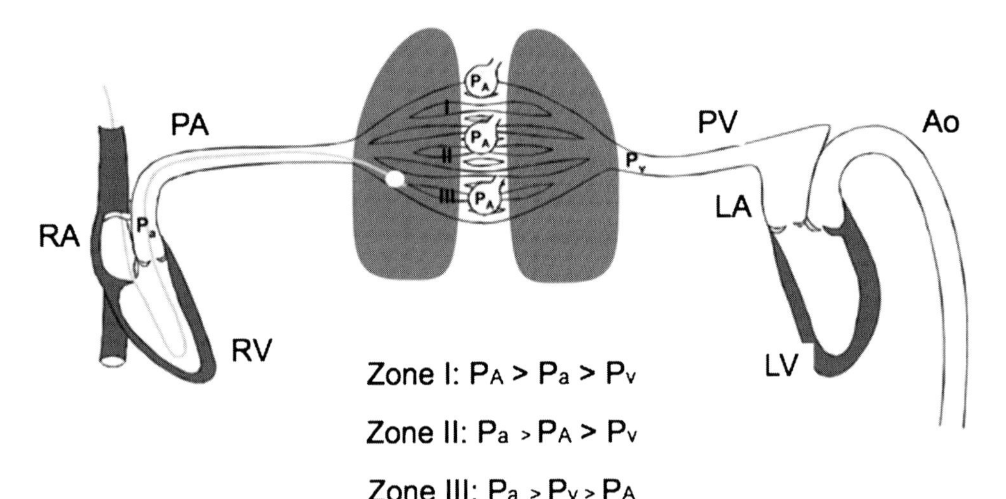

Figure 12.6 Correct positioning of the PAC in lung zone III according to the West model.

The PCWP curve resembles the CVP curve. However, because atrial depolarization originates in the RA and because the LAP curve has to be transmitted retrogradely through pulmonary veins, capillaries, arterioles and arteries, the PCWP curve shows a characteristic delay in comparison with the CVP curve. For instance, the PCWP a wave (reflecting left atrial contraction) occurs in early ventricular systole. Moreover, and unlike the CVP curve, the PCWP v wave is often taller than the a wave, probably indicating that the left atrium is less distensible than the RA. In addition, a and c waves often fuse to one a to c wave in the PCWP curve, given the shorter atrioventricular conduction in the LV. Characteristic changes in the morphology of the PCWP curve occur in certain LV pathologies. However, these waveform abnormalities are often difficult to interpret and recognize.

Many clinicians still use PCWP as an estimate for LV preload, assuming that the higher the PCWP, the higher LV filling. However, the relationship between PCWP and LVEDV is mainly determined by LV compliance. This is typically decreased in critically ill patients, for example, owing to ventricular hypertrophy, distension, arterial hypertension, myocardial ischaemia, sepsis, pericardial effusion/tamponade or use of catecholamines. Moreover, a variety of other conditions can affect the relationship between LVEDV and PCWP. In addition, PCWP is measured only as intra- and not as transmural pressure, thereby disregarding the influence of juxtacardiac pressure. Particularly in mechanically ventilated patients, this practice invalidates the use of PCWP as a parameter of cardiac preload. Consequently, the overwhelming majority of clinical studies demonstrate that PCWP fails to adequately reflect cardiac preload and to predict the individual patient's response to a fluid challenge. Modern haemodynamic management should base fluid therapy on volumetric parameters (e.g. LV end-diastolic area, global end-diastolic volume) and

Table 12.2 Components of the PCWP curve

Component	Event
a wave	Atrial contraction
c wave	Isovolumic ventricular contraction
x descent	Atrial relaxation
v wave	Atrial filling
y descent	Early ventricular filling

Table 12.3 Waveform abnormalities of the PCWP curve

LV pathology	Waveform abnormality	Mean PCWP
Myocardial ischaemia	Prominent a wave (indicative for increased LVEDP) Prominent v wave (indicative for increased LVEDP and/or for ischaemic mitral regurgitation)	Elevated
MR	Tall regurgitant v wave (starting in early systole); obliteration of x descent	Acute MR: elevated Chronic MR: may be normal
Mitral stenosis	Tall a wave Attenuated y descent (obstruction to transmitral flow)	Elevated
Ventricular septal defect	Giant antegrade v wave (indicative for increased forward flow)	Elevated
Hypervolaemia, congestive heart failure, LA compression	Prominent a wave, tall v wave	Elevated

Abbreviations: LA, left atrium; LV, left ventricle; LVEDP, left ventricular end-diastolic pressure; MR, mitral regurgitation; PCWP, pulmonary capillary wedge pressure.

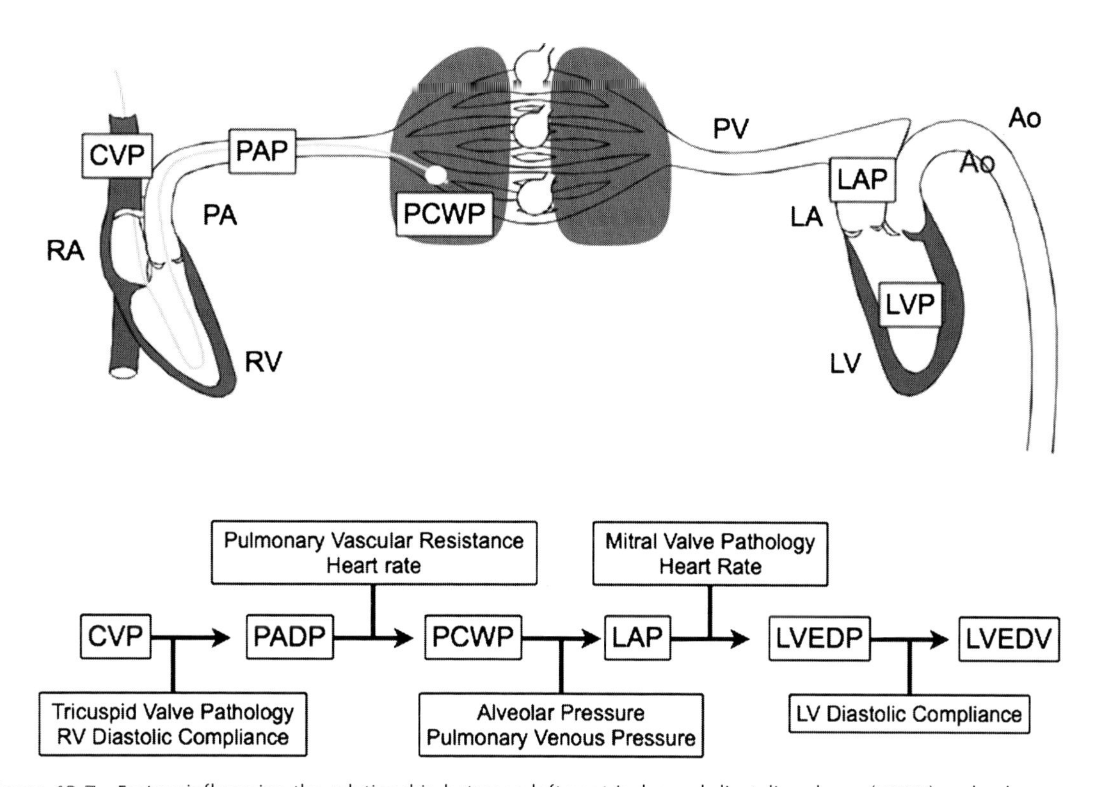

Figure 12.7 Factors influencing the relationship between left ventricular end-diastolic volume (LVEDV) and pulmonary capillary wedge pressure (PCWP).

dynamic preload indicators (e.g. systolic or pulse pressure variation).

Calculated variables

Parameters measured with the PAC can be used to calculate several haemodynamic variables. In particular, vascular resistances are commonly used to describe RV or LV afterload. However, the calculation of vascular resistance is based on a hydraulic fluid model with continuous, laminar flow through rigid pipes. In contrast, the human vascular system consists of collapsible vessels in which blood as a viscous fluid circulates in a turbulent and pulsatile manner. Moreover, the validity of atrial pressures as effective downstream pressures in these calculations has to be questioned; atrial pressures underestimate the critical closing pressure in the end of the circuit. In particular, pulmonary vascular tone cannot be adequately described with these formulas. As a consequence, clinicians should avoid altering haemodynamic management based only on calculated vascular resistance.

Complications

Complications of PAC monitoring can be classified as complications associated with cannulation (similar to the ones with a central venous catheter), catheterization or resulting from the residing catheter.

Arrhythmias

Supraventricular and ventricular arrhythmias are the most frequent complication during the catheterization process (in up to 70% of the patients). As they are caused by the catheter making contact with the endocardium, immediate withdrawal or further advancing the catheter normally results in restoration of regular heart rhythm. In rare cases, ventricular fibrillation can be induced by catheterization, in particular in patients with acute myocardial infarction (risk of 1.1%) and in the subset of patients with RV infarction (risk of 4.5%). Touching the intraventricular septum can induce a transient right bundle branch block in up to 5%. While being of no consequence in the normal patient, this complication can result in complete heart block in patients with preexisting left bundle branch block.

Thromboembolic events

These may be an underestimated problem. Thrombi attached to the PAC can be demonstrated 1 hour after insertion in a significant number of patients, and the incidence of pulmonary embolism is commonly estimated at 1%.

Lung infarction

A lung infarction usually results from obstruction of pulmonary blood flow in a PA branch occluded by a PAC, usually after accidental migration distally into the wedge position. Therefore, every PAC must be connected to a continuous pressure monitoring device to ensure proper position in the proximal PA and prevent 'over-wedging.'

Mechanical complications

These consist of right-sided endocardial lesions (mostly without consequences) and of knot formation around cardiac structures, which should be suspected when difficulties are encountered during withdrawal of the PAC. Confirmation can be obtained by chest radiography. Knots around tricuspid chordae tendineae can lead to severe tricuspid insufficiency by destroying the valve apparatus when removing the catheter. Removing a PAC knotted around another intracardiac catheter can dislocate this device. Knots may have to be removed by interventional radiology or even by open heart surgery. Other mechanical complications, like suturing the PAC to the heart during surgery, are rare.

Infective complications

The incidence of infective complications varies widely. Local infection of the introducer sheath has

Table 12.4 Calculated haemodynamic variables

Variable	Formula	Normal Range
Systemic vascular resistance	(MAP − CVP)/CO [(MAP − CVP)/CO] × 80	10–20 Wood units (mmHg/L per minute) 800–1600 dynes s cm^{-5}
Pulmonary vascular resistance	(MPAP − PAOP)/CO [(MPAP − PAOP)/CO] × 80	0.5–2 Wood units (mmHg/L per minute) 40–160 dynes s cm^{-5}
Stroke volume	CO/HR	60–90 mL
Mixed arterial oxygen content (cao_2)	$(0.003 \times Pao_2) + (1.39 \cdot Sao_2 \cdot Hb)$	16–20 mL/dL
Mixed venous oxygen content (cvo_2)	$(0.003 \times Pvo_2) + (1.39 \cdot Svo_2 \cdot Hb)$	13–15 mL/dL
Arteriovenous oxygen difference ($avDO_2$)	$cao_2 - cvo_2$	3–5 mL/dL
Oxygen delivery (Do_2)	$CO \cdot cao_2 \cdot 10$	600–1400 mL/min
Oxygen consumption (Vo_2)	$CO \cdot avDO_2 \cdot 10$	180–280 mL/min
Oxygen extraction rate (ERo_2)	Vo_2/Do_2	20–30%

been reported in up to 22% of cases, and PAC tip colonization may also occur in 22%, depending mainly on duration of catheter placement. When the PAC is left in situ for more than 72 hours, PAC-related bloodstream infections increase substantially, favouring early removal. Because PAC colonization mostly originates from the introducer sheath, changing the PAC means inserting a new venous access sheath, which can cause further complications in itself and may not be technically easy.

Pulmonary artery rupture

Inflation of the balloon in a PA smaller than the balloon diameter can result in PA rupture. It occurs in 0.02% to 0.20% of patients monitored with a PAC and results in a mortality of up to 50%. Special 'wedge syringes' are used to limit the injected volume of air to 1.5 mL. The wedge trace has to be carefully observed to prevent 'over-wedging,' which can be identified by an abrupt increase in wedge pressure. Other mechanisms of PA rupture include chronic erosion by the catheter tip, eccentric inflation of the balloon forcing the PAC tip into the vessel wall and brusque positioning manoeuvres at excessive insertion depths. A PA rupture usually causes haemoptysis, which can lead to hypoxaemia and/or severe bleeding. Therapy depends on the severity of the bleeding and includes mechanical ventilation or even resection of the involved lung lobe.

Indications

Despite more than 30 years of clinical use, there is still controversy about the value of the PAC in clinical practice. A number of studies have been performed to evaluate the impact of the PAC on mortality and morbidity in different subsets of patients.

In the majority of studies (not specific to cardiac critical care), no change in outcome was observed whether a PAC was used or not. Therefore, PA catheterization is often based on expert opinion rather than evidence-based criteria. It has to be noted that the presence of a monitoring device alone does not alter outcomes when not linking diagnostic results to specific therapies.

Measurement of PAP and CO and calculation of related variables (vascular resistance, oxygen delivery and consumption) is justified if the additional information obtained influences diagnosis and/or therapy. This is particularly true for patients with elevated PAP associated with decreased cardiac performance, for instance during heart or lung transplantation and other cardiac surgical procedures associated with an increased risk of right heart failure (mitral valve surgery and implantation of assist devices).

Key points

- Placement of the PA catheter often leads to self-limiting arrhythmias. More serious complications are rare but may be life threatening.
- Insertion of a PAC should be considered when multiple inotropes are needed or when elevated PAPs are suspected in combination with cardiac failure.
- If the catheter is correctly placed, PCWP may be measured and used as an estimate of cardiac filling.
- Trends rather than absolute numbers should be used to guide therapy.
- The catheter should be removed when the information it provides is no longer valuable; prolonged use increases complications.

FURTHER READING

Harvey S, Harrison DA, Singer M, *et al.* Assessment of the clinical effectiveness of pulmonary artery catheters in management of patients in intensive care (PAC-Man): a randomised controlled trial. *Lancet* 2005;366:472–477.

Naeije R. Pulmonary vascular resistance. A meaningless variable? *Intensive Care Med* 2003; 29:526–529.

Pulmonary Artery Catheter Consensus Conference: consensus statement. *Crit Care Med* 1997;25:910–925.

Sandham JD, Hull RD, Brant RF, *et al.* A randomized, controlled trial of the use of pulmonary-artery catheters in high-risk surgical patients. *N Engl J Med* 2003;348:5–14.

Swan HJ, Ganz W, Forrester J, *et al.* Catheterization of the heart in man with use of a flow-directed balloon-tipped catheter. *N Engl J Med* 1970;283: 447–451.

Chapter 13

Minimally invasive methods of cardiac output and haemodynamic monitoring

M. THAVASOTHY

Introduction

Minimally invasive haemodynamic monitoring devices are increasingly being used in cardiac critical care. Their advantages include ease of set-up, continuous measurement of stroke volume (SV) and cardiac output (CO) and the ability to provide other haemodynamic data to assist circulatory management.

Arterial pressure monitors

LiDCO and PiCCO (Pulse Contour Cardiac Output) monitors use a modified form of the Fick principle to analyse the arterial pressure waveform and calculate specific data based on this. They both allow calculation of CO and preload responsiveness, a useful measure of intravascular volume.

Cardiac output

THE LIDCO

The LiDCO (Lithium Dilution Continuous Cardiac Output) monitor detects changes in the concentration of a fixed dose of lithium. Lithium is chosen because of its low toxicity and high signal-to-noise ratio. Lithium is injected via a central venous line and sensed via a radial or other systemic arterial line every time the monitor is calibrated. This allows measurement of CO using the Fick principle and calibrates the instrument for further readings. Calibration is recommended when the monitor is first connected to a patient, and then every 24 hours. This method uses a characteristic of the arterial pulse waveform known as the pulse power. Pulse power analysis makes use of the law of mass conservation, and assumes that within a fixed circulatory system, any acute changes in that system are due to changes in SV input. Hence, it converts a pulsatile pressure–time trace into a pulsatile volume–time trace via a simple algorithm that uses a nomogram for arterial compliance. It incorporates the actual measure of SV determined by lithium dilution. This volume–time trace is then given a numerical value to describe its 'power,' an attribute that is related to, but not dependent on, the wavelength and frequency of the waveform. This makes pulse power analysis less vulnerable to arterial pulse transduction problems. The pulse power is finally calibrated to an actual measurement of SV and CO determined by the aforementioned lithium transpulmonary dilution technique. Following this, any changes in pulse power determined solely from the arterial trace can be correlated with changes in CO and SV continuously.

THE PICCO

Pulse contour analysis derives information from the actual pressure trace to calculate changes in SV. The technique breaks down the pulse contour into systolic and diastolic fractions, separated by the dicrotic notch. The area under the systolic fraction (A_{sys}) bears an indirect relationship to SV. This relationship varies over time and is dependent on a number of variables. To help quantify these variables and thus calculate actual SV, pulse contour analysis effectively 'translates' the arterial circuit into an analogous electrical circuit. This circuit contains a battery (pulse pressure), current (CO), capacitor (aortic compliance) and resistor (systemic vascular resistance [SVR]). Aortic compliance is calculated from the rate of decline of the diastolic downslope on the arterial trace, which also provides a measure of pulse pressure. It is calibrated against the ratio of thermodilution-derived SV to pulse pressure. Transpulmonary dilution using a thermal dye instead of lithium, injected via a large central vein and detected via a femoral arterial line, is used to give an absolute measure of CO, again determined using the Fick principle. This is then not only used to give an absolute calibration for A_{sys}, but also to calculate SVR, once the gradient between arterial and central venous pressure (CVP) is known (SVR = pressure gradient ÷ CO). Once all three variables are known, CO can be calculated on a beat-to-beat basis. However, SVR requires transpulmonary thermodilution for independent estimation (unlike aortic compliance and pulse pressure, which can be measured from the arterial trace itself). Therefore, any significant change in SVR after, for example, a large change in vasopressor dose, means the device requires recalibration to maintain accuracy.

Preload responsiveness

Preload responsiveness reflects the likelihood that a fluid challenge (increase in preload) will result in an increased SV. Arterial pressure monitors are able to provide an index of this by measuring the degree of arterial 'swing' in response to intermittent positive pressure ventilation. An increase in intrathoracic pressure inhibits venous return to the right ventricle. The effect of this reduction in preload on the left ventricle depends on its position on the Starling curve. On the plateau part of the curve, such a reduction has a minimal effect on SV. However, on the ascending part of the curve, this gives rise to a significant reduction in SV, manifested as a fall in both systolic and pulse pressure (termed systolic pressure variation [SPV] and pulse pressure variation [PPV]). Both SPV and PPV are far more sensitive and specific indicators of preload responsiveness than absolute values for CVP and pulmonary artery wedge pressure (PCWP). The PPV appears to be the more sensitive of the two, because it is less affected by the direct transmission of changes in intrathoracic pressure to the aorta, and is the index most frequently quoted (normal value, $<10\%$). For the index to provide relevant information clinically, the patient must be fully ventilated with a tidal volume of at least 8 mL/kg ideal body weight, and must also be in sinus rhythm. Both spontaneous ventilation and patient-triggered ventilation invalidate the index. A 'pseudonormal' PPV is seen in patients with pericardial tamponade, severe cardiac failure and ventricular outflow obstruction.

Other haemodynamic indices measured using transpulmonary thermodilution

VOLUMETRIC INDICES

Right and left atrial pressure monitoring has traditionally been used to reflect the likely distending pressures and hence infer the likely end-diastolic volumes of the right and left ventricles. These pressures, however, are susceptible to changes in both intrathoracic pressure and ventricular compliance (secondary to ventricular hypertrophy or severe sepsis). These factors may help account for the fact that CVP and PCWP are such poor indicators of preload responsiveness. Volumetric indices, however, more accurately reflect end-diastolic volumes, and hence the likely SV response to a fluid challenge. The volumes measured are deduced from the mean transit time (MTT) of the initial thermodilution curve measured by the PiCCO. This represents the time taken for half the thermal tracer to pass from the venous circulation, through the heart and lungs, to the arterial circulation.

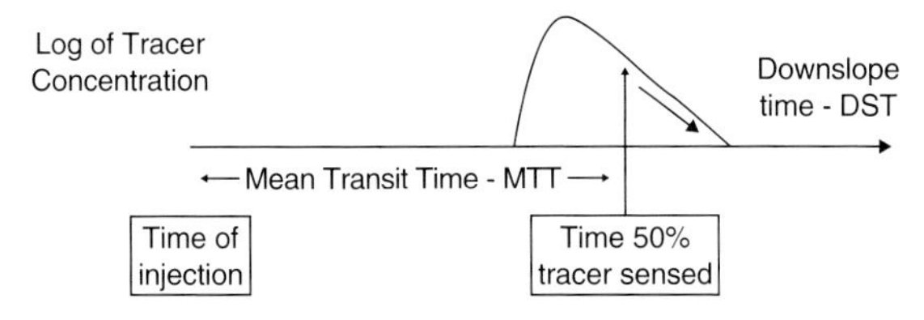

Figure 13.1 Mean transit time.

The product of this time interval and the CO, representing the sum of both intrathoracic blood volume (ITBV) and extravascular lung water (EVLW), is termed the intrathoracic thermal volume (ITTV). The downslope time, on the other hand, represents the time it takes for the thermal tracer to be eluted from the largest 'chamber' in the circuit, the pulmonary chamber. This consists of both the pulmonary blood volume and the EVLW volume, and is termed the pulmonary thermal volume (PTV). Subtraction of PTV from ITTV gives a measure of the volume in both right and left atria and ventricles, termed the global end-diastolic volume (GEDV). Because the size of the pulmonary circulation is thought to bear a fixed relationship to this volume, ITBV can also be calculated (ITBV $= 1.25 \times$ GEDV $- 28.4$).

EXTRAVASCULAR LUNG WATER

The transpulmonary thermodilution calibration method used in the PiCCO can also give an indication of EVLW. This relies on the subtraction of calculated ITBV, as derived above from GEDV, from the ITTV, derived from the MTT, which includes EVLW. This in vivo technique has been validated against gravimetric measures of lung water in post mortem specimens. It is used in some centres as the basis for their haemodynamic therapy algorithms, particularly in patients with significant respiratory compromise. However, another more accurate, although far less user-friendly in vivo, method of measuring EVLW exists. It employs two dyes, one of which remains within the intravascular compartment alone, and the other of which equilibrates with both the intravascular and extravascular compartments to give a measure of extravascular volume. When compared with this double-indicator method, the single-dye transpulmonary thermodilution technique seems to overestimate EVLW at higher values.

Advantages and disadvantages

PULSE POWER (LIDCO)

Advantages

Because it does not rely on the contour of the waveform, it is relatively immune to transduction problems caused by over- or underdamping. This also means that the site of arterial pressure monitoring is less important; thus, it can be used with a radial arterial line.

Disadvantages

Although lithium as the transpulmonary calibration dye gives a good signal-to-noise ratio, it cannot be used in patients who are taking lithium therapeutically. Also, certain muscle relaxants such as atracurium can interfere with its measurement, and cause the arterial sensor to drift.

PULSE CONTOUR (PICCO)

Advantages

Use of a thermal 'dye' for calibration also allows estimation of intrathoracic and global end-diastolic blood volumes, which appear to correlate with preload better than traditional pressure-based measurements. They also allow estimation of EVLW, particularly useful in patients with acute respiratory distress syndrome and acute lung injury.

Disadvantages

The continuous measurement of SV and CO is dependent on accurate transduction of the pressure waveform, which leaves the system vulnerable to unrecognized damping errors, and necessitates the use of a femoral arterial line to ensure optimal waveform acquisition. In addition, accurate transmission of the pressure wave from the aorta to distal vessels may be compromised under certain conditions, particularly after cardiopulmonary bypass. Finally, there have been some reports of occasional calibration inaccuracies using transpulmonary thermodilution.

The oesophageal Doppler

This monitor uses a probe that is inserted into the oesophagus. It measures the change in frequency of an ultrasound beam transmitted and received from the probe to the descending aorta. The descending aorta is posterolateral to the oesophagus in the thorax and in close proximity to the probe. The probe itself is usually inserted blindly into the oropharynx. It is relatively stiff and so follows the curvature of the oropharynx into the oesophagus, although accidental tracheal insertion may occur. Oropharyngeal insertion is not tolerated by awake patients, although a new, softer, probe for nasopharyngeal insertion in awake patients is now available. The advantage conferred by its stiffness is that rotational movements of the probe applied near the mouth are accurately transmitted to the tip of the probe in the oesophagus. This makes obtaining an optimal trace easier. It also means that small movements at the mouth such as rotation greatly affect the position and orientation of the probe. The frequency change measured (Doppler shift) directly correlates with the speed of blood travelling through the aorta.

The integral of the blood velocity–time waveform (area under the curve) then represents stroke distance. This waveform is displayed on the monitor and, in addition to the associated sound of the waveform, can help to guide manipulations of the probe to obtain the most accurate trace. If the aortic diameter is known, the product of stroke distance and aortic cross-sectional area gives the SV. Different monitors evaluate aortic diameter in different ways. The CardioQ uses a cadaveric nomogram of aortic diameters that is then cross-referenced against the patients' weight, height and age to give an estimation of the likely aortic diameter. The Hemosonic, on the other hand, uses M-mode echocardiography directly to measure aortic diameter in vivo.

Specific aspects of the velocity–time waveform correlate with changes in preload, afterload and contractility. Their interpretation can aid haemodynamic manipulation. Peak velocity and mean acceleration are both influenced by the contractility of the ventricle, as well as the afterload against which the ventricle has to pump. Corrected flow time refers to the duration the ventricle spends in systole, as a fraction of the total cardiac cycle, corrected to a heart rate of 60 bpm to give an actual time in milliseconds. It is inversely proportional to pulse pressure and hence SVR. Increases in SVR leave the heart with less time to contract before LV outflow tract pressure equilibrates with aortic pressure, resulting in closure of the aortic valve. Corrected flow time correlates to a degree with changes in preload. It is used in several algorithms to optimize fluid management.

The oesophageal Doppler has demonstrated good accuracy and minimal bias when compared to thermodilution-derived CO. Ease of set-up and insertion has lent itself to intraoperative use. A number of studies have shown that fluid therapy guided by the oesophageal Doppler can lead to improvements in both surgical morbidity and hospital length of stay. There is a small learning curve associated with both the placement of the probe and interpretation of the waveform. However, in some patients it can prove difficult to obtain an accurate trace from the descending aorta. Also, probe

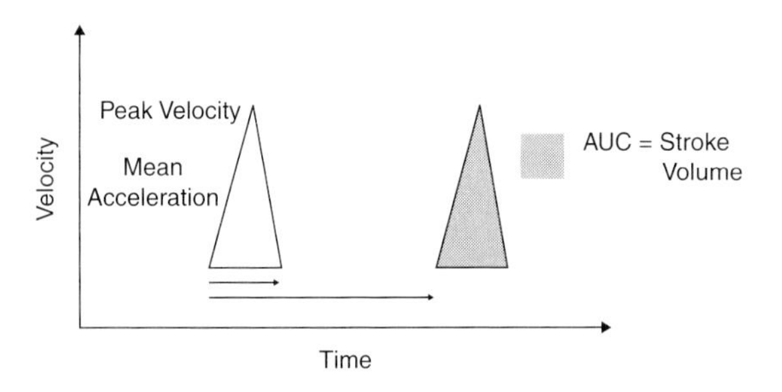

Figure 13.2 Oesophageal Doppler waveform.

Table 13.1 Contraindications to the use of oesophageal Doppler.

Absolute
Postoesophagectomy
Oesophageal trauma or other pathology
Variceal bleed
Base of skull fracture
Maxillofacial trauma
Relative
Intraoperative use of aortic cross-clamp
Significant aortic valve disease
Thoracic aortic aneurysm

movement during the time the probe is in position may lead to inaccuracy in data acquisition without frequent, expert analysis of the waveform.

In addition, two assumptions on which the calculation of SV and CO are based can give rise to inaccuracies. The first assumption is that aortic diameter is fixed throughout the cardiac cycle, when in reality it changes, particularly during systole. The second assumption is that 70% of CO from the heart is delivered to the descending aorta (the other 30% going to the head and arms), and so a fixed scaling factor of 70:30 is used to calculate total CO. However, this ratio can change, depending on a number of factors including how sedated the patient is, and whether the patient is in shock. Despite these limitations, of all the minimally invasive CO monitors currently on the market, the oesophageal Doppler has the longest history of clinical use and the most extensive evidence base.

THE NICO

The NICO also employs the Fick principle to calculate CO. Instead of using an intravascular marker, it uses a noninvasive intrapulmonary marker, CO_2, to calculate transpulmonary blood flow and thus CO. It can only be used in intubated patients. The monitor is attached to the inspiratory and expiratory limbs of the breathing circuit. It records both

$$CO = \frac{V_{CO_2}}{PaCO_2 - PvCO_2}$$

Figure 13.3 NICO equation. Pa_{CO_2}, pulmonary arterial CO_2; Pv_{CO_2}, pulmonary venous CO_2; V_{CO_2}, total volume of CO_2 exhaled over a defined period.

end-tidal CO_2 (ET_{CO_2}) and total CO_2 within the circuit. From these, it calculates CO.

Because venous CO_2 capacity is so large, a small increase in total volume of CO_2 exhaled over a defined period (V_{CO_2}) produced by a fixed degree of rebreathing within the ventilator circuit gives rise to a significant increase in pulmonary venous CO_2 (Pv_{CO_2}), but an insignificant increase in pulmonary arterial CO_2 (Pa_{CO_2}). Hence the formula can be simplified to remove the necessity to measure Pa_{CO_2}. Although the calculation appears relatively simple, a number of prerequisites are necessary to maintain accuracy.

- Minute ventilation must remain fixed, and CO should remain fairly stable during measurement.
- Compensation for shunt fraction needs to be made. This is a measure of the volume of blood that does not take part in pulmonary gas exchange and so is not measured in the equation above. Shunt fraction is determined from the O_2 saturation: fraction of inspired oxygen (Fi_{O_2}) ratio (although greater accuracy is obtained if arterial partial pressure of oxygen (P_{O_2}) from a blood gas is substituted for O_2 saturation).
- In the presence of significant physiological dead space, ET_{CO_2} does not equate to Pv_{CO_2} and so arterial P_{CO_2} may need to be measured directly to compensate for this.

Although easy to set up and use, the NICO is limited by the fact that it can only be used in patients who are both intubated, fully ventilated and, for maximal accuracy, relatively haemodynamically stable. Additional sources of inaccuracy, such as the presence of significant shunt or dead space, may account for some of the variable results seen in a few validation studies comparing CO_2-based CO measurements with thermodilution-derived CO.

Key points

- Minimally invasive monitors of CO are increasingly popular, primarily because of their ease of set-up and use.
- Each monitor has advantages and disadvantages regarding accuracy, ease of set-up, ease of interpretation and utility in specific patient groups. These mainly relate to the strengths and weaknesses inherent in the different methodologies used. As long as these are understood, such monitors can be used to assist haemodynamic management.
- Indicators of preload responsiveness, derived from the arterial pressure trace, are far more accurate at predicting the likely effects of fluid administration than standard pressure indices such as CVP and PCWP.
- The oesophageal Doppler currently has the largest evidence base regarding both its benefits and use in various patient subgroups.

FURTHER READING

Cholley BP, Singer M. Esophageal Doppler: noninvasive cardiac output monitor. *Echocardiography* 2003;20:763–769.

Combes A, Berneau JB, Luyt CE, *et al.* Estimation of left ventricular systolic function by single transpulmonary thermodilution. *Intensive Care Med* 2004;30:1377–1383.

Katzenelson R, Perel A, Berkenstadt H, *et al.* Accuracy of transpulmonary thermodilution versus gravimetric measurement of extravascular lung water. *Crit Care Med* 2004;32:1550–1554.

Mielck F, Buhre W, Hanekop G, *et al.* Comparison of continuous cardiac output measurements in patients after cardiac surgery. *J Cardiothorac Vasc Anesth* 2003;17:211–216.

Rex S, Brose S, Metzelder S, *et al.* Prediction of fluid responsiveness in patients during cardiac surgery. *Br J Anaesth* 2004;93:782–788.

Rocco M, Spadetta G, Morelli A, *et al.* A comparative evaluation of thermodilution and partial CO_2 rebreathing techniques for cardiac output assessment in critically ill patients during assisted ventilation. *Intensive Care Med* 2004;30:82–87.

Chapter 14

Echocardiography and ultrasound

S.T. RUNNELS, K. VALCHANOV AND R. HALL

Introduction

Monitoring and diagnostics in the critical care unit are gradually becoming more complicated and more accurate. This in turn increases the demand for medical training and ability to interpret data. In this setting, ultrasound is becoming an important diagnostic tool. The ultrasound modalities used are body surface scans and semi-invasive scans.

Body surface scans, like ultrasound, for venous access, assessment and drainage of pleural collections, urinary bladder scans, and transthoracic echocardiography (TTE) are practically devoid of direct complications. However, like all diagnostic imaging, they still carry risks of poor image acquisition and incorrect data interpretation. In contrast, the semi-invasive scans like transoesophageal echocardiography (TOE) offer better image quality but also carry risks of direct injury.

Ultrasound

Modern ultrasound machines are small, portable and provide excellent resolution and image quality if set up correctly. With training and experience, portable ultrasound in critical care is an important and often used tool. Many units want their own equipment to allow them to carry out bedside assessment on a 24-hour basis, and staff working in critical care should ensure they are trained in both use and interpretation. Particular uses include the following.

- Identification of central veins and confirmation of patency, to guide central venous access. This is particularly important because patients may have had multiple lines inserted and may be coagulopathic, which may make blind insertion of lines difficult and dangerous.
- Diagnosis of pleural collections. This allows safe drainage by guiding passage of the needle/drain.
- Verification of full urinary bladder, directing suprapubic catheterization.

Transthoracic echocardiography

For a long time, TTE has been a conventional diagnostic modality in cardiovascular medicine. Technological improvements have improved image quality and made machines smaller and more portable. Poor image acquisition is still, however, a common problem owing to air, bone, calcium and foreign bodies impeding the visualization of heart structures. Critical care patients often have overinflated lungs as a result of mechanical ventilation with positive end-expiratory pressure, mediastinal air, tissue oedema, chest drains and dressings; these combine to reduce the quality of the acoustic window and may make accurate use impossible. Therefore, the rate of failure to perform an adequate examination may be as high as 30% to 40%, particularly in mechanically ventilated patients.

Despite this, because of its noninvasive nature, TTE is often employed first in critical care. Because the probe is placed directly on the chest wall it is nearer structures such as the right ventricle and the aortic valve than the transoesophageal probe; therefore, these structures are better examined. It is also able to identify pericardial collections and estimate size relatively accurately; therefore, if cardiac tamponade is suspected, TTE may be a valuable diagnostic tool. Extensive training and experience is required to enable accurate use of TTE, the process of which is very similar to TOE (see below).

Transoesophageal echocardiography

Transoesophageal echocardiography has become a routine diagnostic tool in cardiothoracic critical care. It may be used to guide therapy as well as diagnose conditions, and repeated scans may allow assessment of change. It is the investigation of choice if a patient has an endotracheal tube in situ.

Safety

Because TOE is a semi-invasive tool, minor complications may occur in up to 2% of patients. The incidence of oesophageal perforation is estimated at 1 in 5,000, and mortality 1 in 10,000, although this may be higher in critical care because of factors such as steroid use and coagulopathy, making significant oesophageal injury more likely.

Table 14.1 Common indications for performing transoesophageal echocardiography in the critically ill patient

Haemodynamically unstable patient
Suspected cardiac tamponade or pericardial effusion
Assessment of ventricular performance/function
New murmur
Sepsis of unknown origin (? endocarditis)
Suspected aortic dissection
Mechanically ventilated multiple trauma or chest trauma patient
Widening of the mediastinum on chest radiograph, suspected aortic injury
Potential catheter, guidewire, pacer electrode or pericardiocentesis needle injury with or without signs of tamponade

Table 14.2 Complications of transoesophageal echocardiography

Minor

- Dislodgment of endotracheal or nasogastric tube
- Transient haemodynamic instability during insertion of probe
- Lip, tooth or oropharyngeal injury
- Transient dysphagia after the study
- Effects of sedation or anaesthesia (hypotension, compromise of airway)

Major

- Oesophageal or gastric injury, including perforation or tear

Transoesophageal echocardiography use

Transoesophageal echocardiography allows rapid assessment, diagnosis, documentation and review of most cardiovascular pathology in the cardiothoracic intensive care unit. Because of the position of the probe, it is particularly suited to imaging structures nearest the oesophagus. This includes the left atrium, mitral valve and descending thoracic aorta.

ASSESSMENT OF VENTRICULAR FUNCTION

Left heart

An examination of the left ventricle is quick to perform and can answer many key questions in the unstable patient. It allows assessment of left ventricular systolic function, measurement of ejection fraction and detection of regional wall motion abnormalities. Ejection fraction and fractional shortening are commonly used as estimates of contractility, but multiplane studies should be used for assessment of global function. Stroke volume may also be measured as an accurate estimate of CO. Regional wall motion abnormalities have been shown to allow

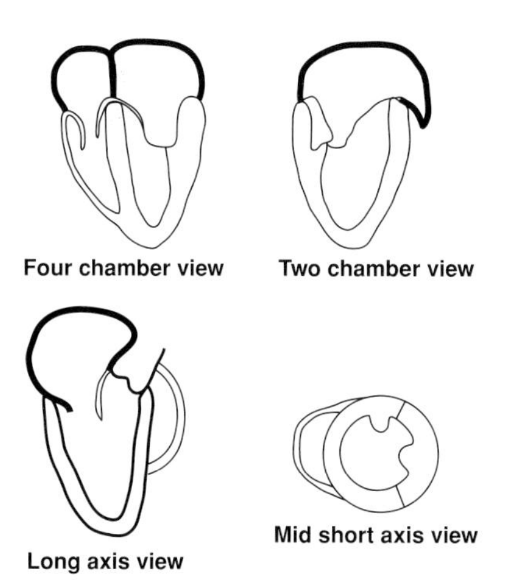

Figure 14.1 Common TOE views used in critical care.

more accurate and rapid diagnosis of ischaemia than electrocardiographic changes. They also allow identification of ischaemia due to particular coronary artery pathology and may guide surgical or percutaneous treatment. The TOE findings that are consistent with myocardial ischaemia include:

- new regional wall motion abnormalities;
- decreased ventricular wall shortening (hypokinesia, akinesia, dyskinesia);
- ventricular diastolic dysfunction;
- ischaemic mitral regurgitation via annular dilation or papillary muscle rupture/dysfunction; and
- ventricular mural thrombus.

Transoesophageal echocardiography is also particularly useful for assessment of left ventricular filling and guiding medical therapy based on this.

Right heart

Right ventricular (RV) failure is not uncommon after cardiac surgery, and TOE allows assessment of RV function and dilatation by demonstrating pressure or volume loading, hypokinesia or bulging of the interventricular septum into the LV. Pulmonary artery pressure may be estimated by Doppler interrogation of the velocities of regurgitant jets through the tricuspid and pulmonary valves.

PERICARDIAL COLLECTIONS AND TAMPONADE

Pericardial effusions are commonly present after cardiac surgery. Whether the fluid collection leads to significant haemodynamic compromise and tamponade is determined by the volume and rate of accumulation as well as location of the collection. The heart can tolerate collections of up to 1 L if they accumulate slowly, however, as little as 50 to 100 mL can lead to compromise if accumulated rapidly in a sensitive location. Pericardial collections can readily be seen during either TTE or TOE examination. Assessment of transtricuspid and transmitral flow may help to assess the haemodynamic significance of the effusion, as well as the need and urgency of surgery. The origin of noniatrogenic collections may also be identified, such as aortic dissection.

Tamponade

It is important to appreciate that cardiac tamponade is a clinical diagnosis and TOE findings alone cannot rule out the diagnosis. If no pericardial effusion is seen on TOE but the patient remains unstable, reexploration must still be considered. The TOE findings that are suggestive of tamponade include:

- echolucent space adjacent to the cardiac structures;

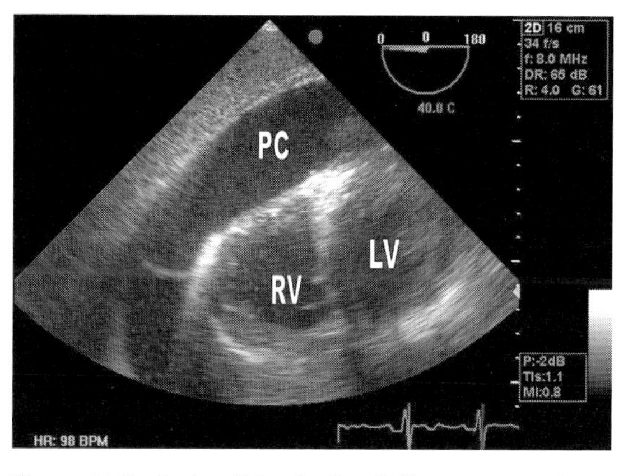

Figure 14.2 Pericardial collection (PC) on transgastric view, mostly posterior to the heart.

- atrial systolic collapse (94% sensitive, 100% specific);
- ventricular diastolic collapse (60%–90% sensitive, 85%–100% specific);
- respiratory changes in the ventricular diastolic filling patterns; and
- paradoxical ventricular septal wall motion with respiration.

ASSESSMENT OF VALVULAR FUNCTION

Assessment of native valves

Stenotic or regurgitant defects may be identified and the severity estimated. The detailed anatomical defect and associated pathophysiology may also be seen. In the setting of haemodynamic instability after valve surgery, systolic anterior motion of the anterior mitral leaflet may be seen, but this is a rare postoperative complication after mitral valve repair or aortic valve replacement. Fluid loading, avoidance of inotropes and slowing the heart rate all improve systolic anterior motion of the anterior mitral leaflet, but further surgery may be required if haemodynamic instability persists.

Assessment of prosthetic valves

Assessment of implanted prosthetic valves is routinely done intraoperatively. However, the prosthesis may still malfunction for some time after surgery. Common problems include paravalvular leak, thrombosis and endocarditis, which may be diagnosed by TOE.

Endocarditis

Endocarditis is a not infrequent diagnosis in the intensive care unit, and TOE plays a central part, guiding the extent and direction of therapy. The diagnosis of endocarditis cannot be made or excluded based solely on TOE findings, but should be made in conjunction with pathological and clinical data. Transoesophageal echocardiography should allow identification of the exact structures involved, assist in estimation of the severity of the disease and allow identification of associated regurgitant lesions and abscess formation.

Table 14.3 Transoesophageal echocardiography findings suggestive of endocarditis

Irregularly shaped mass: attached most often to the upstream side of the valve, with motion, classically described as 'dependent on, but more chaotic than' the underlying valve
Valve leaflet perforation
Chordal rupture
Valvular regurgitation
Prosthetic valve dysfunction/rocking/perivalvular leak
Myocardial/perivalvular abscess
Intracardiac fistula

AORTIC PATHOLOGY

Thoracic aortic pathology that may be identified by TOE includes aortic aneurysm, aortic dissection and traumatic aortic rupture. Patients may be transferred into critical care with suspected aortic lesions after an abnormal chest radiograph or computed tomography, and TOE allows definitive diagnosis; however, surgery should not be delayed and echocardiographic examination is often carried out in theatre after induction of anaesthesia. A TOE examination allows evaluation of the aortic valve, most of the ascending aorta and arch and the entire descending thoracic aorta. It also allows evaluation of myocardial function giving clues to coronary artery involvement.

TRANSOESOPHAGEAL ECHOCARDIOGRAPHY FOR THE HAEMODYNAMICALLY UNSTABLE PATIENT

Haemodynamic compromise in critical care must be managed expeditiously and the cause identified. A TOE examination may allow rapid diagnosis and observation of effects of treatment in real time. In this setting, TOE allows identification of pericardial effusion, estimation of biventricular filling and rapid assessment of right and left ventricular function. The TOE result is often used to assist in making the decision to return to theatre, although resternotomy should never be delayed if cardiovascular instability persists. Transoesophageal echocardiography may also be indicated in pulmonary oedema leading to hypoxia as systolic or diastolic left ventricular failure, mitral stenosis or mitral regurgitation may be contributory.

TRANSOESOPHAGEAL ECHOCARDIOGRAPHY FOR INTRACARDIAC SHUNTS

Unexplained shunts and hypoxia are not infrequent in critically ill patients and echocardiographic examination can readily demonstrate interatrial or interventricular communications by two-dimensional or Doppler examination.

TRANSOESOPHAGEAL ECHOCARDIOGRAPHY FOR HEART FAILURE PATIENTS

Transoesophageal echocardiography is often used to guide medical therapy and assess mechanical support in cardiac failure. The competency of the aortic valve may be confirmed before intra-aortic balloon pump placement, and the correct position of the balloon below the left subclavian artery confirmed. After ventricular assist device placement, TOE is particularly useful to confirm correct placement and orientation of the pipes and rule out pericardial collections affecting flow.

Echocardiography training and accreditation

Echocardiography requires skill to perform and interpret. The accreditation process may require the candidate to pass a written examination and submit a logbook within a 2-year period. The written examination is composed of theoretical multiple choice questions and a practical interpretation of echocardiographic images. Accreditation or certification in echocardiography is not compulsory, but is highly recommended.

Short but specific critical care echocardiography courses also exist. These are designed to train personnel to perform abbreviated, but focused echocardiography with the aim of a quick diagnosis in an unstable patient. These may allow studies to be done after a shortened period of training, but even straightforward conditions may be misdiagnosed or misinterpreted, leading to inappropriate management or interventions; therefore, proper accreditation should be the aim.

Quality assurance may also become an issue. Critical care personnel making diagnoses require sufficient assessment of echocardiography skills, continuing medical education and maintenance of competency.

Key points

- Ultrasound in critical care may facilitate venous cannulation and drainage of fluid collections, as well as its diagnostic capabilities.
- Transthoracic echocardiography often provides poor image quality, making interpretation difficult in mechanically ventilated patients.
- Transoesophageal echocardiography is the investigation of choice in haemodynamically unstable patients in critical care.

FURTHER READING

Sidebotham D, Merry A, Legget M. *Practical perioperative transoesophageal echocardiography*. Philadelphia: Butterworth Heinemann; 2004.

Chapter 15

Central nervous system monitoring

M. LEEMANS AND C.R. BAILEY

Introduction

Patients undergoing cardiothoracic surgery risk significant perioperative neurological dysfunction. This includes stroke, short- and long-term neurocognitive dysfunction, depression, delirium and confusion. The reasons for such injury are multifactorial, and include hypoperfusion, macro- and microemboli, effects of general anaesthesia, initiation of inflammatory pathways and metabolic derangement. Postoperative monitoring is aimed at identifying abnormalities arising from a primary injury and/or preventing further neurological injury.

In addition, neurological monitoring is useful for assessing sedation levels; patients on the critical care unit should ideally be lightly sedated, readily rousable and cooperative. Most drugs are given using standard dosing guidelines without applying knowledge of their pharmacokinetics and dynamics, and large variability is found when studying population pharmacology. Sedation and analgesia should be individualized and goal directed; therefore, appropriate monitoring is crucial.

Clinical monitoring

For the majority of patients in a cardiothoracic critical care unit, the central nervous system (CNS) is currently monitored clinically by means of regular neurological examination and sedation scores only.

Neurological examination

A physical examination forms the basis of any assessment of the CNS. However, because most patients are recovering from the effects of general anaesthesia or continue to receive a combination of sedatives and analgesics, only simple examination is possible and hence only gross neurological deficits elicited.

Sedation scores

Most patients in a cardiothoracic critical care unit receive sedation, anxiolysis and analgesia during their admission. Achieving an optimum level of sedation is challenging and has far-reaching implications. Incorrect levels of sedation have significant consequences in terms of morbidity, mortality and financial cost.

Optimal sedation levels target patient comfort, anxiolysis, analgesia, tolerance of endotracheal tubes, mechanical ventilation and allow therapeutic interventions to be undertaken. To achieve this, numerous drugs are in common usage. The choice of agent is less important than the correct titration of the chosen drug. Sedation scoring systems have been implemented to guide drug administration to ensure patient comfort while avoiding the hazards of oversedation. Many different systems are in use, but little work has been carried out to establish their reliability and validity. Such scoring systems include the Ramsay score, Addenbrooke's score and Newcastle scoring system.

Table 15.1 Potential consequences of incorrect sedation

Oversedation	Undersedation
Hypotension	Agitation
Pneumonia	Poor pain control
Deep vein thrombosis	Accidental extubation
Prolonged ventilation	Accidental loss of vascular catheters
Prolonged intensive care admission	Increased oxygen requirements
Increased diagnostic procedures	Myocardial ischaemia
Increased cost of care	Raised intracranial pressure
	Posttraumatic stress disorder

RAMSAY SCORING SYSTEM

This scoring system was initially designed in 1974 to assess sedation and rousability following administration of alphaxalone-alphadolone. In addition to the critical care environment, it can be used in any situation where sedatives or opioids have been given. Ramsay sedation scores correlate reasonably well with both the bispectral index (BIS) and evoked potentials. It depends, however, on the patient's ability to respond and cannot be used if muscle relaxants have been administered.

CAMBRIDGE (ADDENBROOKE'S) SEDATION SCORE

This system was developed specifically for use in neurocritical care. It is simple and allows a score to be measured even if muscle paralysis is employed.

NEWCASTLE SEDATION SCORE

This complex system was devised for patients being mechanically ventilated and is based on the Glasgow Coma Scale. There are five aspects, each of which is scored separately. These are then added together and the total value calculated, falling into six scoring levels. The complexity of the system precludes this from popular use.

Table 15.2 Ramsay sedation score

Score	
1	Anxious, agitated, restless
2	Cooperative, orientated
3	Responds to command only
4	Brisk response to light glabellar tap or loud auditory stimulus
5	Sluggish response to light glabellar tap or loud auditory stimulus
6	No response

Noninvasive monitoring

In addition to clinical assessment, the following provide noninvasive ways of monitoring the CNS.

Electroencephalogram

The electroencephalogram (EEG) provides information on the spontaneous electrical activity of the cerebral cortex, which is recorded from electrodes placed on the head according to the International

Table 15.3 Cambridge sedation score

Level	
1	Agitated
2	Awake
3	Roused by voice
4	Roused by tracheal suction
5	Unrousable
6	Paralysed
7	Asleep

Table 15.4 Newcastle sedation score

Eyes open	Spontaneously	4
	To speech	3
	To pain	2
	None	1
Response to nursing procedures	Obeys commands	4
	Purposeful movement	3
	Nonpurposeful movement	2
	None	1
Cough	Spontaneous strong	4
	Spontaneous weak	3
	On suction only	2
	None	1
Respirations	Extubated	5
	Intubated, spontaneous respiration	4
	Synchronized mandatory ventilation/pressure-support ventilation	3
	Respiration against ventilator	2
	No respiratory effort	1
Spontaneous communication		2

Score	Grades of sedation	Sum
1	Awake	17–19
2	Sleep	15–16
3	Light sedation	12–14
4	Moderate sedation	8–11
5	Deep sedation	5–7
6	Anaesthesia	4

Ten-Twenty Electrode System. This is a standardized electrode positioning system that allows reproducibility and valid comparisons between individuals. The recorded signal is amplified and filtered to give an accurate reflection of the electrical activity of the cerebral cortex.

The EEG is used extensively for diagnosis and classification of seizure activity. In critical care, it may also be used to detect ischaemic cerebral events, focal neurological disease, vasospasm after subarachnoid haemorrhage (SAH) and elevated intracranial pressure (ICP). When maximal suppression of electrical activity is required, the EEG guides administration of intravenous drugs to achieve burst suppression or isoelectricity. However, the EEG is cumbersome, generates large amounts of paper and expertise is required for data interpretation.

Developments have been made to condense and simplify the information generated from the EEG to facilitate data interpretation, with the BIS and evoked potentials being the most commonly used.

Bispectral index

The BIS was originally developed in 1992 as a tool to monitor the depth of anaesthesia and its most important function is to help prevent awareness during surgery. Although this is not a problem in the critical care environment unless the patient is fully paralyzed, it is increasingly used to provide information on the level of sedation. Electrodes are integrated into one sensor to obtain the electroencephalographic signal from the forehead.

Electrical activity undergoes Fourier analysis and information is combined to produce a dimensionless number from 0 to 100. Acquisition of the signal in the critical care unit is challenging, because the electrodes must be placed correctly and stay in place for long periods. Although the details of the algorithm are proprietary and not published, the basic principles have been described. The BIS integrates several disparate descriptors of the EEG into a single variable based on a large volume of clinical data to synthesize a combination that correlates with behavioural assessments of sedation and hypnosis. Most sedative and anaesthetic agents produce a characteristic increase in β EEG activity between 13 and 30 Hz. To prevent this pattern of EEG activation being reported as arousal, a β activity subvariable is included in the BIS algorithm.

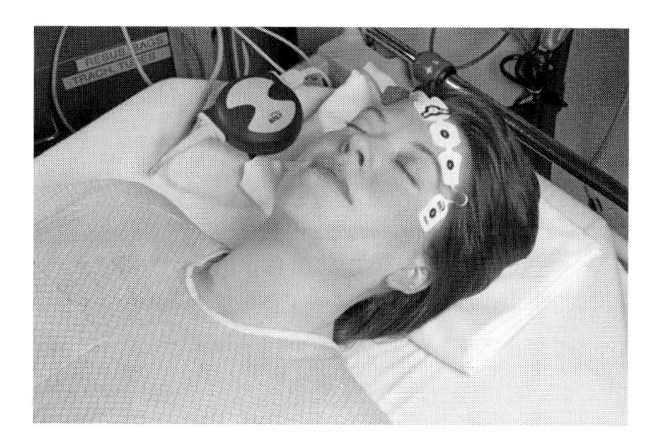

Figure 15.1 BIS monitoring.

Table 15.5 The bispectral index

Value of BIS	Clinical state of patient
85–100	Awake
65–85	Sedation
40–65	General anaesthesia
30–40	Deep hypnosis
0–30	Burst suppression

Burst suppression represents a benign pattern frequently seen in healthy brain at deep levels of anaesthesia. It can be identified in the raw EEG and is composed of episodes of electrical quiescence ('suppression') alternated with high-frequency, high-amplitude electrical activity ('bursts'). Increasing anaesthetic drug concentration causes increased duration of the suppression periods and to avoid a paradoxical increase in the presence of burst suppression the BIS includes a burst suppression subvariable. The BIS correlates well with effect site concentration of inhalational or hypnotic drugs; data has been verified by repeated testing on large population groups. There are, however, large variations between and within population groups.

Its use has been extended into the critical care environment to provide information on levels of sedation, but it has not been validated in this environment and in the absence of a surgical stimulus.

The BIS does not reflect the effect of opioids or their synergistic effect with hypnotics. This is a major drawback; opioids are commonly used in conjunction with hypnotic drugs in critical care. The BIS therefore appears to reflect the state of hypnosis rather than analgesia.

There are also several sources of inaccuracy in BIS values. The BIS does have the advantage of being a

Table 15.6 Sources of potential inaccuracy of BIS

Sweating	Age
Electromyographic activity	Deranged glucose levels
Drugs such as ketamine	Liver impairment
Electrolyte imbalance	Renal impairment
Deranged arterial CO_2 levels	Extremes of temperature

Table 15.7 Auditory evoked potential index

Score	Clinical state
60–100	Awake
40–60	Sedation
30–40	Loss of consciousness
20–30	General anaesthesia
10–20	Deep hypnosis
0–10	Burst suppression

simple and portable bedside device and does not need in-depth expertise for interpretation.

Auditory evoked potentials

Auditory evoked potentials (AEP) are a further derivation of the EEG developed to assess depth of anaesthesia and may additionally be used to monitor sedation levels.

The electrical activity in the brain in response to stimulation of specific sensory pathways is measured. The AEP, particularly midcortical AEP (MCAEP), are used to discriminate between the awake and the unconscious state. A repetitive auditory stimulus, 9.3 Hz and 70 dB above the hearing threshold, is applied to cranial nerve VIII. This generates a reproducible sequence of waveforms. These are detected from EEG electrodes placed on the mastoid process, the midline and a ground electrode. A waveform arises sequentially from the brainstem (BAEP), the auditory radiation, auditory cortex and associated areas of the cortex. The waves following the BAEP are termed the MCAEPs. These are sensitive to intravenous induction agents and volatile anaesthetics. The waves generally increase in latency and decrease in amplitude with increasing hypnotic drug concentration.

To facilitate interpretation, the AEP index has been developed. This is based on the wave amplitude of successive segments of MCAEP recordings. The use of MCAEP as an aid to assessing sedation in a critical care environment is limited because of interference. In addition, opioids and midazolam have little effect on MCAEP and ketamine has no effect. As these drugs are commonly used in critical care, AEP has not been widely applied.

Somatosensory evoked potentials

Operations on the descending aorta and thoracoabdominal aneurysm surgery run a significant risk of postoperative paraplegia. This may be the result of global spinal cord hypoperfusion or the failure to successfully reimplant segmental spinal arteries.

Somatosensory evoked potentials (SSEPs) are used to monitor the integrity of the ascending neural pathways and as a guide to cerebrospinal fluid (CSF) lumbar drainage. An electrical stimulus, typically over a peripheral nerve, generates a potential difference that is measured by electrodes placed over the scalp, spine and peripheral nerve proximal to the stimulation site. Abnormal SSEPs may result from dysfunction of the peripheral nerve, plexus, spinal cord, spinal root, cord, brainstem, somatosensory pathways or somatosensory cortex. Alterations in amplitude and latencies of the recorded response may indicate disruption of neural transmission.

The usefulness of SSEPs for detecting paraplegia is limited by signal interference from various anaesthetic drugs, including volatile anaesthetics and nitrous oxide. In addition, it does not monitor motor function; thus patients with normal SSEPs may awaken with significant motor deficits.

Motor evoked potentials

Motor evoked potentials (MEPs) are used to assess the integrity of descending motor pathways. They may be used in conjunction with SSEPs to assess spinal cord function. The primary motor cortex or spinal cord may be activated by an electrical stimulus, which is transmitted through cutaneous electrodes, or a magnetic stimulus in the form of a changing magnetic field. A neurogenic potential may be recorded in the distal spinal cord or peripheral nerve or as a myogenic potential difference from the innervated muscle. Myogenic MEPs are affected by muscle relaxants and volatile anaesthetics. Both SSEPs and MEPs are not in regular use.

Transcranial Doppler

Transcranial Doppler (TCD) provides an indirect method of measuring cerebral blood flow (CBF) in the major vessels supplying the brain. A 2-MHz ultrasound beam is transmitted, usually through the temporal bone, to a depth of 5 to 6 cm and directed at the middle cerebral artery (MCA). By applying the Doppler principle to the reflected ultrasound wave, red cell flow velocity is measured. There is a linear relationship between mean blood flow velocity and CBF and thus adequacy of blood flow can be established.

Theoretically, flow through any large vessel may be assessed; however, the MCA and basilar arteries are most frequently used. In addition to measuring red blood cell velocity, TCD can be used to provide further information on the cerebral circulation. The ultrasound beam measures flow throughout the cardiac cycle. The peak systolic and end-diastolic flow are known as the waveform pulsatility. In the absence of vessel stenosis or vasospasm, the waveform pulsatility can be used as an indirect measure of cerebrovascular resistance.

The TCD also can be used to differentiate between vasospasm and hyperaemia after SAH. In both these situations, flow through the MCA is high ($>$120 cm/s). The flow through the extracranial internal carotid artery is measured and then compared with flow through the MCA. If the ratio of MCA flow to extracranial internal carotid artery flow is more than 3, vasospasm is present. If the ratio of MCA flow to extracranial internal carotid artery flow is less than 3, hyperaemia is present. This is known as the Lundeburg ratio.

In addition to this information, work is being carried out to investigate the use of the TCD in measuring cerebral perfusion pressure (CPP) and ICP monitoring.

The benefits of the TCD include the fact that it is easily performed by the bedside, noninvasive and relatively inexpensive. However, accuracy depends on operator expertise and technique.

Near infrared spectroscopy

Near infrared spectroscopy is a noninvasive method of measuring regional changes in cerebral oxygenation. Light in the infrared range (700–1,000 nm) is passed through the skin, skull and brain. Oxygenated and deoxygenated blood absorbs light within this range. The absorption spectra for these two substances are different and in accordance with the Beer–Lambert law, the amount of light absorbed by these two substances is dependent on the respective concentrations of each. Thus, the amount of oxygenated blood passing through different regions of the brain can be quantified. To assess only the intracranial tissues, a dual detector system is used. It is assumed that the detector closest to the light source depicts light passing through the skull and extracranial tissues. The distal detector depicts light passing through the skin, skull and brain. The difference between these signals reflects light absorbed by brain tissue only.

Advantages include the ability to assess regional differences in cerebral oxygenation and the noninvasive nature of the device. Inaccuracies may occur when differentiating between intra- and extracranial changes in blood flow.

Invasive monitoring

In patients at high risk for neurocognitive dysfunction or known brain injury, invasive methods of monitoring the CNS should be considered.

Jugular bulb oximetry

Jugular bulb oximetry ($Sjvo_2$) gives an indication of global cerebral oxygen delivery and consumption.

A retrograde catheter is inserted into the internal jugular vein. The tip of the catheter is ideally placed at the level of the jugular bulb, which corresponds with the mastoid process externally and C1 /C2 intervertebral space on a lateral neck radiograph. Venous blood from the brain drains directly into the jugular bulb and accurately reflects mixed cerebral venous blood. Sampling blood from this area gives an indication of global oxygen delivery compared with oxygen consumption.

The normal range of $Sjvo_2$ is 55% to 70%. A lower $Sjvo_2$ may indicate poor oxygen delivery or a high oxygen extraction ratio owing to increased oxygen demand. To differentiate between these two states, a specimen of arterial blood is taken simultaneously. A difference in arterial and venous blood of more than 9% reflects increased oxygen utilization. An $Sjvo_2$ below 50% has been associated with a poor neurological outcome.

Supranormal oxygen levels may indicate supranormal oxygen delivery or may suggest minimal cerebral oxygen utilization, the likely outcome of which is very poor. Only global cerebral oxygenation is reflected; differences at regional levels cannot be detected.

Inaccuracies may occur owing to incorrect catheter placement, protein deposition on the catheter tip or too rapid sampling, which may aspirate blood from extracranial sources. In addition, frequent recalibration is necessary.

Table 15.8 Causes of abnormal $Sjvo_2$

Low $Sjvo_2$	High $Sjvo_2$
High extraction ratio decreased cerebral blood flow	Supranormal O_2 delivery
Elevated intracranial pressure	Poor oxygen utilization
Seizures and pyrexia Decreased oxygen delivery	

Intracranial pressure monitoring

The importance of measuring ICP relates to the Kellie–Monroe principle. This states that the skull is a rigid vault and contains brain parenchyma, blood and CSF. In health, these three constituents remain balanced in a state of dynamic equilibrium and the ICP remains stable. In disease states, for example, haematoma, cerebral oedema, or tumour, there is limited compensatory capacity for the increasing volume within the intracranial cavity. To preserve normal ICP, the volume of CSF is reduced. Decreased production of CSF is coupled with shunting of CSF into the dural sac surrounding the spinal cord. The cerebral blood volume also decreases, to maintain normal ICP values. Once these mechanisms are exhausted, autoregulation is lost and ICP rises rapidly. This accounts for the nonlinear shape of the pressure–volume curve. Normal ICP is between 7 and 15 mmHg, fluctuating with posture, cardiac and respiratory cycles. The ICP also correlates with MAP and CPP (MAP − ICP = CPP).

Decreased CPP results in cerebral hypoperfusion and ischaemia, and is termed secondary brain injury. A persistently elevated ICP is an indicator of poor outcome; thus, treatment is aimed at keeping the ICP below 20mmHg. There are numerous

Table 15.9 Methods of intracranial pressure monitoring

Placement	Advantages	Disadvantages
Intraventricular	Allows drainage of CSF	High infection rate Most invasive Can be difficult to insert Cannot drain CSF and monitor waveform simultaneously
Intraparenchymal	Low infection rate	Measures local ICP Recalibration difficult
Subarachnoid	Low infection rate No brain penetration	Limited accuracy
Epidural	Low infection rate Easy to insert	Limited accuracy
Lumbar drain	Easy to insert Can be used for CSF drainage after thoracic aortic surgery	Limited accuracy Cannot be used if ICP elevated
Transcranial Doppler	Noninvasive	Limited accuracy

Abbreviations: CSF, cerebrospinal fluid; ICP, intracranial pressure.

devices available for monitoring ICP, although the ideal monitor is yet to be devised

In addition to pressure readings, the ICP waveform can also be analysed. The frequency of the waveform relates to heart rate and the three phases of the waveform relate to certain physiological variables, namely, P1, the 'pressure' wave (arterial pressure transmitted from choroid plexus); P2, 'tidal' wave (owing to brain compliance); and P3, the closure of the aortic valve (dicrotic notch).

Table 15.10 The 'ideal' ICP monitor

Accurate global pressure readings
Simple to calibrate
Allows ICP waveform analysis
Noninvasive
Low infection rate
Allows aspiration of CSF

Abbreviations: CSF, cerebrospinal fluid; ICP, intracranial pressure.

In health, P2 is smaller than P1. In disease states, as compliance decreases, P2 increases in amplitude. With continuous ICP monitoring, three slow waveforms may be evident. A waves are 'plateau' waves and a steep increase in ICP to 40 mmHg or more is always pathological and occurs with intact autoregulation but reduced compliance. They persist for 5 to 20 minutes. B waves occur at 0.5 to 2.0 waves/min and are related to the vascular tone. C waves occur at 4 to 8 waves/min and are of little pathological significance.

Microdialysis

Microdialysis can be used to analyse the extracellular biochemical environment of the brain. This includes metabolites (glucose, lactate, pyruvate, adenosine), neurotransmitters (glutamate, aspartate, γ-aminobutyric acid), inflammatory markers (cytokines) and drugs.

A fine-bore, double-lumen catheter is inserted into the brain parenchyma. An isotonic solution is slowly infused (0.1–0.2 mL/min) through the outer lumen which has an outer semipermeable membrane. Substances small enough to pass through the pores of this membrane diffuse down their concentration gradient into the lumen. This fluid then moves into the return lumen of the catheter by mean of hydrostatic pressure through an opening in the distal tip of the return lumen. The fluid is then collected and analysed at 10- to 60-minute intervals.

Changes in concentrations of substances reflect alternative pathways of metabolism, cell ischaemia and cell death. Microdialysis provides information on the local biochemical environment; thus, accurate catheter placement is essential.

The use of microdialysis is currently restricted to specialist centres.

Brain tissue oximetry

Cerebral tissue oximetry measures levels of oxygen, carbon dioxide and pH in a localized area. A sensor is inserted into the brain tissue, preferably the prenumbral area. There are presently two types of sensors available, a polarographic Clarke electrode, which measures brain oxygen tension and a multiparameter sensor, which can measure oxygen, carbon dioxide, pH and temperature using a fibreoptic probe. It has potential benefits as it monitors regional oxygenation, but the technique is invasive and there is yet to be any conclusive data as to its validity. At the moment it remains largely a research tool.

Multimodal monitoring

As there is no ideal CNS monitoring device currently available, the concurrent use of two or three CNS monitoring techniques has been recommended. This attempts to compensate for shortfalls and limitations of one device compared with another, thus generating a more comprehensive reflection of CNS status. Unfortunately, this is expensive and may produce conflicting information, making interpretation and decision making challenging.

Key points

- Simple neurological examination and sedation scores continue to form the cornerstone of CNS assessment.
- The BIS provides a noninvasive and objective means of assessing depth of anaesthesia.
- Invasive monitoring should be considered in patients at high risk of developing neurological deficits or with known brain injury.
- Multimodal monitoring provides the most accurate assessment of CNS function.
- Many monitors are not yet in regular clinical use, but remain a research tool.

FURTHER READING

Bruhn J, Myles PS, Sneyd R, *et al.* Depth of anaesthesia monitoring: what's available, what's validated and what's next? *Br J Anaesthesia* 2006;97:85–94.

Nortje J, Gupta AK. The role of tissue oxygen monitoring in patients with acute brain injury. *Br J Anaesthesia* 2006;97:95–106.

Schulte-Tamburen AM, Scheier J, Breigel J, *et al.* Comparison of five sedation scoring systems by means of auditory evoked potentials. *Intensive Care Med* 1999;25:377–382.

Steiner LA, Andrews PJ. Monitoring the injured brain: ICP and CBF. *Br J Anaesthesia* 2006;97:26–38.

Chapter 16

Point of care testing

C.H.A. WILLMOTT AND J.E. ARROWSMITH

Introduction

Point of care (POC) testing is rapidly expanding. It can be defined as an analytical test undertaken in a setting distinct from a normal hospital laboratory; other synonyms include near patient testing, bedside testing and remote (as in, remote from a laboratory) testing. It encompasses a variety of testing media, ranging from single reagent strips to handheld electronic devices and bench-top analysers, which may be used to test virtually any body fluid. This chapter concentrates on POC testing of blood samples only.

Implementation

The concept of POC testing is not new; mediaeval medics relied on the observation of blood, urine and stool to assess the balance of humours (phlegmatic, choleric, sanguine and melancholic), in the presence of the patient (or victim!). Although some tests have continued to be carried out in this manner, the days of physicians counting red cells down the microscope have long gone.

Although pneumatic sample transportation systems and the automation of many clinical laboratory analytical methods have undoubtedly reduced the time from sampling to result (the 'turn-around time'), the trend toward centralized services may, paradoxically, slow down receipt of results.

Despite the demand for rapid test results, particularly when it is perceived that these may dictate a change in or initiation of a new therapy, there is little evidence that this has any significant impact on clinical outcomes. Impact on overall running costs is also unknown.

Blood gas analysis

One of the most commonly performed POC tests in the critical care setting is blood gas analysis, whether it be arterial blood gases for assessment of gas exchange, or mixed venous gases as a marker for adequacy of cardiac output/tissue perfusion.

Bench-top analysers

Initially, the same devices used in clinical laboratories were simply relocated to the critical care unit. As the devices have become more sophisticated, technological advances have also allowed them to become smaller, and dispensed with the need for additional cumbersome equipment. Furthermore, a wide range of tests may now be performed (e.g. basic blood gas and acid–base analysis, lactate, Na^+, K^+, Ca^{2+}, Mg^{2+}, haematocrit, haemoglobin and co-oximetry) that are as accurate and reliable as their clinical laboratory counterparts.

Handheld devices

Some devices combine a handheld console with multifunction, single-use cartridges capable of analysing samples as small as two drops of blood. Each cartridge contains a sample well and transit pathway, a pouch of buffered calibration fluid and a series of thin film semiconductor biosensors.

Table 16.1 The arguments for and against POC testing.

Cost	On a per unit basis, POC testing is almost always more expensive than the same test in a centralized laboratory. As with all new technologies, the cost of hardware is initially high, while life expectancy can be limited. Over time, this situation is likely to be reversed, as hardware prices fall and hardware becomes more robust – e.g. measurement electrodes in bench-top blood gas analysers.
Accuracy	Early POC testing devices were often less accurate than their laboratory-based counterpart. With increasing experience of miniaturization, this gap has now effectively been closed.
Reliability	POC testing devices, just like their laboratory-based counterparts, require regular servicing, calibration and QC testing to maintain reliable and uninterrupted function. The issue of reliability is significant in clinical areas where there is no identified body responsible for POC testing equipment upkeep.
Storage and handling	Many POC testing devices rely on liquid or dry strip media for either calibration or measurement purposes. The provision of inadequate facilities for media storage (e.g. areas exposed to extremes of temperature), or inadequate training in media handling, can lead to unrecognized system errors. The shelf-life of some media is limited, and tests conducted using out-of-date media for QC, calibration or measurement purposes could also lead to errors which may not be detected by internal QC protocols.
Data quality	Provision: The result of a test may be shown as a change in the colour of a reagent strip, displayed on a local screen, or printed on paper. Transcription: Transferring the result obtained from a POC device typically involves manually copying or transcribing the information into the patient record. Any time results are transcribed there is potential for human error, which may not be noticed. Storage: Most laboratories provide a permanent, centralized electronic record of test results that can be accessed from multiple remote centres simultaneously. Early POC devices provided only a real-time, local readout of results. Newer devices are capable of internally storing individual patient data and transferring it to a centralized electronic patient record.
Legal	As in all areas of medicine, mishaps occur when treatment is determined based on the outcome of POC testing. In these situations, it is important to be able to show that an identified person or group has responsibility for each of the following: Sourcing POC testing material, including devices and all related media required for QC, calibration and sample testing Acquisition of POC testing material Servicing of POC testing devices QC of POC devices Training of end-users Data collection and storage Interpretation of collected data

Abbreviations: POC, point of care; QC, quality control.

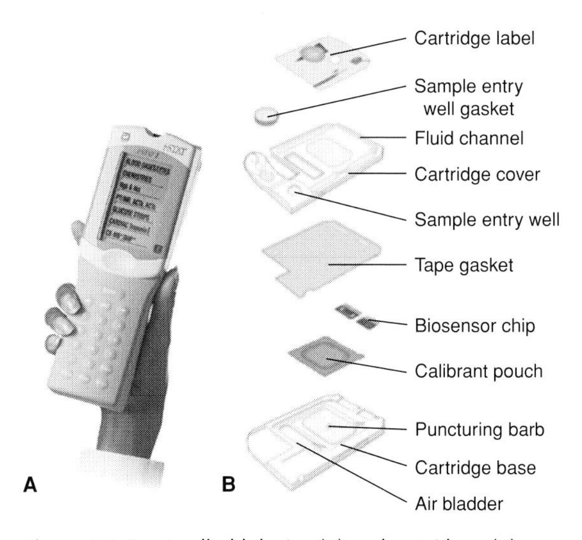

Figure 16.1 Handheld device (*A*) and cartridges (*B*) allowing coagulation testing at the bedside.

Currently available cartridges permit analysis of blood gases, biochemistry, coagulation and cardiac markers.

At the start of the test cycle, an integral barb punctures the calibration fluid pouch allowing the solution to pass over the biosensors. The activation of a small air bladder then forces the calibration fluid into a waste reservoir while moving the blood sample from the sample well to the biosensors.

In-line testing

Fluorescent optode technology consists of a fibreoptic bundle combined with a substrate-specific fluorescent dye. The intensity of light emitted by the dye, as electrons return to their ground state, is proportional to the concentration of substrate within the sample. This allows ex vivo in-line monitoring, which provides analysis of blood drawn into a sampling reservoir incorporated into a standard pressure monitoring transducer. After analysis, the sample is returned to the patient, eliminating loss of blood through repetitive sampling. Sterility is maintained because the sampling system remains closed throughout the testing procedure. Despite its many practical advantages, the small number of available analytes (e.g. Po_2, Pco_2, pH, glucose) and high unit cost has limited uptake of the technology.

Tests of coagulation

Prothrombin time

The prothrombin time (PT) is the time taken for citrated whole blood to clot following addition of thromboplastin (phospholipid combined with tissue factor) in the presence of calcium, a test of both the extrinsic and common pathways of the coagulation cascade. Because of the varying sensitivities of the reagents used for PT analysis, it is more common to report the International Normalized Ratio, calculated from the test PT result and the International Sensitivity Index of the reagent used.

Prolongation of the PT indicates a problem in either or both of the extrinsic and common pathways. Common causes include warfarin (coumadin) therapy, hepatic dysfunction, vitamin K deficiency and specific clotting factor deficiencies (e.g. I, II, V, VII, IX, and X).

Point of care PT testing may be useful during major haemorrhage, and elevated PT may indicate the need for fresh frozen plasma administration. Most devices rely on the impedance of movement of either the blood itself, or an object within the blood to determine the onset of clot formation.

Partial thromboplastin time

The partial thromboplastin time (PTT) is the time taken for citrated whole blood to clot following exposure to phospholipid without tissue factor (hence the term 'partial') – a test of both the intrinsic and common pathways of the coagulation cascade. Calcium is used as an activator of coagulation, hence the use of the term *activated* PTT (aPTT). Common causes of a prolonged aPTT include unfractionated heparin therapy, hepatic dysfunction, factor IX deficiency and the presence of the lupus anticoagulant. The aPTT is not a useful test for monitoring fractionated (low-molecular-weight) heparin therapy, a more direct measure of anti-factor Xa activity is more appropriate.

As with PT, samples have traditionally been sent to central laboratories for analysis. However, POC testing may allow more accurate titration of intravenous heparin therapy and may be particularly useful to monitor infusion during renal replacement therapy.

Activated coagulation time

As with PTT, activated coagulation time (ACT) measures the integrity of intrinsic and common pathways. It is used almost exclusively for assessment of heparin therapy during acute medical interventions such as cardiopulmonary bypass (CPB) or extracorporeal membrane oxygenation (ECMO). High doses of heparin are given during these interventions, to prevent blood clotting when in almost constant contact with foreign antigen, in the form of the CPB/ECMO circuit. Such high doses render the sample unclottable on the PTT test methodology; it should be noted that ACT is much less sensitive than PTT, and, as such, should not be used in place of PTT for routine management of prophylactic heparin infusions.

For ACT, activators such as celite (diatomaceous earth) or kaolin, are added to whole blood to initiate coagulation. Typically an ACT of at least 350 to 400 seconds is considered necessary before initiating CPB. Because of the critical nature of a short ACT and the speed with which it must be corrected while on extracorporeal circuits, these tests are almost universally done at the bedside. Results are sensitive to temperature (among other things); typically, the device warms the sample or collection media to 37°C before analysis. Aprotinin (a serine protease inhibitor sometimes used during CPB to limit bleeding due to fibrinolysis) prolongs ACT when celite is used as the activator.

Heparin management test

Proposed as an alternative to ACT testing for adequate heparin anticoagulation and reversal in the setting of CPB, clotting is activated by aluminium magnesium silicate in presence of calcium and buffer. Clot formation is detected by reduction of movement of paramagnetic iron oxide particles in an oscillating magnetic field. It must always be remembered that the heparin dose–response curve is nonlinear, and heparin effect, rather than concentration, is the more important factor.

Thromboelastography

Thromboelastography (TEG) assesses the viscoelastic properties of whole blood to provide information on a range of variables involved in haemostasis, including clotting factors, platelets and the fibrinolytic system. A small sample is placed into a warmed cup, which oscillates over a given angle. A pin is introduced into the sample from above, suspended by a torsion wire. As clot formation occurs, the oscillation of the cup is increasingly transmitted to the pin, and hence the torsion wire. As the clot lyses, fibrin strands linking the pin to the cup break down, and the movement of pin and wire is correspondingly reduced. Change of torsion over time is depicted graphically, and analysis to provide commonly used variables is usually performed by integrated software.

Because it provides information regarding the various stages of coagulation and fibrinolysis, TEG is commonly used to guide therapy for excessive blood loss. Institutions have devised their own protocols

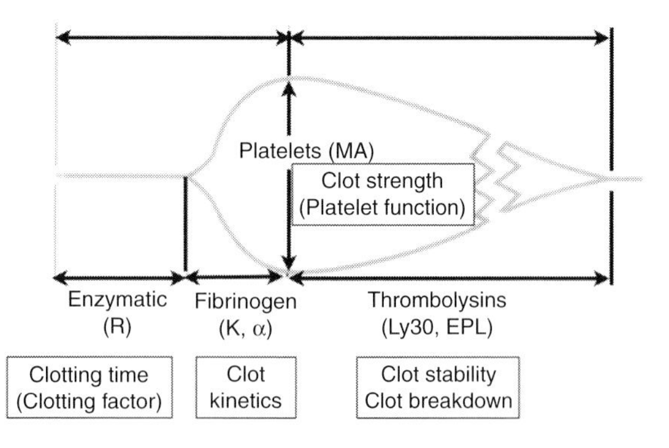

Figure 16.2 Components of the TEG traces.

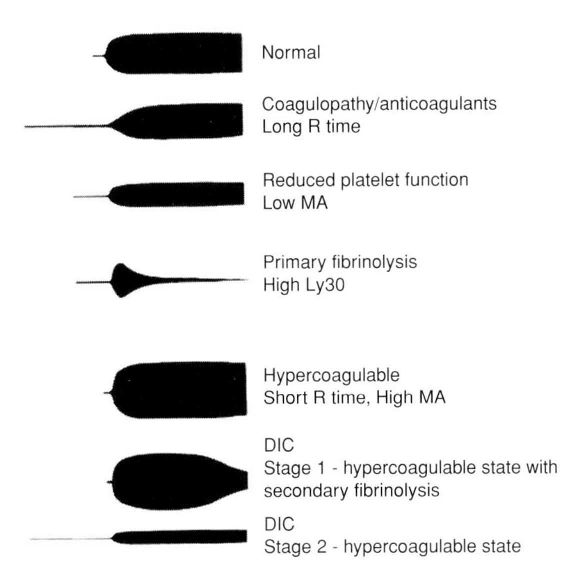

Figure 16.3 The TEG traces in various clinical scenarios.

to determine when TEG is appropriate, and to guide response to results.

Heparinase cups are available, allowing neutralization of the effect of heparin on coagulation. When compared with the standard test, any residual heparin effect is easily seen and this may be used to guide further protamine administration. Standard TEG is also insensitive to the antiplatelet effects of both aspirin and clopidogrel; however, cups containing specific reagents for these drugs are now available. For these reasons, TEG should be used as an adjunct to, rather than replacement for, traditional coagulation tests.

Rotational thromboelastometry

Rotational thromboelastometry utilizes similar methodology to TEG. The torsion wire is replaced by a firmer strut, held in place by a ring of ball bearings. Rather than change in torsion, data on pin rotation are generated by an optical sensor detecting light reflected from a mirror attached to the pin.

Sonoclot

This device assesses the viscoelastic properties of whole blood during coagulation, producing results similar to TEG. Clot formation is analysed by the varying impedance to ultrasonic probe vibration owing to formation of fibrin cross-links.

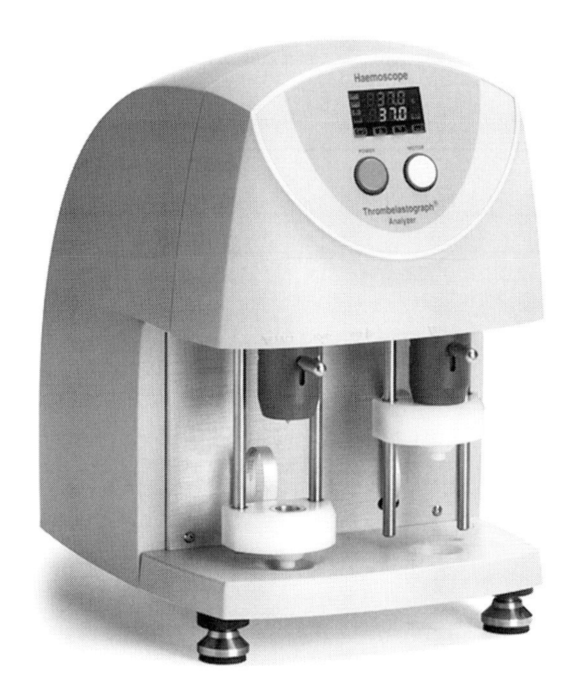

Figure 16.4 The TEG machine, with two incubators.

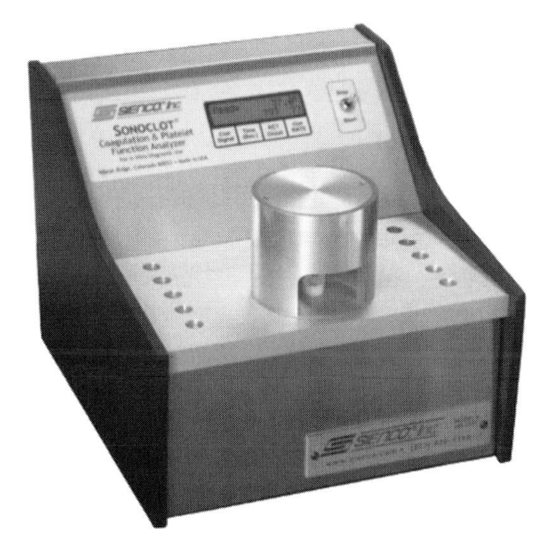

Figure 16.5 Sonoclot machine.

Platelet function analysis

Traditionally performed in the laboratory by light transmittance aggregometry, POC devices are now available to assess platelet function and the effects of antiplatelet therapy. The Platelet Function Analyzer (PFA-100; Dade Behring, Frankfurt, Germany) assesses the function of platelets based on the speed with which they are able to occlude a hole of specific dimensions. Sample blood is drawn across the membranes by vacuum to create high shear stress, simulating conditions in vivo.

Prolonged occlusion time is related to platelet dysfunction, but results may be affected by anaemia or thrombocytopenia. Although aspirin effects will be detected, this method may not be suitable for identifying clopidogrel effects. The VerifyNow Ultegra (Accumetrics Inc, San Diego, CA) system is a POC version of the laboratory test, using a turbidimetric optical detection system. It may be used for a variety of situations, including monitoring of both aspirin and clopidogrel treatment regimes.

Glucose monitoring

Glucose monitoring is the most widely used POC test applied to blood, with handheld glucose meters commonplace in hospitals, primary care practices and in the homes of millions of diabetics. There are many devices in the marketplace, although most now rely on enzymatic degradation of glucose to produce a result; either a colour change, measured by spectrophotometry, or production of electrons, measured by amperometry.

Whole blood is used in almost all POC devices, which may affect accuracy:

- Most devices prevent the passage of red cells into the analysate by allowing the plasma portion to diffuse through multiple absorbent layers.
- Some devices contain agents to lyse erythrocytes to allow analysis of the entire sample.
- Samples measuring only the plasma fraction tend to read about 10% to 12% higher than those analysing whole blood, simply as a function of the red cell mass in the whole blood sample.

Many of these devices use 'haematocrit compensation'; most devices assume a haematocrit of around 40%. Variations in haematocrit affect the result. This can have significant impact in situations where haematocrit may differ from the norm, or may change rapidly. In essence, a more accurate device may be needed in certain specialized situations, whereas a more robust but less precise device may be useful for home testing.

Key points

- Accurate calibration, quality control and result transcription is essential whenever POC is used.
- Increased cost must be offset by accuracy and clinical advantages before implementation.
- The laboratory should be involved in purchase, implementation and maintenance of POC testing.

FURTHER READING

Despotis GJ, Joist JH, Hogue CW, *et al.* The impact of heparin concentration and activated clotting time monitoring on blood conservation. *J Thorac Cardiovasc Surg* 1995;110:46–54.

Shore-Lesserson L. Evidence based coagulation monitors: heparin monitoring, thromboelastography, and platelet function. *Semin Cardiothorac Vasc Anesth* 2005;9:41–52.

Shore-Lesserson L. Platelet inhibitors and monitoring platelet function: implications for bleeding. *Hematol Oncol Clin North Am* 2007;21:51–63.

Chapter 17

Importance of pharmacokinetics

F. PEA AND M. FURLANUT

Introduction

Pharmacokinetics can be defined as the study of drug and drug metabolite concentrations within the body. It describes how drug concentrations may vary over time owing to the different phases after drug administration, namely absorption, distribution, metabolism and elimination. Knowledge of changes in critical illness and after major surgery may allow prediction of the correct dose and regime to ensure therapeutically effective levels at the site of action. In critical care, the pathophysiological changes over the course of the illness may significantly alter the pharmacokinetic behaviour of drugs. Therefore, changes may need to be made at different times to prevent over- or underdosing.

Pathophysiology

To understand the correct principles of drug administration in critical illness, it is necessary to identify which pathophysiological changes occur at what point during critical illness.

Gastrointestinal absorption

Drug absorption in the gastrointestinal tract after oral administration is a kinetic process, which may be reduced by an unpredictable amount in the early postoperative period after major surgery. It is reduced due to gastric stasis, metabolic imbalance or reduced splanchnic blood flow associated with hypotension and use of inotropic agents. Therefore, the intravenous route may be preferable until enteral/oral feeding is established, to ensure therapeutic levels are achieved. However, not all drugs are formulated for intravenous administration, so they may have to be omitted for a period of time, usually 24 to 48 hours. Gastric motility and absorption is worsened by opioid administration (and severe pain), and gastrointestinal ileus after surgery may be prolonged for some days, especially during prolonged administration of inotropic agents. Nausea and vomiting obviously preclude oral administration of drugs, as does oesophageal surgery or injury.

Systemic cyclosporine levels, after oral administration after organ transplantation, demonstrate the reduced absorption seen after surgery. In these patients, total body exposure to cyclosporine (in terms of area under the concentration–time curve) administered via nasogastric tube is very low immediately after transplantation, but significantly improves within the first 5 days after surgery. Therefore, oral administration immediately after heart transplantation may result in inadequate immunosuppression and intravenous dosing is recommended.

Distribution

Fluctuation in the extracellular fluid content as a response to the trauma of surgery may significantly increase the volume of distribution of some drugs. This may be especially the case for hydrophilic antimicrobials, namely β-lactams, aminoglycosides and glycopeptides, whose distribution is limited to the extracellular compartment. These agents are unable to move intracellularly by passive diffusion, so that the presence of extra volume in the interstitium may result in significant dilution and lower drug concentrations. The dose (and loading dose in particular) may therefore have to be increased until this fluid is redistributed and extracellular volume is decreased again. Additionally, drug loss may occur by loss from chest drainage, which may also contribute to alterations in the volume of distribution of hydrophilic antibiotics.

Metabolism

Alterations in liver function, common in critical illness, may affect drug metabolism, especially when phase I mechanisms are involved. However, this rarely contributes to major intra-individual pharmacokinetic variations after cardiac surgery.

A number of drugs competing for liver metabolism, however, do significantly alter drug clearance in critically ill patients, especially when multiple agents are administered. This may be of particular interest after transplantation, with respect to immunosuppressive therapy. Cyclosporine, sirolimus and tacrolimus are all metabolized by the cytochrome microsomal system isoform 3A4 (CYP3A4), whose activity may be significantly reduced or increased by the simultaneous administration of other drugs acting as inhibitors or inducers.

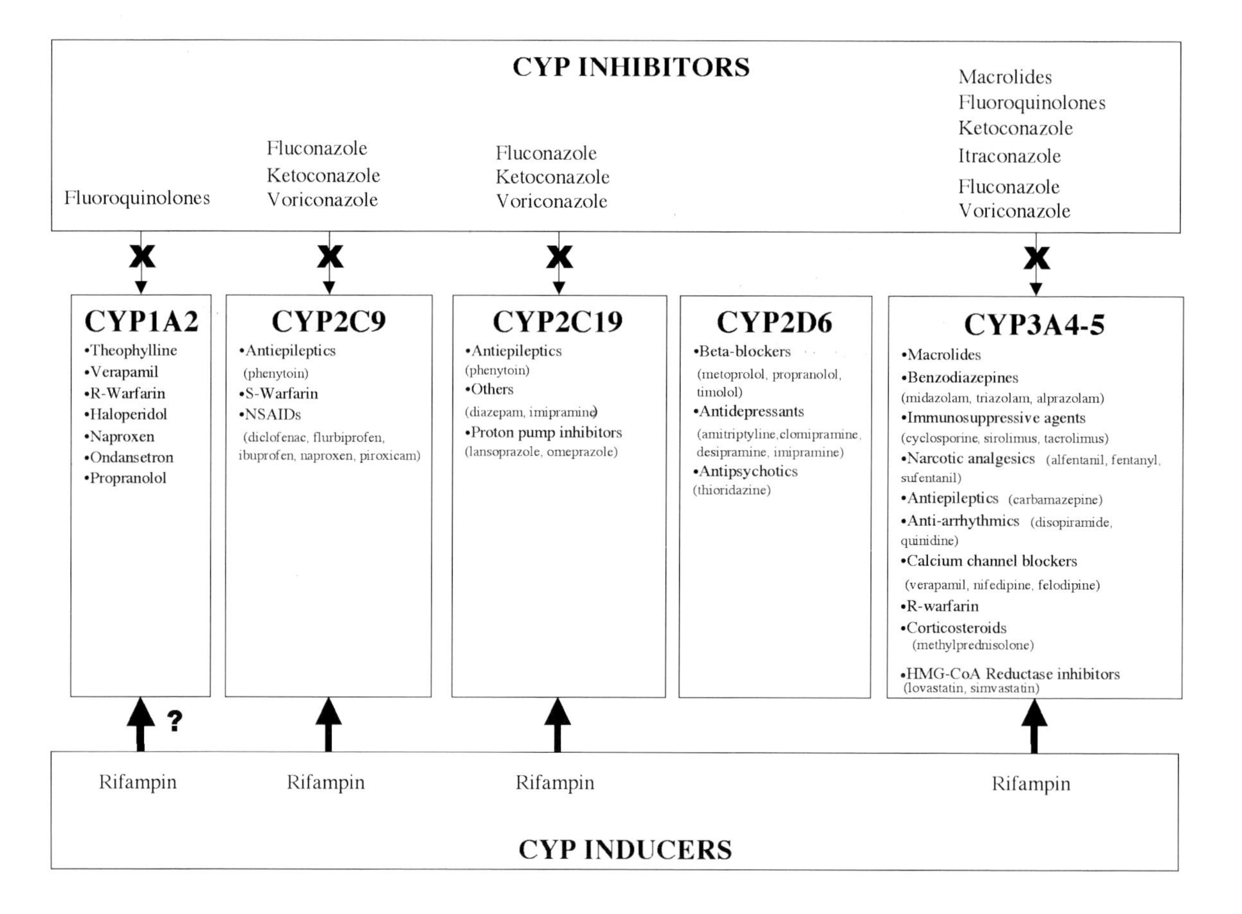

Figure 17.1 Cytochromes inhibitions/induction by various drugs.

Table 17.1 Pathophysiological or iatrogenic conditions affecting renal clearance of drugs

Causes of increased renal clearance	Causes of decreased renal clearance
Hypertension	Hypotension
Use of haemodynamically active drugs (furosemide, dopamine, dobutamine)	Renal dysfunction
Hypoalbuminaemia	Dialysis

The metabolic activity of CYP3A4 is consistently inhibited by macrolide antibiotics, especially erythromycin and clarithromycin, and azole antifungal agents, especially itraconazole and voriconazole, but also fluconazole. Therefore, administration of these antibiotics and immunosuppression must be undertaken with great care. On the other hand, co-treatment with the CYP3A4 inducer rifampicin may cause a significant increase in the total body clearance of cyclosporine, tacrolimus and sirolimus. Therefore, drug levels should be regularly monitored to guide dose adjustments, when such combinations of drugs are administered.

Elimination

Reduced renal function leading to impaired drug elimination is the most common and relevant pathophysiological mechanism affecting drug concentration in critically ill patients. Increased drug levels may occur after only a short period of renal dysfunction, which is common after cardiac surgery because of fluctuating blood pressure and renal perfusion. Worsening renal function leads to even poorer drug elimination, which may be estimated by a rising serum creatinine. The dose of drugs may need to be altered to take this into account. The requirement for renal replacement therapy also has a significant effect on drug dosage, particularly sedatives, analgesics and some antimicrobials.

Positive inotropes (such as dopamine and dobutamine) and diuretics may actually enhance the clearance of drugs eliminated by the renal route. Most hydrophilic antimicrobials (namely, β-lactams, aminoglycosides and glycopeptides) are almost completely excreted by the kidney; therefore, therapeutic drug monitoring is essential in critical illness, often on a daily basis.

Receptors

Receptor numbers and function may alter in critical illness. *Tolerance*, the decreased effect after a number of doses in the absence of changes in elimination, may occur to sedatives and analgesics. The density of catecholamine receptors may also decrease owing to changes in plasma adrenaline and noradrenaline concentrations.

Pharmacokinetics and pharmacodynamics of drugs during cardiopulmonary bypass

Extracorporeal circulation (CPB or ECMO) may significantly alter drug elimination and concentration. Acute haemodilution leads to a significant decrease of plasma concentrations of almost any drug. This is rapidly corrected in the case of drugs which are accumulated intracellularly (namely, those with a high volume of distribution [>1 L/kg]), owing to the redistribution from the intracellular to the extracellular compartment. However, the concentration of hydrophilic drugs whose distribution is extracellularly limited is permanently reduced.

Additionally, haemodilution, by causing hypoalbuminaemia, may increase the free moiety of normally highly protein-bound drugs; because it is this that is biologically active, an increased pharmacodynamic effect should be expected. The free fraction of normally highly protein-bound drugs may be further increased as a consequence of the effect of heparin administration on plasma protein binding. Heparin, by promoting the hydrolysis of plasma triglycerides, favours the competitive binding of free fatty acids to plasma protein,

Table 17.2 Factors affecting drug pharmacokinetics during cardiopulmonary bypass

Causes	Possible pharmacokinetic effect
Haemodilution	Total drug concentration
Heparin administration	Free drug moiety because of displacement from plasma protein binding
Hypothermia	Hepatic drug clearance
Sequestration in cardiopulmonary bypass equipment	Total drug concentration

which may result in displacement of bound drugs. Hypothermia may reduce the metabolic activity of the liver, so that the hepatic clearance of drugs may be decreased. Finally, significant amounts of drugs may be sequestered in bypass equipment owing to adsorption (e.g. insulin). It has been shown that CPB reduces the efficacy of antimicrobial prophylaxis with hydrophilic antibiotics (ceftazocine and vancomycin), so that higher doses are recommended, with repeated administration after conclusion of CPB.

Key points

- Gastrointestinal drug absorption in critical care patients may be erratic and unpredictable in the early postoperative period.
- Concentrations of hydrophilic antimicrobials may be reduced as a consequence of fluid accumulation in the interstitial space.
- Routine therapeutic drug monitoring should be used to guide dosage of immunosuppressive agents after transplantation, especially when antibiotics are coadministered.
- Drug monitoring of glycopeptides and aminoglycosides is also required owing to haemodynamic instability and renal dysfunction in critical illness.

FURTHER READING

Pea F, Furlanut M. Pharmacokinetic aspects of treating infections in the intensive care unit: focus on drug interactions. *Clin Pharmacokinet* 2001;40:833–868.

Pea F, Viale P, Furlanut M. Antimicrobial therapy in critically ill patients: a review of pathophysiological conditions responsible for altered disposition and pharmacokinetic variability. *Clin Pharmacokinet* 2005;44:1009–1034.

Chapter 18

Radiology

N.J. SCREATON AND E.P. SMITH

Introduction

The portable chest radiograph is the primary imaging modality on the critical care unit. Daily physical examination of sedated, intubated patients may be difficult and new or rapidly evolving changes in cardiorespiratory status may only be appreciated on chest radiography.

The routine chest radiograph

The efficacy and accuracy of the portable anteroposterior (AP) chest radiograph in assessing cardiopulmonary or pleural complications in critical care and its role in detecting malpositioned monitoring devices have been evaluated in many studies. Although undoubtedly the chest radiograph is valuable in the assessment of complications after intervention or change in clinical status, the role of the 'routine' daily radiograph is more controversial. Although not specifically recommending against routine radiography, one should emphasize the value of more targeted investigations.

Technical considerations

Technique

Optimal radiographic technique is essential to maximize the efficacy and accuracy of bedside radiography. The AP chest radiograph should be obtained with the patient upright using a film-to-focus distance (FFD) of 1.8 m and 5 degrees caudal angulation of the x-ray beam. In supine patients, the FFD should be 1.1 m with a perpendicular x-ray beam. Consistency in technique and positioning is critical for optimal evaluation on serial examinations. Whenever possible, care should be taken to remove extrinsic tubing and objects from the patient's chest before exposure.

The development in recent years of digital alternatives to conventional x-ray films (computed radiography and direct radiography) provides wide exposure latitude, enabling image manipulation and reducing the need for reexposures. Although the spatial resolution of digital images is slightly inferior to conventional radiographs, this is generally considered insignificant in situations requiring portable radiography.

Image viewing

Prompt availability of images and reports are essential to maximize the efficacy of bedside radiography. Digital imaging and Picture Archiving and Communication System networks (PACS) have become commonplace in recent years. The PACS systems should significantly reduce the time between request and image availability on critical care, but this does not necessarily have a measurable impact on the time clinical actions are initiated. This may be because of organizational factors, such as timing of ward rounds, rather than image availability, particularly for 'routine' examinations.

Optimal viewing of conventional films requires bright light boxes; however, typical high-resolution

Table 18.1 Uses of chest radiographs in critical care

Cardiac and mediastinal silhouettes
Pulmonary parenchyma
Pneumothorax
Effusion
Indication of fluid balance

PACS monitors have a lighting output of one tenth of that of a conventional light box. Therefore, the relative balance between monitor light output and background lighting plays an important role in image interpretation in the critical care environment. Lack of control over ambient lighting means it may not be optimal for image interpretation. Ideally, PACS monitors should be in an area with adjustable, glare-free, indirect lighting. Blinds and shades should be used to control outside lighting where necessary. Walls should be painted dark to avoid reflection and improve contrast.

The top edge of the display terminal should be no higher than eye level. The current recommendation is for the top edge to be 15 to 50 degrees below eye level. The eye-to-screen distance should be at least 25 inches (62.5 cm) and preferably greater, so that the focusing muscles of the eye are not strained. The top of the monitor should be slightly farther from the eyes than the bottom of the monitor. Sequential films should be available for review. A combination of high- and medium-resolution dual-monitor display stations are recommended. The implementation of a continuing quality improvement to facilitate PACS training, workflow modifications, quality assurance and clinical acceptance are essential.

Interpretation of critical care chest radiographs

An appreciation of normal postoperative findings after cardiothoracic surgery is essential when interpreting critical care films. A systematic approach to the portable radiographs is required. It is good practice to check the position of all lines, tubes and intravascular catheters before evaluating the heart, mediastinum, lungs and pleural space. Knowledge of their normal position and recognition of abnormal positioning is essential when interpreting postoperative chest radiographs.

Lines and tubes

VENTILATORY SUPPORT

Endotracheal tube malposition is a frequent complication in patients receiving respiratory support. Studies have shown that the endotracheal tube tip may move on average 1.9 cm toward the carina with head flexion and 1.9 cm away from the carina on extension. Optimal endotracheal tube position is with the tip in the mid trachea, approximately 5 to 6 cm above the carina with the head in the neutral position. This ensures safe positioning independent of neck position. If the carina is not clearly visible on the radiograph, its position may be estimated by comparison with previous portable chest radiographs or from the knowledge that the carina is usually at the level of the fifth or sixth thoracic vertebral body. On digital radiographs, adjusting the window setting may facilitate identification of the carina. Radiographic assessment may be more accurate than clinical examination, because of unpredictable differences in anatomy and difficulty in auscultation of breath sounds.

A well-placed tracheostomy tube should lie parallel to the tracheal long axis and be approximately one half to two thirds the tracheal diameter; the cuff should hug but not distend the tracheal wall. The tip should be located one half to two thirds the distance between tracheal stoma and carina, at approximately the level of the third thoracic vertebral body. Neck flexion and extension do not affect the position of the tracheostomy tube.

VASCULAR ACCESS, MONITORING AND SUPPORT

To reliably reflect central venous pressure, the central venous catheter tip should lie between right atrium and the most proximal venous valves, which are found in the subclavian and internal jugular veins approximately 2.5 cm from their confluence. On chest radiographs, both line position and line-related complications may be assessed. The catheter tip should be visualized between the origin of the superior vena cava (SVC), medial to the anterior portion of the first rib, and the right atrium.

The pulmonary artery catheter (PAC) tip should be 5 to 7 cm distal to the main pulmonary artery bifurcation. Ideally, the tip of the PAC should reside within a large pulmonary artery and should not be located peripheral to the interlobar pulmonary artery that forms the hilum of each lung. An upper lobe PAC can result in an inaccurate wedge pressure measurement. A coil of the PAC in the heart may cause arrhythmias or cause subsequent balloon migration into a segmental vessel.

The balloon of the intra-aortic balloon pump (IABP) has a radiopaque tip, which should be positioned just distal to the origin of the left subclavian artery at the level of the aortic knob.

PACING DEVICES

Temporary epicardial pacing wires are seen as fine radiopaque wires adjacent to the right atrial and right ventricular margins on postoperative radiographs.

During single-chamber ventricular pacing, the tip of a transvenous pacing device should lie within the right ventricle; during biventricular pacing, the distal tip of the right ventricular lead should lie within the right ventricular apex and the left ventricular lead in the coronary sinus.

MEDIASTINAL AND PLEURAL TUBES

Mediastinal drains are generally manufactured with radiopaque stripes to allow radiographic identification. If the chest tube has side holes, these should lie within the pleural space.

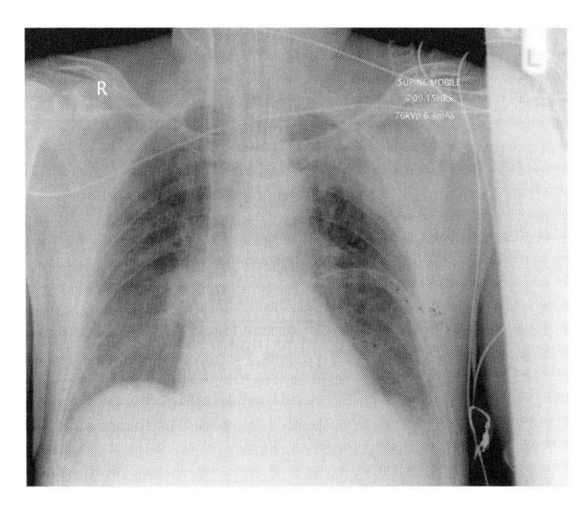

Figure 18.1 Supine chest radiograph showing a malpositioned IABP. The tip is projected too proximally over the aortic knob. The PAC is coiled across the tricuspid valve, with the tip in the right ventricle. The endotracheal tube and intercostal drains are correctly positioned.

NASOGASTRIC TUBES

Nasogastric tubes may easily be identified, and their tip is also radiopaque.

CORONARY ARTERY BYPASS GRAFT MARKERS

The location of the vein graft anastomoses may be marked with either large wire circles around the ostia or small, washer-like markers. Such markers are useful to the cardiologist when localizing grafts for catheterization during subsequent angiography. Haemostatic clips, used to ligate intercostal arteries when the internal mammary artery is used for bypass grafting, are commonly seen on follow-up chest radiographs and should not be confused with the IABP catheter tip.

Cardiopulmonary abnormalities

ATELECTASIS

Atelectasis is a common finding after cardiothoracic or abdominal surgery. When atelectasis is due to multiple peripheral mucus plugs, pulmonary

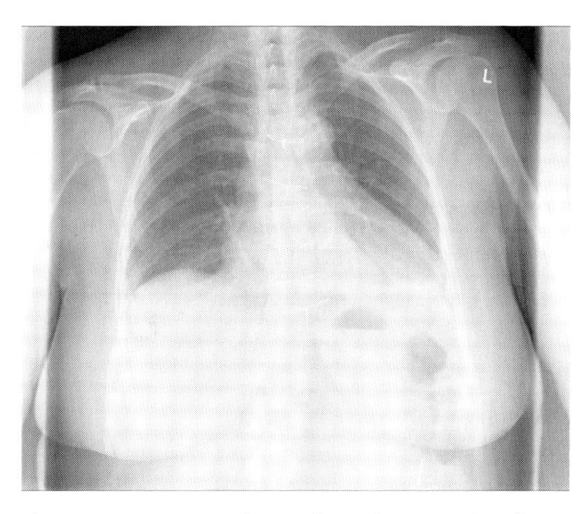

Figure 18.2 Erect PA chest radiograph post aortic valve replacement demonstrates a left lower lobe collapse as a triangular density behind the heart ('sail sign') obscuring the medial aspect of the left hemidiaphragm and descending aorta.

consolidation rather than volume loss may be the dominant radiologic feature. Areas of atelectasis tend to change rapidly and often clear rapidly after suctioning or physiotherapy. In ventilated patients, atelectasis occurs more frequently in the left lower lobe (66%) than the right lower (22%) or right upper lobes (11%).

Although a chest radiograph may be normal in the presence of mild atelectasis, typical radiographic features include the presence of opaque, linear bands or plate atelectasis, which usually predominates in the lower lobes. Patchy, segmental or complete lobar consolidation is less common. Lobar atelectasis, defined by complete lobar collapse and mediastinal shift, represents one extreme form of postoperative atelectasis. Increased density behind the heart and loss of the normal silhouettes of the left hemidiaphragm and descending aorta are common radiographic features of significant left lower lobe collapse.

ASPIRATION PNEUMONITIS

Radiographic sequelae develop within hours of the aspiration of gastric contents and consist of infiltrates, which are usually bilateral patchy and diffuse or mainly right sided, and often progress over the first 24 to 48 hours. In the uncomplicated case, there is usually evidence of stability or regression by 72 hours with complete clearing within 1 week. Predominant involvement of the dependent lung regions results in consolidation in the lower zones and medially in the mid zones owing to involvement of the apical segments of the lower lobes.

PNEUMONIA

The radiographic features of progressive air–space consolidation may not be reliable in the critical care setting and, although the pulmonary findings may progress rapidly over several days, the temporal appearance is seldom as rapid as that seen with atelectasis, aspiration pneumonitis or pulmonary oedema. Clinical correlation can be difficult; cavitation and effusion are frequent in nosocomial pneumonia.

PULMONARY OEDEMA

Portable radiography in the critical care setting may be unreliable in differentiating increased permeability oedema (sepsis, acute lung injury [ALI]) from hydrostatic pulmonary oedema (left ventricular failure, fluid overload). The distribution of pulmonary vascularity on chest radiographs is determined by the position of the patient and intravascular volume. The normal vascular pattern in the erect patient is that the lower lung zone vessels carry greater blood flow than the upper zone vessels because of the effect of gravity and are therefore visibly larger. In the supine patient, pulmonary vascular redistribution to the upper zones is a normal finding.

Hydrostatic pulmonary oedema

This is manifested by decreased flow through the dependent microcirculation secondary to interstitial oedema, coupled with shunting of flow to the nondependent lung zone vessels. In the erect position this results in 'upper lobe redistribution,' or an inverted blood flow pattern compared with normal. However, preexisting pulmonary disease, such as emphysema or pulmonary fibrosis, can significantly alter the pulmonary vascularity and compromise the ability to correctly determine vascular pattern on the chest radiograph.

Features on the supine radiograph that may facilitate the detection of volume overload include change in the heart size, vascular pedicle or vessel calibre on serial radiography obtained using the same technique. Determination of changes in cardiac size on serial portable chest radiographs can be hazardous but, in general, there should be no more than 2 cm variation in transverse cardiac diameter. The vascular pedicle width is typically normal or narrowed in capillary permeability oedema or acute cardiac failure and widened in volume overload, renal failure and cardiac failure. However, the vascular pedicle width is also affected by rotation, supine position and ventilatory pressure.

In hydrostatic pulmonary oedema as the left atrial pressure increases (18–22 mmHg), interstitial oedema develops resulting in thickening of the walls and ill-definition of the bronchi and vessels (peribronchial cuffing). Kerley B or septal lines represent thickening of the interlobular septa and are seen as fine linear structures lying perpendicular to and extending to the pleural surface. Kerley B lines are common in hydrostatic pulmonary oedema, but uncommon in capillary permeability oedema. As the left atrial pressure increases beyond 25 mmHg, alveolar oedema develops. Radiographically this is characterized by ill-defined, air space opacities in the perihilar or lower lung zones. Pleural effusions that accompany congestive cardiac failure are frequently bilateral, but larger on the right. When an effusion associated with hydrostatic pulmonary oedema is unilateral, it is usually – but not always – on the right.

Pulmonary oedema may also have an asymmetrical distribution owing to positioning of the patient (e.g. decubitus position). Oedema may be inhomogeneous in patients with chronic pulmonary disease or pulmonary emboli.

Capillary permeability oedema

The characteristic radiographic pattern follows a predictable sequence mirroring the histopathological changes of exudative, proliferative and repair phases. Initially in the first 24 hours after insult, when there is little alveolar oedema, the chest radiograph is generally normal with the exception of ALI secondary to direct lung injury (e.g. aspiration pneumonia). As ALI evolves, widespread ground glass opacification with increased lung density obscuring lung markings becomes apparent and during the next 36 hours, with greater exudation of inflammatory fluid into the interstitium and air space, there is frank consolidation on the chest radiograph. Airspace opacification on the chest radiograph is a typical but not pathognomonic feature of ALI.

The radiographic changes of uncomplicated ALI usually plateau after the initial bilateral airspace consolidation and remain unchanged for a variable time. Awareness of this radiographically stable phase is important and sequential review of serial critical care chest radiographs can aid diagnosis. Any new focal areas of consolidation raise the possibility of nosocomial pneumonia. In the final phase, the chest radiograph abnormalities begin to resolve.

PULMONARY EMBOLISM

The diagnosis of pulmonary embolism in the critical care environment is difficult. Radiographic findings may include a normal chest radiograph, peripheral wedge-shaped pulmonary opacities, atelectasis, elevation of the diaphragm, pleural effusions and focal oligaemia. Computed tomography pulmonary angiography is the imaging modality of choice in establishing the diagnosis or making an alternative diagnosis.

PLEURAL EFFUSION

Pleural effusions are common in patients who have undergone thoracotomy or median sternotomy. Large pleural effusions or those that increase rapidly in size may be due to haemorrhage or empyema. Portable ultrasound is a valuable bedside tool and can demonstrate loculation and guide drainage. Pleural effusion persisting beyond the third postoperative day in cardiac patients may signal the onset of a postpericardiotomy syndrome and can be accompanied by a pericardial effusion and pulmonary parenchymal opacity. Pleural effusion secondary to subdiaphragmatic abscesses rarely appears until the second postoperative week. The radiographic manifestations of pleural fluid on supine radiographs include homogenous increased density of the affected hemithorax without obscuration of the vascular markings, loss of the silhouette of the hemidiaphragm, decreased visibility of the lower lobe vasculature, apical capping and thickened horizontal fissure.

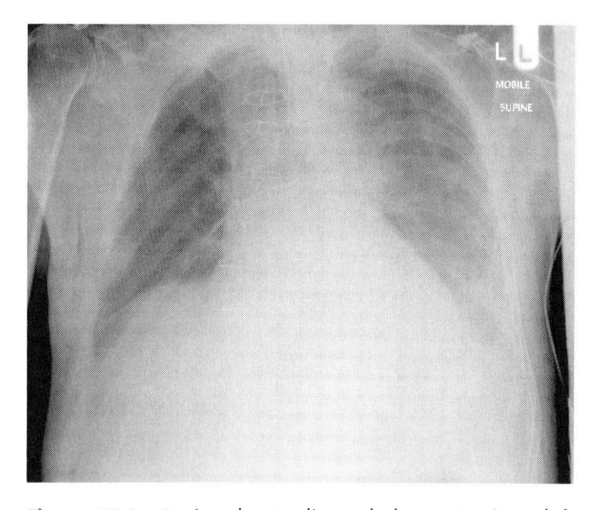

Figure 18.3 Supine chest radiograph demonstrating a left pleural effusion and a malpositioned Swan-Ganz catheter. There is homogenous increased density of the left hemithorax with obscuration of the left hemidiaphragm and of the pulmonary vasculature. The tip of the Swan-Ganz catheter is located in the right interlobar artery and, therefore, should be withdrawn 3 to 4 cm.

ABNORMAL AIR COLLECTIONS

Pneumothorax, pneumomediastinum and subcutaneous emphysema are frequently present after median sternotomy or can occur as a complication of mechanical ventilation. In the ventilated patient, once an air leak has developed, it can rapidly increase in size with the development of a tension pneumothorax. Size measurements of pneumothorax on chest radiographs correlate poorly with measurement obtained by computed tomography. Shift of the mediastinum to the contralateral side of a pneumothorax is suggestive of tension on radiological grounds. However, particularly in patients with ALI or pleural adhesions, the diagnosis of tension pneumothorax is primarily based on clinical findings because there may be little or no shift of the mediastinum. In these patients, the most specific sign (albeit insensitive) is flattening of the heart border and other vascular structures such as the SVC and IVC, reflecting impairment of venous return.

In the supine patient with pneumothorax, air rises anteriorly and medially within the pleural space. This may be difficult to appreciate on the supine chest radiograph or may mimic a pneumomediastinum or pneumopericardium. A deep lateral costophrenic angle, the 'deep sulcus sign,' on the involved side with crisp outlines to the diaphragm and heart border may be the only radiographic findings on the supine chest radiograph.

Artefacts such as skin folds, bandages or superimposition of the arms may all mimic pneumothorax. Pneumopericardium is manifested by a lucent rim around the heart, extending only as high as the main pulmonary artery on the upright radiograph. On the supine radiograph, however, pneumopericardium can be misinterpreted as a pneumothorax or pneumomediastinum; air cannot be seen entirely around the base of the heart. A decubitus film usually resolves the problem. In patients who have a pericardial–pleural window, an ipsilateral pneumothorax may result in pneumopericardium.

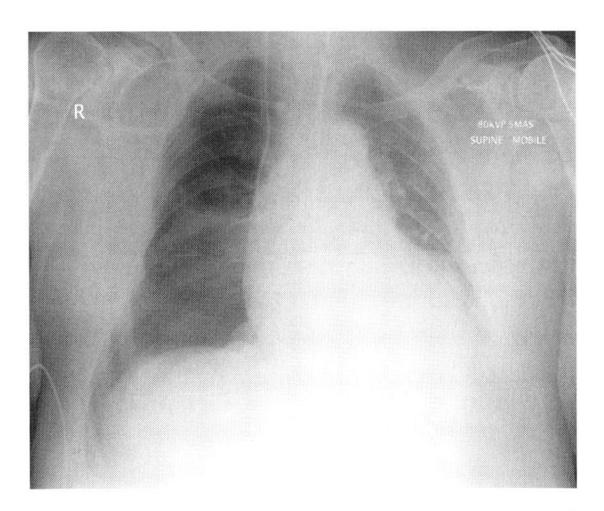

Figure 18.4 Supine right pneumothorax. The mediastinal contours, right atrial border and anterior aspect of the right hemidiaphragm are crisp, consistent with an anterior pneumothorax. A deep lateral costophrenic angle ('deep sulcus sign') is present.

Shifting pneumothorax is a specific complication in lung and heart transplant recipients owing to disruption of the normal anatomy. After bilateral lung transplantation (and occasionally after heart transplant), the two hemithoraces are in continuity so pneumothoraces are commonly bilateral. In this situation, a pneumothorax can shift from side to side on sequential chest radiographs.

A benign, self-limiting pneumoperitoneum may occasionally occur after cardiac surgery as a result of a long median sternotomy incision extending below the diaphragm or after subxiphoid tunnelling of epicardial pacing wires postoperatively or insertion of mediastinal drains.

CARDIOMEDIASTINAL OUTLINE

The initial postoperative film is the best baseline for subsequent change in mediastinal width. The mean increase in mediastinal width from preoperative posteroanterior to postoperative AP supine radiograph may be up to 35% in stable patients without evidence of bleeding. Massive haemorrhage is often associated with an increase in mediastinal width of more than double the baseline, but occasionally the width may remain within the normal range. Additional signs of mediastinal haemorrhage include apical soft tissue and pleural effusions.

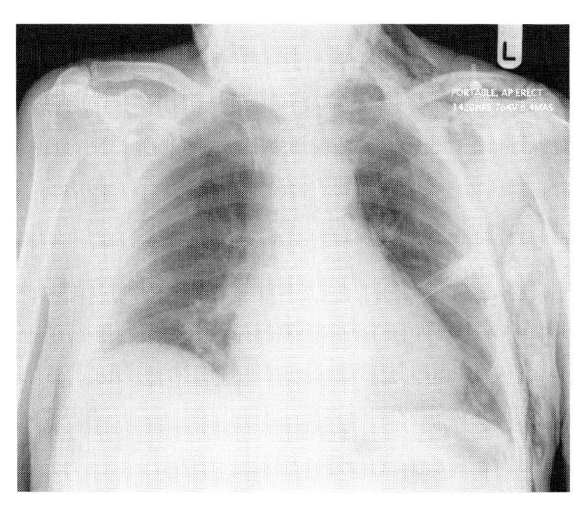

Figure 18.5 An AP erect chest radiograph post double lung transplant showing extensive pneumomediastinum, with a lucent rim around the left heart border and aortic knob. There is a left intercostal drain and no pneumothorax. Extensive surgical emphysema is present in the subcutaneous tissues over the left chest and supraclavicular fossae.

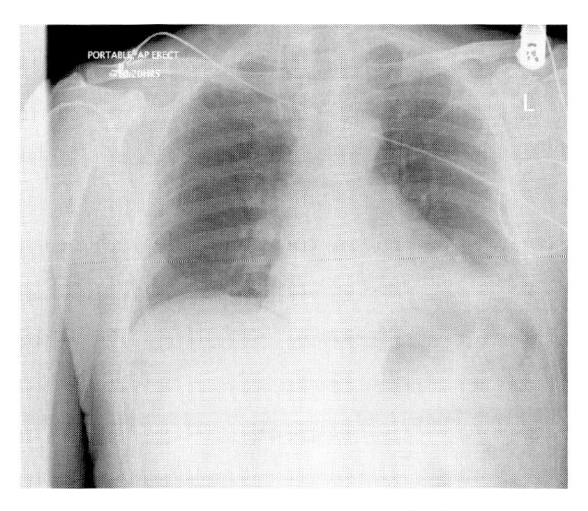

Figure 18.6 An AP erect chest radiograph after coronary artery bypass grafting demonstrates a lucent rim beneath the right hemidiaphragm, consistent, in the absence of abdominal signs or symptoms, with a benign pneumoperitoneum.

Key points

- Optimal radiographic technique is essential to maximize the efficacy and accuracy of bedside radiography.
- Appropriate viewing conditions and review of the film series improve diagnostic interpretation.
- A systematic approach to the portable chest radiograph is important and appreciation of the normal vascular redistribution pattern and the distribution of pleural fluid and air in the supine patient is essential.
- Alternative imaging techniques are useful, including bedside ultrasound to determine the presence and size of fluid collections and identify a safe site for drainage.

FURTHER READING

Aberle DR, Wiener-Kronish JP, Webb WR, *et al.* Hydrostatic versus increased permeability pulmonary edema: diagnosis based on radiographic criteria in critically ill patients. *Radiology* 1988;168:73–79.

Krivopal M, Shlobin OA, Schwartzstein RM. Utility of daily routine portable chest radiographs in mechanically ventilated patients in the medical ICU. *Chest* 2003;123:1607–1614.

Making the Best Use of a Department of Clinical Radiology: Guidelines for Doctors. The Royal College of Radiologists; 2003. Available at: www.rcr.ac.uk.

Watkins J, Weatherburn G, Bryan S. The impact of a picture archiving and communication system (PACS) upon an intensive care unit. *Eur J Radiol* 2000;34:3–8.

SECTION 3 System Management in Cardiothoracic Critical Care

3.1 *Cardiovascular System in Cardiothoracic Critical Care*

Chapter 19

Rhythms

L.S. RING AND S.P. FYNN

Introduction

Arrhythmias are a common problem in the cardiothoracic critical care unit. Although a broad spectrum of arrhythmia types and mechanisms are possible, atrial fibrillation (AF) and ventricular tachycardia (VT) are the commonest tachycardias encountered. Bradycardias, such as atrioventricular block (AV block) or sinoatrial disease, can also be problematic. These rhythm disturbances often require prompt recognition and treatment. Failure to do so may result in life-threatening cardiac events.

Atrial arrhythmias

Atrial fibrillation

The most common postoperative arrhythmia, AF usually happens within the first 4 to 5 days after cardiac surgery. It occurs in approximately 30% of all postcardiac surgical patients, although up to 60% of those undergoing valve repair or replacement may be affected. The risk of developing postoperative AF depends on a number of preexisting and perioperative factors.

The mechanism of postoperative AF is unknown. However, inflammation has been shown to play a role. Patients with higher C-reactive protein levels after cardiac surgery have a greater chance of developing AF. There is some evidence that off-pump surgery reduces inflammation and postoperative AF, although this has not been confirmed in randomized controlled trials. The development of AF in the early postoperative period has an adverse effect on prognosis, with a threefold increase in risk of stroke, plus an increased incidence of myocardial infarction, ventricular arrhythmias, cardiac failure and the need for mechanical circulatory support. Postoperative AF increases the overall hospital stay by an average of 3 days, and recurrent AF is the commonest cause of hospital readmission after discharge after cardiac surgery.

PREVENTING POSTOPERATIVE ATRIAL FIBRILLATION

Although AF may occur in the postoperative setting without any obvious precipitating factors, the chances of developing this arrhythmia can be reduced by ensuring that there are no significant electrolyte abnormalities (especially hypokalaemia), and that hypoxia, acidosis and infection are treated promptly.

β-Blockers are widely used to prevent postoperative AF and can be administered very soon after surgery. If patients are taking β-blockers before cardiac surgery, withdrawal of these drugs results in a significantly increased risk of AF. Some clinicians advocate the routine administration of magnesium plus β-blockers after cardiac surgery because this combination may be significantly more effective than β-blockade alone.

There is some evidence that sotalol and calcium channel blockers can also be effective in preventing AF, although the most effective drug currently available is amiodarone. However, amiodarone has

Table 19.1 Risk factors for developing postoperative AF

Preoperative	Intraoperative	Postoperative
Elderly	Mitral valve surgery	Hypoxia
Chronic airway disease	Cardiac venting via right superior pulmonary vein	Acidosis
Bradycardia	Prolonged cross-clamping time	Electrolytes abnormalities (hypokalaemia, hypomagnesaemia)
Hypertension		

limitations as it requires a period of loading before it reaches a therapeutic level. The drug is also associated with an array of side effects. For these reasons, it is recommended that the use of amiodarone for the prevention of postoperative AF should be for the short term only. There is no evidence to support the use of digoxin to reduce the risk of AF. In fact, its use before cardiac surgery has been associated with an increased risk of postoperative AF.

The administration of statins perioperatively has been shown to reduce the incidence of AF, as well as the incidence of major adverse cardiac events. Their mechanism of action is unknown, although an anti-inflammatory action has been postulated.

Epicardial pacing wires are routine after cardiac surgery and they may be used to prevent AF. Atrial overdrive pacing (atrial pacing above the intrinsic sinus rate) may be effective. Initial studies had shown that biatrial pacing may be the best approach, although this method has not gained widespread acceptance. Asynchronous ventricular pacing is known to increase the chance of developing postoperative AF.

TREATING POSTOPERATIVE ATRIAL FIBRILLATION

Any precipitating factors, as described, should be identified and treated if possible. Consideration must be given to the need for anticoagulation. Left atrial thrombus can form within 24 to 48 hours of the onset of AF; therefore, heparin or warfarin must be started. This may need to be continued for some time, particularly if the patient is deemed to be at risk of further AF and has other risk factors for thromboembolic disease (advanced age, cardiac failure, diabetes, hypertension and previous stroke).

RESTORING SINUS RHYTHM

Generally, at least one attempt to restore sinus rhythm should be made if postoperative AF develops. This can be done either in the acute setting of the critical care unit (especially if the patient is haemodynamically compromised) or at a later date. Restoration of sinus rhythm is most effectively achieved through synchronized DC cardioversion. This approach results in sinus rhythm in at least 80% of cases. If there is significant haemodynamic compromise, emergency cardioversion is required.

Chemical cardioversion, using pharmacological agents, is an alternative to the electrical approach. The most effective drug is amiodarone, which if started soon after the onset of AF, may restore sinus rhythm in 60% to 90% of cases. Other antiarrhythmic drugs such as sotalol, β-blockers and calcium channel blockers can be used in an attempt to restore sinus rhythm, although they are less effective than amiodarone. Class I antiarrhythmic drugs (e.g. flecainide, propafenone) are very effective at chemically cardioverting acute-onset AF but may be proarrhythmic and therefore should be avoided.

VENTRICULAR RATE CONTROL IN ATRIAL FIBRILLATION

If an attempt to restore sinus rhythm is unsuccessful, it is important to control the heart rate in AF. This minimizes the haemodynamic consequences and symptoms associated with AF. The drugs of choice in this setting include β-blockers, calcium blockers and digoxin.

Atrial flutter

Atrial flutter is commonly seen after cardiac surgery and the precipitating factors are the same as those that cause AF. The usual type of atrial flutter (so-called typical flutter) is a macroreentrant circuit involving the tricuspid annulus. The waveform rotates around the annulus at approximately 300 times per minute, although, because of this rapid rate of depolarization, only alternate waveforms are able to conduct through the AV node, giving rise to a ventricular rate that is regular and usually at 150 or less commonly at 75 beats per minute. The electrocardiographic (ECG) pattern of atrial flutter has a characteristic appearance

TREATMENT

The management of atrial flutter is similar to that of AF and anticoagulation is required. An attempt at restoring sinus rhythm is usually appropriate and synchronized DC cardioversion is the most effective method. Pharmacological agents (amiodarone, sotalol) are far less effective and the class IC antiarrhythmic drug group are contraindicated. These drugs (flecainide, propafenone) can slow the

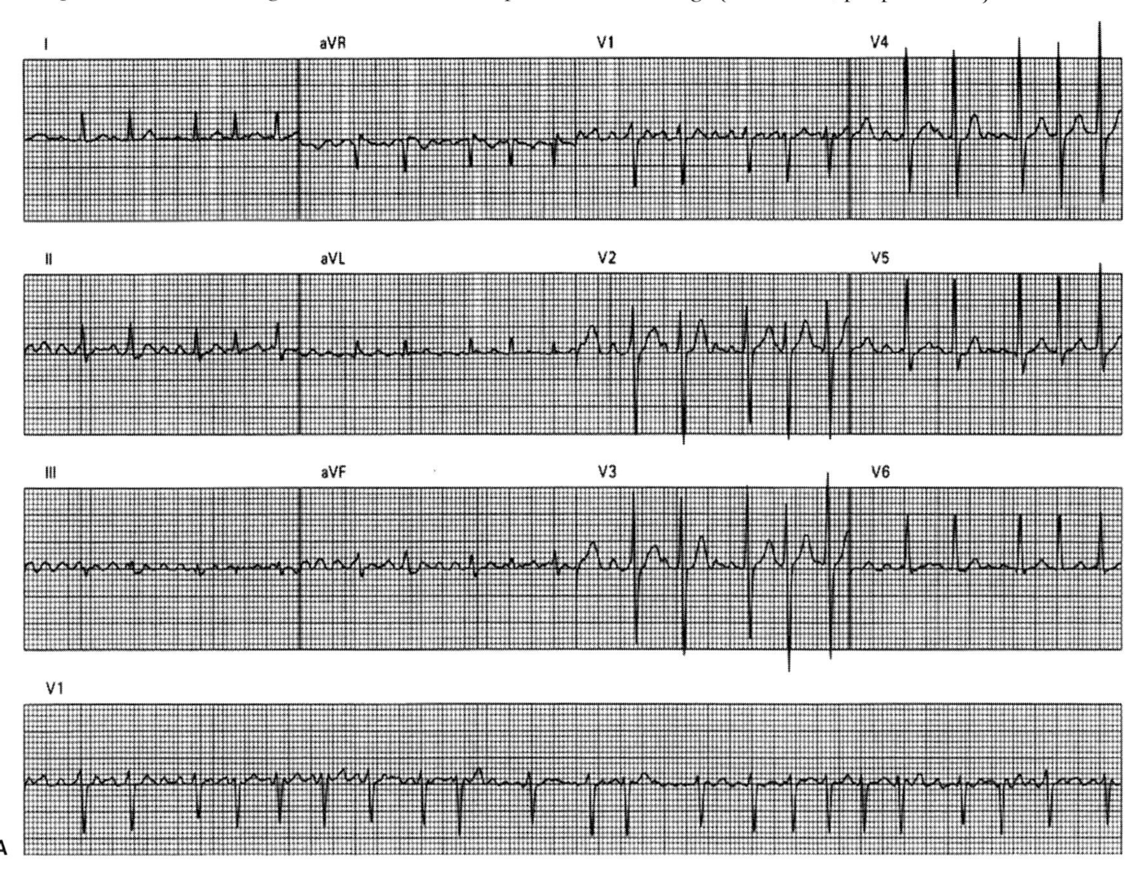

Figure 19.1 The ECG recordings of (*A*) AF and (*B*) atrial flutter. (*A*) Atrial fibrillation results in an irregularly irregular ventricular rate. Atrial fibrillatory waves can be seen between the QRS complexes. Although in some leads these waves appear coarse, they are clearly different to the regular atrial activity seen in atrial flutter. (*continued*)

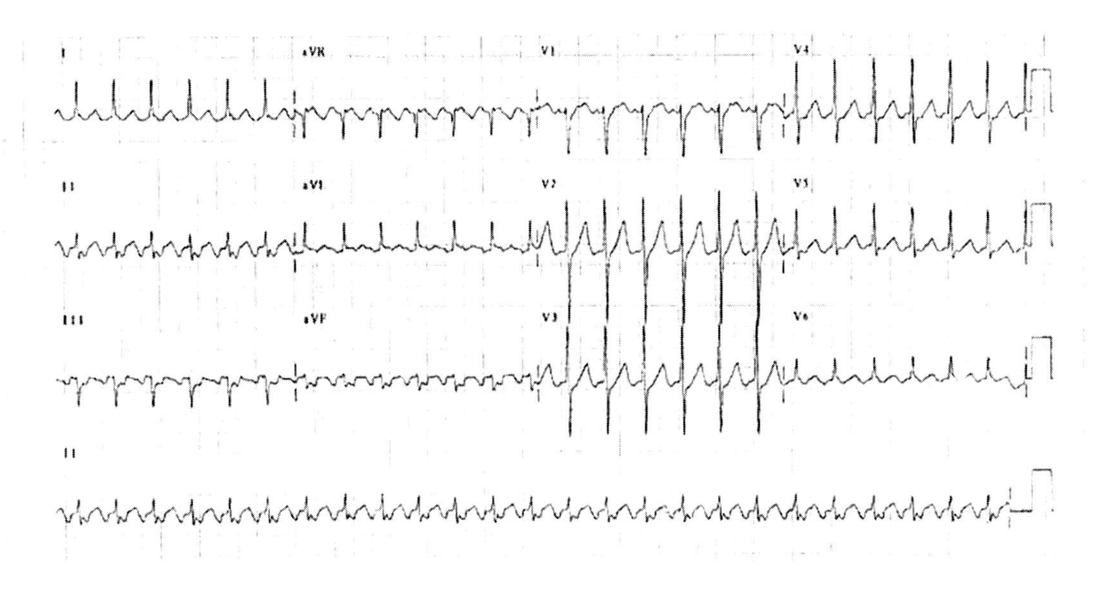

Figure 19.1 (*B*) An ECG of atrial flutter with 2:1 conduction block to the ventricles giving rise to a regular ventricular rate of 150 bpm. The atrial activation appears as a characteristic 'saw-tooth' pattern in leads II, III and aVF.

rate of the flutter circuit around the annulus, potentially allowing the AV node to conduct each flutter waveform through to the ventricles, resulting in heart rates of 250 to 300 bpm. In contrast to AF, overdrive atrial pacing (atrial pacing at a rate slightly faster than the flutter rate) can occasionally terminate atrial flutter. However, this may result in the atrial flutter degenerating into AF.

In the unusual case of atrial flutter not responding to these approaches and causing significant haemodynamic effects in the critical care unit, consideration can be given to percutaneous radiofrequency catheter ablation. Radiofrequency energy is delivered at the cavotricuspid isthmus to prevent the flutter circuit forming around the tricuspid annulus. This procedure, which is now a routine, first-line approach for many patients with atrial flutter in the 'nonacute' setting, has a success rate of more than 90% with a complication rate of less than 1%.

Ventricular arrhythmias

Ventricular arrhythmias after cardiac surgery can be life threatening. Prompt recognition and treatment of these arrhythmias are essential. Any causative factors must also be identified and rectified to reduce early postoperative mortality.

Ventricular tachycardia

Ventricular tachycardia is a broad complex rhythm (QRS width $\geq$120 ms) at a rate of at least 120 bpm, and is defined as sustained if lasting longer than 30 seconds. Ventricular tachycardia increases myocardial oxygen demand and can 'degenerate' into ventricular fibrillation. If the QRS morphology is constant, the VT is classed as monomorphic. However, there may be a beat-to-beat variation in the QRS axis during VT, so-called polymorphic VT.

POLYMORPHIC VENTRICULAR TACHYCARDIA

This can be due to ischaemia (e.g. graft occlusion, incomplete revascularization) or extreme electrolyte imbalance. Other potentially reversible causes of VT should also be considered.

If the VT is due to abnormal repolarization of the myocardium (manifest on the ECG as prolongation

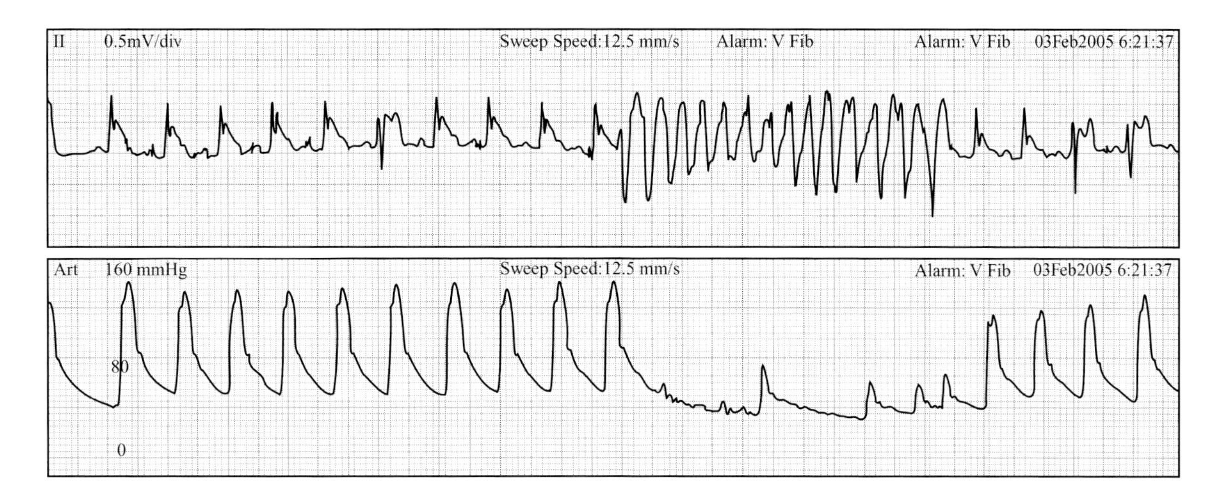

Figure 19.2 Polymorphic VT. These recordings are taken from a cardiac monitor in a patient 2 days after CABG. The upper tracing is an ECG showing a nonsustained episode of polymorphic VT. In sinus rhythm, significant ST segment elevation can be seen. The lower tracing is a simultaneous pressure waveform from an arterial line and shows severe hypotension during the VT. Angiography revealed an occluded bypass graft to the right coronary artery.

of the QT interval), it is termed *torsade de pointes*. This type of VT can also be caused by ischaemia or electrolyte imbalance, but is more often due to the proarrhythmic effects of drugs, particularly antiarrhythmic drugs. The mechanism of action is usually via inhibition of potassium channel (K^+) function. However, there is an increasing recognition that other 'noncardiac' drugs can also affect K^+ channel function.

Treatment

Sustained polymorphic VT is life threatening and requires immediate defibrillation. The treatment of nonsustained polymorphic VT may simply involve the recognition of the causative factor and its subsequent withdrawal (e.g. antiarrhythmic drugs causing QT prolongation on the ECG) or correction (e.g. electrolyte abnormalities). If ischaemia is suspected, early consideration should be given to

Table 19.2 Postoperative causes of ventricular tachycardia

Hypoxia	Acidosis	Ischaemia
Hypovolaemia	Antiarrhythmics*	
Hypothermia	Antibiotics*	
Hypo/Hyper K^+*	Antidepressants*	
Hypomagnesaemia*		
Hypocalcaemia*		

**Can prolong the QT interval on the ECG and cause torsades de pointes.*

Table 19.3 Differential diagnosis of broad complex tachycardia

Favours VT	Favours supraventricular tachycardia with bundle branch block
AV dissociation	Marked irregularity in the heart rate
Fusion and capture beats	QRS morphology identical to that in SR
Extreme cardiac axis deviation	Terminates with adenosine
QRS duration >150 ms	
Concordance of QRS across praecordium	

Abbreviations: AV, atrioventricular; VT, ventricular tachycardia.

coronary and graft angiography. There is some evidence that intravenous magnesium may be effective in the acute setting. If the VT is bradycardia-dependent, pacing the right ventricle (either through epicardial wires placed at the time of surgery or transvenously) may be antiarrhythmic.

MONOMORPHIC VENTRICULAR TACHYCARDIA

This form of VT is usually in the setting of an existing myocardial scar from previous infarction. Monomorphic VT is initiated by trigger beats, usually ventricular ectopics, which are common after cardiac surgery. The scar provides a barrier around which a stable electrical wavefront can rotate. Modulating factors such as electrolyte abnormalities, acidosis and hypoxia can increase the frequency of ectopy and alter the electrical properties of the myocardium to increase the likelihood of VT being initiated and maintained. In patients undergoing coronary artery bypass grafting (CABG), revascularizing areas of previous infarction or peri-infarction can itself be arrhythmogenic. In patients undergoing cardiac surgery with previous myocardial infarction and impaired left ventricular function, there is a 30% incidence of postoperative VT.

Treatment

Monomorphic VT causing haemodynamic compromise requires prompt electrical cardioversion. Any electrolyte and metabolic abnormalities should be corrected; if ischaemia is suspected, coronary and graft angiography should be considered. Concomitant antiarrhythmic drug therapy is usually also necessary. Cardioselective β-blockers can be effective for ischaemic VT, although the drug now generally used as first-line therapy for VT is amiodarone. This needs to be given through a large vein and often higher doses are required than for atrial arrhythmias (5–10 g, at 1.2 g/d). Lidocaine works more quickly than amiodarone and can be effective in terminating an acute episode of VT. However, unlike amiodarone, this drug has significantly negative inotropic effects and is contraindicated in patients with impaired cardiac function. Although very effective at suppressing ventricular ectopy, class I antiarrhythmic drugs should be avoided if possible in patients with VT and ischaemic heart disease. Class IC drugs (e.g. flecainide) are absolutely contraindicated, whereas the class IA drugs (e.g. procainamide) may be used if β-blockers and amiodarone are ineffective.

Temporary ventricular pacing may be used either to prevent the onset of bradycardia-dependent VT, or to terminate recurrent sustained VT by 'overdrive' pacing. Where VT persists despite antiarrhythmic drugs, more aggressive strategies may be considered. Percutaneous radiofrequency catheter ablation has a greater than 75% success rate in the

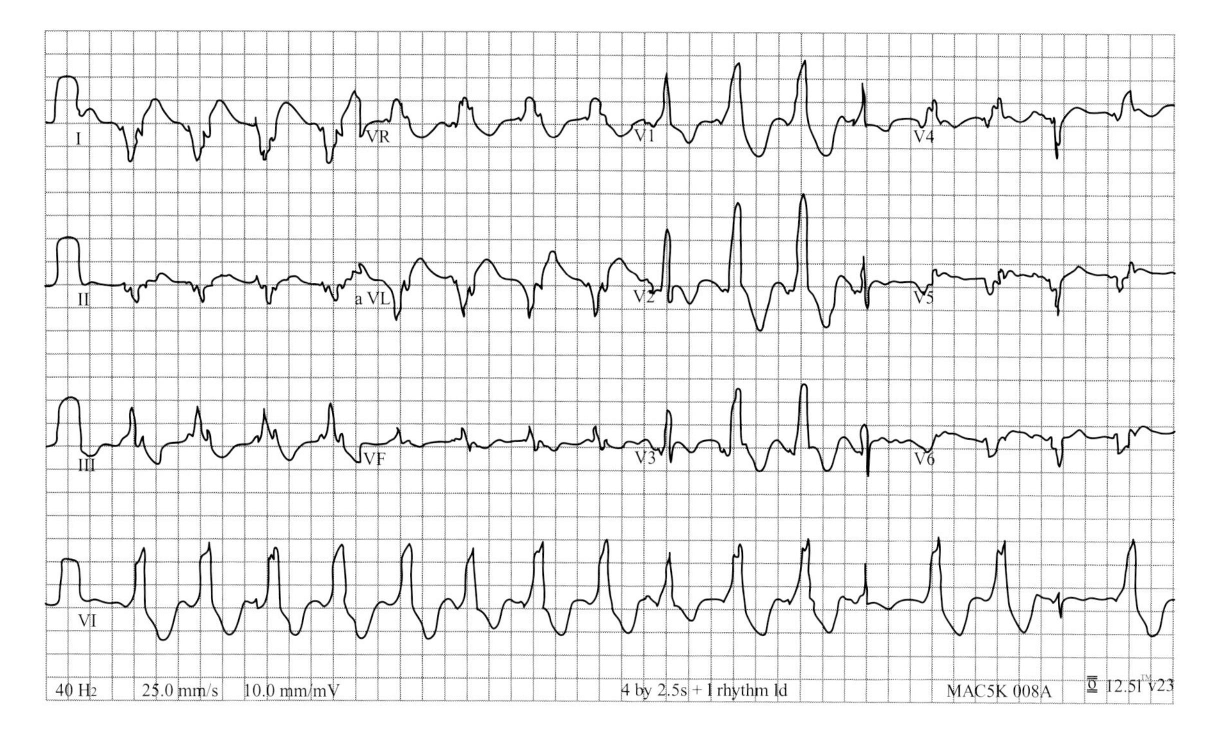

Figure 19.3 Monomorphic VT. An ECG of broad complex tachycardia with extreme axis deviation. The 9th and 12th QRS complexes are 'fusion' beats, in which the resultant QRS morphology is due to a combination of ventricular depolarization, partly via the tachycardia circuit and partly via the AV node. The penultimate (narrow) beat is a 'capture' beat, in which the ventricle is depolarized purely via the AV node. These ECG appearances are pathognomic for VT.

setting of haemodynamically stable and well-tolerated monomorphic VT. However, such an approach carries with it a 5% risk of serious complication (cardiac tamponade, stroke).

Implantable cardiac defibrillators (ICDs) have no role in the acute management of VT after cardiac surgery. However, new-onset VT after cardiac surgery can recur in up to 35% of patients within the first year. In this cohort of patients who also have significantly impaired left ventricular function, ICDs are far more effective than antiarrhythmic drugs at preventing late sudden cardiac death.

ELECTROCARDIOGRAPHIC DIAGNOSIS OF VENTRICULAR TACHYCARDIA

In the majority of cases, broad complex tachycardia is due to VT. However, on occasion the underlying arrhythmia may be supraventricular tachycardia, which is being conducted with bundle branch block and thus manifesting as a broad complex tachycardia on the ECG. Clues may exist on the ECG to help differentiate this, although if there is any doubt, the default diagnosis is VT.

Bradyarrhythmias

Excessively slow heart rates can be a problem after cardiac surgery. Although these can usually be managed effectively (by cardiac pacing if necessary), sinoatrial arrest or high-grade AV block can result in profound haemodynamic compromise, collapse and even death on occasion.

The mechanism of postoperative bradycardia is often related to the nature of the cardiac surgery that has been undertaken. Furthermore, the underlying

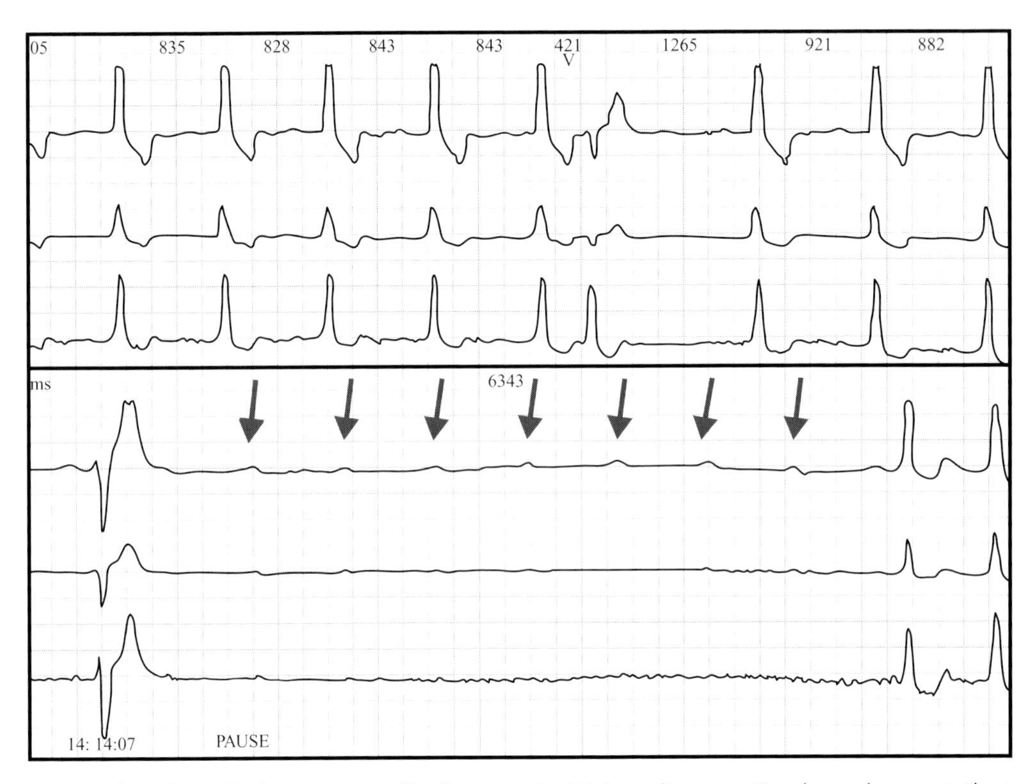

Figure 19.4 High-grade AV block. An ECG recording from a patient 5 days after an aortic valve replacement. The top tracing shows sinus rhythm with a prolonged PR interval and broadened QRS complexes. In the lower tracing, there is a sudden complete failure of AV conduction resulting in a 7-second pause before an escape beat appears. The arrows mark the continuing atrial activity (nonconducted p waves) during the pause. A permanent pacemaker was subsequently implanted.

pathology may itself have caused preoperative, subclinical conduction system disease that is merely exacerbated by surgery. In practice, however, all patients who undergo any form of cardiac surgery should be considered at risk of any type of bradycardia in the early postoperative phase.

Sinoatrial disease

Dysfunction of the sinus node can manifest as sinus bradycardia, sinoatrial exit block ('dropped' p waves) or sinus arrest (long pauses). The latter can predispose to junctional escape rhythms or tachycardia (atrial or ventricular). Surgery involving the right atrium, such as repair of atrial septal defects, carries with it the highest risk of postoperative sinus node dysfunction.

Atrioventricular block and His–Purkinje conduction disturbances

The severity of AV block is generally divided into three degrees, each with their own characteristic ECG pattern. First-degree block usually represents slowing of conduction in the AV node (long PR interval on ECG) and is not clinically significant. Second-degree AV block manifests as occasional failure, usually of the AV node, to conduct to the ventricles, whereas with third-degree (or complete) AV block there is total conduction block between the atrium and ventricles. With the latter the level of conduction failure may be at the AV node or in the more distal His–Purkinje system. Although electrolyte abnormalities, such as hypokalaemia, can affect the conduction properties of the AV node, the aetiology of postoperative AV block is closely linked with the nature of the cardiac surgery. Those patients undergoing either surgery for congenital heart defects or valve surgery are at the highest risk.

The commonest manifestation of conduction system disease after CABG is a combination of block (or slowed conduction) in the right bundle branch and left anterior fascicle of the left bundle branch (so-called bifascicular block). These components of the conduction system are closely approximated after the division of the His bundle, and share the same blood supply. Both structures are therefore often damaged by the same insult, and this manifests on the ECG as right bundle branch block with a leftward cardiac axis.

TREATMENT

Reversal of any electrolyte abnormalities or withdrawal of rate slowing drugs should be simple first-line measures. It is now routine for most cardiac surgical patients to have epicardial temporary pacing wires attached at the time of surgery, which can be removed percutaneously several days later. These wires provide a means by which the heart rate can be increased if necessary in the early postoperative phase. If epicardial wires are not present, temporary transvenous cardiac pacing can be used. The decision to implant a permanent pacemaker can de difficult as it is well recognized that AV block after cardiac surgery may be transient. Guidelines recommend a waiting period of up to 2 weeks postoperative, although nearly all of those patients who regain normal AV conduction usually do so within 9 days of surgery. However, even in these patients there remains a risk of 'late' AV block, which can have potentially catastrophic consequences. Therefore, because permanent pacing generally has a low complication rate, it is reasonable to have a lower threshold for implanting pacemakers in patients with transient complete AV block after cardiac surgery.

Key points

- The most common postoperative arrhythmia, AF may be related to electrolyte disturbance or underlying inflammation.
- Anticoagulation should always be considered if atrial arrhythmias persist or recur.
- Ventricular arrhythmias can be life threatening and must be treated immediately. Underlying ischaemia should be considered.
- Bradyarrhythmia after cardiac surgery usually resolves within 2 weeks and temporary pacing is normally effective until heart rate recovers.

FURTHER READING

Dunning J, Treasure T, Versteegh M, *et al;* EACTS Audit and Guidelines Committee. Guidelines on the prevention and management of de novo atrial fibrillation after cardiac and thoracic surgery. *Eur J Cardiothorac Surg* 2006;30:852–872.

Chapter 20

Basic haemodynamic support

C.J. BROOMHEAD

Introduction

Cardiac surgical patients often present for surgery with impaired ventricular contractility owing to chronic ischaemia or valve lesions. The heart is then subjected to a surgical procedure, which produces a period of global ischaemia and a massive, whole-body inflammatory response. The deleterious effects of cardiopulmonary bypass (CPB) are due to activation of the coagulation, fibrinolytic and complement pathways. This may lead to postoperative adverse effects, including extravascular fluid accumulation or 'third spacing,' coagulopathy and haemorrhage, and pulmonary, renal, cardiac and vasomotor dysfunction.

The perioperative period is often a time of significant haemodynamic and vasomotor instability. Ventricular contractility is usually impaired for up to 24 hours, which may respond to simple supportive measures such as fluid administration. When more severe, there may be a reduction in blood pressure and cardiac output (CO) associated with end-organ dysfunction. Under these circumstances, haemodynamic support is required.

Optimize the heart rate

The CO is a product of stroke volume (SV) and heart rate (HR). Generally, a postoperative HR of 80 to 100 beats per minute is regarded as optimal. The most frequent postoperative rhythm problem is bradycardia. This may be related to preoperative β-blockade or postoperative nodal dysfunction.

Increasing the HR in bradycardic patients improves CO. In addition, by decreasing diastolic filling time and reducing the end-diastolic volume (EDV), left ventricular (LV) wall tension is reduced and the perfusion of the subendocardium is improved, reducing the potential for ischaemia.

The HR is usually increased by epicardial pacing, using wires placed at the time of surgery. Atrial or dual chamber pacing are preferable because they maintain the atrial contribution to CO. If pacing is not an option, isoprenaline, a β2-agonist, may be used.

The infusion rate is increased gradually until the desired increase in HR is achieved. Isoprenaline is generally a well-tolerated chronotrope, and the most common side effect is tachycardia, which is easily treated by reducing the infusion rate. The other common effect of β2-agonism is a reduction in the peripheral vascular resistance owing to vasodilatation (particularly of the skeletal muscle bed), causing hypotension. Often this responds to simple fluid administration, but pharmacological vasoconstriction may be required. Pulmonary vasodilatation is often also produced. This may improve CO by offloading the right ventricle, which is very sensitive to pulmonary hypertension.

Optimize the rhythm

Postoperative dysrhythmias are common after cardiac surgery and these are reviewed in Chapter 19. Ventricular and supraventricular dysrhythmias

Table 20.1 Isoprenaline

Actions	Synthetic catecholamine Direct β1- and β2-agonist
Cardiac effect	Inotropic and marked chronotropic effects
Vascular effects	Marked vasodilation
Advantages	Effective direct β1-agonist Increases CO by increasing HR and contractility and reducing afterload Potent bronchodilator
Disadvantages	Tachycardia – dysrhythmias – dose related and severe Hypotension is common owing to the reduction in SVR Nonselective vasodilation may redirect blood flow to skeletal muscle and skin Myocardial ischaemia possible owing to increased oxygen consumption and hypotension
Indications	Bradycardia unresponsive to atropine when pacing not available Patients with low CO and fixed SV (i.e., LV aneurysm resection) Status asthmaticus β-Blocker overdose
Administration	Central intravenous infusion is optimal May be infused via peripheral line owing to lack of vasoconstriction
Metabolism	Liver conjugated with glucuronide and local metabolism by enzymes. Short half-life (2 min)
Dosage	Infusion at 0.02–0.05 μg/kg per minute

Abbreviations: CO, cardiac output; HR, heart rate; LV, left ventricular; SV, stroke volume; SVR, systemic vascular resistance.

that cause significant cardiovascular compromise should be corrected urgently, either by chemical or electrical means. If the preoperative rhythm was sinus rhythm, then the optimal postoperative rhythm must also be sinus. Loss of sinus rhythm leads to a reduction in ventricular filling of approximately 30% in normal hearts, and up to 50% in noncompliant ventricles. This is not well tolerated in the postoperative period, because the reduction in LV function associated with poor contractility and reduced compliance leads to dramatic reduction in CO.

Optimize the preload

Optimizing LV preload increases SV, and hence CO, with minimal increase in myocardial oxygen consumption. Therefore, this should always be achieved before increasing contractility by drug therapy. The relationship between preload, measured by cardiac filling pressures, and force of cardiac contraction is described by the Frank–Starling curve.

As preload increases, so SV increases until maximal ejection is achieved (inflexion point). From this point on, the ventricle is unable to respond to further filling and SV falls as the ventricle is overdistended. In patients with preexisting cardiac disease, the Frank–Starling curve may be flattened preoperatively, and further flattened by the effects of CPB. As a result, increases in preload produce smaller increases in CO and care must be taken not to fill beyond the point of maximal efficiency.

In practical terms, optimizing the preload is best achieved by repeated administration of small fluid

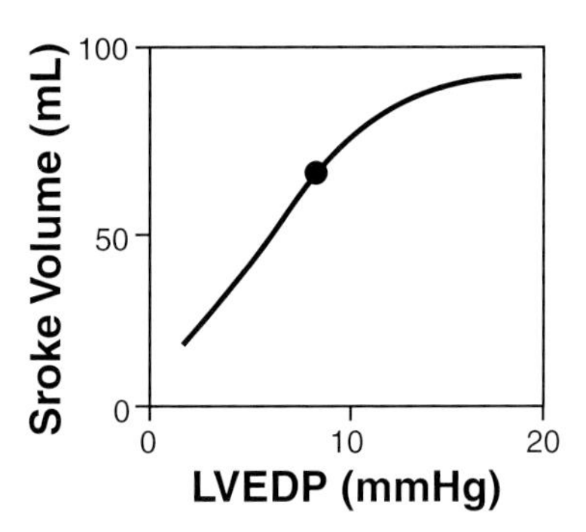

Figure 20.1 Frank–Starling mechanism. Increasing venous return to the LV increases end-diastolic pressure and volume, thereby increasing ventricular preload. This results in an increase in SV. 'Normal' operating point is a left ventricular end-diastolic pressure of 8 mmHg and SV of 70 mL/beat.

challenges, typically 200-mL boluses, and observing the response. Initially, the fluid challenge produces an increase in EDV (observed by preload pressures such as central venous pressure or pulmonary artery occlusion wedge pressure), and a commensurate increase in SV. When further fluid challenge no longer produces an increase in SV, the patient is optimally filled.

Optimize contractility

If, after optimizing all these parameters, the patient remains in a low CO state, then consideration should be given to starting inotropic treatment. A low CO state may be defined as a cardiac index of less than 2.4 L min^{-1} m^{-2}, with evidence of organ dysfunction such as elevated serum lactate or urine output below 0.5 mL/kg per hour. Steps should be taken to exclude cardiac tamponade as a cause of low CO state, and consideration should also be given to instituting mechanical support such as an intra-aortic balloon pump (see Chapter 21). Low CO state reduces oxygen delivery to vital organs, and if it persists, leads to multiple organ failure. Early intervention to improve CO by inotropic or mechanical support reduces complications, allowing faster recovery and improved survival.

At present, commonly used inotropes fall into two groups: catecholamines and phosphodiesterase (PDE) inhibitors. Despite the development of a large variety of inotropes, there is no consensus about which are best used to treat low CO state, and there is little evidence to support any particular choice. It is disappointing that there are no trials demonstrating that any one agent has an increased beneficial effect. There is also inconsistent evidence showing improvement of regional perfusion between agents.

β-Agonists are certainly potent inotropes and chronotropes, and increase CO compared with placebo; however, there are serious disadvantages to using these drugs. Myocardial oxygen consumption is increased owing to increased contractility and afterload, tachycardia is common and tachyarrhythmias (particularly atrial fibrillation) may result. These effects may worsen myocardial ischaemia. With long-term administration or in patients with preexisting cardiac failure, β-adrenergic receptor downregulation may occur, reducing the response to these drugs.

The PDE inhibitors act beyond the cell-surface receptor by inhibiting the breakdown of cyclic adenosine monophosphate (cAMP) by PDE III in cardiac and peripheral smooth muscle. The elevated cAMP levels produce augmented myocardial contractility and peripheral arterial and venous dilatation, with relatively little change in HR. In pulmonary hypertension, this has been shown to reduce mean pulmonary arterial pressure and improve right ventricular function. In contrast to catecholamines, PDE inhibitors produce improved diastolic relaxation (lusitropy).

The PDE inhibitors have a minimal effect on myocardial oxygen consumption; the lack of tachycardia and systemic vasodilatation offsets the increased inotropic action. However, they can produce such marked systemic vasodilatation that the addition of a vasopressor may be required to maintain blood pressure, making it likely that the

Table 20.2 Comparative properties of inotropes

Inotrope	Significant comments
Catecholamines	
Adrenaline (epinephrine)	Marked inotropic actions with minimal chronotropic actions
	May produce a raised serum lactate
Dobutamine	Marked inotropic and chronotropic actions
	Tachycardia, tachydysrhythmia and AF are common
Dopamine	The least effective inotrope
	Marked vasoconstriction at modest doses
	No evidence of renal or splanchnic benefits
	High level of adverse events – ischaemia, tachydysrhythmia
Dopexamine	Modest inotropic action
	Significant incidence of tachydysrhythmia
	No evidence of renal or splanchnic benefits
Phosphodiesterase inhibitors	
Enoximone	Marked inotrope with minimal chronotropic actions
	Marked vasodilatation
Milrinone	Marked inotrope with minimal chronotropic actions
	Marked vasodilatation
	No evidence of acute tolerance
	Reduced tachydysrhythmia compared to catecholamines
	Effective in pulmonary hypertension
	Lusitropic

Abbreviation: AF, atrial fibrillation.

beneficial effects on myocardial oxygen consumption will be not be observed. The half-life of PDE inhibitors is measured in hours rather than minutes, so a loading dose is required before starting an infusion and the onset of activity will be slower. Administering the loading dose on CPB has been shown to improve the ability to wean from CPB and reduce the need for postoperative catecholamine support. The PDE inhibitors have the potential to accumulate in renal failure, but acute tolerance is not observed. Unlike catecholamines, PDE inhibitors have been shown to improve flow through arterial grafts.

Choice of agent

Deciding which catecholamine to use is difficult. Adrenaline improves SV with little increase in HR, but may worsen metabolic acidosis.

Dobutamine appears at least as effective as adrenaline as an inotrope, but has a greater incidence of tachycardia and tachydysrhythmia, as well as systemic vasodilatation and hypotension. Dopamine may produce pulmonary and systemic vasoconstriction at modest doses (5 μg/kg per minute) and can also cause tachycardia. Dopexamine is a more effective inotrope than dopamine, but less so than dobutamine. There is no good evidence that dopamine or dopexamine can produce an improvement in splanchnic blood flow or renal function. This suggests that dobutamine or adrenaline may be the most appropriate choices.

The evidence is less clear with PDE inhibitors. Milrinone has been more extensively studied, confirming group-specific actions such as lusitropy. There is

Table 20.3 Adrenaline

Actions	Naturally occurring catecholamine produced by the renal medulla Direct agonist at α- and β-receptors
Cardiac effect	Marked $\beta 1$ agonist with inotropic actions
Vascular effects	Dose-dependent, low doses dilate $\beta 2$, higher doses constrict α
Advantages	Effective direct inotrope May have greater maximal effect than dobutamine Effective bronchodilator and mast cell stabilizer Shortens systole, improving diastolic myocardial blood flow (in absence of tachycardia)
Disadvantages	Tachycardia and dysrhythmias may occur Myocardial ischaemia owing to increased contractility and heart rate Pulmonary vasoconstriction may impair RV function Elevated plasma glucose and lactate Hyperkalaemia owing to hepatic release Organ ischaemia owing to vasoconstriction
Indications	Situations with low CO due to reduced contractility As part of the cardiac arrest protocol Treatment of anaphylaxis Treatment of bronchospasm
Administration	Central intravenous infusion Vasoconstriction may produce tissue necrosis if infused via peripheral line May be administered via endotracheal tube
Metabolism	Offset due to neuronal uptake and metabolism by MAO and COMT Short half-life (2 min)
Dosage	Low infusion rate <0.01 $\mu g/kg$ per minute produces vasodilatation Higher infusion rates 0.01–0.20 $\mu g/kg$ per minute produces inotropism and vasoconstriction Maximal rate 0.5 $\mu g/kg$ per minute

Abbreviations: CO, cardiac output; COMT, catechol-O-methyltransferase; RV, right ventricular; MAO, monoamine oxidase.

little to choose, however, between different drugs in terms of efficacy. Milrinone has a half-life of 60 minutes compared with 120 minutes for enoximone, but may inhibit platelet aggregation.

Optimize the afterload

Should the patient remain hypotensive after all these steps have been completed, and cardiac index is greater than 2.4 L min^{-1} m^{-2}, then it is likely that there is excessive vasodilatation. Correction of this can be achieved by adding an α-agonist, classically noradrenaline, which increases systemic vascular resistance (SVR) and thus blood pressure (especially diastolic). This leads to an increase in LV intracavity pressure and cavity radius. By Laplace's law, this increases LV wall tension, and hence myocardial oxygen consumption. At the same time, an increase in SVR may also lead to a reduction in CO. Because these are unlikely to be beneficial effects in the early postoperative recovery period, care should be taken to optimize all other parameters and ensure that CO is adequate before

Table 20.4 Dobutamine

Actions	Synthetic analog of dopamine β1-Agonist, less β2 and α actions
Cardiac effect	Inotropic with minor chronotropic effects
Vascular effects	Primarily vasodilatation
Advantages	Effective direct inotrope Less tachycardia than dopamine Afterload reduction may improve LV function Reduced pulmonary vascular resistance may improve RV function
Disadvantages	Tachycardia and dysrhythmias are dose related and may be severe at higher doses Hypotension may occur if reduction in SVR is not offset by increased CO Nonselective vasodilatation may redirect splanchnic flow to skeletal muscle Tolerance occurs within 72 hours owing to receptor downgrading
Indications	Low CO states, particularly if SVR and PVR are increased, such as cardiogenic shock
Administration	Central intravenous infusion is optimal May be infused short term via peripheral line owing to lack of vasoconstriction
Metabolism	Liver conjugated with glucuronide and local metabolism by enzymes. Short half-life (2.4 min)
Dosage	Infusion rate 2.5–10.0 μg/kg per minute Maximal rate 40 μg/kg per minute

Abbreviations: CO, cardiac output; LV, left ventricular; PVR, pulmonary vascular resistance; RV, right ventricular; SVR, systemic vascular resistance.

instituting a vasoconstrictor. Whenever vasopressors are required, it is worth considering invasive monitoring of the circulation, which has traditionally been achieved by the use of a Swan-Ganz pulmonary artery catheter (see Chapter 11).

It is important to decide on the optimal blood pressure for each individual patient. In general this is the minimum pressure needed to restore end-organ function and reverse metabolic derangement, such as acidosis and elevated serum lactate levels. The exact pressure needed to achieve this depends, in part, on the patient's normal preoperative blood pressure. If preexisting hypertension was present, then higher postoperative pressures should be the aim.

The vasoplegic syndrome

Arterial hypotension despite normovolaemia with vasopressor dependence has become an increasing problem after cardiac surgery. First described in 1994, vasoplegic syndrome is a post CPB phenomenon, generated by a profound inflammatory response, and characterized by marked vasodilatation unresponsive to usual doses of noradrenaline. It is widely quoted as having an incidence of approximately 10%. Although it may occur in patients with normal ventricular function, a reduced ejection fraction is known to be a major predisposing factor. In patients with both a poor ejection fraction and prolonged CPB, the incidence rises to as high as 50%.

Table 20.5 Dopamine

Actions	A catecholamine precursor of noradrenaline in nerve terminals and adrenal medulla Multiple and variable – $\alpha 1$, $\beta 1$, $\beta 2$ and DA actions
Cardiac effect	Inotropic and chronotropic effects
Vascular effects	Systemic and pulmonary vasoconstriction
Advantages	None
Disadvantages	Least effective inotrope Less maximal inotropic effect than adrenaline Tachycardia and dysrhythmias are dose related and often severe at higher doses Splanchnic blood flow decreases at doses >2.5 μg/kg per minute Pulmonary and systemic vasoconstriction severe at modest doses >5 μg/kg per minute Renal and splanchnic ischaemia at high doses (>10 μg/kg per minute) Marked increases in myocardial oxygen consumption produces myocardial ischaemia
Indications	Hypotension owing to low SVR, in patients without tachycardia or ventricular irritability Safe use requires invasive monitoring due to multiple actions (except at low doses)
Administration	Central intravenous infusion Vasoconstriction may produce tissue necrosis if infused via peripheral line
Metabolism	Reuptake into nerve terminals and local metabolism by COMT and MAO. Short half-life (2.4 min)
Dosage	Infusion rate 1–20 μg/kg per minute Consider switching to adrenaline if little benefit by 10 μg/kg per minute

Abbreviations: COMT, catechol-O-methyltransferase; DA, dopaminergic; MAO, monoamine oxidase; SVR, systemic vascular resistance.

The increased incidence of vasoplegic syndrome may be related to the widespread use of angiotensin-converting enzyme (ACE) inhibitors. The renin–angiotensin system is known to play an important part in the postoperative control of vasomotor tone. Long-term administration of ACE inhibitors leads to tissue accumulation, reducing the levels of the vasoconstrictor angiotensin II and increasing the levels of the vasodilator bradykinin. This effect is accentuated by CPB because the lungs are the major site of bradykinin catabolism and are excluded from the CPB circuit.

The vasoplegic syndrome is important because it is associated with a poor outcome. When it persists for longer than 48 hours, mortality after cardiac surgery may be as high as 25%. Furthermore, the duration of noradrenaline refractory vasoplegia appears directly proportional to the outcome. Therefore, it has been suggested that early, aggressive treatment of the vasoplegic syndrome may reduce morbidity and mortality.

THE ROLE OF VASOPRESSIN

Early work suggested an association between vasoplegic syndrome and a relative or absolute deficiency of vasopressin. The major physiological role of vasopressin is water regulation, and it has little role in normal vasomotor control. However, in shock states, there is rapid and marked endogenous release of vasopressin and it assumes an

Table 20.6 Milrinone

Actions	Synthetic bipyridine phosphodiesterase III inhibitor Inhibits the breakdown of cAMP
Cardiac effect	Augmented contractility, lusitropy and chronotropy
Vascular effects	Peripheral arterial and venous dilatation
Advantages	Less prodysrhythmic than catecholamines Tachycardia rarely a feature Minimal increase in myocardial oxygen consumption Pulmonary vasodilatation improves RV function Intracellular action means efficacy retained when receptors downregulated Does not induce tachyphylaxis Synergistic actions with β-agonist catecholamines
Disadvantages	Vasodilatation and hypotension
Indications	Low cardiac output syndromes Facilitate weaning from CPB
Administration	Central intravenous infusion May be infused short term via peripheral line owing to lack of vasoconstriction
Metabolism	Major route of elimination is renal (80%), with minor hepatic metabolism. Moderate half-life (30–60 min)
Dosage	Loading dose 25–50 mcg/kg over 10 minutes, often on CPB Infusion rate 0.375–0.750 μg/kg per minute Reduce dose in renal impairment

Abbreviations: cAMP, cyclic adenosine monophosphate; CPB, cardiopulmonary bypass; RV, right ventricular.

important role as a vasoconstrictor. Reduced systemic blood pressure is registered by the aortic and carotid baroreceptors, stimulating vasopressin release from the posterior pituitary gland via the sympathetic nervous system. Prolonged hypovolaemia, sepsis and CPB have all been demonstrated to produce inappropriately low levels of vasopressin (a relative deficiency). This is probably due to impaired autonomic function in septic shock and after CPB. Administration of exogenous high-dose vasopressin in these situations has been shown to markedly increase blood pressure.

The direct vasopressor effects of vasopressin are produced by constriction of capillaries and arterioles, increasing SVR. This is mediated via the V1 receptors in vascular smooth muscle cells located throughout the body but particularly in skin, adipose tissue and skeletal muscle. At the doses used in vasoplegic syndrome, vasopressin produces less vasoconstriction in the coronary, splanchnic and cerebral circulations than noradrenaline. At higher doses, such as those used to treat bleeding oesophageal varices, there is marked vasoconstriction in all vascular beds.

Although vasopressin produces classical direct vasoconstriction like noradrenaline, it also has other unique actions, which are thought to explain its efficacy in vasoplegic syndrome:

Table 20.7 Characteristics of vasoplegic syndrome

Despite noradrenaline infusion of >0.5 μg/kg per minute, findings are typically	
	MAP <50 mmHg
	Cardiac index >2.5 L min^{-1} m^{-2}
	Right atrial pressure <5 mmHg, left atrial pressure <10 mmHg
	Low SVR <800 dynes s cm^{-5}
Risk factors	Preoperative intravenous heparin
	Preoperative angiotensin-converting enzyme inhibitors
	Calcium channel blockers
	Reduced preoperative ejection fraction
	Prolonged CPB
	Elevated IL-1, -6
	Diabetes
	Protamine
Complications	Prolonged critical care stay
	Acute renal failure/longer time on ventilator/increased need for inotropes and vasopressors/increased transfusion
	Increased mortality

Abbreviations: CPB, cardiopulmonary bypass; IL, interleukin; MAP, mean arterial pressure; SVR, systemic vascular resistance.

- It inhibits ATP sensitive potassium channels in vascular smooth muscle, which mediate vasodilatation.
- It inhibits the release of the proinflammatory cytokine interleukin-1, which produces vasodilatation by stimulating endothelial nitric oxide production.
- It has sympathomimetic actions, enhancing the sensitivity of the peripheral vasculature to pressor agents including noradrenaline.

Table 20.8 Endogenous vasopressin concentrations (pg/mL)

Normal hydrated human	<5
Dehydrated human	5–10
Post cardiopulmonary bypass	100–500
Haemorrhagic shock	≤1,000

There are numerous small clinical studies demonstrating the beneficial effects of vasopressin use in vasoplegic syndrome, and it has replaced noradrenaline in many centres. However, caution is advised; there are no large studies to support its use or to demonstrate improved patient outcome. Vasopressin has many side effects,

Table 20.9 Adverse effects of vasopressin

Decreased cardiac output	Gastric infarction
Myocardial ischaemia	Bronchoconstriction
Ventricular dysrhythmia	Tremor
Metabolic acidosis	Vertigo
Cardiac arrest	Water intoxication
Abdominal cramps	Venous thrombosis
Nausea and vomiting	Local tissue necrosis owing to extravasation

although none have been described in vasoplegic syndrome studies so far. This may be due to the small size of the studies, and care should be taken during its administration.

THE ROLE OF METHYLENE BLUE

After the discovery of the role of nitric oxide in the vasodilatation of sepsis, it was suggested that there may be a role for nitric oxide as a mediator in vasoplegic syndrome. Inducible nitric oxide synthase is found in vascular smooth muscle and cardiac myocytes. Inflammatory mediators induce the synthase, increasing nitric oxide production. Nitric oxide then activates soluble intracellular guanylate cyclase, increasing intracellular cyclic guanosine monophosphate, so producing vascular smooth muscle relaxation and decreased myocardial contractility. However, it has not been possible to demonstrate elevated nitric oxide levels after CPB, suggesting that, although nitric oxide may play a part in vasoplegic syndrome, it is not the critical pathway.

Table 20.10 Adverse effects of methylene blue

Cardiac arrhythmias	Haemolytic anaemia and Heinz body anaemia
Coronary vasoconstriction	Green–blue discolouration of urine and skin
Angina	Gas exchange deterioration
Decreased cardiac output	Increased pulmonary vascular resistance
Decreased splanchnic and renal blood flow	Headache, dizziness, confusion
Nausea, vomiting and abdominal pain	Profuse sweating
Hyperbilirubinaemia	

Table 20.11 Methylene blue administration

Available as 100-mg methylene blue in 10-mL ampoules (1% w/v)
Store <25°C; protect from light
Treatment of hypotension in patients with sepsis or vasoplegic syndrome who are unresponsive to vasopressor catecholamines (an unlicensed indication)
Dilute the required dose to 100 mL of sodium chloride 0.9%
Infuse 1–2 mg/kg over 20 minutes
Dose for identification of parathyroids 5–7 mg/kg
Lethal dose 40 mg/kg

The focus has now moved to non-nitric pathways. Cardiopulmonary bypass elevates the levels of many inflammatory mediators such as interleukin-1, atrial natriuretic peptide, bradykinin and oxygen free radicals. These are capable of activating of guanylate cylcase, producing vascular hyporeactivity. There is also some evidence that this pathway of vasodilatation cannot be reversed by the administration of noradrenaline.

Methylene blue is a competitive inhibitor of guanylate cylcase. In studies of vasoplegic syndrome, it has usually been administered by infusion as a single dose of 2 mg/kg over 20 minutes. It has a rapid onset of action, with a maximal effect at approximately 2 hours after the infusion. Methylene blue is reduced in erythrocytes to leukomethylene blue and eliminated in bile, faeces and urine. Although methylene blue has serious side effects, these are dose related and have not been reported in vasoplegic syndrome studies, which use low doses compared with those used to identify the parathyroid glands before surgery.

Key points

- Early recognition of patients with low CO states and vasoplegic syndrome is important.
- Early institution of appropriate treatment may reduce complications and length of critical care and hospital stay, and improve survival.
- Optimize HR, rhythm and preload, and exclude cardiac tamponade.
- Institute invasive monitoring of haemodynamics.
- Start inotropes for low CO states. Be prepared to change drug if it appears not to improve haemodynamics.
- If hypotension and low organ perfusion persists, consider vasoplegic syndrome and add vasopressors, generally noradrenaline or vasopressin.

FURTHER READING

Albright TN, Zimmerman MA, Selzman CH. Vasopressin in the cardiac intensive care unit. *Am J Crit Care* 2002;11:326–330.

Gillies M, Bellomo R, Doolan L, *et al.* Bench-to-bedside review: Inotropic drug therapy after adult cardiac surgery – a systematic literature review. *Critical Care* 2005;9:266–279.

Levy JH, Bailey JM, Deeb GM. Intravenous milrinone in cardiac surgery. *Ann Thorac Surg* 2002;73:325–330.

Shanmugam G. Vasoplegic syndrome – the role of methylene blue. *Eur J Cardiothorac Surg* 2005;28: 705–10.

Chapter 21

Mechanical circulatory support

S.S.L. TSUI AND J. PARAMESHWAR

Introduction

A left ventricular assist device (LVAD) was first successfully used to bridge a patient with postcardiotomy shock to recovery in 1966; 2 years later, a patient in cardiogenic shock was salvaged with an intra-aortic balloon pump (IABP). Research on the total artificial heart also commenced in the late 1960s. Today, we have a wide range of options for circulatory support.

The decision whether to institute mechanical support depends on the aetiology of heart failure and on the likely long-term treatment strategy. Which method is deployed is determined by the acuteness of onset of heart failure, its potential reversibility and severity, local availability as well as the duration of support required.

Invasive haemodynamic monitoring is indispensable and provides the best evidence for the requirement and the adequacy of circulatory support. The pulmonary artery catheter provides important information, including left ventricular (LV) preload, LV afterload, right ventricular (RV) afterload and cardiac output (CO) as well as providing information on the adequacy of systemic oxygen delivery.

Intra-aortic balloon pump

The IABP is the most common form of circulatory support and is used in response to many different clinical situations. The balloon catheter has two channels: one for the passage of helium gas used to inflate and deflate the balloon, the other for direct monitoring of intra-aortic blood pressure. It is commonly inserted in a retrograde fashion via the femoral artery. Occasionally, in surgical patients with severe aortoiliac disease, it is inserted antegrade via the ascending aorta. The balloon is positioned in the descending thoracic aorta with the balloon segment of the catheter distal to the origin of the left subclavian artery.

The balloon is rapidly inflated at the end of ventricular systole, just as the aortic valve closes, generating a surge in the aortic pressure during ventricular diastole. Just before ventricular systole, the balloon is rapidly deflated, reducing the aortic pressure against which the LV has to eject. The timing of balloon inflation and deflation is triggered automatically by the patient's electrocardiogram (ECG) or arterial waveform.

Management of the patient with an intra-aortic balloon pump

The frequency and intensity of balloon augmentation can be controlled on the balloon pump console. The inflation ratio refers to the number of balloon inflations to the number of QRS complexes and can be set at 1:1, 1:2 or 1:3. The augmentation percentage (from 10% to 100%) determines how fully the balloon is inflated. During normal use, IABP support is initiated with a 1:1 inflation ratio at 100% augmentation. The timing of the inflation/deflation triggers should be checked regularly

Table 21.1 Types of mechanical circulatory support

Cardiopulmonary bypass (CPB)
Extra corporeal membrane oxygenation (ECMO)
Intra-aortic balloon pump (IABP)
Ventricular assist devices (VAD)
Total artificial hearts (TAH)
Cardiac compression devices
Aortic compression devices

and adjusted when required to optimize the support provided.

To reduce thromboembolic risks associated with an IABP, systemic anticoagulation with heparin infusion is advised, aiming for an activated partial thromboplastin time ratio of at least 1.5. Distal limb perfusion must be assessed regularly and distal pulses checked either by palpation or with a hand-held Doppler probe.

The effectiveness of IABP augmentation is diminished when there is excessive tachycardia (>120 bpm) or when the cardiac rhythm becomes irregular, as in atrial fibrillation. Therefore, inotropic support should be moderated to minimize the occurrence of such rhythm disturbances. As cardiac function begins to recover, and provided the IABP is well tolerated and there is no risk of ischaemic injury to the limb, the inotrope dose should ideally be reduced before IABP support is weaned (e.g. dopamine infusion down to ≤ 5 g/kg per minute). If the cardiac index is maintained above 2.2 L min^{-1} m^{-2} with acceptable preload (pulmonary artery occlusion wedge pressure <15 mmHg), attempts can be made to wean the IABP. First, the IABP augmentation can be reduced to 50% for 2 to 4 hours. Next, the inflation ratio reduced from 1:1 to 1:2 for another 2 to 4 hours followed by 1:3 before the balloon catheter is removed. Heparin can be discontinued at the start of IABP weaning so that coagulation is normalized by the time the IABP is removed.

Table 21.2 Indications for IABP

Ischaemic myocardium
  Unstable angina despite maximal medical therapy
  Ischaemia-induced ventricular arrhythmia
  Elective support in high-risk percutaneous coronary interventions

Structural complications of acute myocardial infarction
  Ventricular septal defect
  Acute mitral valve regurgitation

Cardiogenic shock
  After myocardial infarction
  Acute myocarditis
  Acute deterioration of chronic heart failure
  After cardiotomy
  Acute donor organ failure

Table 21.3 Beneficial effects of the intra-aortic balloon pump

Balloon deflation during ventricular systole
  Reduces left ventricular afterload
  Reduces peak LV wall stress and LV stroke work
  Decreases myocardial oxygen demand
  Reduces mitral valve regurgitation
  Increases LV ejection

Balloon inflation during ventricular diastole
  Increases coronary perfusion pressure
  Augments coronary blood flow
  Improves myocardial oxygen delivery

Overall effects
  Augments CO
  Reduces pulmonary capillary wedge pressure
  Relieves pulmonary congestion

Abbreviations: CO, cardiac output; LV, left ventricular.

Complications

Major vascular complications can occur in up to 15% of patients treated with an IABP. Femoral insertion of an IABP may not be possible in 5% of

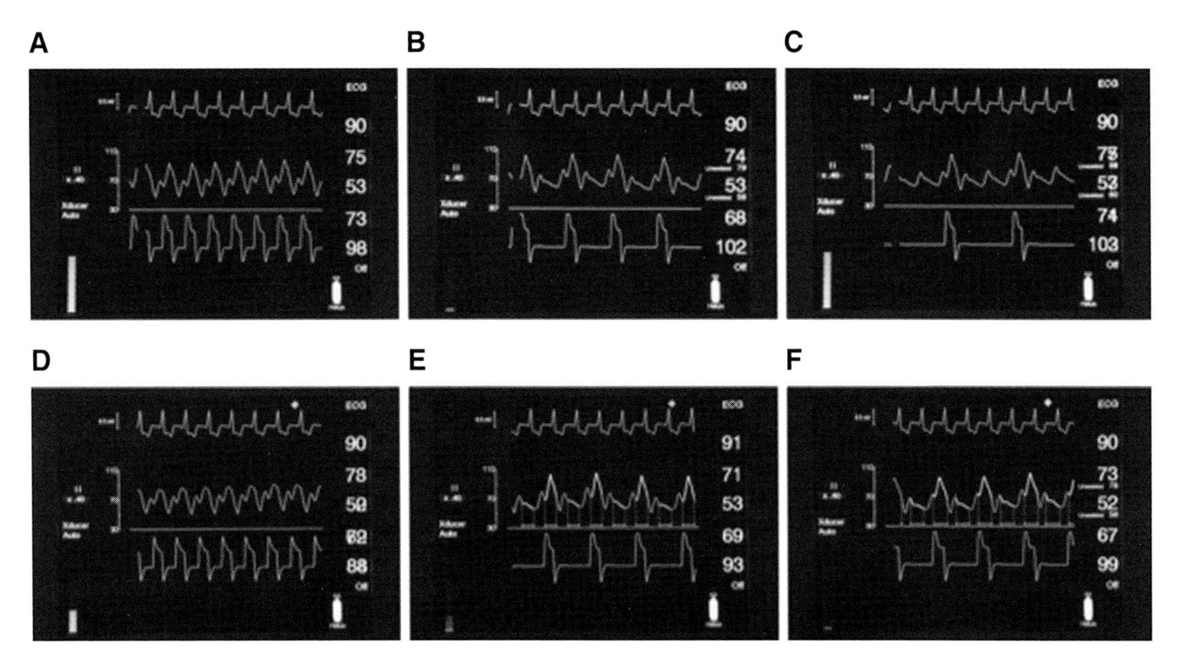

Figure 21.1 Intra-aortic balloon console tracings. The screen displays ECG at the top, aortic pressure waveform in the centre and balloon inflation/deflation at the bottom. (*A–C*) Full IABP augmentation with inflation ratio of 1:1, 1:2 and 1:3, respectively, showing augmentation of the aortic pressure during diastole and transient reduction of aortic pressure just before systole and cardiac ejection. (*D*) Balloon augmentation set at 50%. (*E*) Inflation ratio set at 1:2 and inflation interval highlighted showing correct balloon inflation trigger at the dicrotic notch. (*F*) Incorrect balloon setting with balloon inflation triggered too early.

patients because of a tortuous or diseased iliofemoral system. During insertion, vascular injury can lead to dissection, rupture or haemorrhage. Once in situ, distal limb ischaemia can result from thromboembolism or a combination of peripheral vasoconstriction and low CO state. Malpositioning of an IABP may result in obstruction of visceral or renal arteries.

Other complications include infection, thrombocytopenia and rupture of the balloon. When the latter occurs, blood is seen to track down the gas channel of the balloon driveline. Whenever this is observed, the balloon must be immediately deflated and the catheter removed.

Ventricular assist devices

Severe heart failure refractory to medical management and IABP support has an appalling prognosis. Inadequate forward perfusion gives rise to end-organ dysfunction and metabolic acidosis, and excessive backpressure results in pulmonary oedema and systemic venous congestion. Ventricular assist devices (VADs) can be used to augment perfusion and relieve congestion, potentially reversing the physiological derangement. The VADs are mechanical blood pumps that work either in parallel (atrial cannulation) or in series (ventricular cannulation) with the native ventricle. A LVAD withdraws oxygenated blood from the left atrium or left ventricle, and returns it to the aorta; a RVAD draws venous blood from the right atrium or right ventricle, and returns it to the pulmonary artery. In general, it is preferable to cannulate the ventricle for VAD inflow because this provides superior ventricular decompression, avoids ventricular stasis and affords higher VAD flow rates.

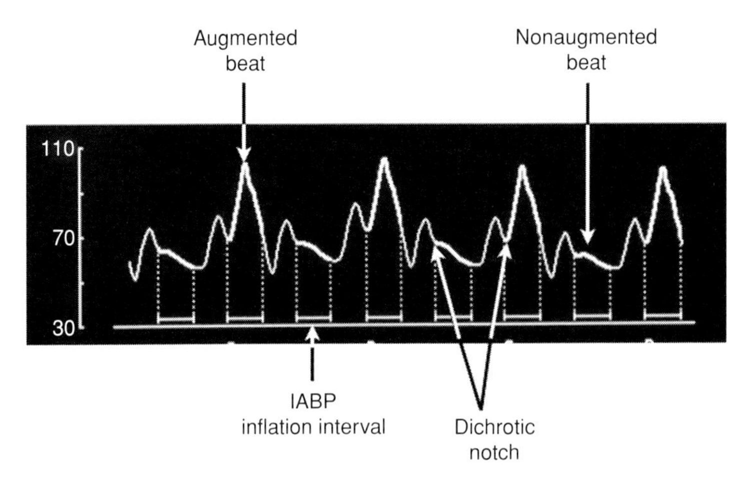

Figure 21.2 Aortic pressure trace with IABP inflation ratio set at 1:2. The IABP inflation interval has been highlighted to show IAB inflation at the dicrotic notch and deflation just before cardiac systole.

The output of a LVAD depends on adequate RV function to deliver sufficient blood flow across the lungs into the left heart chambers for the LVAD to pump. Likewise, a RVAD can only provide benefit if the native LV can generate enough stroke work to cope with the pulmonary blood flow produced by the RVAD. If both native ventricles are failing, two VADs are required to provide biventricular assistance (biVAD) to support the circulation.

In its simplest form, emergency short-term VAD support can be provided by any blood pump and two vascular cannulae: one for inflow from the heart to the VAD, the other for outflow return from the VAD to the aorta. In the absence of specialized VAD equipment, such a set-up can be lifesaving and maintain the circulation for hours or days while a more suitable alternative is sought.

There is a growing number of pump systems specifically intended for use as a VAD. These systems consist of blood pumps that are less traumatic to blood components, and have cannulae designed to provide more secure attachment to the heart chambers with superior flow characteristics. Temporary VAD systems are intended for short-term circulatory support in critical care (days or weeks). Long-term VAD systems are designed to provide circulatory support for months or years. Patients with implanted long-term VAD systems can often be discharged from hospital and treated as outpatients.

The fate of patients receiving a VAD depends on the underlying cause of the cardiac dysfunction and its reversibility. In some cases of postcardiotomy shock and fulminant myocarditis, cardiac function recovers after a period of circulatory support and the VAD can be weaned and removed, a process known as 'bridging to recovery.' Unfortunately, in the majority of cases of chronic heart failure, such as ischaemic or dilated cardiomyopathies, the myocardial dysfunction is unlikely to be reversible. Occasionally, a VAD is required for these patients who are already waiting for a heart transplant because of deteriorating cardiac status. Here, the VAD is used to buy time for the patient until a suitable donor heart can be found, a process called 'bridging to transplant.' For a selected few patients with advanced heart failure who are not transplant candidates, VAD support can be offered as a permanent implant, a process called 'destination therapy.'

Ventricular assist devices: Decision-making process

The questions, 'Which patient to support with a VAD?'; 'When to insert a VAD?'; 'Does the patient require LVAD alone or BiVAD?'; and 'Which VAD

Table 21.4 Categories of patients considered for ventricular assist device insertion

	Groups	Description
I	Precarious	Severe heart failure with borderline haemodynamics requiring inotropic therapy with or without IABP
II	Decompensated	Untransplantable owing to acute end-organ failure or chronically raised pulmonary vascular resistance (>6 Wood units)
III	Failure to wean from CPB	Postcardiotomy shock or acute donor organ failure after heart transplantation
IV	Salvage	Cardiac arrest massaged onto CPB

Abbreviations: CPB, cardiopulmonary bypass; IABP, intra-aortic balloon pump.

system to use?' are often difficult to answer. The decisions are influenced by a number of factors including patient comorbidities, transplant waiting times, resource availability, institutional experience and device availability. In general, patients who are considered for VAD support belong to one of the following four categories.

Group I consists of transplant-eligible patients with precarious haemodynamics who are managed on the critical care unit. They are the most challenging group of patients to make a decision on because a rush to implant a VAD too early may 'deny' them a more straightforward course of heart transplantation without mechanical bridging, whereas waiting too long for a donor heart may result in end-organ failure or worse still, cardiac arrest and death. In these cases, it is important to monitor the trends in haemodynamics as well as inotrope requirements. Adequacy of end-organ function is best assessed with hourly urine output, arterial oxygenation, prothrombin time and acid–base balance. In the United Kingdom, where the median waiting time for an 'urgent' donor heart is approximately 1 week, most of these patients can be transplanted without needing VAD support. In other countries, where the minimum waiting time for an 'urgent' heart runs into many months, most of these patients are treated with a VAD. Ventricular tachyarrhythmia is an ominous sign and should prompt an earlier decision for VAD insertion. Because the 'bridging' period to a transplant can range from months to sometimes over a year, these patients should be implanted with a long-term VAD so that they can be discharged home. Currently, there are several wearable or portable VAD systems that allow patients independent mobility during VAD support with reasonable quality of life. Patients in this category have an 80% to 90% chance of being successfully bridged to a heart transplant if treated with a VAD.

Group II consists of patients who are otherwise transplant candidates except for one or more serious, but potentially reversible, complications of advanced heart failure, such as acute end-organ failure or pulmonary hypertension. Unless such complications can be reversed, these patients are not transplantable and they will invariably die from their heart failure. Acute end-organ failure secondary to a low CO state sometimes recovers when the systemic circulation is mechanically augmented; elevated pulmonary vascular resistance owing to LV failure and pulmonary venous congestion often decreases with mechanical unloading of the LV. These patients are sick and those who survive the surgery of VAD implant often require weeks or months of VAD support to reverse their end-organ failure before they can be rehabilitated for a heart transplant. It is therefore most appropriate to consider a long-term VAD system in these cases. Operative risks are higher in this decompensated group and only 60% to 70% survive to receive a heart transplant.

Group III consists of patients who, after heart surgery, could not be weaned from cardiopulmonary bypass (CPB) despite maximal inotropic therapy and IABP. This includes patients with postcardiotomy shock and those with acute donor organ failure after heart transplantation. In the absence of contraindications, a short-term VAD may be considered to enable weaning from CPB. Alternatively, a venoarterial extracorporeal membrane oxygenation (ECMO) circuit may be used to support the circulation (for more on this topic see Chapter 28). Injured hearts that are likely to recover tend to do so within 5 to 7 days. If weaning from mechanical support cannot be accomplished after this period because of ongoing poor ventricular function, a decision has to be made between device removal and death, or continued support and bridging to transplantation (or retransplantation). Occasionally, it may be felt appropriate to switch over to a long-term device to wait for a suitable donor heart. Overall survival rate for the postcardiotomy group is poor at 40% to 50%, whereas those treated for acute donor organ failure may achieve 60% to 70% survival.

Group IV consists of patients with catastrophic heart failure and cardiac arrest, who have been massaged onto CPB or ECMO for resuscitation. These patients tend to be young, previously fit and would normally be good candidates for heart transplantation. The main uncertainty that exists here is the neurological status after a period of cardiopulmonary resuscitation. Again, a short-term VAD or venoarterial ECMO may be used to support the circulation until neurological assessment can be performed. Severe neurological injury usually becomes obvious within 48 hours of circulatory support, facilitating the decision to withdraw treatment. Otherwise, consideration may have to be given to bridging to transplantation or switching to a longer term device.

Table 21.5 Contraindications to using ventricular assist devices postcardiotomy
Age >60 years
Uncontrollable bleeding
Intractable metabolic acidosis
Other comorbidities
Preexisting neurological impairment
Severe cerebral vascular disease
Severe peripheral vascular disease
Advanced chronic pulmonary disease
Chronic renal failure
Chronic liver disease
Recent malignancy

Preoperative management

Patients requiring a VAD implant are probably amongst the sickest patients to undergo cardiac surgery. They have severe heart failure and are either in impending or established end-organ failure. A low CO state coupled with systemic venous congestion results in compromised organ perfusion. The kidneys become refractory to diuretic therapy and hepatic dysfunction manifests as coagulation abnormalities. The lungs are stiff from pulmonary congestion, increasing the work of breathing and many patients are grossly fluid-overloaded.

If the stability of the patient permits, a period of preoperative optimization in the critical care unit before VAD implant can be highly beneficial. Inotropic therapy should be rationalized to reduce the risk of arrhythmias and a period of IABP support helps to augment end-organ perfusion. Vitamin K can normalize an elevated prothrombin time, which in turn reduces the risk of postoperative haemorrhage.

Continuous venovenous haemofiltration (CVVH) is the most expeditious way of reducing excessive intravascular volume and total body water content (for more on this topic see Chapter 30). Patients with chronic heart failure with a central venous pressure (CVP) below 20 mmHg are often also grossly oedematous. The aim is to normalize the preload and bring the CVP towards 10 to 12 mmHg. In practice, CVVH can be used to give a negative balance of up to 500 mL/h (as tolerated) until the target CVP is reached. In these patients, it is not uncommon to remove 7 to 10 L of fluid in the first 24 hours of CVVH. As the venous pressure begins to normalize, excessive fluid from third spaces also returns to the intravascular compartment and peripheral oedema resolves. Finally, by normalizing an elevated preload, overstretched ventricles and atrioventricular valves reduce in size, often resulting in functional improvement.

Perioperative management

The perioperative strategy should be aimed at minimizing further insult to these sick patients during VAD implantation, targeting those areas that are known to result in serious morbidities and mortality. Perhaps the most unpredictable and dangerous complication after LVAD implantation is RV failure. The other commonly encountered problem is early postoperative haemorrhage.

Broad-spectrum prophylactic antibiotics, full-dose aprotinin and normothermic CPB are used for all VAD implants. Transoesophageal echocardiography (TOE) is carried out to confirm aortic valve competence and exclude the presence of a patent foramen ovale or an atrial septal defect. If present, they require surgical closure at the time of VAD implant to prevent a right-to-left shunt after decompression of the left-sided chambers with a LVAD. The lungs are kept ventilated throughout the bypass period with the addition of nitric oxide at 10 parts per million to minimize atelectasis and pulmonary vasoconstriction. Ultrafiltration is used to maintain haemoglobin above 10 g/dL and base excess within 2 mEq. The VAD is implanted on a beating heart, avoiding aortic cross-clamp and cardiac ischaemia. The pericardial space is flooded with carbon dioxide so that gas bubbles entrained into cardiac chambers can dissolve more readily. The RV is supported with an infusion of dopamine at 5 μg/kg per minute. Heart rate is optimized with temporary pacing at 90 to 100 bpm. Systemic vascular resistance is maintained between 800 and 1000 dynes s cm^{-5} using an infusion of vasopressin or with an α-agonist. Thorough de-airing of the heart is confirmed with TOE before finally attempting to wean from bypass.

Postoperative management

At the end of the procedure, haemostasis is crucial to minimize haemorrhage. An effective closed drainage system should prevent mediastinal and pump pocket collections. Some surgeons close the pericardial sac or place a surgical membrane between the sternum and the mediastinum to facilitate subsequent resternotomy and reentry. The percutaneous cannulae or drivelines must be secured to minimize movement and trauma to the exit sites. This is the best way to encourage tissue healing onto the driveline and minimize exit site infections.

Once returned to the critical care unit, VAD patients must be closely monitored for early complications.

Antibiotic prophylaxis is continued for 48 hours. Coagulation defects should be corrected without waiting for signs of significant bleeding. Right ventricular function often remains precarious in the early days after LVAD implantation. Right ventricular failure can be precipitated by excessive LVAD flows or elevated pulmonary vascular resistance. Therefore, it is advisable to limit the LVAD flow rate in the first few days to avoid overwhelming the RV. Furthermore, it is essential to avoid factors that may

Table 21.6 Early complications of ventricular assist device support

Perioperative haemorrhage
Right ventricular failure
Cerebral vascular events
Metabolic
Embolic
Haemorrhagic
Infectious
Haemolysis
Thromboembolism
Mechanical pump failure

precipitate increases in pulmonary vascular resistance such as hypoxia and acidosis.

Anticoagulation is usually omitted in the first 24 hours and is only started when the patient has stopped bleeding (<30 mL/h for 3 consecutive hours). Most units begin with an infusion of unfractionated heparin and this is continued for 5 to 7 days before warfarin is commenced. The actual anticoagulation/antiplatelet regime is device specific as well as unit specific.

Rising right atrial pressure coupled with a fall in pump flow should alert to impending RV failure. This can be confirmed with TOE, which demonstrates full right-sided cardiac chambers with empty left-sided chambers. The atrial and ventricular septa are seen to bulge towards the left and these are often accompanied by tricuspid valve regurgitation. Under these circumstances, it is important not to increase the preload further with more fluid transfusions. Immediate treatment consists of a combination of inotropic support for the RV and pulmonary vasodilators. These may include adrenaline (up to 0.1 μg/kg per minute), enoximone (5 μg/kg per minute), nitric oxide (up to 20 parts per million) and/or nebulized iloprost (9.9 μg every 3 hours). If the patient does not respond readily to these measures, early consideration should be given to returning the patient to the operating room for the addition of a RVAD.

Types of ventricular assist devices

Technical developments in mechanical circulatory support have progressed rapidly over the last 10 years. There is now a large range of systems available for clinical use. These can be classified into temporary and long-term systems. Within each group, they can be subdivided into volume displacement devices (or pulsatile devices) and continuous flow devices. A full description of all available devices is beyond the scope of this book. A few selected examples of commonly available VADs that are in clinical use are briefly described below.

Table 21.7 Classification and examples of ventricular assist device systems

Temporary devices
Volume displacement
Abiomed BVS 5000
Medos
Continuous flow
Impella
Levitronix Centrimag*
Long-term devices
Volume displacement
HeartMate I
Novacor
Thoratec PVAD
Thoratec IVAD
Continuous flow
Micromed DeBakey
Jarvik 2000
HeartMate II
Berlin Incor*
Ventracor VentrAssist*
Terumo Duraheart*

**Denotes the latest bearing-less designs. All names are trademarked.*

LEVITRONIX CENTRIMAG

This is an extracorporeal system that is designed for up to 14 days of circulatory support. A single system can provide either LV or RV support. A second system can be used simultaneously to provide biventricular support. The inflow and outflow cannulae can be rapidly inserted into the heart and great vessels with or without CPB. Other clinical equipment such as a membrane oxygenator or haemofilter can be spliced into the system. Although patients supported with the Centrimag are kept on the critical care unit, they can be allowed to move around the bed space and can undergo physiotherapy. Because of its simplicity and versatility, the Centrimag is becoming rapidly adopted by many cardiac surgical centres.

HEARTMATE I

This is an implantable, pulsatile LVAD that is designed for long-term circulatory support. The pump consists of an electrically actuated pusher plate, a blood sac and two porcine valves, one for inflow, one for outflow. It has a uniquely textured blood-contacting surface made up of scintillated titanium microspheres, which encourages the formation of a neointima once implanted, providing low thrombogenicity. The VAD is surgically implanted in the abdomen with the inflow connected to the LV apex and the outflow to the ascending aorta.

The percutaneous driveline is connected to a wearable controller and rechargeable battery system. The HeartMate I is a large device and is designed to provide LV support of up to 10 L/min. However, patients with the device only require low-dose aspirin and generally do not need systemic anticoagulation with warfarin.

THORATEC SYSTEM

The Thoratec system was originally designed as a pulsatile paracorporeal ventricular assist device (PVAD), which can be used as either LV or RV support. Two units can be used simultaneously to provide biventricular support. The inflow and outflow cannulae are passed across the abdominal wall and the pump unit rests in front of the abdomen. The VAD is connected to an external pneumatic drive console via a gas line and can provide pulsatile support of up to 6.5 L/min.

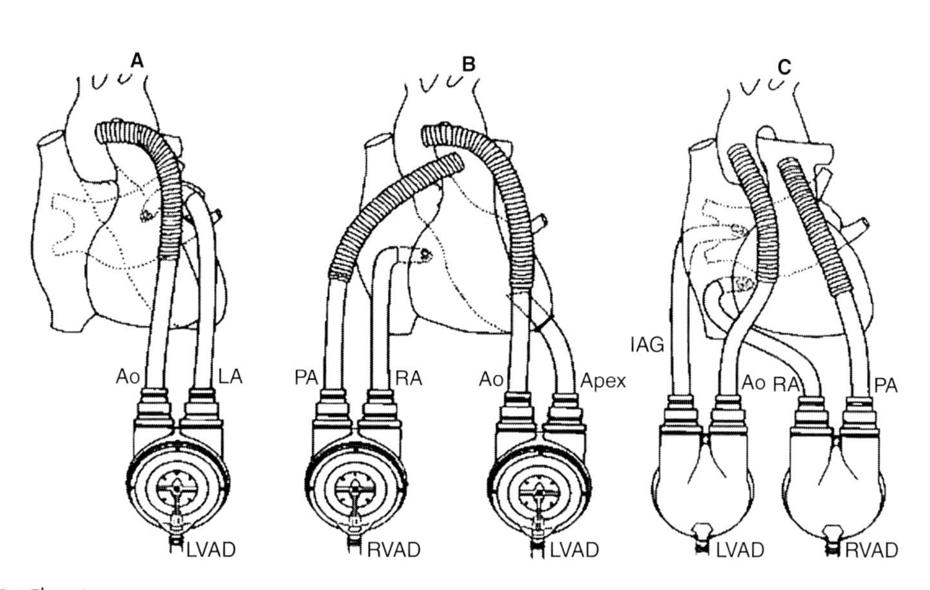

Figure 21.3 Thoratec.

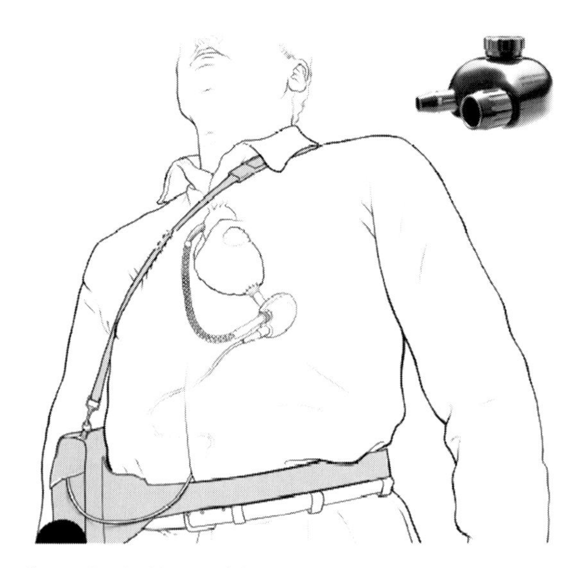

Figure 21.4 Ventrassist.

More recently, Thoratec has adapted the PVAD into an implantable ventricular assist device. It can be used as LV or RV support as well as biventricular support using two complete units. This makes the system much more acceptable for patients and their carers; it is currently the only implantable VAD that can provide support for either ventricle.

VENTRACOR VENTRASSIST

This is one of the latest generations of long-term LVADs consisting of a small implantable titanium centrifugal pump, percutaneous driveline, portable controller and rechargeable battery packs. When activated, the impeller is hydrodynamically suspended on a thin film of blood and requires no conventional bearing. By eliminating the potential for mechanical wear and tear, these pumps are designed for maximum durability. Continuous flow devices tend to be smaller than pulsatile devices, and are quiet in operation, making them less intrusive to live with. It is hoped that these pumps can provide long-term circulatory support with lower morbidity and mortality.

Key points

- Invasive haemodynamic monitoring provides the best assessment for the requirement and the adequacy of circulatory support.
- Although IABP support can improve both left and right heart function, careful monitoring is required to prevent serious complications such as limb ischaemia.
- Temporary VADs may be used if there is a chance of cardiac recovery or if neurological status is uncertain.
- More permanent VADs are most commonly inserted to manage heart failure until transplantation, but destination therapy may be feasible in the future.
- Haemorrhage, RV failure and infection are the most common serious postoperative complications.

FURTHER READING

Frazier OH, Kirklin J. *Mechanical circulatory support.* ISHLT Monograph Series; 2006.

Goldstein D, Oz MC. *Cardiac assist devices.* London: Blackwell Publishing Ltd; 2002.

Samuels L, Narula J. Ventricular assist devices and the artificial heart. *Cardiol Clin* 2003;21.

Chapter 22

Systemic hypertension

R. FENECK

Introduction

Haemodynamic control is an essential component of safe perioperative care. The importance of hypertension in the perioperative period has long been recognized and it is known that sympatho-adrenal activation and perioperative hypertension may lead to adverse effects, particularly myocardial ischaemia and haemorrhage. These adverse events are themselves linked to poor outcomes, yet they may be prevented by good cardiovascular control.

Even in those patients who are normotensive before surgery, perioperative surgical stress may have an adverse effect. This is particularly true of cardiac surgery, where the impact of sternotomy and handling the great vessels in the phase before cardiopulmonary bypass (CPB) may be provocative in many patients.

Preoperative management

Many patients who present for coronary revascularization do not demonstrate adequate blood pressure control according to current recommendations, despite these having been validated by observed reductions in morbidity and mortality.

Effects of hypertension

Primary or essential hypertension may result from a complex interaction of renal, neurogenic, endocrine and cardiovascular factors, particularly alterations in the activity of the vascular endothelium. Specific conditions may also be responsible. These causes of secondary hypertension are important because they may have implications for other aspects of perioperative care. However, the effects of hypertension, particularly when longstanding, may precipitate significant problems in the perioperative period. Renal disease may be associated both with the development of high blood pressure and adverse effects resulting from established hypertension. Longstanding hypertension has been associated with an increased incidence of renal dysfunction, and numerous studies have identified renal dysfunction as a determinant for cardiovascular morbidity and mortality and an outcome determinant for patients undergoing cardiac surgery.

Hypertension has a significant adverse effect on the autoregulation of blood flow in many vascular beds including the cerebral circulation, where the curve is shifted to the right. As a result, a fall in blood pressure may result in a reduction in cerebral blood flow greater than would be seen in normotensive patients.

Hypertension represents a significant increase in left ventricular (LV) afterload, which may lead to LV hypertrophy and in due course, to LV dilatation and failure. The association between hypertension and the development of coronary artery disease is clear and many, perhaps most, patients presenting for coronary revascularization have hypertension as a significant comorbidity.

Table 22.1 Classification and management of blood pressure

BP classification	Systolic BP (mmHg)		Diastolic BP (mmHg)	Initial drug treatment
Normal	<120	and	<80	None
Prehypertension	120–139	or	80–89	None
Stage 1 hypertension	140–159	or	90–99	Thiazide diuretic Consider ACE inhibitor, ß-blocker, CCB
Stage 2 hypertension	>160	or	>100	Two-drug combination – thiazide + ACE or ARB or ß-blocker or CCB

Abbreviations: ACE, angiotensin-converting enzyme; ARB, angiotensin receptor blocker; BP, blood pressure; CCB, calcium channel blocker.
Adapted from the 7th Joint National Committee report on prevention, detection, evaluation and treatment of high blood pressure.

Significance of perioperative hypertension

Factors determining the development of perioperative hypertension in cardiac surgery patients are numerous. In these patients, even isolated systolic hypertension has been shown to be associated with adverse outcomes, including an increased risk of bleeding and blood transfusion. However, although good blood pressure control is ideal in every patient, there is little evidence that poor control of systemic hypertension preoperatively should be a reason for cancelling surgery.

PERIOPERATIVE BLOOD PRESSURE CONTROL

Recommendations for patients undergoing noncardiac surgery suggest that the patient's blood pressure should be kept within 20% of the baseline value. These values are inappropriate for cardiac surgery. Cardiac surgery involves delicate suture lines to arterial structures, including coronary artery bypass grafts and the aorta. It is necessary to minimize the risk of these being disrupted, and this means controlling blood pressure during the pre- and post-CPB phases of cardiac surgery. In addition, increased LV wall stress may provoke myocardial oxygen imbalance and ischaemia in individuals at risk for ischaemia. The highest permissible blood pressure after CPB depends on the nature of the surgery. It is rare to justify mean pressures above 80 mmHg immediately after CPB, but in certain types of surgery, for example, major aortic reconstruction, much lower values (55 mmHg mean) may be required, particularly for the first 1 to 2 hours.

In the early postoperative period, continuing antihypertensive control is often necessary. Numerous factors may interact to provoke ongoing vasoconstriction and hypertension. Controlling the blood pressure significantly below the patient's normal level may cause organ hypoperfusion, particularly of the kidneys. On the other hand, high pressure may contribute to excessive haemorrhage, leading to transfusion and/or chest reopening, both of which are clearly associated with an increased risk of adverse outcome.

An acceptable compromise may be to control the blood pressure to the lowest level associated with an adequate urine output, although this in turn may not be simple in a patient with renal dysfunction.

MAINTENANCE OF PREOPERATIVE TREATMENT

Early studies suggested that continuation of angiotensin-converting enzyme (ACE) inhibitors

Table 22.2 Factors influencing the development of perioperative hypertension

For	Against
Preoperative	Preoperative
Preexisting hypertension	Normotensive
Poor preoperative blood pressure control	Continuing antihypertensive medication
Discontinuing antihypertensive medication	ACE inhibitors
Intraoperative	Intraoperative
Inadequate anaesthesia and analgesia	Adequate anaesthesia (volatiles, high-dose opioid analgesia, epidural analgesia)
Surgical stress, especially sternotomy, mechanical stimulation of the aorta	Avoiding CPB (i.e., OPCAB surgery)
Nonpulsatile CPB	Vasodilators
Hypothermia	
Prolonged CPB (increased circulating pressor amines)	
Postoperative	Postoperative
Inappropriate or poorly controlled use of inotropes and vasopressors	Vasodilator use
Inadequate anaesthesia/analgesia	Full rewarming
Inadequate rewarming	

Abbreviations: ACE, angiotensin-converting enzyme; CPB, cardiopulmonary bypass; OPCAB, off-pump coronary artery bypass.

and angiotensin II inhibitors up to the day of surgery was associated with an unacceptable degree of hypotension on induction of anaesthesia. Although this may be successfully managed with crystalloid transfusion, occasionally vasopressor treatment is necessary, and this in turn may be more complex due to variable responsiveness to α-agonists. Thus, the initial recommendation was to discontinue treatment at least 24 hours preoperatively, more recently modified to 10 hours. In addition, hypotension and difficulty in weaning from CPB was also noted, presumably owing to the accumulation of bradykinin, a compound normally metabolized by ACE, resulting from the inflammatory cascade induced by CPB. Other work has challenged these recommendations, although some centres still recommend withdrawing ACE inhibitors in the days before cardiac surgery.

Controlling hypertension

General measures

The importance of general measures in controlling perioperative hypertension cannot be overstated. Hypertension occurring during surgery is most properly managed by attention to the adequacy of analgesia and anaesthesia. The antihypertensive effects of modern volatile anaesthetics are frequently used first to control blood pressure before any specific therapy is given. In the postoperative period, adequate analgesia and/or anxiolysis may also preclude the need for specific antihypertensive treatment.

In perioperative hypertension, therapy should be directed towards correcting the physiological abnormality. This is most frequently related to sympathoadrenal activation, resulting in an increase in resting arteriolar tone, venoconstriction with reduced pooling of venous blood and an enhanced inotropic state. Logically, appropriate therapy would result in arteriolar dilatation, a mild reduction in venous tone and a mild to moderate reduction in contractility.

Drugs

α2-RECEPTOR AGONISTS/IMIDAZOLE RECEPTOR AGONISTS

α2-Agonists possess properties of sedation, analgesia and blood pressure control. The cardiovascular effects are typified by clonidine, and are best described as a biphasic response. At lower doses, the predominant effect is sympatholysis mediated by agonist activity at the α2-adrenoreceptor. At higher doses, a peripherally mediated hypertensive effect is seen owing to activation of α2B-adrenoceptors, thought to be located on smooth muscle cells in arteriolar vessels. Most cardiovascular studies with clonidine have been more concerned with its sympatholytic effects rather than simple blood pressure lowering. Clonidine has been shown to improve circulatory stability, including heart rate (HR) control and baroreflex activity. Recent data have suggested that perioperative administration of clonidine to patients at risk for coronary artery disease significantly reduces the incidence of perioperative myocardial ischaemia and postoperative death.

Dexmedetomidine, an isomer of medetomidine, has greater selectivity and specificity for α2-adrenoreceptors than clonidine. Its properties of providing sedation, analgesia without respiratory depression (albeit with a clear ceiling effect) and sympatholysis with effective blood pressure control would seem to be highly desirable. Dexmedetomidine is associated with a mild reduction in blood pressure, such as would be required for good haemodynamic control after surgery, and studies before and after surgery suggest a blood pressure controlling effect. α2-Adrenoceptor agonists produce highly desirable effects; however, their effectiveness at controlling acute severe systemic hypertension has not been studied.

α-Adrenoceptor blockers

α1-Antagonists can be divided into selective (doxazosin, indoramin, prazosin, terazosin) and nonselective compounds (phentolamine). For acute perioperative blood pressure control, these drugs have their limitations.

Only phentolamine can be regarded as suitable for use in the cardiac surgical patient. It is usually used as a short-term treatment for perioperative vasoconstriction and hypertension. Tachyphylaxis, reflex tachycardia and increased circulating noradrenaline levels limit its use for prolonged blood pressure control in the perioperative period. The effective dose may vary, but it is rare to need more than 1 mg intravenously at a time, although repeated dosing is usual.

β-Adrenoceptor blockers

Although β-blockers are no longer considered essential first-line drugs in the management of hypertension in the community, many cardiac surgical patients, and almost all who are undergoing coronary revascularization, will be taking β-blockers preoperatively. Patients chronically taking β-blockers should not have these withdrawn before surgery, and continued use of β-blockers may have beneficial effects on the incidence of perioperative hypertension, atrial fibrillation and adverse myocardial outcomes. β-Blockers have the advantage not only of blood pressure control, but also of HR control, the importance of which has been convincingly advocated.

They are important agents for the treatment for perioperative hypertension, particularly in patients with both hypertension and tachycardia. They reduce the HR and contractile power and therefore tend to reduce blood pressure.

The choice of β-blocker is likely to be guided by pharmacokinetic considerations, including the speed of onset and duration of action, as well as by the side effects. β2-Receptor antagonists may provoke bronchospasm, which may limit their use in susceptible patients. They also have effects on atrioventricular (AV) conduction, causing a prolongation of conduction time through the AV node. This may be a disadvantage to their postoperative use, particularly if the patient has an intracardiac conduction abnormality.

Esmolol, metoprolol and labetalol are the most commonly used intravenous β-blockers for perioperative β-blockade for blood pressure control. Esmolol is 60% protein bound, and undergoes renal excretion. It has a half-life of approximately 9 minutes, owing to its rapid metabolism by esterase hydrolysis. As a result, esmolol has been used in the management of acute hypertensive events at induction and endotracheal intubation, during surgery, during emergence and endotracheal extubation and during the postoperative period both as prophylaxis and as therapy.

Metoprolol is a cardioselective compound. Intravenously, 1 to 5 mg may be given for blood pressure control with the initial dose usually at the lower range. An effect is usually seen within 2 to 3 minutes, and may last for up to 4 hours. Labetalol has selective, competitive, α1-adrenergic blocking and nonselective, competitive, β-adrenergic blocking activity. In man, the ratio of α-:β-blockade has been estimated to be approximately 1:7 after intravenous administration, in contrast to a ratio of 1:3 after oral dosing. Labetalol may be given both by bolus administration and by continuous infusion.

Dopaminergic agonists

Fenoldopam is a synthetic dopaminergic agonist without agonist adrenergic effects, although there is evidence of a mild adrenoceptor blocking effect. It may be particularly suited to controlling blood pressure in the perioperative period. Fenoldopam does not cross the blood–brain barrier and is a selective agonist at peripheral DA1 receptors. Vascular effects include dilatation primarily of the renal, mesenteric and coronary vasculature. There is also an increase in glomerular filtration rate and an increase in sodium and water excretion. Fenoldopam undergoes hepatic conjugation with no active metabolites and no adverse effects on cytochrome P450. Fenoldopam seems to be one of a small number of vasodilators with a highly favourable profile for use in the perioperative period.

Calcium channel blockers

In vascular smooth muscle, calcium channel blockade and the resulting reduction in calcium influx into the smooth muscle cell results in vasorelaxation and a fall in blood pressure. The dihydropyridines are used for blood pressure control. They interact with the dihydropyridine receptor on the L-type or T-type calcium channel, suggesting that an endogenous vasopressor might have an effect at this site. The effect of blocking this receptor is to render the channel more likely to be in the closed state, with resultant reduction in calcium influx and vasodilatation.

Systemic and coronary vascular resistance are reduced, blood pressure falls, cardiac filling pressures are maintained and cardiac and stroke output are increased. The lack of venodilatation and thus maintenance of preload is responsible for increasing stroke output and preserving pulmonary artery and pulmonary capillary wedge pressure. However, in patients with primary pulmonary hypertension, there is evidence to suggest a therapeutically useful pulmonary vasodilator effect.

Isradipine, nicardipine and nifedipine may be used as systemic vasodilators by the intravenous route. Intranasal nifedipine has been described as safe and effective, although some strongly question its use. Clevidipine is a new compound with an ultrashort duration of action owing to its metabolism by tissue esterases similar to esmolol. Clevidipine has a half-life of approximately 1 minute in cardiac surgery patients and a context-sensitive half-time of less than 2 minutes for up to 12 hours of administration; therefore, it is administered by infusion.

Other agents

Angiotensin-converting enzyme inhibitors reduce the generation of angiotensin II and thus reduce the effects of vasoconstriction, aldosterone secretion and sympathetic activation. Angiotensin-II (A-II) receptor antagonists act by binding to specific membrane-bound receptors that displace A-II from its type 1 receptor subtype. These drugs therefore function as selective blockers. Both groups of drugs have been shown to be highly effective in the management of chronic hypertension and chronic heart failure, and many cardiac surgery patients may be taking either ACE inhibitors or antithrombin receptor antagonists preoperatively.

Hydralazine has an uncertain mechanism of action. Hyperpolarization of muscle cells, probably through the opening of potassium channels, inhibition of the release of calcium from the sarcoplasmic reticulum in smooth muscle, reduction in calcium stores in the sarcoplasmic reticulum and stimulation of the formation of nitric oxide (NO) by the vascular endothelium have all been implicated. Its use in the preoperative period is now rare.

NITRIC OXIDE DONORS

Nitric oxide is an endogenous compound normally secreted by the vascular endothelium in response to a number of stimuli. These may activate receptors coupled to phospholipase C, producing an increase in inositol triphosphate, which results in an increase in calcium release from the sarcoplasmic reticulum. This, once linked to the binding protein calmodulin, activates NO synthetase and leads to the conversion of L-arginine to citrulline with the liberation of NO.

A number of drugs act as a source of NO promoting vasorelaxation. Nitric oxide gas is given by inhalation, but it is rapidly scavenged by haemoglobin and is quickly deactivated, with a half-life of less than 1 minute. As a result, it causes selective pulmonary vasodilatation and is unsuitable for systemic blood pressure control.

NITRITES

Sodium nitroprusside (SNP) is arguably the most effective vasodilator in both arterial and venous vasculature in clinical use, and is almost invariably effective, provided steps are taken to control a reflex increase in HR. Simultaneous administration of a β-blocker is therefore commonplace. Sodium nitroprusside is a highly unstable molecule. It is light-sensitive and the formulation must be provided and administered using light-protected equipment.

The molecule is broken down in erythrocytes with the consequent liberation of cyanide ions and NO. The cyanide ions are converted in the liver by rhodonase to thiocyanate, a reaction dependent on a sulphur donor such as thiosulphate. Thiocyanate undergoes renal excretion, and the presence of thiosulphate or other sulphur donor is an important factor in preventing the build up of cyanide ions and cyanide toxicity.

Sodium nitroprusside has a rapid onset and ultra-short duration of action. Its half-life is of the order of 2 to 4 minutes, although the metabolite thiocyanate has a half-life of several days. It is recommended that the duration of treatment should not exceed 72 hours.

NITRATES

In common with other nitrates, nitroglycerin (GTN) must be denitrated to produce NO, the active component. A number of denitration mechanisms have been proposed, including reaction with sulphydryl groups, or consequent on the actions of glutathione S transferase, cytochrome P450 and xanthine oxidoreductase. More recent evidence suggests that the conversion of GTN to 1,2 GDN and NO is catalysed by mitochondrial aldehyde dehydrogenase.

The primary use of GTN and other nitrates, including isosorbide mononitrate, is as antianginal agents. They have a beneficial effect on coronary blood flow via selective vasodilatation of epicardial coronary arteries and by venorelaxation and consequent reduction in LV end-diastolic pressure and hence subendocardial compression. Myocardial demand is also reduced consequent on a reduction of LV wall stress.

Nitrates are commonly used for perioperative blood pressure control, particularly in the setting of cardiovascular surgery. Step increases in an intravenous infusion of GTN cause a reduction in venous tone and central venous pressure, with a gradual reduction in systemic pressure. Bolus doses, on the other hand, cause an immediate and significant reduction in arterial pressure. The greater effect on the venous side of the circulation may be a reflection of different background rates of NO production in the vascular endothelium of veins and arterioles.

Key points

- Surgical stress and the effects of CPB combine to produce vasoconstriction and systemic hypertension in the intraoperative and early perioperative periods.
- Adequate preoperative control may reduce fluctuations in blood pressure perioperatively.
- Most patients need intravenous medication to control blood pressure during and immediately after surgery. The most commonly used agents are GTN and SNP.
- β-Blockade may be associated with decreased incidence of atrial fibrillation and adverse myocardial outcomes, and β-blockers should not be acutely withdrawn.

FURTHER READING

Chobanian AV, Bakris GL, Black HR, *et al.* Seventh report of the Joint National Committee on Prevention, Detection, Evaluation and Treatment of High Blood Pressure. *Hypertension* 2003;42:1206–1252.

Howell SJ, Sear JW, Foex P. Hypertension, hypertensive heart disease and perioperative cardiac risk. *Br J Anaesth* 2004;92:570–583.

Vuylsteke A, Feneck RO, Jolin-Mellgard A, *et al.* Perioperative blood pressure control: a prospective survey of patient management in cardiac surgery. *J Cardiothorac Vasc Anesth* 2000;14:269–273.

Chapter 23

Pulmonary hypertension

E. LIN AND A. VUYLSTEKE

Introduction

Pulmonary hypertension (PHT) can be associated with a variety of both pulmonary and extrapulmonary diseases. Acute PHT in critical care may often be secondary to conditions such as acute respiratory failure, left heart failure and pulmonary embolism, or due to decompensation of chronic PHT by concurrent pulmonary or cardiovascular disease. Patients with chronic PHT can also be admitted to critical care for the treatment of other conditions, or as part of their perioperative management. Some are admitted because they have benefited from a specific operation to treat the underlying pulmonary condition (lung transplantation, pulmonary endarterectomy).

Definition

Pulmonary arterial hypertension (PAH) is a term used to classify a variety of conditions that share in common an injury to the pulmonary vasculature that produces elevations in pulmonary arterial pressure. It is noteworthy that the definition of PHT has been the subject of heated debates for many years, and various numbers or indices have been proposed to define it.

It is now accepted that PHT can be defined as a sustained elevation of pulmonary arterial mean pressure to more than 25 mmHg at rest or 30 mmHg with exercise. It is defined as PAH if in addition the mean capillary wedge pressure and left ventricular end-diastolic pressure are less than 15 mmHg.

Clinically, PHT is a condition in which an increase in the right ventricular (RV) afterload leads to organ damage, either as a consequence of hypoxia or decreased blood flow. Treating PHT is ultimately taking care of the RV because it is the integrity of RV function, rather than the degree of vascular injury, that is the major determinant of symptoms and survival in PHT.

Classification

Pathophysiology

Regardless of its aetiology and presentation (acute or chronic), PHT is usually accompanied by RV dysfunction owing to increased afterload as a result of the increased pulmonary pressures. The RV failure (acute cor pulmonale) occurs when increased pulmonary vascular resistance overwhelms the ventricular compensatory mechanisms, either abruptly or gradually in the case of chronic cor pulmonale.

Ventricular interdependence (the way RV failure greatly affects diastolic and systolic function of the left ventricle [LV]), progressive RV ischaemia (the end stage of RV failure) and systemic organ hypoperfusion (caused by antegrade and retrograde heart failure) progressively causes multiorgan dysfunction and ultimately failure.

Table 23.1 Clinical classification of pulmonary hypertension

1. Pulmonary arterial hypertension	1. Idiopathic 2. Familial 3. Associated with a. Collagen vascular disease b. Congenital systemic-to-pulmonary shunts c. Portal hypertension d. HIV infection e. Drugs and toxins f. Other (thyroid disorders, glycogen storage disease, Gaucher disease, hereditary haemorrhagic telangiectasia, haemoglobinopathies, myeloproliferative disorders, splenectomy) 4. Associated with significant venous or capillary involvement a. Pulmonary veno-occlusive disease b. Pulmonary capillary haemangiomatosis
2. PHT with left heart disease	1. Left-sided atrial or ventricular heart disease 2. Left-sided valvular heart disease
3. PHT associated with lung diseases and/or hypoxaemia	1. Chronic obstructive pulmonary disease 2. Interstitial lung disease 3. Sleep disordered breathing 4. Alveolar hypoventilation disorders 5. Chronic exposure to high altitude 6. Developmental abnormalities
4. PHT due to chronic thrombotic and/or embolic disease	1. Thrombotic obstruction of proximal pulmonary arteries 2. Thrombotic obstruction of distal pulmonary arteries 3. Nonthrombotic pulmonary embolism (tumour, parasites, foreign material)
5. Miscellaneous	1. Sarcoidosis, histiocytosis X, lymphangiomatosis, compression of pulmonary vessels (adenopathy, tumour, fibrosing mediastinitis)

Abbreviations: HIV, human immunodeficiency virus; PHT, pulmonary hypertension.

Although PHT itself is a process initially thought to be driven by vasoconstriction, it now appears that pulmonary vascular proliferation and remodelling occur, involving a complex and heterogeneous constellation of multiple genetic, molecular and humoral abnormalities that interact in a complicated manner, with fibroblasts, smooth muscle, endothelial cells and platelets all playing a role. In a nutshell, the pathophysiology of PHT can be simplified to this: vasoconstriction, thrombosis and remodelling of the pulmonary vasculature.

Diagnosis

The diagnosis of PHT involves detection, characterization and assessment of the severity. This allows prognosis estimation and assessment of the therapeutic options. Most patients are diagnosed as the result of an evaluation of symptoms (such as some unstable patients in cardiothoracic critical

Table 23.2 Clinical symptoms and signs of pulmonary hypertension

Symptoms	Signs
Dyspnoea	Normal to low blood pressure (occasionally high)
Fatigue	Jugular venous distension with prominent a and v waves
Lower limb oedema	Lung changes
Weakness	RV heave
Palpitations	RV 4th and/or 3rd heart sound
Abdominal fullness	Loud P2
Angina	Ascites
Syncope and presyncope	Hepatomegaly (often pulsatile)
Cyanosis	

Abbreviation: RV, right ventricular.

care); whereas others are diagnosed during screening of asymptomatic populations at risk. Right heart catheterization (using a Swan–Ganz catheter) is mandatory to establish the diagnosis.

Treatment

Chronic medical therapy

Although there is no universal cure for chronic PHT, newer medical therapies have been shown to improve a variety of clinically relevant endpoints, including survival, exercise tolerance, functional class, haemodynamics, echocardiographic parameters and quality-of-life measures. Insights into the pathophysiology of PAH have supported the use of various therapeutic targets for treatment.

Surgical therapy

Surgical and interventional therapies for PAH in appropriately selected patients have the potential to dramatically improve or, in some cases, cure PAH. The radical option is to replace the diseased lung (by transplantation). Another option is atrial septostomy despite the fact that there is no definite evidence that it is worthwhile. It may be used as a bridge to transplantation. The artificial right-to-left shunt increases cardiac output, augments systemic oxygen transport (despite the fall in systemic arterial oxygen saturation) and decompresses the right heart. Pulmonary endarterectomy is the definitive treatment for those patients suffering from chronic thromboembolic hypertension and amenable to surgery (see Chapter 53).

Acute medical therapy

The first aim in critical care is to reduce RV afterload and improve oxygen delivery to tissues.

OXYGENATION

Treatment with 100% oxygen is a selective pulmonary vasodilator in patients with PHT, regardless of primary diagnosis, baseline oxygenation or RV function.

ANTICOAGULATION

Anticoagulation is desirable (as with any low cardiac output state) and should always be considered

UNDERLYING CAUSE

Attempts should be made to improve the underlying disease process. This may include optimization

Table 23.3 Diagnostic tools for pulmonary hypertension

Detection	Physical examination Chest radiograph Electrocardiogram Echocardiogram
Characterization	Essential testing Pulmonary function tests Overnight oximetry V/Q lung scan Connective tissue disease screen HIV serology Full blood count Liver function tests Antiphospholipid antibodies Confirmatory RHC with acute vasodilator testing Supplementary tests Transoesophageal echocardiography Spiral CT/pulmonary angiography Clotting studies Polysomnography Lung biopsy Oxygen saturation, uric acid, troponin
Assessment of severity	WHO functional class Six-minute walk test

Abbreviations: CT, computed tomography; HIV, human immunodeficiency virus; RHC, right heart catheterization; V/Q, ventilation/perfusion; WHO, World Health Organization.

of left heart failure therapy, optimization of gas exchange in chronic obstructive pulmonary disease or acute respiratory distress syndrome and antibiotics if an infective process is suspected.

Regardless of the aetiology, attention should be paid to avoiding respiratory acidosis and correcting metabolic acidosis. Measures to maximize recruitment of lung alveoli thereby reducing ventilation/perfusion (V/Q) mismatch and pulmonary vascular resistance should be employed, such as patient positioning and optimization of ventilation and positive end-expiratory pressure. Catecholamine use should be avoided if possible and endogenous release minimized by ensuring adequate analgesia and sedation and avoiding shivering.

DIRECT CONTROL

As the ultimate goal is to improve RV function, all key therapies are listed in the Management of the right ventricle paragraph!

Management of the right ventricle

The RV is a thin-walled, highly compliant but poorly contractile chamber. It is dependent on the function of the LV and in particular the septum. The blood supply to the RV depends on whether the coronary supply is right or left dominant (or balanced). In most cases, the right and left anterior descending coronary arteries both supply the interventricular septum and the majority of the RV free wall is supplied by the right coronary. Unlike the LV, which receives perfusion predominantly during diastole, the RV is perfused throughout the cardiac cycle, and is dependent on the perfusion pressure (systemic pressure) and RV pressure. Therefore, RV performance is directly related to systemic pressure during PHT. Additionally, the RV is very sensitive to increased RV preload or afterload, septic shock, coexistent LV dysfunction or right coronary artery disease.

PHARMACOLOGICAL SUPPORT

Numerous medications have been suggested and trialled in an attempt to:

- decrease preload: vasodilators such as glyceryl trinitrate;
- increase RV contractility: inotropes such as adrenaline;
- decrease afterload: inhaled nitric oxide, nebulized prostacyclin; and
- combine all these effects: phosphodiesterase inhibitors to decrease preload, increase contractility and decrease afterload

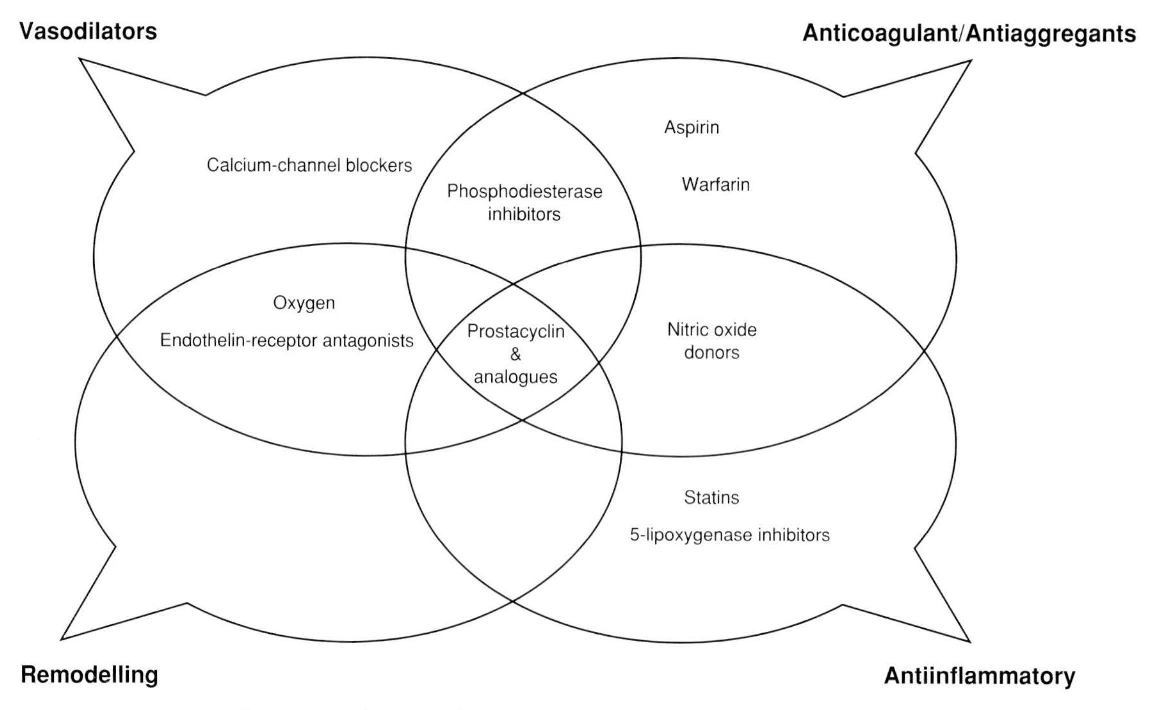

Figure 23.1 Treatment for PHT according to pathophysiology.

However, none is easy to use and their mechanism of action may be more complex than previously thought. Table 23.14 shows a brief overview of the main medications used in critical care to treat PHT, with some of their benefits and/or limitations. In clinical practice, these medications are used in combination and guided by careful monitoring.

In the acute setting in critical care, nebulized prostacyclin may be the best option to reduce pulmonary pressure and offload the RV. This may be administered via the endotracheal tube or a facemask, and can be weaned gradually, although it will need to be administered every 3 hours because of its short half-life.

In the context of more long-term treatment, oral sildenafil can be started and may have significant beneficial effects. Oral bosentan or an intravenous prostacyclin infusion may also be used to control longstanding PHT, but this may not alter the overall prognosis. This is nearly universally poor unless the primary cause can be corrected.

MECHANICAL SUPPORT

Mechanical support may be beneficial in life-threatening disease, but is usually only tried in specialized units:

- intra-aortic balloon pump: mode of action not understood but increased coronary blood flow, increased systemic arterial pressure and altered ventricular interaction are probably responsible;
- extracorporeal circulation (or oxygenation): can be used as a bridge to definitive intervention;
- rapid fluid removal by aggressive diuresis or renal replacement therapy: allows drastic reduction of ventricular preload; and
- artificial lung perfused by the RV and applied in parallel with the pulmonary circulation: could reduce ventricular load and improve cardiac efficiency in the setting of PHT (but this is not yet available!)

Table 23.4 Medical treatment of pulmonary hypertension

	Benefits	**Disadvantages**
Inhaled nitric oxide	Rapid onset of action No acute systemic effects therefore hypotension not a concern	Expensive Continuous administration Requires intubation for optimal delivery Difficult to wean – rebound Absence of evidence of benefit
Inhaled prostacyclin (and analogues)	Good clinical effec Relatively easy to wean No systemic effects at low dose	Requires specific nebulizers to avoid intolerance (facial flushes) Systemic effect observed at higher doses Must be administered regularly and frequently
Standard intravenous vasodilators (e.g. glyceryl trinitrate, sodium nitroprusside)	Good clinical effect	Marked systemic effect therefore hypotension a problem
Intravenous prostacyclin	Many studies and clinical reports Antiaggregant Potentially antiproliferative	Systemic vasodilatation Needs to be given by infusion owing to short half-life
Phosphodiesterase inhibitors (i.e., sildenafil)	Safe Multiple actions Can be given orally or intravenously	Systemic vasodilatation in the acute setting Many side effects Ceiling effect limits benefit
Endothelin receptor antagonists (e.g. bosentan)	Oral administration Well tolerated	Effects take time to be established and may not be significant in all patients

Key points

- Pulmonary hypertension is usually secondary to other conditions.
- Right ventricular strain and failure due to increased afterload causes the clinical syndrome.
- Management of the underlying cause should accompany pharmacological treatment.

FURTHER READING

Fischer LG, Van Haken H, Bürkle H. Management of pulmonary hypertension: physiological and pharmacological considerations for anesthesiologists. *Anesth Analg* 2003;96:1603–1616.

Klepetko W, Mayer E, Sandoval J, *et al.* Interventional and surgical modalities of treatment for pulmonary arterial hypertension. *J Am Coll Cardiol* 2004;43(12 Suppl S):73S–80S.

Simonneau G, Galie N, Rubin LJ, *et al.* Clinical classification of pulmonary hypertension. *J Am Coll Cardiol* 2004;43(12 Suppl S):5S–12S.

3.2 *Respiratory System in Cardiothoracic Critical Care*

Chapter 24

Noninvasive ventilation

C. MORO AND F. FALTER

Introduction

Noninvasive ventilation (NIV) is the delivery of ventilatory support without the need for an invasive artificial airway. It has a role in the management of acute or chronic respiratory failure and is increasingly being established in the treatment of patients with heart failure. Noninvasive ventilation is advocated in a range of acute and chronic conditions as well as home ventilation.

Modes

Continuous positive airway pressure

Continuous positive airway pressure (CPAP) provides a pneumatic splint that holds the upper airway open. It provides positive airway pressure throughout all phases of the ventilatory cycle, but does not provide any inspiratory support. End-expiratory pressure is usually limited to 5 to 10 cmH_2O; higher pressures tend to result in gastric distension.

Bi-level positive airway pressure

Bi-level positive airway pressure ventilation provides two preset levels of positive pressure, the lower at the end of expiration and the higher during inspiration. Ventilatory support is delivered by the transition between these two pressure levels; initiation of inspiratory pressure rise may be patient triggered or mandatory.

Pressure-limited ventilation

Ventilators are set to deliver inspiratory support up until a preset airway pressure is reached. Inspiration and expiration are triggered by the patient.

Mechanism of action

Noninvasive ventilation decreases the work of breathing by assisting with the respiratory effort and decreasing the amount of negative pressure needed to generate a breath. It improves pulmonary mechanics and oxygenation by increasing functional residual capacity, decreasing transdiaphragmatic pressure and decreasing diaphragmatic electromyographic activity. This leads to an increase in tidal volume, a decrease in respiratory rate and an increase in minute ventilation.

Application

A fundamental requirement for NIV is the ability of the patient to cooperate with treatment. Confusion or disorientation lead to poor results owing to displacement of the mask and noncoordination with the ventilator. For most patients, there is only a relatively small window of opportunity to initiate NIV. Increasing acidaemia, haemodynamic instability and exhaustion with decreased levels of consciousness make NIV likely to fail and endotracheal intubation necessary. Although the best starting point can only be judged clinically, the following are predictive of successful NIV:

Table 24.1 Advantages and disadvantages of noninvasive ventilation

Advantages	Disadvantages
Preservation of airway defence mechanism	Difficulty setting up
No sedation required	Discomfort, pressure sores on face
Avoiding complications of endotracheal tube	Air leak at higher pressures
Ability to communicate, eat and drink	Restriction of ambulation
Cooperation with physiotherapy	Possibility of aspiration (airway not protected)
Reduced dead space	Claustrophobia (especially hood)
Ease of application and removal	Demands on staff time to adjust
Availability on the ward or at home	Lack of access to bronchial tree for suction

- moderate hypercapnia ($Paco_2$ between 6 and 12 kPa);
- moderate acidaemia (pH between 7.10 and 7.35); and
- improvement in gas exchange, heart rate and respiratory rate within 2 hours of starting NIV.

Indications

Obstructive disease

Chronic obstructive pulmonary disease (COPD) remains the commonest indication for NIV and has been most studied. Reduced rate of intubation, mortality and length of hospital stay have been demonstrated, along with fewer complications. Noninvasive ventilation is not frequently used in the treatment of asthma; however, bi-level pressure has been shown to improve lung function more rapidly when compared with conventional treatment.

Table 24.2 Indications for noninvasive ventilation

Exacerbation of COPD
Acute cardiogenic pulmonary oedema
Weaning from invasive ventilation
Poor respiratory effort after tracheal extubation
Postoperative support, especially sleep apnoea and obesity (hypoventilation)
Hypoxia despite high Fio_2

Abbreviation: COPD, chronic obstructive pulmonary disease.

Cardiogenic pulmonary oedema

Continuous positive airway pressure has been shown to rapidly improve gas exchange, reduce dyspnoea and reduce intubation rates. Controversy remains regarding the use of bi-level positive airway pressure ventilation because it reduces inspiratory work even further and delivers additional tidal volume, but it may be associated with increased myocardial ischaemia.

Pneumonia

Despite doing little to facilitate the clearance of secretions, NIV is associated with reduced intubation rates and length of critical care stay in patients with severe community-acquired pneumonia. It is particularly effective in pneumonia complicating COPD, the immunocompromised state and after lung transplantation.

Weaning

Noninvasive ventilation can be an adjunct in weaning patients from invasive ventilation.

Table 24.3 Contraindications for noninvasive ventilation

Facial trauma/burns
Recent facial, upper airway, or upper gastrointestinal tract* surgery
Fixed obstruction of the upper airway
Life-threatening hypoxaemia*
Haemodynamic instability*
Severe comorbidity*
Impaired consciousness*
Confusion/agitation*
Vomiting
Bowel obstruction*
Copious respiratory secretions*
Focal consolidation on chest radiograph*
Undrained pneumothorax*

**Noninvasive ventilation may be used, despite the presence of these contraindications, if it is to be the "ceiling" of treatment.*
Adapted with permission from the British Thoracic Society Guidelines on NIV.

Failure of extubation

Noninvasive ventilation can be applied early in the development of postextubation respiratory failure, and CPAP followed by bi-level positive airway pressure ventilation is commonly attempted before reintubation. Caution should, however, be exercised because the benefit from such intervention is unclear.

Setting up noninvasive ventilation

The success of NIV depends on four crucial factors:

- comfortable patient–ventilator interface,
- optimal ventilator settings,
- appropriate monitoring, and
- a skilled and attentive care team.

Mask selection

Nasal, oronasal (full-face) masks, mouth pieces and an inflatable hood resembling a space helmet are currently available. They are usually made from a nonirritant material such as silicon rubber. The main characteristics to achieve comfort and safety are:

- minimal dead space and a soft inflatable cuff to provide a close seal with the skin,
- good fit along the contour of the face to minimize air leaks, and
- ease of removal, in case fast access to the airway is required.

Although there is little difference in efficacy, the nasal mask may be more comfortable than the full-face mask because it is applied to a smaller part of the face, but coordination with the ventilator is more difficult if the mouth is not covered, and greater patient cooperation and education are required. An adequate seal may be difficult to achieve, but it is important to apply the minimum strap tension despite these difficulties to avoid pressure sores. Different sizes and shapes of masks may provide a better fit. The nasal mask may make communication and oral intake easier. Either mask may be removed for short periods during treatment to allow patients a rest and facilitate speech, oral intake and expectoration.

Helmets are becoming more popular because of improved comfort and tolerability, although claustrophobia is a common complaint initially. The helmet has been shown to achieve comparable improvement in oxygen saturations and rate of reintubation with decreased facial skin breakdown; however, $Paco_2$ during the use of the helmet may remain elevated.

Ventilator selection and settings

Noninvasive ventilation can be delivered by conventional critical care machines or purpose-designed, smaller, more portable ventilators. The latter are able to provide synchronized NIV with automatic compensation for leaks.

Set volume NIV is often not successful owing to mask leakage and failure to deliver the selected tidal volume, leading to frequent triggering of alarms. Therefore, set pressure ventilators are usually used. These provide a high-flow CPAP or cycle between high inspiratory and low expiratory pressures (bi-level positive airway pressure generators) and thus are more leak tolerant and improve synchrony.

The following initial settings can be suggested for bi-level positive airway pressure ventilation:

- FiO_2 as in place before NIV;
- inspiratory pressure, 12 to 15 cmH_2O;
- expiratory pressure: 4 to 5 cmH_2O;
- trigger pressure: −2 cmH_2O;
- V peak%: 40%;
- inspiratory time: 1 to 1.5 seconds;
- rise time: 0.5 seconds;
- backup rate: 15 breaths/min; and
- backup inspiratory/expiratory ratio: 1:3.

The ideal inspiratory pressure should then be determined by gradually increasing inspiratory pressure as tolerated until adequate tidal volumes are achieved.

Table 24.4 Factors associated with success or failure of noninvasive ventilation in chronic obstructive pulmonary disease exacerbations

Success	Failure
High $PaCO_2$	High APACHE score
pH 7.25–7.35	Pneumonia
Low A–a gradient	Copious secretions
Improvement in $PaCO_2$, pH and respiratory rate after 1 hour	Edentulous
Normal conscious level	Poor nutritional status
	Confusion/impaired consciousness

Abbreviation: APACHE, Acute Physiology and Chronic Health Evaluation. Adapted with permission from British Thoracic Society Guidelines on NIV.

Complications

Complications of NIV include the following:

- local damage to facial tissue because of the pressure effects of the mask and straps;
- mild gastric distension;
- eye irritation;
- sinus pain or congestion; and
- barotrauma.

Adverse haemodynamic effects resulting from NIV are unusual, although preload reduction and hypotension may occur. Close monitoring is essential, and respiratory rate, comfort and synchrony with ventilation as well as oxygen saturation should be recorded.

Delays in recognizing NIV failure (seen as increasing respiratory acidosis, inability to maintain adequate oxygen saturation, increasing haemodynamic instability or development of arrhythmias, rising respiratory rate) delay intubation. This might be a cause of increased mortality.

Practical considerations

Commencing noninvasive ventilation

A full explanation and demonstration is required, and patient position should be optimized. The appropriately sized mask should be chosen and fitted, allowing the patient time to familiarize themselves with it. It is often easiest to commence NIV by the nurse holding the mask in place for the first few minutes before it is secured using straps or other headgear. These may need to be adjusted several times until comfortable. Arterial blood gas analysis is required soon after commencing NIV and at regular intervals or whenever settings are changed.

Troubleshooting

If the patient does not synchronize with the ventilator:

Table 24.5 Initiation process for noninvasive ventilation

Explain process to patient.
Select interface (usually face mask) and ventilator.
Fit the interface.
Silence ventilator alarms (if present).
Initiate noninvasive ventilation while holding mask in place (patient to hold mask if possible).
Start with expiratory positive airway pressure of typically 3–5 cmH_2O.
Titrate IPAP to patient comfort: start low (5–8 cm H_2O) and increase gradually up to 20 cmH_2O (usually 12–16).
Avoid IPAP >20 cmH_2O.
Set back up rate to 15 breaths per minute and back up I:E ratio to 1:3.
Secure mask: avoid excessive strap tightening.
Monitor Spo_2 and add entrained oxygen to achieve Spo_2 88%–92%.
Check for air leaks into eyes, around nose and sides of face.
Coach, encourage and reassure.
Monitor and check patient frequently.
Project an optimistic and confident attitude.

Abbreviations: I:E, inspiration:expiration; IPAP, inspiratory positive airway pressure.

- check mask fit for excessive leakage,
- adjust inspiratory time, and
- adjust inspiratory trigger.

If the patient is uncomfortable:

- adjust patient posture/position,
- adjust straps, change mask size/type, and
- try nasal mask.

If the patient feels next breath coming in before they have breathed out:

- reduce the rate.

If the patient feels breath is being delivered too forcefully:

- increase the rise time.

If the patient's respiratory rate is high and they feel breaths are not being delivered quickly enough (air hunger):

- decrease the rise time.

If the $Paco_2$ remains elevated:

- check circuit and connections for leaks,
- assess whether patient is rebreathing,
- check patency of expiratory valve,
- consider increasing expiratory pressure, and

Table 24.6 Factors to consider in adjusting failing noninvasive ventilation

Ensure prescribed medical therapy still being given (nebulized bronchodilators).
Consider adding IV aminophylline.
Consider need for physiotherapy and mucolytics.
Ensure no complications of NIV (e.g. pneumothorax or aspiration, check with radiograph).
If $Paco_2$ still elevated: Ensure oxygen in target range 88%–92% (or lower if necessary) to avoid worsening V/Q mismatch. Check for mask leakage; adjust straps or change mask size/type if necessary. Check circuit for leaks and patency of expiratory valve. Check synchronization with the ventilator. Adjust trigger sensitivities. Consider increasing EPAP if high PEEP suspected. Check chest wall movement. Consider increasing inspiratory positive airway pressure or inspiratory time. Consider adding doxapram.
Pao_2 low, but $Paco_2$ improved. Increase entrained oxygen.
Consider increasing EPAP.

Abbreviation: EPAP, expiratory positive airway pressure; NIV, noninvasive ventilation; PEEP, positive end-expiratory pressure.
Adapted with permission from the British Thoracic Society Guidelines for NIV.

- check patient synchronization with ventilator.

If ventilation is inadequate:

- consider increasing inspiratory pressure,
- consider increasing inspiratory time,
- consider increasing rate, or
- consider a different mode of ventilation.

Key points

- Noninvasive ventilation may provide respiratory support without the need for endotracheal intubation and the associated complications.
- Tight-fitting face masks may be very uncomfortable and poorly tolerated; nasal masks and hoods may be preferable.
- Setting up and frequently adjusting NIV is time consuming but necessary.
- Noninvasive ventilation may be continued in specialist wards or at home after discharge from critical care.

FURTHER READING

Caples SM, Gay PC. Noninvasive positive pressure ventilation in the intensive care unit: a concise review. *Crit Care Med* 2005;33:2651–2658.

Ferrer M, Esquinas A, Arancibia F, *et al.* Noninvasive ventilation during persistent weaning failure: a randomized controlled trial. *Am J Respir Crit Care Med* 2003;168:70–76.

Liesching T, Kwok H, Hill NS. Acute applications of noninvasive positive pressure ventilation. *Chest* 2003;124:699–713.

Masip J, Roque M, Sanchez B, *et al.* Noninvasive ventilation in acute cardiogenic pulmonary edema: systematic review and meta-analysis. *JAMA* 2005;294:3124–3130.

Chapter 25

Invasive ventilation

A.J. DAWSON AND A. VUYLSTEKE

Introduction

In cardiothoracic critical care, the vast majority of patients require mechanical ventilation at some point in time. It is therefore important to have a good understanding of the underlying mechanical technology of ventilators and the physiological effects of mechanical ventilation.

Mechanics of ventilation

All ventilators require five key components:

- a power source (pneumatic, electrical or combined);
- a drive mechanism, which transforms the energy source into direct gas flow to the patient;
- the ability to generate a pressure gradient (positive or negative) for flow delivery;
- control mechanisms (mechanical, pneumatic, electrical – closed or open loop); and
- a pneumatic circuit, which directs gas flow within the ventilator (internal circuit) and from the ventilator to the patient (external circuit).

Basic components of breath delivery

All breaths delivered by the ventilator can be broken down into four parts:

1. the end of expiration and beginning of inspiration;
2. the delivery of inspiration;
3. the end of inspiration and beginning of expiration; and
4. the expiratory phase.

Transition between the phases is controlled by ventilator settings known as '*phase variables*,' which are responsible for each part of the breath.

TRIGGERING PHASE

The triggering variable that begins the inspiratory gas flow can be time, pressure, flow or volume. The patient may control the beginning of inspiration (patient triggering). This usually requires the operator to set a 'trigger sensitivity' level. When time is the trigger variable, the breath is considered mandatory.

LIMITING PHASE

The limiting phase is the variable that places a maximum value on a control setting (e.g. pressure, volume, flow or time) during breath delivery. The type of waveform produced for pressure, flow and volume defines a breath delivery. Breaths may be:

1. *Volume-controlled*: a constant volume and constant flow waveform; the pressure waveform varies depending on lung characteristics.
2. *Pressure-controlled*: the pressure waveform has a preselected specific pattern, but volume and flow vary depending on lung characteristics.
3. *Time-controlled*: pressure, volume and flow waveforms all vary depending on lung characteristics.

CYCLING PHASE

The cycling phase ends inspiratory gas flow. This may also be pressure, volume, flow or time. For example, the ventilator may cycle to the expiratory phase when pressure reaches a certain set maximum during inspiration or cycle to the expiratory phase when flow falls to a set level (commonly 5 L/min) or percentage (commonly 25%) of peak flow.

EXPIRATION

Expiration is usually a passive process. However, it is possible with some ventilators to generate a negative end-expiratory pressure, by using the venturi effect and actively drawing airflow from the upper airway. Negative end-expiratory pressure helps to offset the increased mean intrathoracic pressure caused by positive-pressure ventilation and allows more rapid respiratory rate delivery. This technique is more commonly seen in paediatric critical care with the use of high-frequency oscillatory ventilation.

Advanced components of breath delivery

PAUSES

Two types of pause can be applied to the breath phases:

1. *Inspiratory pause*: this can be applied at the end of inspiration by delaying the opening of the expiratory valve preventing gas flow from leaving the circuit. Also called an 'inflation hold' or 'inspiratory plateau,' this manoeuvre prolongs the inspiratory time. This allows calculation of static compliance and airway resistance for respiratory dynamics, but more importantly provides extra time for lung compartments with a prolonged time constant to be adequately ventilated.
2. *An end-expiratory pause or expiratory hold*: this can be applied at the end of expiration, to assess pressure buildup within the patient's lungs and ventilator circuit owing to air trapping ('auto-positive end-expiratory pressure'). Both inspiratory and expiratory valves are closed at the end of expiration, allowing equilibration of the pressure within the patient's lungs and airways with the ventilator circuit. This manoeuvre requires complete absence of respiratory effort from the patient.

POSITIVE END-EXPIRATORY PRESSURE

Positive end-expiratory pressure is provided by the characteristics of the expiratory valve during mechanical ventilation. Positive pressure on exhalation can be achieved by either flow resistance or threshold resistance. Flow resistors direct expiratory flow through an orifice area or 'resistor' and act as an expiratory retard device. Pressure across the resistor therefore varies with flow. In comparison, threshold resistors allow expiratory flow to continue unimpeded until pressure within the circuit drops to that equal to the threshold value (the PEEP value). True threshold resistors are therefore unaffected by flow rate and are the expiratory valve of choice; they help to reduce expiratory resistance and reduce the risk of barotrauma.

Intrinsic PEEP, defined as an elevation of the static recoil pressure of the respiratory system at end expiration, may develop in patients with some form of airway obstruction or 'resistance' when incomplete exhalation occurs. The patient's own airways or inserted airway devices therefore act as flow resistors.

The application of PEEP may potentially improve patient ventilation and oxygenation in a number of ways. These include:

- recruitment of collapsed alveoli;
- increasing the functional residual capacity (FRC) and alveolar oxygen reservoir;
- minimizing intrapulmonary shunt; and
- encouraging redistribution of lung water from the alveoli to the interstitium.

Types of breaths

Distinction must be made between a mandatory breath, an assisted breath and a spontaneous breath. A mandatory breath is one in which the ventilator does all the work of breathing and controls the transition between phases of the breath. An assisted breath is one where the patient begins or "triggers" inspiration but the ventilator controls the inspiratory phase and the cycling of inspiration to expiration. A spontaneous breath is one in which the patient controls the transition between all breath phases.

Basic modes of ventilation

Terminology has become confusing when describing modes of ventilation. Each manufacturer has a different term for various types of ventilation and even different terms between newer generations of ventilator. We review the most commonly used terms.

CMV: CONTROLLED MECHANICAL VENTILATION OR CONTINUOUS MANDATORY VENTILATION

This is a mandatory mode of ventilation with no ability to sense patient respiratory effort. Sedation and/or paralysis of the patient is generally required. Breaths will be time triggered, volume or pressure limited and time or volume cycled. CMV is commonly selected as the default mode of ventilation after patient admission.

ACV: ASSIST/ASSIST-CONTROL VENTILATION

This mode of ventilation incorporates sensing mechanisms to assess patient respiratory effort. A drop in pressure, flow or volume within the circuit when the patient actively inspires is sensed by the ventilator and triggers the beginning of inspiration. When all breaths are patient triggered, the mode is referred to as an assist mode; when a backup rate is set and some breaths are time triggered, the mode is called assist control.

IMV: INTERMITTENT MANDATORY VENTILATION

Similar to CMV, IMV also allows spontaneous breathing between mandatory breaths. A minimum respiratory frequency is set by the operator that determines the time between mandatory breaths. Spontaneous breaths may be assisted with pressure support.

SIMV: SYNCHRONIZED INTERMITTENT MANDATORY VENTILATION

This modification of IMV allows the delivery of a mandatory breath to be triggered by patient inspiratory effort if it occurs in the appropriate time frame. When the time comes for mandatory breath delivery, the ventilator waits briefly to see if any patient inspiratory effort occurs to trigger the breath delivery. If triggering occurs, the ventilator delivers the set pressure or volume in response to the patient's effort, an assisted breath. Otherwise, a mandatory breath is triggered instead. The set SIMV rate determines the SIMV cycle (the time period between mandatory breaths). The set respiratory rate determines the SIMV period (the time allowed for mandatory breath delivery). The spontaneous breathing period is the time in between.

PCV: PRESSURE-CONTROLLED VENTILATION

Also called pressure-targeted or pressure-limited ventilation, in this mode of ventilation a peak target pressure, an inspiratory time, inspiration:expiration (I:E) ratio and respiratory rate are set to establish total cycle time. Often a slope or rise time (default rise time ~0.2 seconds) is also selected to determine the rapidity with which the target peak inspiratory pressure is achieved. Breaths may be patient- or time-triggered, are pressure-limited and may be time- or flow-cycled. Volume and flow delivery vary depending on lung characteristics.

PSV: PRESSURE-SUPPORT VENTILATION

Unlike the modes described, this is a spontaneous ventilation mode designed to support the patient by assisting with the work of breathing. Breaths are always patient-triggered and pressure-limited; they are also generally flow-cycled. Backup pressure and time cycling are often incorporated in case of leaks in the system or active exhalation by the patient during inspiratory pressure delivery. Volume delivery varies depending on the pressure set, the degree of inspiratory effort made by the patient and their lung characteristics.

CPAP: CONTINUOUS POSITIVE AIRWAY PRESSURE

This is a mode of ventilatory support used in spontaneously breathing patients only. It may be delivered from a mechanical ventilator, but is more commonly delivered from a free-standing CPAP unit. These systems may function as demand flow or continuous flow systems. Demand flow systems apply positive pressure during exhalation only utilizing a PEEP device. The patient must drop the pressure in the circuit with inspiratory effort to receive gas flow via a one-way valve device. In comparison, continuous flow systems utilize a threshold resistor and reservoir to maintain the pressure within the circuit at the set level. Source gas flow must be high enough to maintain pressure in the system regardless of the inspiratory flow demanded by the patient. Continuous flow systems are preferred because they avoid the potential for rebreathing and triggering sensitivity issues seen with demand-flow systems and provide the minimum variation in airway pressure throughout the respiratory cycle.

BiPAP: Bi-LEVEL POSITIVE AIRWAY PRESSURE, Bi-LEVEL PRESSURE ASSIST

This mode of ventilation is described in many different ways including, bi-level PEEP, bi-level CPAP, bi-level positive pressure and bi-level pressure support. It is a spontaneous mode of ventilation similar to CPAP where the positive airway pressure level is set individually for the inspiratory (IPAP) and expiratory (EPAP) phases of the breath cycle. The breath is patient-triggered, pressure-limited and flow-cycled between the two set pressure levels. However, some ventilators allow backup time triggering and time cycling to be set in case of patient apnoea. The overall ventilatory effect is very similar to PSV with PEEP.

IRV: INVERSE RATIO VENTILATION

Not a mode of ventilation in its own right, but an adaptation of the usual inspiratory and expiratory time ratios, this technique was primarily introduced to try to improve oxygenation in patients with acute lung injury. Inspiratory time is prolonged relative to the expiratory time, increasing the mean airway pressure and potentially encouraging re-expansion of collapsed, noncompliant lung. The shortened expiratory time tends to add an element of incomplete expiration resulting in auto-PEEP. This in itself may be beneficial as it can increase FRC and oxygenation, but needs to be monitored to ensure avoidance of alveolar barotrauma. Significant degrees of sedation or paralysis are often required to avoid patient dyssynchrony. However, studies have shown that low tidal volume, high respiratory rate and optimum PEEP may be beneficial in acute lung injury, and this is now the preferred primary mode of ventilation.

ASV: ADAPTIVE SUPPORT VENTILATION

This mode of ventilation utilizes the waveforms for pressure, volume and flow to calculate the dynamic compliance and expiratory time constant for the ventilator–patient circuit. From this, the respiratory rate and tidal volume that will minimize the work of breathing for the patient are determined depending on the set target parameters. Patient-triggered breaths are supported with PSV and the ventilator adjusts the pressure delivery to keep the respiratory rate and tidal volume in the optimal calculated range. When the patient is apnoeic breaths are time-triggered, pressure-limited and time-cycled.

HFV: HIGH FREQUENCY VENTILATION

As the name implies, this mode of ventilation uses much higher respiratory rates, and as a consequence much lower tidal volumes, than conventional mechanical ventilation. The mechanism of action of ventilation and oxygenation are not clearly understood. Alveoli located close to the airways are thought to be ventilated by convection as usual. However, it is unclear how more distant alveoli are ventilated and a number of gas mixing theories have been proposed. These include 'Pendelluft,' gas streaming and helical diffusion, Taylor dispersion, molecular diffusion and 'Spike' formation. Discussion of these theories is beyond the scope of this chapter.

The primary purpose for the use of HFV is to minimize the mean airway and intrathoracic pressures while maintaining ventilation and oxygenation in patients in whom conventional mechanical ventilation has failed. There are five different types of high-frequency ventilation:

- high frequency positive pressure ventilation (HFPPV);
- high frequency jet ventilation (HFJV);
- high frequency oscillatory ventilation (HFOV);
- high frequency flow interruption (HFFI); and
- high frequency percussive ventilation (HFPV).

High frequency positive pressure ventilation uses conventional volume- or pressure-limited ventilation with a low compliance circuit and respiratory rates of 60 to 110/min, but is not often employed because of concerns about inadequate tidal volume delivery and air trapping.

High frequency jet ventilation uses an attachable catheter or specialized endotracheal tube to deliver pulses (20–30 msec) of high-pressure gas flow into the airway at a rate of 100 to 600/min. The actual tidal volume delivered is dependent on the length of the pulsation, the driving pressure of the jet, the jet orifice size and the lung characteristics. Exhalation is passive. The HFFI system is actually very similar to HFJV in practice. Instead of an intermittently delivered gas jet, a constant high-pressure gas flow is interrupted by a control mechanism at frequencies up to 15 Hz.

High frequency oscillatory ventilation uses a reciprocating pump mechanism to generate an oscillating pressure wave within the circuit. Pressure in the airway is positive during the inspiratory phase and negative during the expiratory phase. Rates of 60 to 300/min are used.

High frequency percussive ventilation incorporates characteristics of conventional positive pressure ventilation with jet ventilation. High frequency (1.7- to 5-Hz) jet pulses are continuously delivered during the set inspiratory time, each jet pressure limited to the set peak airway pressure.

CLOSED LOOP/SERVO-CONTROLLED MODES

Closed loop/servo-controlled modes use feedback monitoring systems within the ventilator to assess breath delivery, compare and contrast the actual breath delivered with the set target parameters and then adjust subsequent breath delivery to match these set parameters more closely. Commonly used closed loop/servo-controlled modes include mandatory minute ventilation (MMV) and pressure-regulated volume-controlled ventilation (PRVC).

MANDATORY MINUTE VENTILATION

Overall minute ventilation is assessed and compared with the set minimum minute ventilation. Any spontaneous ventilation performed by the patient is 'counted' towards the target minute ventilation. This allows the patient's spontaneous ventilatory pattern to fluctuate while guaranteeing set minimum minute ventilation. This mode may be used as part of a weaning protocol.

PRESSURE-REGULATED VOLUME-CONTROLLED VENTILATION

The target tidal volume is produced over several breaths as the ventilator adapts the inspiratory time and/or flow to deliver the target volume within the set pressure limit.

Physiological effects of mechanical ventilation

Effects on the circulation

Positive pressure ventilation causes an increase in intrathoracic pressure. This impedes venous return to the heart by decreasing the pressure gradient from the peripheral venous system to the right atrium and reduces right ventricular preload. Pulmonary vascular resistance and therefore right ventricular afterload are also increased. The left ventricular preload is reduced owing to the interdependence of the ventricular systems with an ultimate decrease in cardiac output (CO). Increased pressure around the great vessels of the heart can also affect baroreceptor activity. Oscillations of systolic arterial blood pressure owing to fluctuations in CO may be seen between the inspiratory and expiratory phases of mechanical ventilation. Usually the magnitude of these oscillations is small (~10 mmHg), but may be marked in the setting of hypovolaemia, high inspiratory pressures, reduced chest wall compliance and atrioventricular dyssynchrony. Detrimental effects on splanchnic blood flow, renal blood flow, fluid retention and intracranial pressure have all been reported with positive pressure ventilation.

Effects on the respiratory system

The potential damage owing to the requirement for some form of intubation aside, mechanical ventilation has a number of detrimental effects on the respiratory system that should be considered.

Table 25.1 Detrimental effects of ventilation on the respiratory system

Detrimental effects
VALI/VILI: thought to be due to diffuse lung injury caused by regional overdistension of lung compartments and/or repeated alveolar recruitment and collapse during tidal volume delivery
Overt barotrauma and the risk of pneumothorax and/or tension pneumothorax
Potential oxygen toxicity from the application of high F_{IO_2}
Patient–ventilator dyssynchrony with increased work of breathing and respiratory fatigue
Mucosal drying, ulceration, bleeding and secretion retention
Impairment of the mucociliary escalator and increased infection risk

Abbreviations: VALI, ventilator-associated lung injury; VILI, ventilator-induced lung injury.

Possible effects on other physiological systems

- Gut distension and dysmotility owing to air swallowing, requirement for sedative/narcotic medication and feeding tubes.
- Gastrointestinal ulceration, bleeding, infection, inflammation and ischaemia. The mechanism remains unclear, but may be secondary to venous congestion of the mucosal wall, inadequate mucosal oxygen delivery and development of ischaemia with bacterial translocation.
- Sleep disturbance, agitation and fear.
- Difficulty communicating.
- Neuropsychiatric complications including critical care neuropathy and critical care psychosis.

Physiological effects

Both applied and intrinsic PEEP increase alveolar and intrathoracic pressure throughout the respiratory cycle. This reduces CO and elevates central venous and pulmonary artery pressures. This may have effects on intracranial pressure and splanchnic and renal blood flow.

The effects of PEEP on oxygenation of the patient are complex. It may be seen to increase or decrease intrapulmonary shunt, depending on the characteristics of the patient's lungs and pulmonary vasculature. Positive end-expiratory pressure may increase ventilation of alveolar dead space and increase shunt by recruiting alveoli that are not perfused. It may also increase intrapulmonary shunt by diverting blood flow towards nonventilated parts of the lung owing to overexpansion of ventilated lung and the resultant increase in pulmonary vascular resistance in those blood vessels exposed to the elevated airway pressure. On the other hand, PEEP may decrease intrapulmonary shunt by reducing alveolar collapse in dependent parts of the lung where perfusion is greatest, thereby improving oxygenation.

The application of PEEP can increase the work of breathing for the patient if care is not taken with ventilator parameter settings. The decrease in airway pressure required to trigger an assisted breath needs to be larger; therefore, greater work is required by the patient, unless the ventilator is set to trigger on an absolute fall in pressure regardless of the PEEP pressure.

The PEEP influences the distribution of total body water between the intravascular and extravascular fluid compartments. As an impediment to venous return, PEEP encourages movement of fluid out of the vascular space into the peripheries. This may lead to peripheral oedema, inadequate peripheral circulation, tissue ischaemia, infection and necrosis. A decrease in central circulating blood volume may result and the renal compensatory mechanisms of salt and fluid retention worsen oncotic pressure gradients and further encourage the development of oedema.

Oxygenation of the patient only increases if improvements in alveolar recruitment, FRC and intrapulmonary shunt (resulting in increased oxygen content of the blood) outweigh the decline in CO and oxygen transport and delivery that invariably occurs with the application of PEEP. This improvement is seldom seen unless oxygen saturations are below 85% to 90%.

Key points

- Addition of PEEP may improve oxygenation by recruitment of collapsed alveoli, reducing intrapulmonary shunt and increasing FRC; however, this is offset by increased venous pressure and potential reduced CO.
- Synchronized intermittent ventilation and pressure support are most commonly used in lightly sedated patients because they are well tolerated and can be weaned if tolerated.
- Continuous mandatory and pressure-controlled ventilation (especially if inspiratory phase prolonged) is uncomfortable, and relatively deep sedation is required.
- Negative pressure ventilation has numerous deleterious systemic effects, including gastrointestinal ileus and ulceration, and may precipitate hypotension if intravascular filling is relatively poor.

FURTHER READING

Barnes TA. *Core textbook of respiratory care practice.* Mosby; 1994.

Cairo JM, Pilbeam SP. *Mosby's respiratory care equipment.* St. Louis: Mosby; 2004.

MacIntyre NR, Branson RD. *Mechanical ventilation.* Philadelphia: W. B. Saunders; 2001.

Young JD, Sykes K, Hahn CE, *et al. Respiratory support in intensive care.* London: BMJ Publishing Group; 1999.

Chapter 26

Weaning from mechanical ventilation

S.J. ALLEN AND B. McGRATTAN

Introduction

The decision to wean from ventilatory support must balance two opposing concerns: the increased risk of ventilator-associated pneumonia and sepsis with prolonged ventilation versus the increase in morbidity and mortality with premature extubation. The general principle of this chapter is that liberation from the ventilator should commence as soon as possible after the conditions warranting intubation have begun to resolve. The following are considered:

- The physiological effects of weaning from mechanical ventilation.
- Identifying patients ready to commence weaning.
- Methods of weaning.
- Identifying patients ready for extubation or decannulation of tracheostomy.
- Failed extubation and prolonged weaning.
- Emerging techniques.

The cardiovascular pathophysiology of weaning

The withdrawal of mechanical ventilation has the potential to cause cardiovascular instability. This is especially true in cardiac surgery patients.

Increased oxygen demand

The increased respiratory muscle activity of spontaneous ventilation results in increased oxygen demand. This necessitates a rise in cardiac work and myocardial oxygen demand. This may lead to myocardial ischaemia in patients with untreated coronary artery disease, incomplete revascularization or recovering myocardium. Patients with impaired left ventricular (LV) function may be unable to raise their cardiac output sufficiently to meet these demands. They will maintain oxygen supply by either increasing oxygen extraction (noted by falling Svo_2) or by blood flow redistribution, typically away from the splanchnic region. This leads to a fall in gastric pH and a risk of mucosal ischaemia.

Decreased intrathoracic pressure

The reduction in intrathoracic pressure after cessation of mechanical ventilation results in increased venous return. This may lead to LV end-diastolic volume overload and pulmonary oedema (particularly in those with reduced LV compliance). Furthermore, the decrease in intrathoracic pressure surrounding the LV, with no change in the pressure surrounding extrathoracic arteries, effectively increases the afterload of the LV, increasing wall tension and thus myocardial oxygen demand.

Increased sympathetic tone

Weaning to spontaneous respiration may be psychologically and physiologically challenging for the patient recovering in cardiac critical care. Circulating catecholamines increase, predisposing to myocardial ischaemia as a result of increased arterial pressure and tachycardia.

Readiness for weaning

Weaning from ventilation begins with the recognition that factors justifying intubation and ventilation are not present anymore. Some points should be noted.

- These are screening criteria. Some patients never meet all of these criteria before extubation (in one trial, 30% of extubated patients never met weaning readiness criteria) and clinical judgment plays an important role in deciding when and whom to wean.
- Haemodynamic stability has particular importance in cardiac critical care. Attention should be paid to ongoing cardiac issues such as myocardial ischaemia, ventricular dysfunction and the likelihood of their reversibility.
- In patients with severe preexisting respiratory disease, the guidelines on oxygenation may be inappropriate. Target criteria should be reset to reflect baseline gas exchange, meaning that premorbid blood gas results are particularly useful.
- Patients should be actively screened and considered for commencement of weaning at least on a daily basis.
- Ongoing bleeding warrants continuing sedation and ventilation because return to the operating room may be necessary.

Table 26.1 Assessing readiness for weaning

Criterion	Description
Recommendations	Evidence for reversal of underlying cause Adequate oxygenation (P/F ratio >150 mmHg, PEEP ≤5–8 cmH_2O, Fio_2 ≤0.4–0.5, pH >7.25) Haemodynamic stability, not actively bleeding Absence of ongoing myocardial ischaemia Low- to moderate-dose inotropes The ability to initiate respiration
Considerations	Afebrile No significant acidosis Adequate haemoglobin Adequate mentation Stable metabolic status; phosphate, magnesium, etc. Adequate cough and airway protection

Abbreviation: PEEP, positive end-expiratory pressure; P/F, Pao_2/Fio_2.
After McInytre et al. Chest 2001;120;375–396.

Methods of weaning

Spontaneous breathing trial

A spontaneous breathing trial (SBT) may be valuable whenever extubation is considered, and should be considered at least on a daily basis. This should consist of allowing the patient to breathe an appropriate Fio_2 spontaneously through the endotracheal tube.

Studies show that, without SBT, physicians tend to underestimate capacity for weaning; around 80% of general critical care patients tolerate their first SBT and proceed to extubation. However, SBTs should always be properly monitored and discontinued if there is any haemodynamic instability.

Duration of SBT varies, but is usually in the range of 30 to 120 minutes. In general, patient tolerance of SBT is assessed by respiratory pattern, adequacy

Table 26.2 Methods for spontaneous breathing trials

Mode of trial	Comments
T-piece	With 5 cmH_2O CPAP
PSV	PSV 7–10 cmH_2O; CPAP 5 cmH_2O

Abbreviations: CPAP, continuous positive airway pressure; PSV, pressure support ventilation.

Table 26.3 Criteria determining success of weaning

Criterion for assessment	Description
Acceptable gas exchange	Sp_{O_2} >90%; P_{O_2} >8 kPa; pH >7.32
Haemodynamic stability	HR ≤120–140 or changes ≤20%, stable blood pressure, no increase in vasopressor or inotrope dosage
Stable and sustainable respiratory pattern	Rate ≤30–35 breaths min^{-1}
Changes in mental status	No detrimental change (e.g. agitation, confusion)
Patient comfort	No worsening discomfort
Sweating	A marker of increased work of breathing, discomfort
Work of breathing	Use of accessory muscles, laboured breathing

Abbreviation: HR, heart rate.

of gas exchange, haemodynamic stability and subjective evaluation of patient comfort. The associated morbidity of a well-conducted and monitored SBT is low. Tolerance of the trial should lead to a decision regarding removal of mechanical support and the artificial airway. It is the only mode of weaning that has been repeatedly proven systematically to reduce duration of ventilation and length of stay in critical care.

Modes of progressive withdrawal

In those patients who repeatedly fail SBT, there should be a determined effort to establish the reasons and correct these before further weaning. Failure of the SBT is often the sign that a problem has not been corrected; LV failure is a common cause in cardiac surgical patients.

Once these factors are excluded or dealt with, there are two main options. Each has proponents and the debate over which is better is lively. Option one is to maintain a constant background level of adequate respiratory support, and perform regular SBTs (usually once a day). Option two attempts to condition respiratory muscles by gradually increasing the load placed on them through a gradual reduction in the level of mechanical support. This can be accomplished in several ways.

- *Synchronized intermittent mandatory ventilation alone:* This is not recommended because it increases the work of breathing and is less effective than when used in combination with pressure-support ventilation (PSV).
- *Synchronized intermittent mandatory ventilation in combination with PSV:* Once this mode is established, the patient is then weaned by a gradual reduction in the number of controlled breaths delivered. When there are no further controlled breaths delivered, the patient may move on to the stages described next.
- *Gradual reduction in PSV:* The patient is weaned using PSV with a gradual reduction in the level of pressure support applied up to the point where either extubation or SBT can be considered.
- *T-piece/continuous positive airway pressure training:* The patient is maintained on moderate levels of ventilatory support alternating with gradually lengthening periods of unassisted T-piece or continuous positive airway pressure breathing, without PSV support.

There is little consensus in the literature as to which of these techniques is superior. Daily assessment seems to be the major factor in expediting liberation from ventilation.

Readiness for extubation

Patients who have passed a SBT should be considered for extubation. These criteria may not be rigorous enough to be able to recommend decannulation

Table 26.4 Possible factors contributing to ventilatory weaning failure

Respiratory	
Airflow Resistance	Bronchospasm Tube kinking Secretions Airway oedema
Chest wall	Pleural effusion Pneumothorax Obesity Abdominal distension Sternal instability
Parenchyma	Hyperinflation Alveolar oedema Infection
Central drive	Sedation Sleep deprivation Hypothyroidism Metabolic alkalosis
Muscle weakness	Malnutrition Myopathy Hypophosphataemia
Neuromuscular	Critical illness Polyneuropathy Muscle relaxants Phrenic nerve injury
Cardiovascular	LV dysfunction RV dysfunction Myocardial ischaemia Pulmonary hypertension
Psychological	Anxiety Confusion Agitation

Abbreviations: LV, left ventricular; RV, right ventricular.

in patients who have undergone repeated failures of extubation. Such patients may require more detailed assessment, together with planning of postextubation strategies (noninvasive ventilation, preparation for reintubation).

Failed extubation or weaning

The general principle is that failure of weaning or extubation should prompt a rigorous search for the underlying reason, which should then be addressed before further weaning attempts. This is a fundamental part of successful weaning. A strategic, organized and multidisciplinary approach to the patient ensures that:

- reversible factors are identified and treated; and
- all aspects of prolonged weaning are addressed (nutrition, muscle strength, nursing issues, mobilization, etc.) and are reviewed regularly.

The commonest reasons for failure are:

- respiratory load that exceeds the patient's ventilatory capacity;
- cardiovascular limitation; and
- psychological issues.

Table 26.5 Criteria for extubation

Adequate mentation, confusion being a particular challenge
Adequate cough to clear secretions
Minimal secretions, a commonly quoted measure is that they require suctioning less than every two hours
The ability to maintain and protect their own airway
Have passed a spontaneous breathing trial

Tracheostomy

Insertion of tracheostomy can shorten duration of weaning by:

- increasing patient comfort,
- reducing the need for sedatives,
- reducing dead space, and
- improving airway toilet.

The decision to insert a tracheostomy needs to balance risk and benefit (Chapter 9).

Left ventricular dysfunction

Left ventricular dysfunction is a common reason for failed weaning and the considered use of inotropic agents may allow easier extubation. In particular, phosphodiesterase inhibitors (enoximone and milrinone) have been successfully used in this

Table 26.6 Diagnosis and management of left ventricular failure during weaning

Diagnosis	
Clinical	Impaired oxygenation, bilateral rhonchi or crepitations, frank pulmonary oedema
Radiological	Typical radiographic appearance of pulmonary oedema
Haemodynamic	Increased PCWP, decreased Svo_2
Noninvasive	Increased extravascular lung water
Echocardiographic	New segmental wall motion abnormalities (during weaning)
Management	
Reduce preload	Diuresis, haemofiltration
Improve LV contractility	β-Adrenergic agonists (dobutamine, adrenaline) Phosphodiesterase inhibitors (milrinone) Calcium sensitizers (levosimendan)
Reduce afterload	Vasodilators (GTN)
Optimize LV	ACE inhibitors, $\pm$ β-blockers
Mechanical support devices	Rarely consider IABP, if in situ consider leaving in situ
Coronary perfusion	Consider ischaemia, maintain diastolic blood pressure

Abbreviations: ACE, angiotensin-converting enzyme; GTN, nitroglycerin; IABP, intra-aortic balloon pump; LV, left ventricular; PCWP, pulmonary artery occlusion wedge pressure.

setting due to their beneficial inodilatory properties. If an intra-aortic balloon pump (IABP) is in situ, simultaneous weaning of both IABP and ventilation is a recipe for failure. It may be more prudent to leave the IABP until the patient is stable after extubation. Insertion of an IABP may allow successful extubation in certain cases.

Myocardial ischaemia

The diagnosis of myocardial ischaemia should be suspected if the following happen during weaning (usually SBT):

- recurrent episodes of pulmonary oedema;
- electrocardiographic changes (angina);
- rising pulmonary artery pressures; or
- the development of mitral or tricuspid regurgitation.

Echocardiography may allow detection of segmental wall motion abnormalities during the weaning process. Once recognized or suspected, the patient should be managed as for LV dysfunction (which usually accompanies the ischaemia) while considering definitive management of the condition. Options may include IABP support during weaning, angiography, angioplasty or surgical revascularization.

Right ventricular dysfunction

Right ventricular (RV) dysfunction is not infrequently a reason for failure of weaning in cardiac critical care and may cause greater difficulties than LV dysfunction during weaning. The diagnosis of RV dysfunction as a reason for failure can be difficult and is often based on the following:

- preoperative and intraoperative knowledge of the patient's cardiac function;
- rising right atrial pressure;
- increasing tricuspid regurgitation;
- falling Svo_2 and cardiac output;
- deteriorating hepatic function; and
- echocardiography, which may also help to guide treatment.

Management of RV dysfunction should be instituted before further weaning attempts are made.

One of the major causes of RV dysfunction is hypoxia-induced pulmonary hypertension. Of course, the risk of hypoxia is real during attempts at weaning from ventilation. If this occurs and results in a rise in pulmonary artery pressure, the already tired RV fails, hypoxia worsens, the RV fails more and a vicious circle is established in which failure from weaning causes and is caused by RV failure. This can be broken by preventing pulmonary hypertension by judicious use of vasodilators and by ensuring optimal oxygenation. This therapy

Table 26.7 Management strategies for right ventricular failure during weaning

Strategy	Management option
Optimize preload	Guide by echocardiography Often diuresis – sometimes fluid loading
Improve RV contractility	β-Adrenergic agonists (dobutamine) Phosphodiesterase inhibitors (milrinone) Calcium sensitizers (levosimendan)
Reduce RV afterload	Inhaled pulmonary vasodilators (iloprost) Systemic pulmonary vasodilators (GTN) Oral therapy (sildenafil)
Improve coronary perfusion	Vasopressors

Abbreviations: GTN, nitroglycerin; RV, right ventricular.

should be continued for some time after discharge from the critical care area to prevent recurrence and readmission.

Emerging concepts

Noninvasive ventilation

The use of noninvasive ventilation (Chapter 23) shows promise as part of a strategy to assist in weaning by providing planned support following extubation. It can be useful as a rescue technique of failing extubation if applied early but it should not delay reintubation if there is no early evidence of benefit (within 1 hour).

Protocol-based weaning

The evidence on the benefits of protocols for weaning is mixed. The existence of a protocol (irrespective of the specific modes of weaning specified) may improve performance by ensuring regular attention to readiness for weaning and extubation. This may be of particular benefit in units that rely on nonphysician assessment. Remember that guidelines and protocols do not work from a locked filing cabinet! They only succeed if staff are familiar with them and trained and motivated to follow them.

Automated weaning

The use of ventilator-based, computer-driven, automated weaning algorithms has been shown significantly to shorten duration of weaning in both general critical care patients and after cardiac surgery, even when compared with patients weaned according to a standard protocol. Based on respiratory rate, tidal volume and end-tidal CO_2, the algorithm automatically switches from mandatory ventilation to spontaneous respiration and then reduces the level of respiratory support over time, while maintaining the patient in a defined 'physiological comfort zone.' When a specified level of support is reached, the ventilator performs a SBT by reducing support to a minimum. Such systems are now available and may find a place in cardiac surgical critical care.

Key points

- Regular assessment for readiness to wean, together with regular SBT, shortens the duration of ventilation.
- A SBT is a useful way to assess readiness for withdrawal of ventilatory support and provide structure to weaning strategies.
- Failure to wean with SBTs should result in a rigorous search for correctable causes of this failure.
- Progressive weaning, after failure of SBT, can be accomplished equally well by different strategies.
- Noninvasive ventilation, protocol-based weaning and automated ventilatory weaning may shorten duration of mechanical ventilation and length of stay in critical care.

FURTHER READING

Alia I, Esteban A. Weaning from mechanical ventilation. *Crit Care* 2000;4:72–80.

MacIntyre NR, Cook DJ, Ely EW, *et al*. Evidence-based guidelines for weaning and discontinuing ventilatory support: A collective task force facilitated by the American College of Chest Physicians; the American Association for Respiratory Care; and the American College of Critical Care Medicine. *Chest* 2001;120(6 (Suppl):375S–395S.

Chapter 27

Acute lung injury

M. GEORGIEVA, S MORDZYNSKI AND Y.G. WEISS

Introduction

Despite advances in surgical technique, anaesthetic management and postoperative care, acute lung injury (ALI) continues to be a leading cause of morbidity and mortality. In 1994, the American–European Consensus Conference on Acute Respiratory Distress Syndrome (ARDS) Committee defined ALI and ARDS based on three criteria: oxygenation, chest radiograph and pulmonary artery occlusion pressure. ALI and ARDS may be caused by direct injury to the lungs, or by indirect damage via a systemic inflammatory response. It is a severe complication associated with cardiopulmonary bypass (CPB), pulmonary resection and lung transplantation.

Cardiopulmonary bypass–induced lung injury

Reported incidence following CPB ranges from 1% to 3%, with a mortality rate of 30% to 70%.

Pathophysiology

Although not totally clear, it is hypothesized that a systemic inflammatory response is initiated during surgery by a number of processes. These include blood contact with the foreign surface of the CPB apparatus, development of ischaemia–reperfusion injury and endotoxin translocation across the ischaemic gut wall owing to splanchnic hypoperfusion and low cardiac output. The initiating agent triggers complement activation primarily through the alternative pathway, with release of anaphylatoxins C3a and C5a. Neutrophil induction occurs, with subsequent release of lysosomal granular contents such as elastase and myeloperoxidase, production of proinflammatory cytokine factors and induction of nitric oxide synthase with increased production and release of nitric oxide. This leads to endothelial damage, vasodilatation, myocardial depression and lung injury. The coagulation cascade, kallikrein and the fibrinolytic systems are also implicated in the pathophysiology of lung injury.

After CPB, endogenous factors such as interleukin (IL)-10, tumor necrosis factor-a and IL-1 receptor antagonists limit the inflammatory response and prevent organ damage. Protamine may also have a deleterious role to play owing to classical immune- and complement-mediated anaphylactoid reactions.

Pulmonary resection associated lung injury

The prevalence of ALI/ARDS after lung resection ranges from 2.2% to 4.2% with a mortality of 52% to 65%. The highest mortality rates have been associated with right pneumonectomy. Several risk factors have been associated with postpneumonectomy pulmonary oedema.

Pathophysiology

Altered endothelial permeability plays a central role in the pathogenesis of lung injury following

Table 27.1 American–European Consensus Conference on ARDS Committee definition of acute lung injury and adult respiratory distress syndrome

	Timing	Oxygenation	Chest radiograph	Pulmonary artery occlusion pressure
Acute lung injury	Acute onset	$Pao_2/Fio_2 \leq 300$ mmHg, regardless of PEEP level	Bilateral infiltrates on chest radiograph	≤18 mmHg or no clinical evidence of left atrial hypertension
Acute respiratory distress syndrome	Acute onset	$Pao_2/Fio_2 \leq 200$ mmHg, regardless of PEEP level	Bilateral infiltrates on chest radiograph	≤18 mmHg or no clinical evidence of left atrial hypertension

Abbreviation: PEEP, positive end-expiratory pressure.

pulmonary resection, but the exact mechanism remains unclear. Surgical manipulation of the lung, oxygen toxicity owing to high inspired oxygen requirement during single-lung ventilation and the ischaemia–reperfusion injury resulting from collapse and re-expansion of the operated lung all induce production of active oxygen radicals, as well as compromise of endogenous antioxidant systems. Other mechanisms include impaired lymphatic drainage and lung trauma owing to delivery of large tidal volumes with high inspiratory

Table 27.2 Factors associated with development of lung injury

Direct lung injury	Indirect lung injury
Aspiration of gastric contents	Sepsis
Pneumonia	Severe trauma
Pulmonary contusion	Head injury
Drowning	Burns
Toxic inhalation injury	Multiple blood transfusions
Pulmonary resection	Drug overdose
Lung transplantation	Pancreatitis
Following upper airway obstruction	Bone marrow transplantation
Multiple fractures	Leukoagglutinin reactions
	Venous air embolism
	Amniotic fluid embolism
	Cardiopulmonary bypass

Table 27.3 Risk factors associated with postcardiopulmonary bypass lung injury

Age >60
Total volume of blood pumped during bypass >300 L
Smoking
Emergency surgery
Preoperative New York Heart Association classes III and IV
Low cardiac output
Left ventricular ejection fraction ≤40%
Systemic hypertension
Previous cardiac surgery
Shock
Number of blood products received

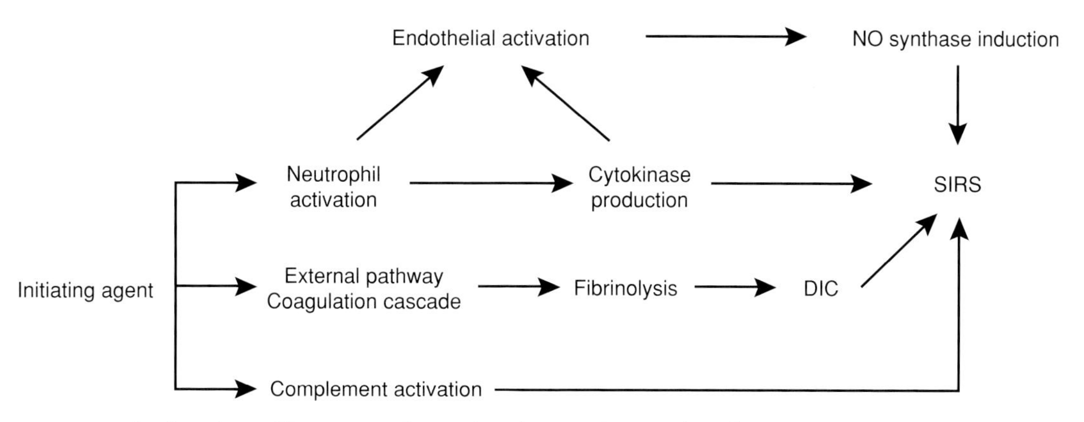

Figure 27.1 Pathophysiology of lung injury after cardiopulmonary bypass: the inflammatory response.

pressures during single-lung ventilation. Elevated pulmonary vascular pressures after pneumonectomy lead to a net increase in capillary filtration pressures, allowing the translocation of fluid and protein to the interstitial pulmonary space and the development of pulmonary oedema. Microembolized particulate matter, such as blood clots, may further elevate pulmonary vascular resistance, thereby worsening lung damage.

Table 27.4 Factors associated with acute lung injury and acute respiratory distress syndrome after lung resection

Preoperative
Age >60
Male gender
Chronic alcohol abuse
Smoking
Concurrent cardiac disease
Prior radiotherapy or chemotherapy
Intraoperative
Pneumonectomy (right > left, carinal > noncarinal)
High intraoperative ventilation pressures
Excessive fluid administration
Extent of tissue resection
Duration of surgery
Reoperation
Administration of blood products
Postoperative
Fluid overload
Nonbalanced drainage of hemithorax with pneumonectomy

Pulmonary injury after lung transplantation

Ischaemia–reperfusion injury is a common cause of respiratory failure in the first 72 hours after lung transplantation, along with haemorrhage, infection, technical problems and acute rejection. It is characterized by the development of airspace disease, progressive hypoxaemia and increases in pulmonary vascular pressures, reflecting both epithelial and endothelial injury. The severe form of ischaemia–reperfusion injury with FiO_2/PiO_2 at 200 mmHg or lower is defined as primary graft failure. The reported incidence is 12% to 25% and it accounts for more than 30% of deaths within the first 30 days after lung transplantation.

Pathophysiology

Three groups of factors are involved in the pathogenesis of ischaemia–reperfusion injury: factors related to the donor, method of graft preservation and effects of implantation and reperfusion after a period of ischaemia.

DONOR FACTORS

Proper organ selection is of great importance with regard to transplant outcome. Lungs from

Table 27.5 Risk factors associated with ischaemia–reperfusion injury after transplantation
Use of cardiopulmonary bypass
Body mass index >25 kg/m^2
Long graft ischaemic time
Immediate postoperative pulmonary hypertension
Primary pulmonary hypertension
Donor age
Donor female gender
Donor African American race

brain-dead patients are exposed to inflammatory events, profound disturbances in endocrine function, episodes of hypotension, prolonged ventilation, trauma, aspiration and infection. This may lead to organ susceptibility to ischaemia–reperfusion injury and alloimmune response following transplantation. It has been shown that IL-8 is upregulated in bronchoalveolar lavage samples and lung tissue from brain-dead donors, and the level correlates significantly with primary graft failure incidence.

GRAFT PRESERVATION

The flush solution – its composition, volume, temperature, and pressure – as well as the inflation and oxygenation of the donor lung and storage temperature are of great importance in organ preservation. Hypothermia is essential for organ storage, but is associated with oxidative stress, intracellular calcium overload, iron release, sodium pump inactivation and induction of cell death. This may induce upregulation of molecules on the cell surface membrane and the release of proinflammatory mediators that will subsequently activate donor and recipient leukocytes after reperfusion. Significant microvascular damage leading to persistent blood flow obstruction can be observed after prolonged ischaemia. This event is known as the 'no-reflow phenomenon.'

REPERFUSION

Reperfusion of the graft leads to a variety of insults, including upregulation of adhesion molecules, cytokines, endothelin, cellular injury from lymphocytes and neutrophils, complement activation, increase in thromboxanes, apoptosis and reduction in endogenous nitric oxide. Endothelin-1 may accumulate before and during the first few hours after reperfusion, which can lead to an increase of vascular endothelial growth factor and subsequently increased vascular permeability.

Clinical course

The clinical course of lung injury is marked by three phases: exudative, proliferative and fibrotic.

Exudative phase

The exudative phase encompasses the first 7 days after exposure to a precipitating agent. Endothelial–epithelial barrier damage occurs and altered endothelial permeability leads to accumulation of protein-rich oedema fluid in the interstitial and alveolar spaces and hyaline membrane formation. Dependent regions of the lungs are predominantly involved. Diminished aeration and atelectasis leads to development of intrapulmonary shunting and consequent hypoxaemia. Pulmonary vascular injury may also occur, with vascular obliteration. This leads to pulmonary hypertension, increased dead space and secondary hypercapnoea.

Proliferative phase

Approximately 7 days after the onset of the pulmonary injury, lung repair processes are started, which heralds the beginning of the proliferative phase.

Fibrotic phase

Lung injury may progress to extensive pulmonary fibrosis with obliteration of normal pulmonary architecture and development of emphysematous regions of the lung. This is the late fibrotic phase.

Diagnosis

Acute-onset shortness of breath and rapidly progressive hypoxaemia are the most important clinical features of the syndrome. Laboratory values are generally nonspecific and reflect underlying clinical disorders. Chest radiography reveals diffuse alveolar and interstitial bilateral infiltrates. Computed tomography demonstrates heterogeneous pulmonary infiltrates with increased density in the dependent regions of the lung. Differential diagnosis includes cardiogenic pulmonary oedema, pulmonary haemorrhage, diffuse pneumonia and acute interstitial and hypersensitivity pneumonitis.

Treatment

The treatment of ALI is predominantly supportive. Lung-protective mechanical ventilation strategies are used and attention to fluid balance is required. Pharmacological therapies studied have been disappointing because of a lack of effect on mortality; however, transient improvements in oxygenation may be achieved by a number of methods.

Ventilator strategies for lung protection

Patients with ALI are prone to ventilator-associated lung injury owing to heterogenic lung involvement and subsequent exposure of a relatively small lung area to positive pressure ventilation. This so-called baby lung leads to volutrauma, barotrauma and release of cytokines with systemic inflammatory response. Lung-protective strategies may prevent worsening of ALI.

Treatment of acute hypoxaemia with high concentrations of oxygen may lead to release of free oxygen radicals with subsequent development of parenchymal injury, hyperoxic tracheobronchitis and absorption atelectasis. The specific threshold for oxygen toxicity is unknown. Keeping the FiO_2 below 0.6 to maintain arterial PO_2 above 60 mmHg may minimize oxygen toxicity and late pulmonary fibrosis.

The use of low tidal volumes ($\leq$6 mL/kg) has been shown to be associated with a decrease in mortality. Other techniques such as the 'open lung approach' (maintaining expiratory plateau pressure $\leq$30 cmH_2O, and keeping the positive end-expiratory pressure [PEEP] above the lower inflection point) or higher PEEP levels are commonly used, but have not been shown to decrease mortality or length of critical care stay.

The static compliance of the respiratory system over the course of lung inflation is well demonstrated by a pressure–volume (P–V) curve. The initial flat portion of the curve shows small increases in lung volume caused by increasing pressure. After this, the increased slope of the curve shows improved lung compliance. The point at which compliance increases significantly is called the lower inflection point or P^{flex}. At higher inflation pressures the slope of the P–V curve again flattens at the upper inflection point. Setting PEEP above the lower, but below the upper inflection point, allows delivery of adequate tidal volumes while limiting repetitive opening and closing of lung units (cyclical atelectasis) and minimizes ventilator-associated lung injury.

Pressure-controlled ventilation may be beneficial by limiting peak and plateau transalveolar pressures. Oxygenation may be improved by using inverse ratio ventilation. Lung-protective ventilation may lead to elevated $PaCO_2$, referred to as *permissive hypercapnia*. Recruitment manoeuvres may be important components of lung-protective ventilation strategies. Recruitment is a dynamic process of reopening collapsed alveoli through an intentional increase in transpulmonary pressure.

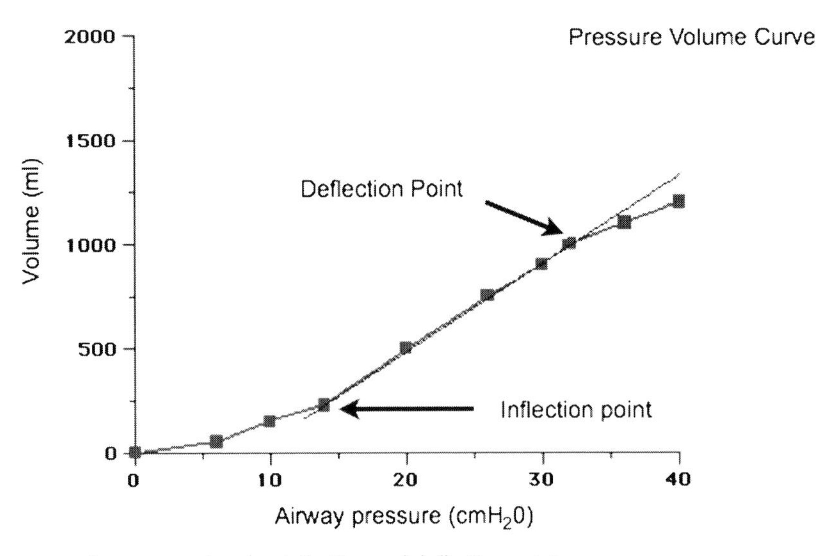

Figure 27.2 Pressure–volume curve showing inflection and deflection points.

Conflicting results mandate further studies evaluating optimal pressure, duration, frequency and outcomes. Side effects such as transient desaturation, hypotension, barotrauma and arrhythmia may occur. The prone position has several physiological benefits – recruitment of dorsal atelectatic lung units, improved respiratory mechanics, decreased ventilation–perfusion mismatch and improved drainage of secretions. The use of prone position transiently improves oxygenation, but has no survival benefit. Complications include retinal damage, nerve compression, pressure sores, vascular catheter dislodgement, limitation of diaphragmatic excursion, venous stasis and loss of artificial airway. Optimal fluid management is of a great importance for proper lung function and adequate tissue perfusion. Two alternative fluid strategies are often used – conservative and liberal. The liberal approach focuses on delivering adequate cardiac output, organ perfusion and oxygen supply. The conservative fluid management strategy prioritizes lung function and gas exchange and has been shown to improve pulmonary function, and shorten the duration of mechanical ventilation and critical care stay without increasing nonpulmonary organ failure. However, studies do not reflect any benefit on mortality. The routine use of the pulmonary artery catheter to guide fluid therapy in the management of patients with ALI is not recommended. It has not been shown to improve organ function or survival, but has been associated with more complications than central venous catheter-guided therapy.

Pharmacological therapy

Acute lung injury is characterized by altered distribution of blood flow in the injured lung with loss of hypoxic vasoconstriction in the nonventilated lung regions and impaired vasodilatation in the aerated lung zones.

Inhaled nitric oxide may provide selective vasodilatation in ventilated lung units, thereby improving ventilation–perfusion mismatch, hypoxaemia and pulmonary hypertension. Inhaled nitric oxide leads to a transient improvement in oxygenation, but does not decrease mortality in published studies. It can be useful as a rescue therapy for severe ARDS with refractory hypoxaemia.

Endogenous surfactant, by lowering alveolar surface tension at the air–fluid interface, is critical in maintaining lung inflation at low transpulmonary pressures. Patients with ALI have complex surfactant abnormalities, such as decreased production, alteration in phospholipid composition, and loss of surfactant protein SP-B and SP-A content. Function is impaired owing to leaked plasma proteins, active oxygen radicals and proteases. Replacement therapy with natural or synthetic surfactant showed no improvement in reducing mortality or ventilator-free days.

Glucocorticosteroids have been studied for some time owing to their anti-inflammatory and antifibrotic properties. No benefits have been proven in prevention and treatment of early phase ARDS. According to the ARDS Network Trial, administration of corticosteroids for persistent ARDS does not reduce mortality, but may increase the number of ventilator- and shock-free days during the first 28 days, in association with an improvement in oxygenation, respiratory system compliance and blood pressure. No increased incidence of infection complications was reported. Initiating steroid therapy more than 2 weeks after the onset of ARDS may increase the risk of death.

Supportive care

Prophylaxis against gastrointestinal bleeding and venous thromboembolism should be considered. Prevention, early recognition and treatment of nosocomial infections are critical because sepsis is a major cause of associated mortality. Adequate nutrition because of increased energy requirements is required; enteral feeding is preferred. Overfeeding should be avoided to prevent excessive carbon dioxide production. Tight glucose control may be associated with a decreased mortality.

Complications

Lung injury is characterized by reduced lung compliance. This, together with positive-pressure ventilation, may cause further lung injury, with development of pneumothorax, pneumomediastinum and emphysema. Prolonged mechanical ventilation and the concomitant use of steroids and neuromuscular blocking agents are associated with neuropathy and myopathy.

One-year outcome in survivors of acute respiratory distress syndrome

Long-term survivors of ARDS have significantly reduced quality of life. They suffer from cognitive impairment such as reduced memory, attention deficit, concentration problems and decreased mental processing speed. Studies report persistent functional disability, muscle wasting and weakness, fatigue, immobility of large joints, finger contracture, foot drop, entrapment neuropathies, alopecia and persistent pain at chest tube insertion sites.

Pulmonary function generally improves considerably after 3 months and reaches the maximum by 6 months after extubation. However, over 50% of ARDS survivors continue to have respiratory abnormalities, including restrictive impairment or decreased diffusion capacity.

Key points

- Lung injury in the cardiothoracic setting contributes to high morbidity, mortality and low quality of life.
- Acute lung injury may follow CPB, lung resection or transplantation, or may present concomitantly with any critical illness.
- The clinical course is characterized by exudative, proliferative and fibrotic phases.
- Treatment is supportive, and a number of measures may be employed to improve oxygenation until the disease improves. Lung-protective ventilation strategies should be used if positive-pressure ventilation is required.
- Long-term lung damage and neurological dysfunction are, unfortunately, common.

FURTHER READING

Cepkova M, Matthay M. Pharmacotherapy of acute lung injury and the respiratory distress syndrome. *J Intensive Care Med* 2006;21: 119–143.

de Perrot M, Liu M, Waddell TK, *et al.* Ischemia-reperfusion-induced lung injury. *Am J Respir Crit Care Med* 2003;167: 490–511.

Grichnik K, D'AmicoT. Acute lung injury and acute respiratory distress syndrome after pulmonary resection. *Semin Cardiothorac Vasc Anesth* 2004;8:317–334.

Hall R, Smith MS, Rocker G. The systemic inflammatory response to cardiopulmonary bypass: pathophysiological, therapeutic, and pharmacological considerations. *Anesth Analg* 1997;85:766–782.

Steinberg KP, Hudson LD, Goodman RB, *et al.* Efficacy and safety of corticosteroids for persistent acute respiratory distress syndrome. *N Engl J Med* 2006;354:1671–1684.

Chapter 28

Extracorporeal membrane oxygenation

R. TIRUVOIPATI AND G.J. PEEK

Introduction

Extracorporeal membrane oxygenation (ECMO) uses cardiopulmonary bypass (CPB) technology to treat potentially reversible cardiorespiratory failure. ECMO involves drainage of venous blood, adding oxygen and removing carbon dioxide and returning the blood to the circulation. The oxygenated blood is returned to a vein in venovenous ECMO and to an artery in venoarterial ECMO.

Extracorporeal membrane oxygenation compared with cardiopulmonary bypass

ECMO differs from CPB in that it can be used for several weeks while awaiting the recovery of heart or lung function. Although superficially similar to CPB, ECMO has certain important differences that are discussed below.

Perfusion technique

The aim of CPB is to facilitate cardiac surgical procedures; it requires total venoarterial bypass (by cannulating aorta and right atrium or inferior vena cava and superior vena cava). This causes stagnation of blood in the pulmonary circulation, some chambers of the heart and some parts of the extracorporeal circuit, such as the venous reservoir. To prevent clotting in these circumstances, total anticoagulation of blood is required.

In contrast with CPB, ECMO involves partial bypass, which is usually established by extrathoracic cannulation with no stagnation of blood in the pulmonary circulation or heart chambers. In addition, there is no direct exposure of blood to air as there would be intraoperatively. The ECMO circuit does not include a large reservoir or the suction apparatus; therefore, partial heparinization provides sufficient anticoagulation. The blood flow of the pump is set at a rate that matches the metabolic needs of the patient; the haematocrit and temperature are maintained in the normal range.

Clinical management

Intraoperative CPB is usually performed for as short a time as possible to minimize systemic complications. ECMO, however, is instituted in the critical care unit with the aim of supporting cardiac or respiratory function for days to weeks (and rarely months). Attention must be given to the use of antibiotics, fluid management, nutrition and general care in the same way as with any critical care patient. Significantly, high-dose inotropes and high-pressure and high oxygen ventilation can be avoided.

Indications

ECMO is indicated in acute cardiorespiratory failure that is potentially reversible. It may also be indicated in some instances of nonreversible cardiorespiratory failure as a bridge to transplantation.

Table 28.1 Differences between cardiopulmonary bypass and extracorporeal membrane oxygenation

	CPB	ECMO
Common cannulation sites	Right atrium or vena cava for venous drainage and aorta for return.	Jugular or femoral vein for drainage and carotid or femoral artery for return in venoarterial ECMO and femoral vein in venovenous ECMO
Heparinization	Full (ACT $\geq$400)	Limited (ACT 160–200)
Hypothermia	Yes	Not usual
Anaemia	Yes	No
Autotransfusion	Yes	No
Arterial filter	Yes	No
Venous reservoir	Yes	No

Abbreviations: ACT, activated clotting time; CPB, cardiopulmonary bypass; ECMO, extracorporeal membrane oxygenation.

Respiratory failure

Reversibility of respiratory failure may be difficult to determine. Most centres exclude patients with chronic lung disease and irreversible pathologies such as pulmonary fibrosis. In addition, patients ventilated with high peak inspiratory pressure (>30 cmH_2O) and high Fio_2 (>0.8) for more than 7 days are usually not suitable for ECMO owing to irreversible lung injury. Acute pneumonia and acute lung injury remain the commonest causes of severe respiratory failure precipitating a requirement for ECMO. Survival following ECMO support is variable, and large-scale studies are ongoing

Cardiac failure

ECMO may be indicated where there is a failure to wean from CPB, cardiogenic shock or cardiac arrest. Other indications include acute myocardial infarction and primary graft dysfunction after cardiac transplantation. The use of ECMO in cardiac failure is increasing, but this is not supported by evidence in the literature at present.

Emerging indications

It has been suggested that ECMO is a potential therapy for a number of other conditions and research has started into the following indications:

- cardiopulmonary resuscitation;
- rewarming in trauma and hypothermia patients;
- hyperthermia for cancer treatment; and
- interval support for organ retrieval.

Mode

The mode of ECMO depends on the indication. The mode of choice for primary respiratory failure is venovenous ECMO; for primary cardiac failure, it is venoarterial ECMO, although some centres use venoarterial ECMO for all patients.

Venovenous ECMO is superior to venoarterial ECMO in primary respiratory failure because it maintains normal pulmonary blood flow; this may allow faster healing of lung injury and reduces the risk of systemic microembolization. It also allows preservation of normal haemodynamics with systemic blood flow being dependent on native cardiac output. In addition, it can be established

Table 28.2 Differences between venoarterial and venovenous extracorporeal membrane oxygenation

	Venoarterial ECMO	Venovenous ECMO
Indication	Primary cardiac failure	Primary respiratory failure
Cannulation sites	Jugular/femoral veins/right atrium for drainage and carotid/femoral artery or aorta for return	Jugular, femoral veins for drainage and return
Circulatory support	Complete	No direct effect, although improved oxygen delivery to coronary and pulmonary circulation does improve haemodynamics
Systemic perfusion	Circuit flow and CO	CO only
Pulse pressure	Reduced	Unaffected
CVP monitoring	Unreliable	Reliable
Arterial $Pa{O_2}$	Unreliable (controlled by circuit)	Reliable
Monitoring of adequacy of systemic perfusion	$SV{O_2}$, lactate levels	Arterial blood gases and lactate levels
Recirculation	No	Yes
Left ventricular emptying and coronary artery blood flow	Could be affected	Not affected
Decrease in initial ventilator settings to 'rest' settings	Rapidly	Slowly

Abbreviations: CO, cardiac output; CVP, central venous pressure; ECMO, extracorporeal membrane oxygenation.

percutaneously (or by the semi-Seldinger technique), thereby avoiding cannulation and ligation of a major artery.

The circuit

The ECMO circuit consists of cannulae, tubing, pump and servo-regulator, membrane lung, heat exchanger and bridge.

Cannulae

The blood flow in the ECMO circuit is proportional to the size of the venous cannula. The size of the arterial cannula is less critical, although it should be able to deliver a predicted blood flow without significantly increasing pressure proximal to the membrane lung. The shortest catheter with the largest internal diameter provides the highest rate of blood flow. The size of the cannulae ranges from 8 to 28 F.

Tubing

The tubing is usually made of polyvinyl chloride (PVC) or silicone except for the portion of raceway (the piece of tubing that goes into the roller occlusion pump), which is Tygon S-65-HL (Norton Performance Plastics, Granville, NY). This is chemically altered PVC material and is more resistant to wear in the roller pump.

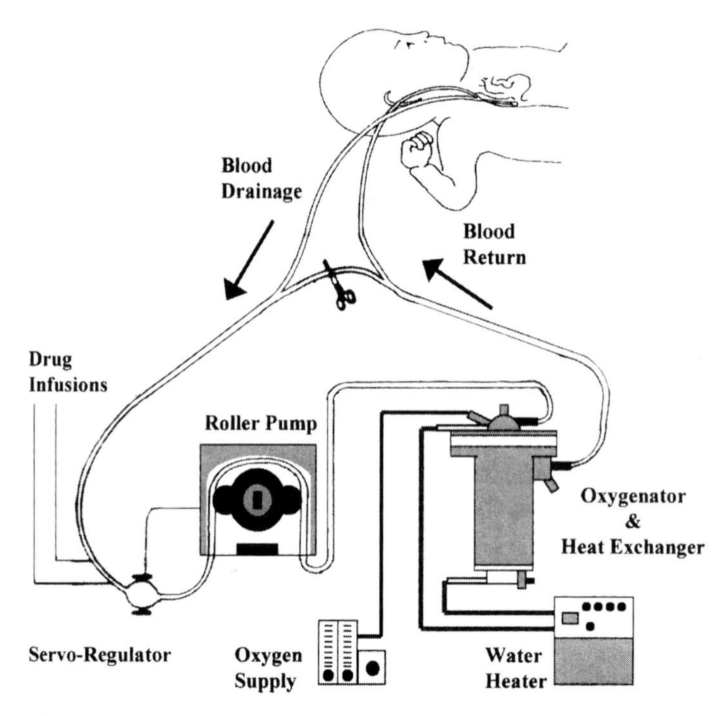

Figure 28.1 Schematic diagram of an ECMO circuit.

Pump and servo-regulator

Roller pumps are most commonly employed, but are safe for prolonged use only if used with a continuous servo-regulator. This prevents the development of high negative pressures, which could lead to haemolysis or damage to vascular endothelium. Roller pumps are reliable and cause little haemolysis.

Centrifugal pumps can be used; they generate flow by a spinning rotor that is magnetically coupled to the motor. Although centrifugal pumps have superior blood handing properties when compared with roller pumps during CPB, these pumps can generate very high negative pressures (up to −700 mmHg) when used without a reservoir during ECMO and this may lead to cavitations and haemolysis.

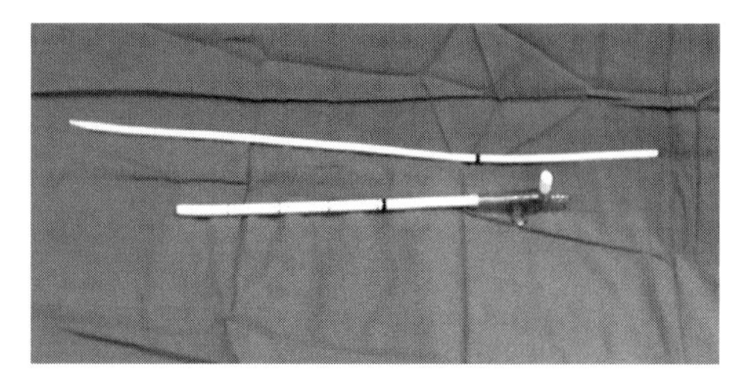

Figure 28.2 Single-lumen ECMO cannula and dilator.

Membrane lung

There are three types of membrane lungs in common usage: silicon membrane oxygenator, microporous hollow fibre oxygenator (polypropylene) and nonporous hollow fibre oxygenator (polymethylpentene). Although diffusion is good in silicon lungs, they have a large surface area without bioactive coating that leads to platelet activation and thrombus formation. Microporous hollow fibre (polypropylene) oxygenators contain tiny pores thorough which gas exchange takes place and can be coated with nonthrombogenic materials. However, they may leak plasma in an unpredictable

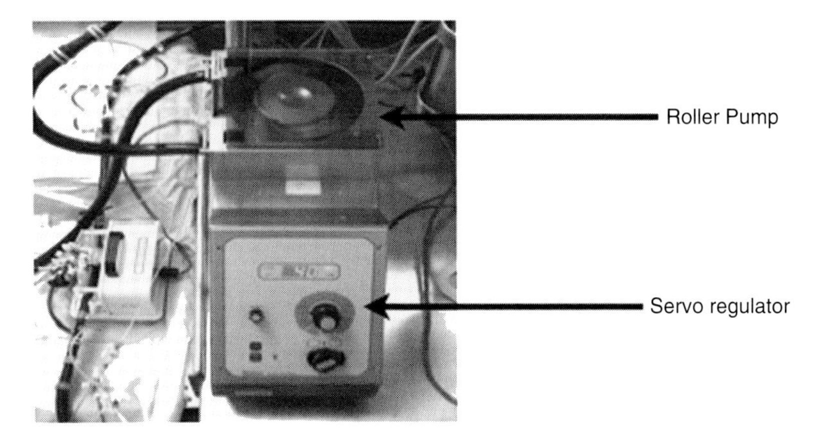

Figure 28.3 Roller pump and servo-regulator.

fashion after a few hours, making them less than ideal for long-term support. The nonporous hollow fibre membrane oxygenator (polymethylpentene) combines the advantages of silicon and hollow-fiber devices, and is the best available oxygenator for long-term support.

Heat exchanger

The large surface of the extracorporeal circuit leads to significant heat loss. To ensure normothermia, a heat exchanger is an essential component of the ECMO circuit. Heat exchangers may be integral to the oxygenator or as a separate device. They can also be used to cool patients if required.

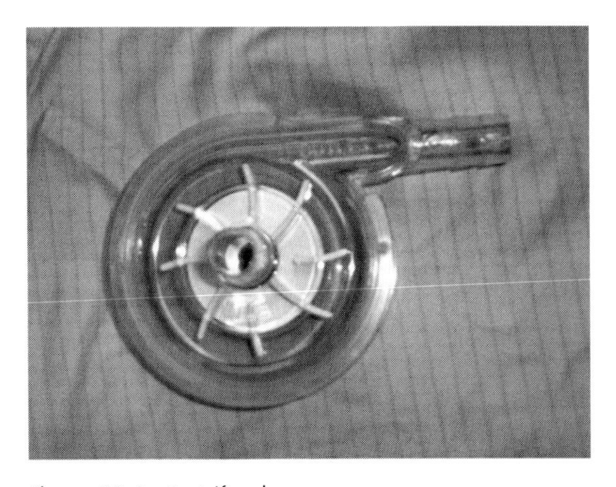

Figure 28.4 Centrifugal pump.

Bridge

The venoarterial ECMO circuit may have a bridge, which allows connection between the drainage and the infusion lines close to the patient and is clamped during ECMO support. It allows temporary separation between the patient and the ECMO circuit during emergencies, such as air in the circuit that could potentially reach the patient, and may make weaning easier (see below). The bridge may have to be unclamped every 15 to 20 minutes for a period of about 5 seconds to prevent clot formation.

Running the device

The aim of ECMO is to maintain adequate systemic oxygen delivery and removal of CO_2. A clear understanding of anticoagulation, cannulation and appropriate management of the ECMO circuit is required.

Anticoagulation

Heparin has several advantages, including immediate onset of anticoagulation, bedside monitoring by activated clotting time (ACT) and swift reversibility with protamine if required. Heparin resistance may occur with prolonged use owing to antithrombin III deficiency and adverse effects such as heparin-induced thrombocytopenia must be considered (see Chapter 34). Heparinization is

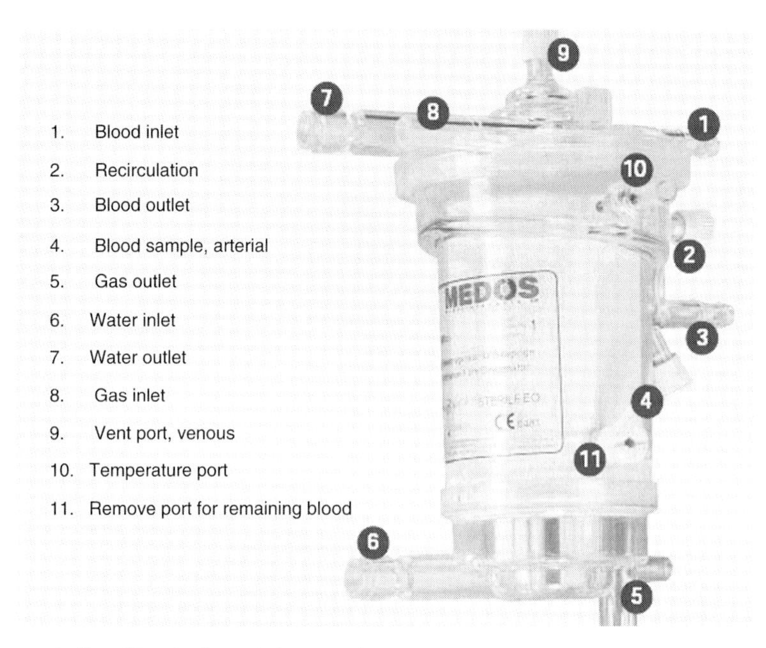

Figure 28.5 Nonporous hollow fiber (polymethylpentene) oxygenator.

established by an initial intravenous bolus of 75 U/kg, followed by an infusion (usually 25–100 U/kg per hour) to achieve an ACT of 160 to 180 seconds. The ACT should be monitored at least hourly initially and the infusion titrated accordingly.

ANTICOAGULATION AND HEPARIN-BONDED CIRCUITS

The use of heparin-bonded circuits allows less intravenous heparin to be given and may provide an increased safety margin when anticoagulation is marginal. Blood may still clot in the circuit or cannula despite the coating if there is low flow or turbulence; therefore, some systemic anticoagulation is still advised.

Cannulation

The site of cannulation may depend on the type of support needed, age and weight of the patient. During cannulation for venoarterial ECMO, arterial ligation is usually required to prevent leakage around the cannula. The right carotid artery or femoral artery may be used. Venous access for venoarterial or venovenous ECMO is via the jugular or femoral veins, almost always by the Seldinger or semi-Seldinger technique. Correct positioning should be confirmed by plain radiographs.

Patient management

The management of patients on ECMO is similar to management of any critical care patient. However:

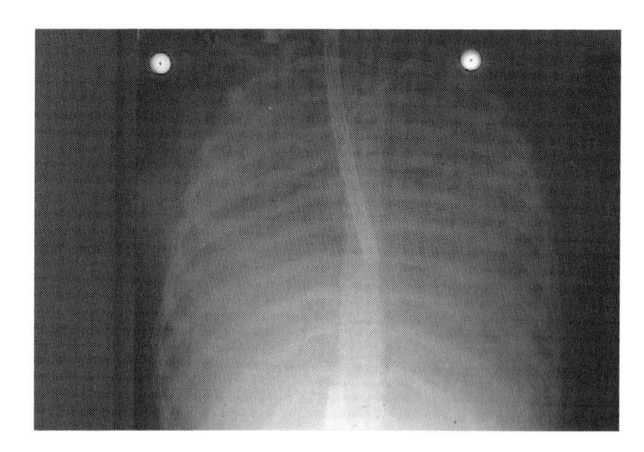

Figure 28.6 Chest radiograph of a patient on ECMO with cannulae in right atrium and in.erior vena cava.

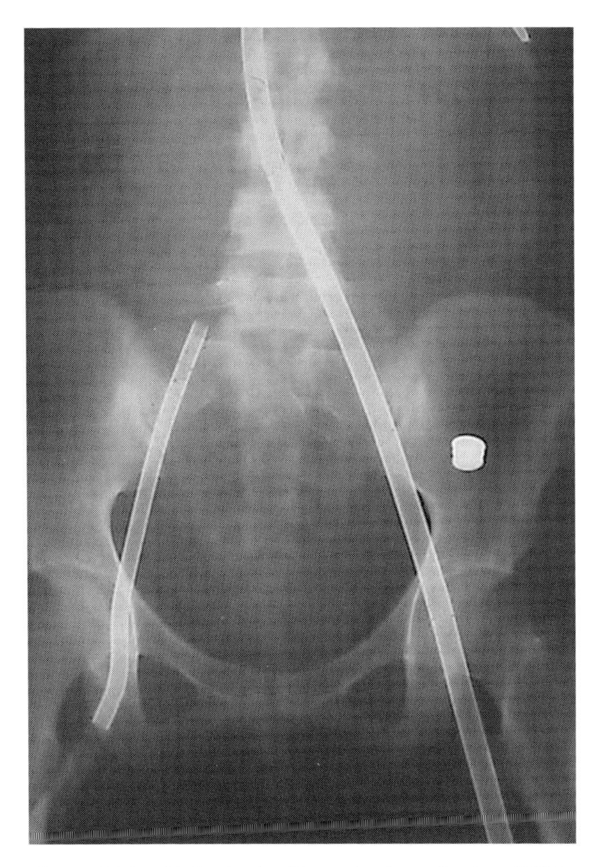

Figure 28.7 Abdominal radiograph of a patient on ECMO demonstrating cannulae in inferior vena cava and iliac veins.

- The ECMO patient should be monitored by a trained ECMO specialist in addition to the critical care nurse looking after the patient. This specialist may be a perfusionist or nurse who has received specialist training and accreditation.
- Ventilator settings should be reduced to 'rest settings' to avoid further damage to the lungs (e.g. 30% inspired oxygen, positive end-expiratory pressure 5–10 cmH_2O).
- Inotropes may often be rapidly weaned to rest the heart.
- Fluid overload should be corrected using either diuretics or filtration.
- If antibiotic treatment is not in progress, the threshold to start and continue antibiotics should be low. The classical signs of sepsis such as temperature, white cell count and C-reactive protein levels may not be as reliable; the circuit acts as an inflammatory stimulus and the temperature is kept constant by the heat exchanger.
- Nutritional requirements should be carefully determined; both underfeeding and overfeeding could be potentially harmful.

Stopping extracorporeal membrane oxygenation

Although ECMO may be continued safely for some time, stopping it when the precipitating pathology has reversed should not be delayed. Lung compliance, changes on chest radiographs and cardiac contractility (which may be best assessed by serial echocardiography) should be regularly monitored. Weaning can be protracted, and there are reports of patients requiring ECMO for weeks and months. However, if complications such as neurological deterioration or end-stage disease such as irreversible pulmonary fibrosis develop, consideration should be given to withdrawal of support.

Weaning and 'trial off'

The ECMO flow rate should be gradually reduced while the response of the patient to the decrease in flow is assessed. This includes monitoring of arterial blood gases in venovenous ECMO and mixed venous saturations in venoarterial ECMO. The minimal flow rate for a 'trial off' or removal of ECMO support without removing the cannulae is usually considered to be 1 L/min for adult patients.

VENOARTERIAL EXTRACORPOREAL MEMBRANE OXYGENATION

Intravenous infusions are disconnected from the circuit and connected to the patient. The heparin infusion should be connected to both the circuit and the patient and half the dose administered to each. The patient is then clamped off from the ECMO circuit while opening the bridge to keep the circuit running. The cannulae are unclamped every 10 minutes to prevent them from clotting.

Careful monitoring over the next 2 hours is required to detect haemodynamic or respiratory deterioration. If stability continues after this time, then the cannulae may be removed.

VENOVENOUS EXTRACORPOREAL MEMBRANE OXYGENATION

Oxygen supply to the oxygenator may be stopped while the patient is placed on 'acceptable' ventilator settings ($Fio_2 \leq 0.6$; peak inspiratory pressure ≤ 30; positive end-expiratory pressure ≤ 10). If arterial blood gases are considered to be inadequate during this time, then the ECMO support should be continued for another 24 to 48 hours before attempting weaning again. When weaning is successfully achieved, the cannulae should be removed promptly.

Decannulation

Venous cannulae can usually be removed without formal surgical exploration (in the critical care unit). A horizontal mattress suture can be placed and the cannula is then clamped and withdrawn by an assistant while the suture is tied. Alternatively, removal followed by a long period of direct pressure may be sufficient. Removal of arterial cannulae usually requires surgical repair of the vessel, which may best be performed in the operating room.

Further care

Heparin anticoagulation is usually not reversed at the time of decannulation unless uncontrollable bleeding ensues. This is because there may be a state of hypercoagulability in the immediate period after ECMO owing to overproduction of clotting factors. It is important to start the patients on standard thromboprophylaxis soon after decannulation.

Transport of patients for extracorporeal membrane oxygenation

ECMO remains a highly specialized service available in only a few centres. The transfer of very sick patients to these centres should be carefully planned and managed. This may be aided by establishing guidelines at referring and receiving centres during the transfer and specialist retrieval teams based at ECMO centres may make the process safer if resources allow.

Carbon dioxide removal devices

These may be an alternative to conventional ECMO in a limited number of patients and trials are currently in progress. However, the available devices do not improve oxygenation and require adequate cardiac output.

Key points

- ECMO may be indicated in patients with severe but potentially reversible respiratory or cardiac failure unresponsive to conventional management.
- The dose of heparin required to anticoagulate patients on ECMO may be very low owing to the properties of the circuit and the oxygenator. This reduces the risk of haemorrhage.
- Patients receiving ECMO require the attention of at least two members of staff continuously.
- Weaning should commence when clinical indices improve, and can be very gradual.

FURTHER READING

CESAR [homepage on the Internet]. Available at: www.cesar-trial.org. *Large randomized trial of ECMO for respiratory failure.*

Extracorporeal Life Support Organization [homepage on the Internet]. Available at: www.elso.med.umich.edu. Provides a registry of all cases of ECMO and has e-book: *ECMO. Extracorporeal cardiopulmonary support in critical care.*

Peek GJ, Firmin RK. Extracorporeal membrane oxygenation for cardiac support. *Coron Artery Dis* 1997;8:371–388.

3.3 *Renal System in Cardiothoracic Critical Care*

Chapter 29

Renal protection and cardiac surgery

S.T. WEBB AND A. VUYLSTEKE

Introduction

There is a wide spectrum of severity of acute renal dysfunction after cardiac surgery, ranging from sub-clinical renal injury to acute renal failure (ARF) requiring renal replacement therapy. The incidence of ARF following cardiac surgery varies depending on the definition, but approximately 5% of cardiac surgical patients require renal replacement for ARF. Acute renal failure is a serious complication; it is associated with increased mortality and prolonged critical care unit and hospital stays.

Measurement of renal function

Although serum creatinine and urine output lack sensitivity and specificity in renal dysfunction, these indices are the most easily measured in clinical practice. Measurement of glomerular filtration rate by creatinine clearance is less straightforward and is of limited value in the absence of steady-state conditions. Other tests of renal function are of questionable clinical use; newer biomarkers are under evaluation and may have greater sensitivity for detecting renal dysfunction.

Definition of acute renal failure

Until recently, there has been no consensus on the optimal measurement of renal function or the definition of ARF. An international interdisciplinary collaborative group, the Acute Dialysis Quality Initiative, has formulated a standard definition of *acute renal dysfunction*, a term that encompasses the range of abnormalities of renal function. The acronym RIFLE defines three grades of increasing severity of acute renal dysfunction (*r*isk; *i*njury; *f*ailure) and two outcome variables (*l*oss; *e*nd stage). Grade of severity of renal dysfunction is based on change from baseline, and may be assessed by the change in glomerular filtration rate (reflected by serum creatinine) or by the change in urine output. The RIFLE classification is being increasingly used to assess the incidence of acute renal dysfunction after cardiac surgery.

Pathophysiology of acute renal dysfunction

Renal blood flow represents a relatively large proportion of total cardiac output (approximately 20%). Oxygen delivery is correspondingly high, whereas overall oxygen consumption is low. However, the kidneys are extremely sensitive to ischaemia and acute renal dysfunction is a frequent complication of hypotension. This apparent paradox is related to the physiological gradient of intrarenal oxygen partial pressures from cortex to medulla. The cortex receives a high percentage of renal blood flow and has a low oxygen extraction, whereas the medulla has a lower physiological blood flow and greater oxygen consumption. The heterogeneous physiology within the kidneys renders the renal medulla particularly vulnerable to hypoperfusion and hypoxia leading

Table 29.1 The RIFLE classification of acute renal dysfunction

Grade	GFR criteria	UO criteria
Risk	Serum creatinine increase ×1.5 or GFR decrease >25%	UO ≤0.5 mL kg^{-1} h^{-1} for 6 h
Injury	Serum creatinine ×2 or GFR decrease >50%	UO ≤0.5 mL kg^{-1} h^{-1} for 12 h
Failure	Serum creatinine ×3 or GFR decrease >75% or serum creatinine >350 μmol/L with acute increase >44 μmol/L per day	UO ≤0.3 mL kg^{-1} h^{-1} for 24 h or anuria for 12 h
Loss	Persistent ARF = complete loss of renal function for >4 weeks	
End-stage	Complete loss of renal function for >3 months	

GFR, glomerular filtration rate; UO, urine output.

to acute tubular necrosis and acute renal dysfunction. Endogenous mechanisms that operate to regulate medullary blood flow in response to ischaemic injury include local vasoactive mediators, the renin–angiotensin–aldosterone system and tubuloglomerular feedback. Acute tubular necrosis results in tubular obstruction by necrotic epithelial debris and leakage of glomerular filtrate into the renal interstitium that is manifest clinically by oliguria.

Aetiology

The aetiology of ARF after cardiac surgery is multifactorial: ischaemia–reperfusion injury, systemic inflammatory response syndrome, embolic injury and drug-related nephrotoxic injury are believed to contribute to its development. Perioperative renal hypoperfusion outside the limits of autoregulatory reserve, particularly during cardiopulmonary bypass (CPB), contributes to renal ischaemia–reperfusion injury. Cardiac surgery triggers systemic inflammatory response syndrome resulting in cell-mediated and cytotoxic injury. Recent evidence suggests that the balance between pro-inflammatory and anti-inflammatory mediators may influence the degree of acute renal dysfunction. Prolonged CPB produces haemolysis and haemoglobinuria that may result in renal tubular injury. Atheroembolism from the ascending aorta during surgical manipulation may result in acute renal dysfunction. Thrombus, air, lipid and tissue may also contribute to the embolic load during cardiac surgery. Exposure to nephrotoxic drugs in the preoperative or postoperative periods may be an additional aetiological factor in the development of ARF.

Risk factors

The cardiac surgical population is getting older, more complex surgery is being performed and more

Table 29.2 Nephrotoxic drugs commonly used in patients undergoing cardiac surgery

Angiotensin-converting enzyme inhibitors
Nonsteroidal anti-inflammatory drugs
Intravenous radiocontrast agents
Aminoglycosides antibiotics
Amphotericin B
β-Lactam antibiotics
Sulphonamides
Cyclosporine
Aprotinin

Table 29.3 Risk factors for acute renal failure after cardiac surgery

Preoperative factors	Intraoperative factors	Postoperative factors
Age	Duration of CPB	Hypovolaemia
Preexisting chronic renal disease	Emergency surgery	LV dysfunction
Diabetes mellitus	Redo surgery	Low CO
LV dysfunction	Combined CABG and valve surgery	Nephrotoxic drugs
Peripheral vascular disease	Ascending aortic manipulation	Mediastinal haemorrhage
Hypertension	Deep hypothermic circulatory arrest	Sepsis
Aortic atheroma	IABP	Abdominal compartment syndrome
Acute endocarditis		Multiple organ dysfunction syndrome
Nephrotoxic drugs		
Genetic predisposition		

Abbreviations: CABG, coronary artery bypass grafting; CO, cardiac output; CPB, cardiopulmonary bypass; IABP, intra-aortic balloon pump; LV, left ventricular.

patients are receiving support for multiple organ dysfunction syndrome. In the future, it is likely that the incidence of perioperative acute renal dysfunction will rise.

Prevention

The identification of high-risk patients and the implementation of potential prophylactic measures are therapeutically attractive strategies for perioperative renal protection. Prevention of acute renal dysfunction may be primary or secondary:

- strategies to reduce the occurrence of renal injury in patients without evidence of acute renal dysfunction referred to as *primary prevention*;
- the avoidance of additional renal injury in the setting of established acute renal dysfunction is termed *secondary prevention*.

The strategies employed in renal protection may be classified as nonpharmacological or pharmacological.

Nonpharmacological strategies

Nonpharmacological renal protection strategies in cardiac surgery include correction of hypovolaemia, maintenance of adequate systemic arterial pressure, avoidance of nephrotoxic drugs, maintenance of glycaemic control, optimal management of CPB and prompt treatment of postoperative complications.

VOLUME STATUS

Intravenous fluids to correct hypovolaemia have been widely used for prevention of renal dysfunction in many different settings. Recent evidence has demonstrated the benefit of isotonic intravenous fluids in the prevention of radiocontrast-induced nephropathy. The ideal composition of fluid and the optimal rate of infusion are not yet clear. Cardiac surgical patients undergoing emergency cardiac catheterization will benefit from the use of low-volume, nonionic, iso-osmolar radiocontrast in conjunction with isotonic intravenous fluids. For fluid resuscitation of the critically ill patient, colloids do not appear to confer an advantage over crystalloids and there is no difference in safety between different colloids.

RENAL PERFUSION PRESSURE

Defense of systemic arterial pressure and maintenance of renal perfusion pressure are essential for the prevention of renal injury. After volume loading to reverse hypovolaemia, vasopressors should be used to support systemic arterial pressure in the management of shock. Despite historic concerns, noradrenaline is an excellent first-line agent. There is no evidence to suggest that it compromises renal or gastrointestinal tract blood flow when used to treat arterial hypotension. Vasopressin is now emerging as a useful agent in catecholamine-resistant shock.

The optimal therapeutic target for systemic arterial pressure to prevent acute renal dysfunction has not been established. A minimum mean arterial pressure of 65 to 75 mmHg is commonly targeted in clinical practice; however, patients with longstanding hypertension may require a higher pressure.

NEPHROTOXIC DRUGS

Minimizing exposure to nephrotoxic drugs is an important strategy to prevent ARF after cardiac surgery. The use of once-daily aminoglycoside dosing and the lipid formulations of amphotericin B have been demonstrated to lower the risk of renal toxicity associated with these drugs.

Antifibrinolytic drugs are commonly used to reduce intraoperative blood loss in cardiac surgery. Both ε-aminocaproic acid and aprotinin affect renal function and there are concerns regarding the risk of renal injury associated with these drugs. Aprotinin in particular is associated with an increased risk of ARF requiring renal replacement therapy. Commonly used nephrotoxic drugs should be avoided in the setting of acute renal dysfunction.

GLYCAEMIC CONTROL

Intensive insulin therapy to maintain glycaemic control reduces the incidence of ARF requiring renal replacement therapy and improves survival in critically ill surgical patients. Intraoperative hyperglycaemia during cardiac surgery is associated with increased morbidity, including ARF, and overall mortality. Ensuring intraoperative glycaemic control with insulin therapy may prove to be renoprotective.

CARDIOPULMONARY BYPASS

The conduct of CPB may affect the incidence of ARF after cardiac surgery. Limiting the duration of CPB and maintaining adequate flow and perfusion pressure are of primary importance to reduce the risk of renal injury. Several other CPB-related strategies may be beneficial, including the use of pulsatile blood flow, leukodepletion during bypass, avoidance of excessive haemodilution and the use of haemofiltration at the end of CPB.

OFF-PUMP CARDIAC SURGERY

Many of the postulated mechanisms of ARF after cardiac surgery relate to the use of CPB; hence, off-pump surgery may offer a theoretical advantage in terms of renal protection. However, the current evidence for off-pump coronary artery bypass graft surgery reducing postoperative renal injury is conflicting. New developments in off-pump minimally invasive surgical techniques that avoid ascending aortic manipulation may prove to be beneficial in reducing renal morbidity.

POSTOPERATIVE COMPLICATIONS

A number of postoperative complications after cardiac surgery are known to be associated with ARF. Timely diagnosis and management of low cardiac output syndrome, mediastinal haemorrhage, sepsis and abdominal compression syndrome are essential to prevent acute renal dysfunction.

Abdominal compression syndrome caused by intra-abdominal hypertension is associated with diminished renal perfusion and may result in ARF (Chapter 38). Acute renal failure in critically ill patients is often part of multiple organ dysfunction syndrome requiring prolonged multiple organ support in the critical care unit. The use of renal replacement therapy for the treatment of ARF is discussed in Chapter 30.

Pharmacological strategies

Theoretically, interventions that optimize renal perfusion and oxygenation during cardiac surgery may prevent ARF. However, the underlying aetiology of acute renal dysfunction is complex and ischaemic injury is only one of several mechanisms of acute renal dysfunction. Hence, pharmacological strategies that are based on increasing renal blood flow or decreasing renal oxygen consumption have been unsuccessful.

Despite extensive investigation, few drug interventions have been demonstrated to be beneficial and some have been clearly shown to be ineffective. A recent systematic review concluded that there is no reliable evidence to suggest that any perioperative pharmacological interventions are beneficial in protecting renal function.

Table 29.4 Potential pharmacological renal protection strategies in cardiac surgery

Vasodilators
Dopamine agonists
Adenosine antagonists
Calcium channel antagonists
Angiotensin-converting enzyme inhibitors
Diuretics
Loop diuretics
Mannitol
Natriuretic peptides
Atrial natriuretic peptide
Urodilatin
B-type natriuretic peptide
Antioxidants
N-Acetylcysteine
Corticosteroids

DOPAMINE AGONISTS

Dopamine acts on a number of receptor types. Renal blood flow is increased by dopaminergic receptor-mediated renal vasodilatation, β-adrenoreceptor stimulation increases cardiac output and α-adrenoreceptor increases renal perfusion pressure.

There is convincing evidence to suggest that dopamine does not prevent ARF, the need for renal replacement therapy nor mortality. Despite its traditional use, there is no role for 'low-dose' dopamine for renal protection. The dopamine analogue dopexamine has been studied in cardiac surgical patients and does not have a beneficial effect on renal function. It is unknown whether fenoldopam, a selective dopamine-1 receptor agonist, has a role in renal protection.

ADENOSINE ANTAGONISTS

Theophylline, an adenosine antagonist, reverses adenosine-mediated renal arterial vasoconstriction in the setting of radiocontrast nephropathy. Further trials are required to determine if theophylline will prove to be useful in preventing radiocontrast nephropathy.

DIURETICS

In the setting of oliguric acute renal dysfunction, diuretics increase urine flow by decreasing tubular reabsorption through several different mechanisms. Increasing tubular flow maintains tubular patency and prevents obstruction and back leak. Loop diuretics inhibit tubular reabsorption in the loop of Henle. There is no evidence to support the use of loop diuretics in the prevention of ARF after cardiac surgery. However, loop diuretics may facilitate the control of fluid balance in critically ill postoperative patients receiving large volumes of fluid. Mannitol acts primarily as an osmotic diuretic and is commonly administered during cardiac surgery as part of the CPB circuit prime. No clear renal protective benefit of mannitol has been demonstrated in cardiac surgical patients.

NATRIURETIC PEPTIDES

Natriuretic peptides induce a natriuretic and diuretic effect by increasing glomerular perfusion pressure and glomerular filtration. Natriuretic peptides have shown conflicting results in the prevention of ARF. However, these agents may be beneficial after cardiac surgery and further studies are awaited.

ANTIOXIDANTS

N-Acetylcysteine is an antioxidant and has been used to prevent ARF in paracetamol-induced liver failure and radiocontrast nephropathy. There is strong evidence to suggest that *N*-acetylcysteine decreases the incidence of radiocontrast nephropathy. To date, the evidence base for the use of this agent in cardiac surgery is inconclusive.

Table 29.5 Perioperative renal protection strategies for cardiac surgery

Preoperative
Administer isotonic intravenous fluids for prevention of radiocontrast-induced nephropathy
Optimize volume status and systemic arterial pressure
Withhold all nephrotoxic drugs
Maintain glycaemic control in diabetic patients
Delay surgery until recovery of preoperative acute renal dysfunction
Arrange preoperative dialysis for patients with dialysis-dependent chronic renal disease
Correct metabolic and electrolyte disturbances associated with renal dysfunction
Intraoperative
Consider off-pump coronary artery bypass surgery
Maintain adequate flow during CPB
Consider maintaining high mean systemic arterial pressure (65–75 mmHg) during CPB
Limit the duration of CPB
Consider using pulsatile flow during CPB
Consider using leukodepletion during CPB
Avoid excessive haemodilution (haematocrit $\leq$0.21) during CPB
Consider using haemofiltration at the end of CPB
Maintain glycaemic control
Avoid nephrotoxic drugs
Avoid aprotinin
Postoperative
Promptly treat postoperative low CO syndrome
Control mediastinal haemorrhage
Avoid nephrotoxic drugs
Maintain glycaemic control
Manage sepsis aggressively
Recognize and treat abdominal compression syndrome
Provide appropriate support for multiple organ dysfunction syndrome
Institute renal replacement therapy for treatment of ARF

Abbreviations: ARF, acute renal failure; CPB, cardiopulmonary bypass; CO, cardiac output.

Key points

- Renal dysfunction is common after cardiac surgery and associated with significant increased morbidity and mortality.
- Prevention can be primary (before the insult) or secondary (after the insult – to prevent further deterioration).
- Correction of hypovolaemia and maintenance of sufficient systemic blood pressure are of paramount importance.
- Pharmacological strategies have not been shown to be effective as yet.

FURTHER READING

Abu-Omar Y, Ratnatunga C. Cardiopulmonary bypass and renal injury. *Perfusion* 2006;21:209–213.

Stafford-Smith M. Evidence-based renal protection in cardiac surgery. *Semin Cardiothorac Vasc Anesth* 2005;9:65–76.

Venkataraman R, Kellum JA. Prevention of acute renal failure. *Chest* 2007;131:300–308.

Zacharias M, Gilmore ICS, Herbison GP, *et al.* Interventions for protecting renal function in the perioperative period. *Cochrane Database Syst Rev* 2005;3:CD003590.

Chapter 30

Renal replacement therapy

Z. RICCI AND C. RONCO

Introduction

Despite advances in the understanding, diagnosis and treatment of acute renal failure, many aspects remain unresolved. Modern technology has provided different modalities to perform extracorporeal renal support, but it is not clear which is superior in terms of efficacy and outcome. Moreover, evidence-based medicine has not yet defined when to start and when to wean off renal replacement therapy (RRT).

Starting renal replacement therapy

Renal replacement is indicated when renal dysfunction leads to one or more of the following:

- severe fluid overload;
- pulmonary oedema;
- hyperkalaemia; and
- metabolic acidosis.

Renal replacement therapy is traditionally considered when all medical treatment (diuretics, bicarbonate administration, fluid restriction and nutritional restriction) have failed. However, greater ease of use and a low associated morbidity has led to RRT being considered earlier in the disease process. This may be related to the perception that maintenance of homeostasis and prevention of complications is increasingly important. There is also some evidence that RRT has some role to play in the management of sepsis and multiple organ dysfunction syndromes, before acute renal failure has ensued. Recent algorithms have placed more emphasis on prevention.

Stopping renal replacement therapy

It is difficult to use biochemical or clinical markers to monitor RRT. Urea concentration should be $\leq$10 mmol/L and creatinine $\leq$221 μmol/L. There is no hard evidence on how and when RRT should be stopped. It is generally accepted, however, that removal of RRT should be considered when the patient demonstrates haemodynamic stability with decreased requirement for vasopressors and improving condition overall. Increasing urine output (in quantity) during RRT is often a signal that the kidneys are improving.

Principles of renal replacement

The kidneys filter the blood to remove excess water and waste products. Renal replacement therapy essentially uses semipermeable membranes to achieve the same result. The membrane may be artificial, as in a filter, or autologous, as in the peritoneum. Many molecules, including water, urea and solutes of various molecular weights, are transported across the membrane by variable combinations of the processes of diffusion, dialysis, convection and ultrafiltration (UF).

During diffusion, the movement of solutes depends on their tendency to reach the same concentration on each side of the membrane; this results in the passage of solutes from the compartment with the higher concentration to the compartment with the lower concentration. Diffusion is affected by characteristics of the semipermeable

Table 30.1 Criteria for starting renal replacement therapy

One criterion: consider RRT; two criteria: why not start RRT?; three criteria: mandate initiation of RRT.
Anuria–oliguria (diuresis ≤200 mL in 12 h)
Severe metabolic acidosis (pH ≤7.10)
Hyperazotaemia (urea ≥30 mmol/L) or creatinine >300 μmol/L
Hyperkalaemia (K^+ ≥6.5 mEq/L)
Clinical signs of uremic toxicity
Severe dysnatraemia (Na^+ ≤ 115 or ≥ 160 mEq/L)
Hyperthermia (temperature >40°C without response to medical therapy)
Severe fluid overload
Multi-organ failure

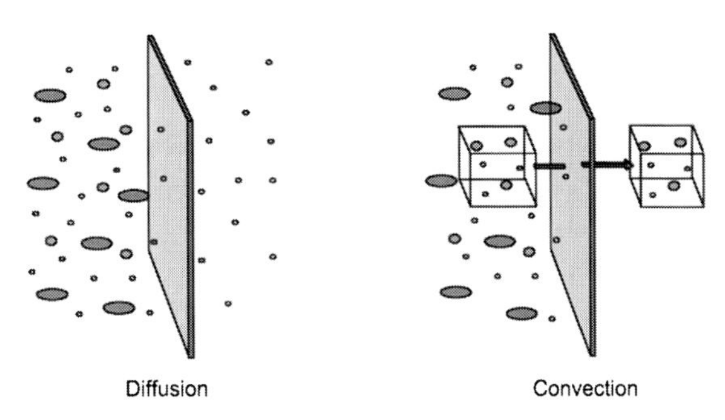

Figure 30.1 Diffusion and convection are schematically represented. During diffusion of solutes, flux (J_x) is a function of solute concentration gradient (d_c) between the two sides of the semipermeable membrane, temperature (T), diffusivity coefficient (D), membrane thickness (d_x) and surface area (A) according to the equation: $J_x = D\,T\,A\,(d_c/d_x)$. Convective flux of solutes (J_f) requires instead a pressure gradient between the two sides of the membrane (TMP), that moves a fluid (plasma water) with its 'crystalloid' content (a process called UF, whose entity is also dependent on membrane permeability coefficient [K_f]). Colloids and cells do not cross the semipermeable membrane, depending on the pores' size. $J_f = K_f \times \text{TMP}$ and $\text{TMP} = P_b - P_d - \pi$, where P_b is the blood hydrostatic pressure, P_d is the hydrostatic pressure on ultrafiltrate side of the membrane and π is the blood oncotic pressure.

membrane including thickness, surface area, temperature and diffusion coefficient. Diffusion can be enhanced by dialysis, in which a solution (the dialysate) flows on the other side of the membrane, countercurrent to blood flow, to maintain a high solute gradient.

In convection, the movement of solute across a semipermeable membrane is a result of transfer of water across the membrane. In other words, as the solvent (plasma water) crosses the membrane, solutes are carried with it if the pore size of the membrane allows. Convection can be enhanced by UF, which creates a transmembrane pressure (TMP) gradient. The UF rate depends on the rate of flow (Q_f), the membrane coefficient (K_m) and the TMP gradient between the pressures on both sides of the membrane:

$$Q_f = K_m \times \text{TMP}$$

The TMP gradient is the difference between the pressure in the blood compartment and filtrate compartment. The blood compartment pressure is directly related to blood flow (Q_b). The filtrate compartment pressure is modulated by suction in modern RRT machines. The machines are designed to maintain a constant Q_f: when the filter is 'fresh' and highly permeable, the pumps retard UF production, generating a positive pressure on the filtrate compartment (TMP is initially dependent only on blood flow). As the membrane fibres become degraded, a negative pressure on the filtrate side is necessary to achieve a constant Q_f. With time, TMP progressively increases to a maximum level at which solute clearance is compromised and clotting of the filter or membrane rupture is possible.

The size of molecules cleared during convection and UF exceeds that during diffusion, because they are physically dragged to the UF side; however, this gradually becomes limited by the protein layer that progressively closes filter pores during convective treatments. In addition, the membrane itself can adsorb molecules, and this is important for higher molecular weight toxins. The membrane adsorptive capacity is generally saturated in the first few hours of filter use and has a relatively minor impact on mass separation processes.

During UF, plasma water and solutes are filtered from blood, leading to a decrease in blood hydrostatic pressure and increase in blood oncotic pressure. The fraction of plasma water that is removed from blood during UF is called the filtration fraction and should be kept in the range of 20% to 25% to prevent excessive haemoconcentration within the filtering membrane. Otherwise, the oncotic pressure gradient could neutralize the TMP gradient resulting in equilibrium.

Haemofiltration

Replacing plasma water with a substitute solution completes the *haemofiltration* (HF) process. The replacement fluid can be administered after the filter (postfilter dilution HF), before (prefilter dilution HF) or both. Postfilter dilution leads to a higher urea clearance (about 2000 mL/h), but prefilter dilution prolongs circuit lifespan by reducing haemoconcentration and protein buildup in the filter fibres. Conventional HF is performed with a highly permeable, steam-sterilized membrane with a surface area of about 1 m^2.

Haemodiafiltration

The addition of convection to the diffusion process allows haemodiafiltration with dialysis and replacement solutions running simultaneously within the same filter to obtain additional solute removal.

Choice of mode

Renal replacement therapy may be intermittent or continuous. In general, intermittent RRT is reserved for haemodynamically stable patients. How effectively RRT is applied may be more important than the method chosen. For example, intermittent peritoneal dialysis (PD) is less effective at clearing urea than haemodialysis, but has comparable patient outcomes. The reason for this difference may be that urea clearance does not accurately represent the clearance of other toxins and solutes. The ideal renal replacement treatment would include:

- efficient solute removal;
- minimum solute disequilibrium;
- low UF rate;
- haemodynamic stability;
- low anticoagulant needs;
- efficiency of resource use; and
- minimal interference with patient mobility.

Indeed, from a critical care perspective, the different possible techniques now resemble the modes of mechanical ventilation, with ventilator settings seamlessly being changed to fit into the therapeutic goals and phases of illness. Renal replacement therapy may be similarly adjusted to fulfill the needs of the individual and the illness.

Practical renal replacement therapy prescription

During RRT, clearance (K) depends on circuit blood flow (Q_b), HF flow (Q_f), or dialysis flow (Q_d), molecular weight of solutes and filter type and size. Circuit blood flow is mainly dependent on vascular access and operational characteristics of the machines.

In HF, Q_f is strictly linked to Q_b by filtration fraction. In dialysis, however, Q_d is not limited by filtration fraction, but when the Q_d/Q_b ratio exceeds 0.3, dialysis is less efficient.

Urea and creatinine are generally used as reference solutes to measure the effectiveness of the RRT prescription, but their clearance is not directly correlated with outcome of chronic renal failure.

Membrane sieving coefficient

During UF, the driving pressure jams solutes, such as urea and creatinine, against the membrane. The sieving coefficient (SC) determines the amount of solute that passes through the pores of the membrane. The SC is calculated by the ratio of the concentration of the solutes in the filtrate divided by that in the plasma. An SC of 1.0, as is the case for urea and creatinine, demonstrates complete permeability and a value of 0 total impermeability. Molecular size ($\leq$12 daltons) and filter porosity are the major determinants of SC. During continuous treatment, a minimum urea clearance of 30 mL h^{-1} kg^{-1} (2.8 L h^{-1} in a 70-kg patient) is required.

Fractional clearance of urea

Efficacy may be defined as the effective solute removal. It can be expressed as a fractional clearance of a given solute

Techniques

Intermittent haemodialysis

Intermittent haemodialysis (IHD) is a mainly diffusive treatment in which blood and dialysate circulate in countercurrent mode on either side of a low permeability, cellulose based membrane. Circuit blood flow is set at around 150 to 300 mL/min and dialysis rate is 300 to 500 mL/min. Dialysate must be pyrogen-free, but not necessarily sterile because dialysate–blood contact does not occur. The UF rate is equal to the scheduled weight loss. This treatment is typically performed for around 4 hours three times a week, but may be required daily. Intermittent haemodialysis is most commonly performed in specialist renal units, using long-term vascular access such as a surgically formed arteriovenous fistula. It is rarely performed in critical care because the rapid fluid shift may cause haemodynamic instability. The machinery required for IHD is large and cumbersome. It is therefore usually located in the renal unit and is unlikely to be moved.

If a patient with chronic renal failure is admitted to cardiothoracic critical care, an intermittent mode of RRT is normally required to maintain homeostasis. Haemofiltration during CPB will normally have been carried out to reduce fluid and solute overload before admission, but further RRT may be needed soon after admission. Suitable temporary vascular access should be secured (often in the operating room) and continuous venovenous haemofiltration (CVVH) is the technique most commonly instituted as a substitute. Once the patient has recovered from the surgery, the continuous treatment may be stopped and the patient transferred from critical care, usually back to the renal unit, on postoperative day 3 or 4. If prolonged critical care is required, continuous RRT will be necessary up to discharge.

Peritoneal dialysis

This is a predominantly diffusive treatment where blood, within the capillaries of the peritoneal membrane, is exposed to dialysate. Access is obtained by the surgical insertion of a peritoneal catheter, which allows the abdominal instillation of dialysate. Solute and water movement is achieved by means of variable concentration and tonicity gradients generated by the dialysate. This treatment can be performed continuously or intermittently. The major complication is infection (peritonitis), which may be asymptomatic and difficult to diagnose. Peritoneal fluid sampling and microscopy and culture should be undertaken whenever infection is suspected.

Peritoneal dialysis is usually carried out in the community in patients with chronic renal failure, and is not as effective as other methods in removing fluid. It is less efficient in critical illness and in the immediate postoperative period owing to reduced abdominal blood flow. It is rarely carried out in critical care, except when long-term patients have recovered from the acute phase of their illness.

Patients who usually receive PD at home but are admitted to cardiac critical care will normally need a continuous mode of RRT (most often CVVH) and therefore require suitable vascular access. In selected cases, when rapid recovery from surgery is expected and HF during CPB has been performed, continuous RRT may not be necessary; PD may be performed the day after surgery. Careful monitoring of electrolytes and fluid balance is required, and hyperkalaemia may limit this treatment option.

Slow continuous ultrafiltration

In slow continuous ultrafiltration, blood is driven by a pump through a highly permeable filter via an extracorporeal circuit, using venovenous access. The ultrafiltrate produced during membrane transit is not replaced and it corresponds to weight loss. It is used only for fluid control in overloaded patients. Circuit blood flow is set at around 100 to 250 mL/min and ultrafiltrate rate is 5 to 15 mL/min.

Continuous venovenous haemofiltration

Continuous venovenous haemofiltration is similar to slow continuous ultrafiltration, except that the ultrafiltrate produced during membrane transit is partly or completely replaced to maintain intravascular volume control. Replacement fluid may be delivered before, after or on both sides of the filter (pre- or postdilution). Clearance for all solutes is convective and equals UF rate. Circuit blood flow is set at around 100 to 250 mL/min and ultrafiltrate rate is 15 to 60 mL/min.

Continuous venovenous haemodialysis

In continuous venovenous haemodialysis, blood is driven through a low-permeability dialyser via an extracorporeal circuit in venovenous mode and a countercurrent flow of dialysate is delivered on the dialysate compartment. The ultrafiltrate produced during membrane transit corresponds with the patient's weight loss. Solute clearance is mainly diffusive and efficiency is limited to small solutes only. Circuit blood flow is set at around 50 to 200 mL/min and ultrafiltrate rate is 10 to 30 mL/min.

Continuous venovenous haemodiafiltration

Continuous venovenous haemodiafiltration is a technique wherein blood is driven through a highly permeable dialyser via an extracorporeal circuit in venovenous mode and a countercurrent flow of dialysate is delivered on the dialysate compartment. The ultrafiltrate produced during membrane transit is in excess of the patient's desired weight loss and replacement solution is needed to maintain fluid balance. Solute clearance is both convective and diffusive. Circuit blood flow is set at around 100 to 250 mL/min, dialysis flow at 15 to 60 mL/min and ultrafiltrate rate is 15 to 60 mL/min.

Haemoperfusion

Blood is circulated on a bed of coated charcoal powder to remove solutes by adsorption. The technique is specifically indicated in cases of poisoning or intoxication with agents that can be effectively removed by charcoal. This treatment may cause platelet and protein depletion.

Plasmapheresis

This uses specific plasma filters. Molecular weight cutoff of the membrane is much higher than that of haemofilters (100,000 to 1,000,000 kilodaltons): plasma as a whole is filtered and blood is reconstituted by the infusion of plasma products such as frozen plasma or albumin. This technique is performed to remove proteins or protein-bound solutes.

High-volume haemofiltration

This treatment uses highly permeable membranes and HF with a high volume setting: Q_b >200 mL/min and Q_f > 45 mL kg^{-1} h^{-1} to increase removal of high-molecular-weight solutes (e.g. sepsis and systemic inflammatory mediators).

Anticoagulation

In many RRT modalities, blood comes into contact with the artificial surfaces and some form of anticoagulation is needed. To reduce the risk of filter clotting, vascular access should to be of adequate size, kinked tubing should be avoided and blood flow

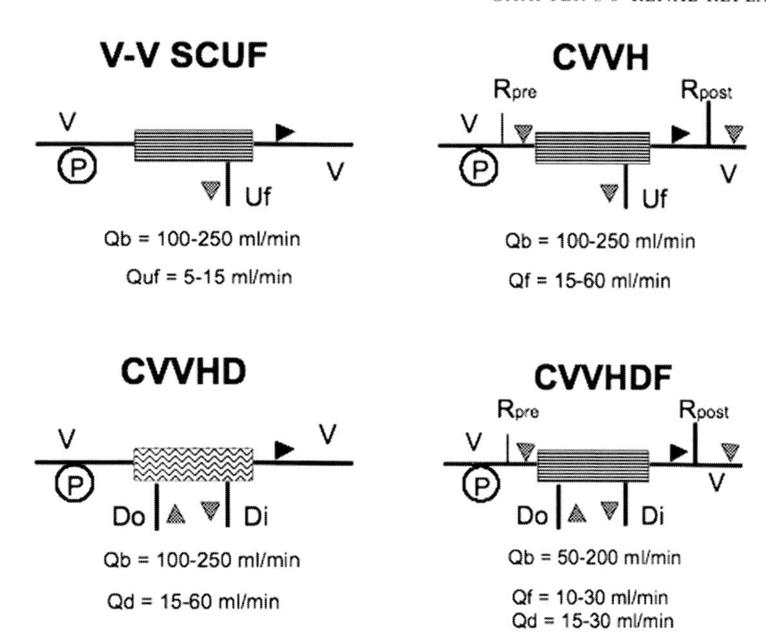

Figure 30.2 Schematic representation of most common continuous RRT set-ups. Black triangle represents blood flow direction; grey triangle indicates dialysate/replacement solutions flows. V-V, venovenous; Uf, ultrafiltration; Rpre, replacement solution prefilter; Rpost, replacement solution postfilter; Do, dialysate out; Di, dialysate in; Qb, blood flow; Quf, ultrafiltration flow; Qf, replacement solution flow; Qd, dialysate solution flow.

Table 30.2 Algorithm for renal replacement therapy prescription

Clinical variables	Operational variables	Setting
Fluid balance	Net UF	Negative balance (100–300 mL/h) is preferred in haemodynamically unstable patients Invasive monitoring of systemic and venous pressures is recommended
Adequacy and dose	Clearance/modality	2,000–3,000 mL/h (or 35 mL/kg per hour) for continuous RRT, consider first CVVHDF. If IHD is selected, an every day/4 hours prescription is recommended.
Acid–base	Solution buffer	Bicarbonate buffered solutions are preferable to lactate buffered solutions in lactic acidosis and/or hepatic failure.
Electrolyte	Dialysate/replacement	Consider solutions without K^+ in case of severe hyperkalaemia. Manage accurately $MgPO_4$.
Protocol	Staff/machine	Well-trained staff should routinely utilize RRT monitors according to predefined institutional protocols.

Abbreviations: CVVHDF, continuous venovenous haemodiafiltration; IHD, intermittent haemodialysis; RRT, renal replacement therapy.

rate should exceed 100 mL/min. Pump flow fluctuations must be prevented (in modern machines this is mainly due to circuit increased resistances rather than flow rate inaccuracies). Venous bubble traps, where air–blood contact occurs, are used to prevent systemic air embolus, and the machine will alarm if bubbles are detected.

There is evidence that, when set-up is optimized, anticoagulants contribute little to the maintenance of circuit patency. When anticoagulants are relatively contraindicated (risk of bleeding, preexisting coagulopathy, thrombocytopenia), RRT can be still be safely performed and filter life may not be compromised.

Unfractionated heparin is the most commonly used anticoagulant. The dose ranges from 5 to 10 IU/kg per hour. In some patients, heparin can also be used in combination with protamine administration postfilter (regional heparinization) with a 1:1 ratio (150 IU of unfractionated heparin per milligram of protamine) and monitoring of prothrombin time (activated partial thromboplastin time). Problems with heparin are relatively unpredictable and include bioavailability, antithrombin III depletion and the risk of heparin-induced thrombocytopenia (HIT).

Low-molecular-weight heparins can be used. Bioavailability is more reliable than unfractionated heparin and the risk of HIT (Chapter 34) is lower. However, the anticoagulant effect cannot be reversed and there may be a higher risk of haemorrhage. They are not better at prolonging circuit life.

Prostacyclin is potentially useful for RRT anticoagulation, being a potent inhibitor of platelet aggregation with a short half-life. It is infused at a dose of 4 to 8 ng/kg per hour with or without the adjunct of low-dose heparin. Hypotension may be induced by higher doses. High costs and the risk of hypotension limit the use of this agent to short-term treatment.

Citrate chelates calcium to prevent clot formation and can produce regional anticoagulation. Administration of calcium chloride may be required to maintain normocalcaemia. This approach is effective in maintaining filter patency and compares favourably with heparin. It also avoids the risk of HIT and does not lead to systemic anticoagulation. However, the risk of hypocalcaemia, metabolic alkalosis, and the cumbersome replacement and dialysate fluid preparation limit its use.

Key points

- New techniques mean that RRT may be instituted earlier in the progression of acute renal failure or congestive cardiac failure, with a lower risk of adverse effects.
- Intermittent techniques are reserved for haemodynamically stable patients, and are rarely used in critical care.
- Venovenous HF is the most commonly used continuous method of RRT.
- Alternatives to anticoagulation with heparin infusion exist, and should be considered if there is haemorrhage or if HIT is suspected.

FURTHER READING

Kellum J, Angus DC, Johnson JP, *et al.* Continuous versus intermittent renal replacement therapy: a meta-analysis. *Intensive Care Med* 2002;28: 29–37.

Tonelli M, Manns B, Feller-Kopman D. Acute renal failure in the intensive care unit: a systematic review of the impact of dialytic modality on mortality and renal recovery. *Am J Kidney Dis* 2002;40:875–885.

Vinsonneau C, Camus C, Combes A, *et al.* Continuous venovenous hemodiafiltration versus intermittent haemodialysis for acute renal failure in patients with multiple-organ dysfunction syndrome: a multicentre randomised trial. *Lancet* 2006;368:379–385.

3.4 *Haematology and Transfusion in Cardiothoracic Critical Care*

Chapter 31

Transfusion

R. ZARYCHANSKI, A.F. TURGEON,
A.A. TINMOUTH AND P.C. HÉBERT

Introduction

Bleeding and the need for transfusion of allogeneic blood products are common during and after cardiothoracic surgery. Despite advances in operative techniques, approximately one third of elective coronary artery bypass grafting procedures require allogeneic blood. As a result, cardiac surgery alone accounts for 10% to 25% of all blood transfused per year within the United States. Although it may be life saving, transfusion of blood components also has associated risks. Before initiating allogeneic transfusion, the expected benefits of a transfusion must therefore be weighed against these risks.

Mechanisms of bleeding in cardiac surgery

A multitude of reasons explain why patients bleed in the context of cardiac surgery. Initially, it is helpful to characterize bleeding as either surgical or coagulopathic in nature. This distinction sounds simple, but is often difficult and is dependent on several factors, including patient characteristics, the operative procedure, surgical technique and the need for transfusion itself.

Surgical causes of excessive bleeding after cardiac surgery account for 50% to 70% of bleeding events. Suggested standard criteria that generally indicate surgical bleeding and mandate surgical exploration can be defined.

The presence of haemodynamic instability (e.g. tamponade) is also important in the decision-making process. In an effort to identify patients requiring surgical reexploration earlier, some units use a blood loss nomogram. This method allows better visualization of bleeding trends and comparison with other patients operated on at the same institution. Reexploration must be considered if haemorrhage rate crosses several centile lines, or if the blood loss exceeds the 95th centile for two consecutive hours.

Many nonsurgical (coagulopathic) causes of bleeding exist and include inheritable bleeding disorders, medications (especially acetylsalicylic acid, clopidogrel, and heparin), hypothermia, renal or liver failure, thrombocytopenia, cardiopulmonary bypass (CPB)-induced platelet dysfunction, dilutional coagulopathy and a hyperfibrinolytic state. Signs indicating coagulopathic bleeding include diffuse microvascular bleeding or oozing, and bleeding from intravenous sites or at locations remote from the operative field.

Approaching and managing excessive bleeding varies considerably among surgeons, anaesthetists and critical care physicians. Although the distinction between surgical and coagulopathic bleeding is challenging, it is critical, given that no amount of excellent medical therapy is likely to attenuate a surgical cause of excessive bleeding.

Predictors of bleeding in cardiac surgery

Regardless of the mechanism of bleeding, anticipating a patient's potential transfusion needs cannot

Table 31.1 Clinical indicators of severe 'surgical' bleeding requiring operative intervention

1. 500 mL of fresh bleeding in first hour
   400 mL per hour for 2 hours
   300 mL per hour for 3 hours
2. >1,000 mL of bleeding in the first 4 hours
3. Sudden massive bleeding
4. Signs of cardiac tamponade

be underscored enough. For those at high risk of bleeding, adequate blood products and equipment must be immediately accessible when needed. Risk factors can be categorized in several domains.

Principles of blood transfusion

Excessive bleeding can be challenging to manage, especially if the cause is uncertain. This complicates decision making with respect to the use of coagulation factors and blood component therapies. The principles of transfusion therapy should always be followed.

The principal objective in managing a bleeding patient is to maintain adequate oxygen delivery. Tissue hypoxia may occur as a result of either decreased circulating volume (stagnant hypoxia) or decreased oxygen-carrying capacity (anaemic hypoxia). Insufficient oxygen delivery results in shock that then leads to metabolic acidosis, cardiovascular instability and worsening coagulopathy.

Maintaining adequate circulating volume is the first essential step. Patients can tolerate considerable reductions in haemoglobin concentration (especially after revascularization) if circulating volume is maintained; either crystalloid or colloid solutions can be used. However, large volumes of starch-containing solutions (e.g. hetastarch or dextran) may exacerbate an existing CPB-induced coagulopathy. A fluid warmer should be used to prevent hypothermia and secondary platelet dysfunction.

The second and related principle of transfusion therapy is the maintenance of tissue oxygenation. Oxygen delivery can be augmented by increasing the cardiac output or the oxygen content of the blood. The latter can be achieved by the administration of oxygen and the transfusion of packed red blood cells (PRBC); however, transfusing stored red blood cells has not consistently been demonstrated to result in acute increases in oxygen delivery.

Once intravascular volume is restored and oxygen delivery is acceptable, the focus shifts to achieving haemostasis. Surgical causes of bleeding need intervention (often reoperation), and nonsurgical causes of bleeding, which are also present in approximately 50% of cases of surgical bleeding, need to be diagnosed and medically treated.

Blood component therapies

It is important that all clinicians understand the indications, risks and recommended usage of component therapies. Because blood components are used to treat or prevent adverse outcomes (generally bleeding), it is helpful to consider each component in the bleeding and nonbleeding patient.

Red cell transfusion

Red cell transfusion remains the cornerstone of blood component therapy. Red cells are necessary for oxygen delivery, but also serve a haemostatic function. Packed red blood cell transfusion increases oxygen delivery and adds to intravascular volume at the expense of increasing blood viscosity. Despite the routine use of red cells in cardiac surgery, there is wide practice variability. Red cell transfusion is indicated in the setting of excessive bleeding and is administered to the nonbleeding, but anaemic postoperative patient. The evidence sustaining both of these uses is discussed below.

Transfusion of PRBCs is also known to be associated with several risks, including transfusion of transmitted infection (viral or bacterial), allergic reactions, transfusion-related acute lung injury

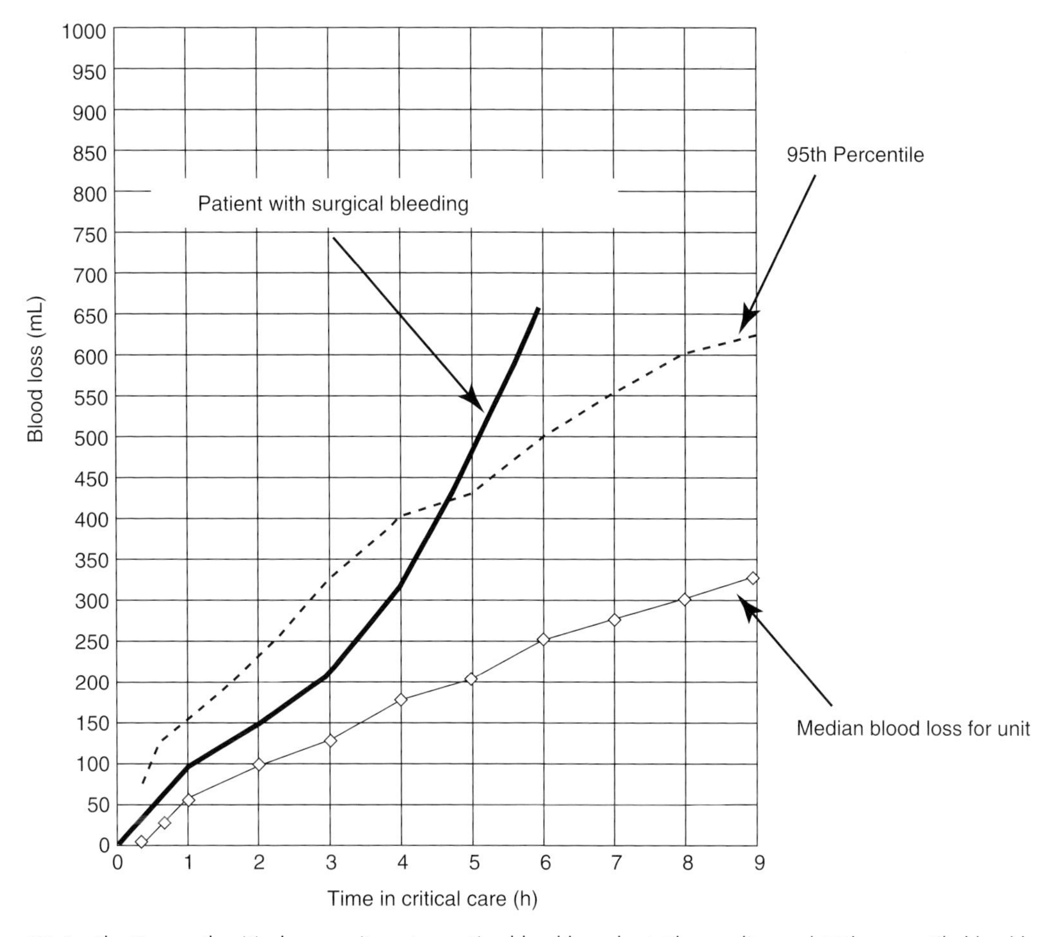

Figure 31.1 The Papworth critical care unit postoperative blood loss chart. The median and 95th percentile blood loss in critical care is plotted against time. In the example shown, an abrupt increase in the expected rate of bleeding for 2 consecutive hours should prompt surgical reexploration.

(TRALI), and transfusion-related immunomodulation. Transfusion of red cells has been independently associated with poorer outcomes, including increased mortality in cardiac surgery. However, a causal relationship has not been proven.

THE BLEEDING PATIENT

The majority of recommendations regarding red cell transfusion in the setting of active bleeding are considered 'expert opinion' and are founded on sound physiologic principles. Volume resuscitation and avoidance of hypothermic shock continues to be the overarching clinical priority. Therefore, in the setting of excessive bleeding, the quantity of red cell units and the rate of transfusion depend on the rate of blood loss. The optimal target haemoglobin in the setting of acute bleeding is unknown.

THE NONBLEEDING PATIENT

Anaemia is common after cardiothoracic procedures, especially after CPB. Moreover, in perioperative and critically ill patient populations, anaemia has been associated with increased mortality in

Table 31.2 Predictors of perioperative bleeding in cardiac surgery

Patient factors
Age >65 years
Female gender
Weight ≤77 kg
Multiple comorbidities
Medications
Antiplatelet agents (e.g. acetylsalicylic acid, clopidogrel, IIb/IIIa inhibitors)
Anticoagulants (e.g. LMWH, warfarin)
Thrombolytics
Preoperative laboratory values
Preoperative anaemia (haemoglobin ≤135 g/L)
Preoperative platelet count (≤150 × 10^9/L)
Increased serum creatinine level
Surgical factors
The individual surgeon
Nonelective surgery
Previous cardiac surgery
Combined procedures
Prolonged CPB time (>2 hours)
Hypothermic circulatory arrest

Abbreviations: CPB, cardiopulmonary bypass; LMWH, low-molecular-weight heparin.

patients with cardiac disease. Given the physiologic importance of red cells to human survival and the known adverse consequences associated with severe anaemia, many studies have focused on the benefits (and potential risks) of red cell transfusion in the setting of anaemia.

Table 31.3 First principles and goals of transfusion

1. Restoration of adequate circulating volume
2. Maintenance of tissue oxygenation
3. To achieve haemostasis
4. Treatment of coagulopathy

Randomized controlled trials specific to cardiac surgery, and meta-analysis of these trials, have been completed and have shown that lower transfusion threshold (transfusion only at lower haemoglobin levels, such as 70 g/L) led to less red cell transfusions, and no difference in clinical outcomes. In fact, mortality was up to 20% lower in a number of studies.

The optimal haemoglobin in postoperative and/or critically ill patients remains undecided. In low-risk patients undergoing revascularization, a conservative transfusion strategy (haemoglobin 70–80 g/L) appears to be well tolerated and results in decreased utilization of scarce donor resources. The optimal haemoglobin concentration in patients undergoing high-risk procedures or in those who have not been fully revascularized remains to be investigated.

Platelets

Thrombocytopenia is frequently encountered in cardiac surgery and a 50% reduction in the circulating platelet concentration is expected after CPB. Platelets are essential for primary haemostasis and the formation of an initial platelet plug upon which cross-linked fibrin is fashioned. In addition to thrombocytopenia, CPB and hypothermia result in substantial platelet dysfunction. Circulating platelets become activated on contact with the CPB circuit, particularly the membrane oxygenator. Once activated, platelets release their internal α granules, which reduces their functional competence. Platelet dysfunction generally persists for several hours post CPB as new platelets are added to the circulation and existing platelets are either cleared from the circulation or regain functionality. Platelet membranes continue to circulate, and can be enumerated by automated haematology analysers, but their functionality remains impaired regardless of the actual count. Therein lies the principal challenge of platelet transfusion immediately following cardiac surgery – the actual platelet count

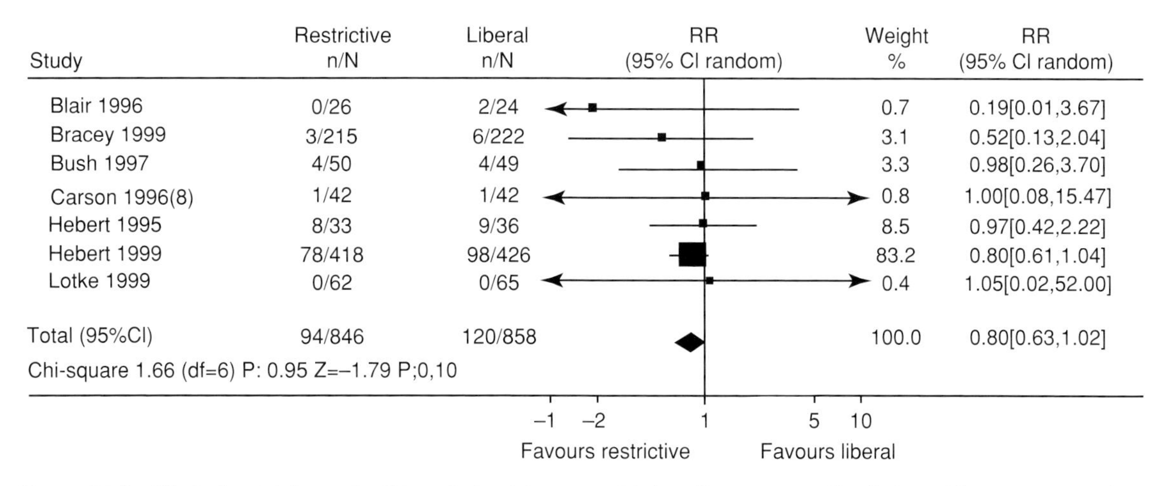

Figure 31.2 Effect of restrictive red cell transfusion triggers on 31-day all-cause mortality. (Adapted from Carson *et al. Trans Med Rev* 2002;16:187–199.)

bears little correlation with platelet function, which makes assessment of the bleeding risk a substantial challenge.

Although platelets are essential to maintain vascular integrity and to decrease bleeding, platelet concentrates are associated with known risks that include TRALI, immunomodulation, anaphylaxis and venous thromboembolism. Because platelets are stored at room temperature in aerated bags, bacterial contamination has also been recognized as an important hazard. Several observational studies have reported increased morbidity and mortality associated with platelet transfusion in cardiac surgery; however, conflicting data exist.

THE BLEEDING PATIENT

The evidence concerning the use of platelet concentrates in the bleeding patient undergoing cardiothoracic surgery and CPB is based largely on the opinion of experts and varies considerably among institutions. Although very few studies have formally addressed this consideration in patients undergoing cardiothoracic procedures, several underlying principles have helped to guide clinical practice.

First, because platelet dysfunction is an expected consequence of CPB, transfusion of allogeneic platelets may be warranted in the bleeding postoperative patient, even in the presence of a normal platelet count. Ideally, a point-of-care test to assess platelet function such as a thromboelastogram would be used to guide platelet therapy. Unfortunately, this test is not routinely available in all centres. As a result, empiric transfusion of platelets may be reasonable provided that blood coagulation parameters (activated partial thromboplastin time [aPTT], International Normalized Ratio [INR] and fibrinogen) are within normal limits. This principle is especially cogent after long CPB times (>2 hours) or should there be preoperative reasons to suspect platelet dysfunction, such as renal failure or the use of aspirin or other platelet inhibitors.

Second, a postoperative platelet count of 70 to 90×10^9/L is adequate to maintain the platelet-dependent portion of coagulation, provided the platelets are functionally competent. Transfusion of platelet concentrates above this threshold is unnecessary and potentially harmful.

Third, to maximize the function of existing and transfused platelets, hypothermia must be actively corrected and avoided with the use of blood warmers and external heating devices. Hypothermia is the only known component of post-CPB platelet dysfunction that can be readily reversed. Although variability exists, it is expected that transfusing one pooled donor platelet unit collected via the buffy coat method (as in the UK), or one apheresis unit, will increase the circulating platelet concentration by ~25 to 50 × 10^9/L. This increase is similar to the transfusion of 4 to 5 random donor units assembled using platelet-rich plasma (as in the United States). Ongoing losses and consumption need to be considered. Adhering to these principles helps to maximize the efficacy of each platelet transfusion and limit exposure to unnecessary blood products.

THE NONBLEEDING PATIENT

The role of perioperative prophylactic or routine platelet transfusions has yet to be defined in cardiac surgery. Several randomized clinical trials in malignancy have demonstrated that a transfusion threshold of 10 × 10^9/L is safe, and is currently recommended. This threshold is rarely reached in cardiac surgery and transfusing platelets at a higher threshold of >50 × 10^9/L is generally recommended in the perioperative management of surgical patients.

Although there is little debate that severe thrombocytopenia is associated with increased surgical bleeding, the optimal threshold platelet nadir is unknown. It is likely that platelet dysfunction is a more significant risk factor than the degree of thrombocytopenia typically encountered. Moreover, the only randomized controlled trial that investigated the role of routine prophylactic transfusion found no differences in bleeding or clinical outcomes. Therefore, most clinicians reserve platelet transfusion for active bleeding or before invasive procedures, when thrombocytopenia is confirmed.

Fresh frozen plasma

Fresh frozen plasma (FFP) is derived from random donor whole blood or apheresis donors and contains near-normal concentrations of all coagulation factors. This includes anticoagulant proteases, immunoglobulins and albumin. In cardiac surgery, deficiencies in multiple coagulation factors develop secondary to haemodilution, bleeding and when large amounts of washed cell saver blood are reinfused. In this setting, haemodilution of coagulation proteins results in a coagulopathy which is further exacerbated by hypothermia. Fresh frozen plasma is indicated for bleeding accompanied by multiple coagulation factor deficiencies or diffuse microvascular bleeding.

Serious consequences are known to be associated with transfusion of FFP. These include allergic and urticarial reactions owing to foreign plasma constituents, anaphylaxis (especially with immunoglobulin A deficiency), transfusion transmitted infections (bacterial and viral) and circulatory overload. One well-recognized risk associated with FFP is the development of TRALI. This risk is thought to be mediated by circulating donor antileukocyte antibodies or biologically active lipids that react with, and consequently 'prime,' the recipient leukocytes. In the setting of CPB or critical illness, these primed leukocytes adhere to the activated endothelium of the pulmonary vasculature and effect a local inflammatory reaction. Given the risks associated with FFP, the use of this product should be based on coagulation testing only.

THE BLEEDING PATIENT

Excessive bleeding associated with multiple coagulation deficiencies is the most frequent indication to consider transfusion of FFP, but randomized trials in this clinical context are lacking. Coagulation testing should guide therapy, but in the setting of diffuse microvascular bleeding and expected coagulopathy, initial empiric use of this plasma fraction may be justified when laboratory delays are unavoidable. Fresh frozen plasma should not simply be used as volume replacement. It is generally recommended in bleeding patients when the INR is, or the aPPT time ratio exceeds, 1.5 the control value. To rule out residual heparin effect, a heparin-neutralized aPTT or a thrombin time should be performed when the postprotamine aPTT is prolonged.

Additional protamine boluses (25–50 mg), or a 4- to 6-hour low-dose protamine infusion (25 mg/h) can be used if heparin rebound is confirmed.

The volume of FFP transfused depends on the rate of continued bleeding and the ability of the patient to synthesize haemostatic proteins. The recommended initial dose is 12 to 15 mL/kg. This dose typically represents 4 U of random donor FFP units (250 mL/U) or 2 U of single donor apheresis FFP (500 mL/U) in an average 70-kg patient. This dose should increase all individual coagulation factors by 25% to 30%, which represents the minimum haemostatic threshold for the individual factors.

THE NONBLEEDING PATIENT

In the nonbleeding patient there is no evidence to suggest that the preemptive administration of FFP is effective at reducing perioperative bleeding or transfusion requirements. Several randomized trials comparing prophylactic FFP with placebo in elective cardiac surgery concluded that FFP has no effect in reducing bleeding or red cell transfusion requirements. Furthermore, liberal use of FFP in critically ill patients with abnormal INRs fails to decrease bleeding and is associated with increased pulmonary oedema and acute lung injury. Despite the lack of benefit and documented risks associated with this product, hospital audits have revealed that

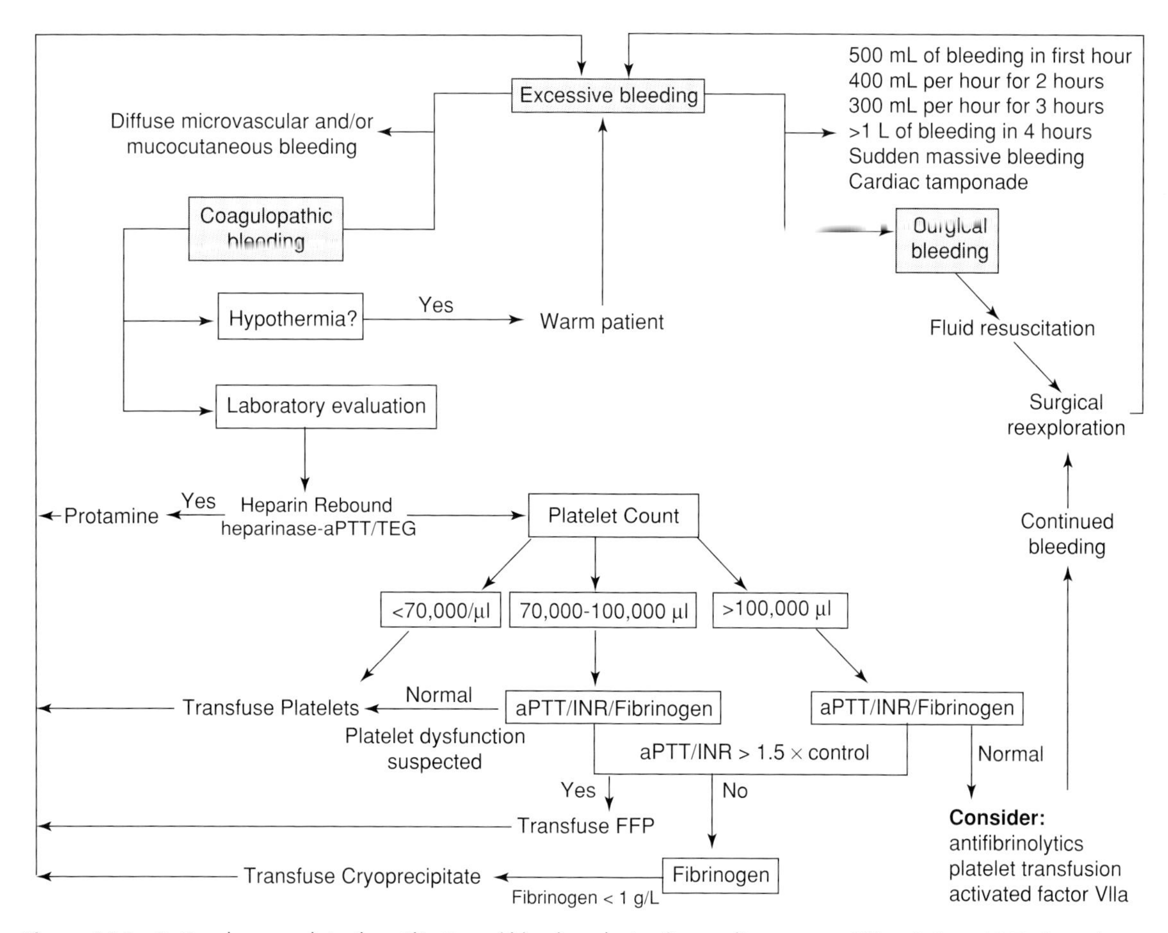

Figure 31.3 Rational approach to the utilization of blood products after cardiac surgery. *Abbreviations*: HNTT, heparin neutralized thrombin time; FFP, fresh frozen plasma; DDAVP, desmopressin acetate; rVIIa, recombinant factor VIIa.

34% to 45% of FFP use is considered 'inappropriate' based on currently published guidelines.

Cryoprecipitate

Cryoprecipitate is obtained by thawing FFP at 4°C, resulting in precipitation of the cryoproteins. After centrifugation, the supernatant is removed and the remaining 'cryoprecipitate' is resuspended in 10 to 15 mL of plasma. Cryoprecipitate is rich in fibrinogen, factor VIII, von Willebrand factor, factor XIII and fibronectin. In this era of recombinant and virally inactivated factor concentrates, the indications for cryoprecipitate have diminished considerably, and now are restricted to microvascular bleeding (coagulopathy), when fibrinogen is ≤ 1 g/L. Each unit of cryoprecipitate contains approximately 150 to 200 mg of fibrinogen and 8 to 12 random donor units should be ordered if the product is deemed necessary. No evidence-based recommendations exist to guide the rational use of this product, and consequently wide practice variation exists.

The rational use of blood products after cardiac surgery

Although no algorithm can encompass the subtleties associated with each clinical scenario, it serves as a starting point from which rational transfusion decisions can be justified. Transfusion decisions based on laboratory data or point-of-care algorithms can reduce exposure to allogeneic blood without increasing bleeding or perioperative complications. The documented strength of such algorithms is to suggest when transfusion will not be beneficial. Their ability to communicate the absolute need for transfusion remains limited.

Key points

- A consistent and ordered approach to excessive bleeding is required to ensure the rational and safe use of allogeneic component therapies.
- Laboratory or point-of-care testing should be used to guide transfusion except in the setting of uncontrolled bleeding.
- Surgical bleeding should always be suspected and resternotomy should not be delayed.
- A regularly updated transfusion algorithm is essential, and compliance should be audited regularly.

FURTHER READING

Bracey AW, Radovancevic R, Riggs SA, *et al.* Lowering the hemoglobin threshold for transfusion coronary artery bypass procedures: effect on patient outcome. *Transfusion* 1999;39: 1070–1077.

Casbard AC, Williamson LM, Murphy MF, *et al.* The role of prophylactic fresh frozen plasma in decreasing blood loss and correcting coagulopathy in cardiac surgery. A systematic review. *Anaesthesia* 2004;59:550–558.

Hebert PC, Wells G, Blajchman MA, *et al.* A multicenter, randomized, controlled clinical trial of transfusion requirements in critical care. Transfusion Requirements in Critical Care Investigators, Canadian Critical Care Trials Group. *N Engl J Med* 1999;340:409–417.

Karkouti K, Wijeysundera DN, Yau TM, *et al.* Platelet transfusions are not associated with increased morbidity or mortality in cardiac surgery. *Can J Anaesth* 2006;53:279–287.

Chapter 32

Blood conservation strategies

A.N.G. CURRY AND R.S. GILL

Introduction

The goal of blood conservation in cardiac surgery is to reduce or avoid patient exposure to allogeneic transfusion. In transfusion situations where the donor and recipient are the same individual, the term 'autologous' is used.

Blood conservation techniques

Techniques for conservation of blood, minimizing the requirement for transfusion, can be subdivided into preoperative, intraoperative and postoperative strategies, and are usually used in combination.

Preoperative phase

Elective surgery allows planning and prevention of common problems that increase the likelihood of a perioperative transfusion.

ANAEMIA

A patient who is anaemic ($\leq$12.5 g/dL) is more likely to be transfused. Any patient referred for elective cardiac surgery should therefore have a full blood count checked in time to detect and treat anaemia. For example, a 4-week course of oral iron supplementation often elevates red cell mass significantly. Other deficiencies, such as folate or vitamin B_{12}, may also be identified and corrected.

CONGENITAL COAGULOPATHIES

Patients presenting for cardiac surgery with inherited coagulation disorders, such as haemophilia, require appropriate perioperative factor replacement. Involvement of a haematologist at an early stage is advisable.

AUTOLOGOUS BLOOD PREDONATION AND ERYTHROPOIETIN

Erythropoietin (EPO) may be used to increase red cell mass alone, or to facilitate autologous blood predonation. Autologous blood predonation involves the patients donating their own blood over a number of weeks with the purpose of retransfusion at the time of surgery. Autologous blood predonation rose in popularity as a technique in the 1980s during the initial phase of the HIV crisis, but is now rarely practiced. Cost and practical issues such as early identification of appropriate patients, blood collection and storage have limited applicability. There also remains concern that:

- the risk of excess thrombosis with EPO has not been excluded;
- autologous blood predonation without EPO does not appear to reduce allogeneic transfusion rate in cardiac surgical patients;
- it is not suitable for urgent or emergency surgical patients;
- autologous blood predonation may be poorly tolerated in patients with significant coronary stenoses or valve lesions restricting cardiac output; and
- the risk of transfusing the wrong unit to the wrong patient is still present.

Table 32.1 Combined strategy for blood conservation

Maximize reserves
Preoperative identification of anaemia
Increasing red cell mass
Minimize losses
Avoiding haemostatic problems
Identification and treatment of preoperative coagulopathy including cessation of antiplatelet agents (where appropriate)
Meticulous surgical technique
Minimizing CPB prime and time
Avoidance of CPB altogether
Intraoperative cell salvage
Antifibrinolytic therapy
Appropriate reversal of heparin
Early intervention for surgical bleeding
Rationalize replacements
Reduction of traditional transfusion threshold
Targeted product replacement

Abbreviations: CPB, cardiopulmonary bypass.

ANTIPLATELET THERAPIES

The vast majority of cardiac surgical patients take antiplatelet drugs. The most frequently encountered agents are aspirin and clopidogrel, but other agents such as abciximab, eptifibatide and tirofiban may be encountered in patients undergoing emergency surgery after incomplete percutaneous coronary revascularization procedures. Nonsteroidal anti-inflammatory drugs (NSAIDS) have also been implicated in increased surgical blood loss.

Many other drugs alter platelet function, but this is usually for a very short time only (e.g. cephalosporins). Platelets contain granules, but lack a nucleus, and hence have no capacity to synthesize new enzymes.

Aspirin causes inhibition of platelet aggregation through irreversibly inhibiting cyclo-oxygenase (COX)-1 both in the platelets (reducing TXA_2) and in the vascular endothelium (reducing PGI_2). The balance is tipped toward inhibition of platelet aggregation by three mechanisms:

- Higher doses of aspirin are needed to inhibit COX-1 in the endothelium than in the platelets (hence low-dose aspirin therapy).
- The vascular endothelium can synthesize new COX-1; platelets cannot.
- Aspirin is subject to first-pass metabolism, giving relative protection to the systemic vascular endothelium, the platelets are exposed to aspirin in the portal blood.

The antiplatelet effect of aspirin only wears off when the affected platelets are replaced, over a 7- to 10-day period.

Clopidogrel also causes irreversible platelet inhibition, but by inhibiting adenosine diphosphate-induced platelet aggregation. Clopidogrel is a prodrug, acting through an active metabolite that circulates at a clinically relevant concentration for around 18 hours after administration. Its effects are additive with aspirin, and the active metabolite permanently inhibits any platelets present, including exogenous transfusion. As such, platelet therapy for clopidogrel-induced blood loss during the time of metabolite circulation is of reduced benefit, and wherever possible, surgery should be delayed until 24 hours after the last dose. Like aspirin, platelet function does not return to normal until new platelets are synthesized in the absence of clopidogrel, over a 7- to 10-day period.

In variable ratios, NSAIDS reversibly inhibit the enzymes COX-1 and -2 and their antiplatelet effects are half-life-dependent, usually wearing off after a few hours.

GpIIb/IIIa inhibitors are the newest and most potent group of antiplatelet agents. The final common pathway in platelet aggregation involves the binding of fibrinogen to activated platelets via the GpIIb/IIIa receptor. By antagonizing the final step of platelet aggregation, all pathways of platelet activation are effectively inhibited.

Table 32.2 Recommended management of preoperative anticoagulant and antiplatelet therapy

Drug	Recommendation
NSAIDS	Avoid preoperatively on day of surgery
Aspirin	Consider stopping 5–10 days before surgery to enable platelet function to return to normal
Clopidogrel	Stop 5–10 days before surgery to enable platelet function to return to normal. Delay urgent surgery for 24 hours after last dose if patient condition permits
Warfarin	Low risk (e.g. AF): Stop 3–5 days before surgery and allow INR to normalize Intermediate risk (e.g. DVT): Convert to s/c heparin, e.g. 5,000 IU twice or three times a day 3–5 days before surgery until 2 hours before surgery, INR allowed to normalize High risk (e.g. mechanical valve): Convert to IV heparin when INR falls ≤2.5, to maintain an aPTT of 2.5–3.5 control values Emergency reversal: vitamin K 5 mg IV, prothrombin complex concentrate (30–50 U/kg) ± FFP 15 mL/kg
Heparin	Stop 6 hours before surgery to allow aPTT to normalize
Abciximab	Delay urgent surgery for 24 hours after dose if patient condition permits
Eptifibatide/ tirofiban	Delay urgent surgery for 4–8 hours after dose if patient condition permits

Abbreviations: AF, atrial fibrillation; aPTT, activated partial thromboplastin time; DVT, deep venous thrombosis; FFP, fresh frozen plasma; INR, International Normalized Ratio.

URAEMIA

Wherever possible, patients with chronic renal impairment should receive preoperative renal replacement therapy to reduce their urea levels because uraemia produces dose-dependent reversible impairment of platelet secretory and aggregatory function and increases surgical blood loss despite a normal platelet count. Desmopressin therapy (DDAVP) increases circulating von Willebrand factor levels and improves platelet aggregation in these patients to a variable degree.

Intraoperative phase

SURGICAL CONSIDERATIONS

Good intraoperative surgical haemostasis reduces blood loss and transfusion requirements. This is not unique to cardiac surgery. Recognition of the coagulopathic consequences of excess transfusion, early control of bleeding points and the use of diathermy reduce surgical bleeding. Shorter CPB time, or avoidance of CPB altogether, helps to preserve platelet function. Topical adjuncts include haemostatic swabs made of cellulose or gelatin, and biological or synthetic glues.

CARDIOPULMONARY BYPASS CONSIDERATIONS

Cardiopulmonary bypass exposes the blood to a foreign surface and results in activation of platelets and the coagulation proteins. Cellular blood components are subjected to physical trauma from the action of the roller pump. Various strategies are available, and of importance to the critical care team:

- *Return to normothermia*: hypothermia-induced coagulopathy can be reduced by sufficient rewarming of core and periphery on CPB.
- *Heparin/protamine interaction*: too little heparin allows coagulation activation and consumption of platelets and clotting factors during CPB. Too much heparin invites heparin rebound after

protamine reversal. Too little protamine leaves residual anticoagulation; too much protamine may exert an anticoagulant effect. Monitoring the degree of anticoagulation, for example using the activated clotting time, permits titration of heparin and protamine doses to confirm adequate anticoagulation and its reversal.

ACUTE NORMOVOLAEMIC HAEMODILUTION

Acute normovolaemic haemodilution involves the removal of a predetermined volume of blood (usually 10 mL/kg) from the patient and simultaneous replacement with crystalloid (3:1) or colloid (1:1, gelatins 1.5:1) to ensure normovolaemia throughout. Reinfusion usually follows CPB and surgical control of bleeding.

INTRAOPERATIVE CELL SALVAGE

Collection and retransfusion of shed blood from the surgical wound is the simplest and most frequently employed blood conservation strategy in cardiac surgery. Blood shed during CPB (while heparinized) is collected via pump suckers into the cardiotomy reservoir. Blood shed before heparinization for CPB and after reversal of the heparin (and in some centres during CPB) is diverted to a cell salvage device for processing.

Studies comparing cell-saved RBCs with circulating blood by labelling red cells with radioisotopes have shown that there is no difference in survival at 24 hours or mean RBC survival rate. Cell-salvaged blood has higher levels of adenosine triphosphate and 2,3-diphosphoglycerate and a greater oxygen carrying capacity than banked blood. Cell-salvaged blood still contains activated polymorphonuclear (PMN) leukocytes and has a very low platelet count ($\sim 10 \times 10^9/\mu L$). The residual platelets have also been activated during blood loss and cell salvage and are degranulated and nonaggregatory. Leukocyte filtration removes the polynuclear neutrophils and their potential role in augmenting inflammation, but induces a significant time delay between blood loss and availability for retransfusion. Shed blood contains low levels of fibrinogen, similar to banked blood, but higher levels of free haemoglobin. Washing by cell salvage machines removes most soluble proteins (e.g. interleukin-6, tumour necrosis factor, thrombin–antithrombin-III complex, plasmin–antiplasmin and free haemoglobin) and nonerythrocyte particulate matter. This has the theoretical disadvantage of removing the coagulation factors; however, postoperative blood loss has been shown to be significantly lower when washed red blood cells (RBCs) are transfused when compared with unwashed RBCs. Once initial equipment outlay costs have been recovered, cell-salvaged blood is cheaper than equivalent volumes of banked blood and is more acceptable to patients. Randomized controlled clinical trials in cardiac surgery have repeatedly shown a reduction in the need for allogeneic transfusion when cell salvage is used.

PHARMACOLOGICAL THERAPIES

The use of pharmacological agents to promote clotting and reduce perioperative blood loss is currently the subject of much debate, and aprotinin is at the centre of this.

The use of prothrombotic drugs seems to be at odds with the usual management strategies of ischaemic heart disease, which revolve around antiplatelet and anticoagulant medications. Pharmacological agents are, however, highly efficacious at reducing blood loss and allogeneic transfusion.

APROTININ

Aprotinin is a basic polypeptide derived from bovine lung. The most frequently employed dose regimen is the Hammersmith or 'high-dose' regimen of 2 MU loading dose, 2 MU to CPB prime and 0.5 MU/h infusion until completion of surgery. A variety of other regimens are used, usually lower doses. Aprotinin inhibits a broad spectrum of serine protease molecules involved in coagulation and fibrinolysis including plasmin, trypsin and kallikrein in a dose-dependent manner. The active forms of factors I, II, VII, IX, X, XI and XII and prekallikrein are all serine proteases. There is no unifying theory to explain the haemostatic action of aprotinin, which is more complex than that of the lysine analogues. Aprotinin is antigenic, and has potential to induce anaphylaxis. This occurs very infrequently in first-time exposure ($\leq$0.1%), but more frequently in reexposure (2.8% overall; $\leq$0.1% first 2 weeks after exposure; 5.0% 2 weeks to 6 months; 0.9% after 6 months). This pattern is consistent with a weak antigen–antibody-mediated response. A test dose of 10,000 KIU (1 mL) 10 minutes before administering a loading dose should be given. Aprotinin is highly efficacious at reducing blood loss and allogeneic transfusion in cardiac surgery, but doubts have been raised regarding its safety. It is now advocated that other agents should be used except in those patients where the bleeding risk is prohibitive.

LYSINE ANALOGUE ANTIFIBRINOLYTICS

Tranexamic acid and ε-aminocaproic acid are synthetic antifibrinolytics. Both agents attach to the lysine-binding site on plasminogen and inhibit binding of plasminogen and plasmin to fibrin. The fibrin polymer formed by coagulation is therefore more resistant to fibrinolysis. The lysine analogues are cheaper than aprotinin and are nearly as effective.

DESMOPRESSIN

A vasopressin analogue, DDAVP does not cause vasoconstriction. It potentiates primary haemostasis at a dose of 0.3 μg/kg through endothelial release of von Willebrand factor and augmentation of factor VIII. It reduces bleeding times in patients with von Willebrand's disease and mild haemophilia. It may have a role in the treatment of the bleeding patient with a functional platelet disorder induced by aspirin or uraemia. Not in widespread use, DDAVP causes a nonsignificant reduction in blood loss and transfusion. There are also reports of up to a 2.4-fold increase in perioperative myocardial infarction rate.

Postoperative phase

Postoperative bleeding is often a combination of failed surgical haemostasis and coagulopathy.

RESULT-BASED PRODUCT TRANSFUSION

Blood product transfusion should be guided by coagulation testing (Chapter 31). Near patient testing of coagulation using thromboelastography (TEG) has been shown to reduce inappropriate platelet and coagulation factor transfusions in complex cardiac surgery. The use of a TEG-guided transfusion policy has been further validated as part of an integrated blood conservation strategy.

CELL SALVAGE

Mediastinal blood shed postoperatively into chest drains can be salvaged and returned to the patient. Like intraoperative cell salvage, this can be either unwashed or washed. Transfusion of unwashed shed mediastinal blood, however, may increase bleeding and wound infection rates. Washed shed mediastinal blood readministration is therefore preferred. Encouraging early results have shown a reduction in allogeneic transfusion and hospital length of stay. The high outlay costs of providing enough processing units, and the lack of a large study demonstrating cost effectiveness has limited the uptake of this technique.

ANTIFIBRINOLYTICS

Starting antifibrinolytics in the postoperative period has no proven advantage. Aprotinin is usually stopped at the end of surgery and there is no proven benefit of continued use in critical care.

RECOMBINANT FACTOR XA

Recombinant factor VIIa has been used in the treatment of haemophiliacs with acquired factor VIII inhibitors since 1996. It is increasingly being used in situations where massive transfusion has precipitated a dilutional coagulopathy resistant to conventional blood product administration and haemorrhage is ongoing. This is at present an off-license indication, but growing numbers of case reports showing control of previously intractable haemorrhage in cardiac surgery have prompted ongoing randomized trials.

Safety profile and the establishment of dosage and timing of administration are the key targets of investigation. At present, the most frequently employed dose is 90 μg/kg (that recommended and validated in haemophilia patients). Factor VIIa has emerged as having a pivotal role in the cell-based model of coagulation, and promotes thrombin generation at the site of blood vessel injury even in the presence of other coagulation factor deficits. It is still too early for the recommendation of recombinant factor VIIa as a universal haemostatic agent, but it clearly shows exciting potential to reduce allogeneic transfusion, especially in complex or revision cardiac surgery.

RED CELL SUBSTITUTES

Red cell substitutes in the form of artificial oxygen-carrying substances are the subject of ongoing research. They take the form of either haemoglobin-based oxygen carriers or perfluorocarbons. Although clearly having great potential to avoid allogeneic transfusion, early results have been disappointing. Short plasma half-lives and significant adverse safety signals have led to all clinical trials being stopped. Further refinement and evidence are required before oxygen carriers are available for use in cardiac surgery.

Key points

- Preoperative identification and treatment of anaemia in elective surgery is simple and effective.
- Antiplatelet agents significantly increase perioperative blood loss, but discontinuation needs to be weighed against risk of thrombosis.
- Intraoperative cell salvage and antifibrinolytic therapies significantly decrease blood loss and transfusion and are widely employed.
- Use of a TEG-guided transfusion algorithm reduces transfusions in complex cardiac surgery.

FURTHER READING

Engoren MC, Habib RH, Zacharias A, *et al*. Effect of blood transfusion on long-term survival after cardiac operation. *Ann Thorac Surg* 2002;74:1180–1186.

Koch CG, Li L, Duncan AI, Mihaljevic T, *et al*. Transfusion in coronary artery bypass grafting is associated with reduced long-term survival. *Ann Thorac Surg* 2006;81:1650–1657.

Ruel MA, Rubens FD. Non-pharmacological strategies for blood conservation in cardiac surgery. *Can J Anesth* 2001;48(4 Suppl):S13–S23.

Shore-Lesserson L, Manspeizer HE, DePerio M, *et al*. Thromboelastography-guided transfusion algorithm reduces transfusions in complex cardiac surgery. *Anesth Analg* 1999;88:312–319.

Chapter 33

Haematological diseases

P. KESTEVEN AND H. POWELL

Introduction

Haematological disease may present de novo in critically ill patients as unexpected haemorrhage or thrombosis. Alternatively, abnormal and unexplained blood results may be seen. More commonly patients with known disease, such as haematological malignancy, present for cardiothoracic surgery and then critical care admission. An understanding of the disease process and its treatment aids in the management of these patients.

Haemorrhage

Disseminated intravascular coagulation

Disseminated intravascular coagulation (DIC) is characterized by systemic intravascular activation of coagulation, leading to widespread intravascular thrombi and bleeding, owing to consumption of platelets and clotting factors. It may present in an acute or chronic form, and is triggered by many clinical conditions including sepsis, malignancy and trauma. Bleeding manifestations include petechiae and oozing from wound sites, intravenous lines, venepuncture sites and mucosal surfaces. Organ failure, secondary to tissue ischaemic injury from intravascular fibrin deposition, is also common. There is no single diagnostic test, but DIC should be considered whenever there is the combination of thrombocytopenia, a prolonged prothrombin time (PT) and activated partial thromboplastin time (aPTT), low fibrinogen levels and evidence of accelerated fibrinolysis from the measurement of D-dimers.

Treatment should be aimed at identifying and removing/treating the underlying condition and providing multiorgan support, plus blood product support if there is active bleeding. In addition, in adults with severe sepsis and multiple organ failure, recombinant human activated protein C may be considered. There is no evidence to support the use of blood products if the patient is not bleeding, whatever the results of the laboratory tests.

Liver dysfunction

Bleeding is a major complication of acute and chronic liver disease. Hepatic cell failure leads to reduced synthesis of all coagulation factors except factor VIII. This results in prolongation of both the aPTT and PT, and reduced fibrinogen concentration. The magnitude of the haemostatic abnormalities correlates with the degree of parenchymal damage and stage of liver disease. The response to fresh frozen plasma in liver disease is unpredictable and, if used, it is advisable to repeat the coagulation screen after the infusion.

Single factor deficiency

Occasionally, individuals with mild congenital bleeding disorders may present with clinical bleeding late in life. Cases of mild inherited or acquired haemophilia may present with postoperative bleeding. The diagnosis is often delayed owing to failure to recognize the significance of a prolonged aPTT.

Table 33.1 Clotting factor deficiencies

Disease	Frequency	Features	Treatment
Haemophilia: factor VIII deficiency or factor IX deficiency	1:5000 to 1:30000	Mild disease may present late in life.	Recombinant factor VIII or IX Prothrombin complex concentrate DDAVP Antifibrinolytics
Factor VII deficiency	1:500,000	Often mild	Factor VIIa
Factor XI deficiency	1:1,000,000	Ashkenazi Jews Variable effect	FFP Factor XI concentrate
Factor X deficiency	1:1,000,000	Can be secondary to amyloid, pneumonia, leukaemia	Prothrombin complex concentrate Factor X concentrate
Factor V deficiency	1:1,000,000	Platelet type bleeding and thrombosis	FFP and platelets
Factor II deficiency	1:2,000,000	Mucosal and deep tissue bleeding.	Prothrombin complex concentrate
Factor VIII deficiency	1:1,000,000	May cause recurrent miscarriage. Can be secondary to gastritis or leukaemia	Factor VIII concentrate FFP

Abbreviations: DDAVP, desmopressin; FFP, fresh frozen plasma;

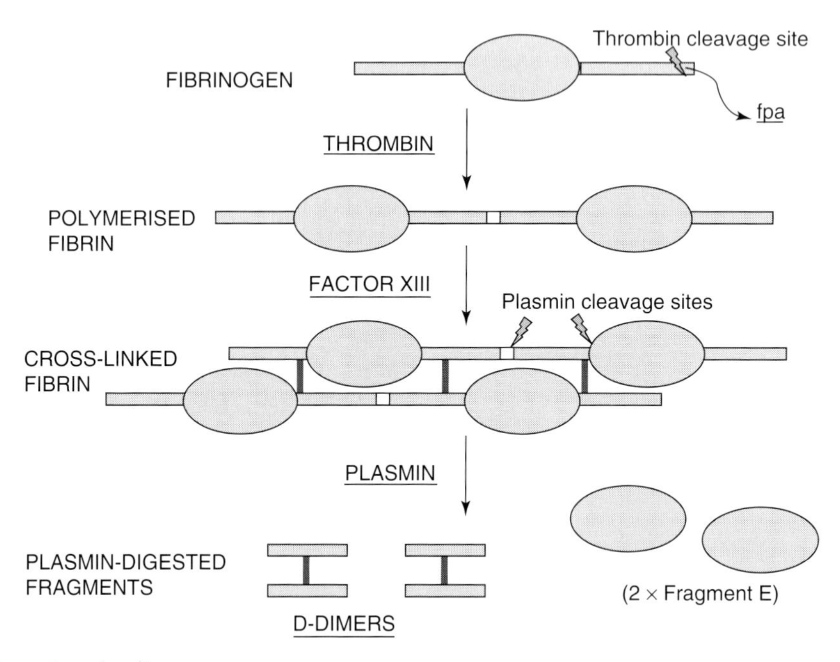

Figure 33.1 Formation of D-dimers.

If an accurate diagnosis of a haemostatic defect is made, treatment is usually self-evident. If specific factors are deficient, concentrate replacements are available. Cryoprecipitate is the treatment of choice for replacing fibrinogen, and this product contains high concentrations of all the 'sticky' proteins, including von Willebrand factor and fibronectin. To replace vitamin K-dependent factors, prothrombin complex concentrate is the treatment of choice.

Dysfibrinogens

Dysfibrinogenaemia is a coagulation disorder caused by structural abnormalities in the fibrinogen molecule resulting in abnormal fibrinogen function. It can be inherited or acquired; the latter usually secondary to liver disease. The inherited form is associated with increased risk of bleeding, thrombosis or both in the same patient or family. Dysfibrinogenaemia should be considered if both the thrombin and reptilase (see below) times are prolonged. Confirmatory tests involve comparisons of fibrinogen clotting activity and fibrinogen antigen levels. Treatment is only necessary if the patient is bleeding and is by transfusion of fibrinogen, usually as cryoprecipitate.

Thrombosis

Pathological clotting may present as arterial thrombosis (coronary or cerebral artery); venous occlusion (deep venous thrombosis [DVT] or central vein catheter-related thrombosis); or most commonly, occlusion of extracorporeal circuits such as haemofiltration filters and cannulae.

Arterial thrombosis

Arterial thrombosis is uncommon and in general occurs as the result of mechanical vessel obstruction leading to sluggish blood flow.

Deep venous thrombosis

Deep venous thrombosis is common in critical care patients and standard thromboprophylaxis measures should be instituted wherever possible. Little has been published concerning the frequency of DVT and pulmonary embolism after coronary artery bypass grafting, but available studies suggest a relatively high rate of DVT (approximately 17%).

Venous thrombosis can also occur as a complication of central venous cannulation in the critical care setting. This is frequently asymptomatic, but can cause upper limb swelling or difficulty in the positioning of new central venous cannulae. The incidence of pulmonary embolism owing to catheter-related central vein thrombosis in critical care patients is unknown.

Thrombosis

Occlusion of haemofiltration circuits and cannulae is the most frequent presentation of thrombosis in cardiac critical care. In such patients undergoing haemofiltration, there is an increase in thrombin–antithrombin complex over the lifespan of the haemofiltration filter, and the rise in thrombin–antithrombin complex levels is inversely correlated with filter lifespan. The mechanisms by which thrombin is generated are likely to be multifactorial. Decreased levels of naturally occurring anticoagulants may reduce the inhibitory capacity against thrombin. Increased activation and reduced inhibition of the tissue factor pathway may contribute to thrombin generation, but it is possible that other atypical stimuli may also be important, such as the activation of coagulation factors on cell surfaces or the direct activation of factor X on the surface of monocytes. In such cases, a careful increase in heparin dose may help.

Pharmacological inhibition of coagulation

Heparin

Incomplete reversal of heparin or heparin rebound (reheparinization owing to heparin molecules moving back into the circulation from the tissues) may exacerbate postoperative haemorrhage. The aPTT and ACT are prolonged; if thromboelastography

(TEG) is available, a heparinase and nonheparinase sample cup should be used, and there will be an obvious difference between the results if heparin effect is persisting. Laboratory testing may involve performing both a thrombin and a reptilase time on the plasma sample. Both thrombin and reptilase (purified enzyme from the venom of *Bothrops atrox* snake; and ancrod, a similar enzyme from *Agkistrodon rhodostoma*) convert fibrinogen to fibrin. However, thrombin is inhibited by heparin and these snake enzymes are not. Consequently, a prolonged thrombin time and normal reptilase time is virtually diagnostic of the presence of heparin. Alternatively, heparin concentration itself may be measured, although this is not common and may be time consuming.

Warfarin

Warfarin inhibits all four vitamin K-dependent factors (II, VII, IX and X) and therefore has a prolonging effect on both intrinsic and extrinsic pathways. However, the PT reagents are most sensitive to its effect, whereas the aPTT reagents are relatively insensitive.

Reversal of warfarin effect may be required, and is usually considered if the International Normalized Ratio (INR) is greater than 2. Rapid reversal may be achieved with a prothrombin complex concentrate, which has high concentrations of all the vitamin K-dependent factors and is presented in a low-volume mix. Fresh frozen plasma is less expensive and equally effective, although it requires larger volumes of replacement fluid and may have side effects such as histamine release and pulmonary hypertension.

In cases requiring elective reversal of warfarin effect, supplementation of vitamin K is sufficient. Provided hepatic function is normal, intravenous vitamin K corrects the INR in approximately 8 hours and oral vitamin K in approximately 24 hours. It should be noted, however, that the INR measures only the extrinsic pathway of the coagulation cascade and factor VII, which initiates this pathway, has a relatively short half-life of approximately 6 hours. Consequently, when reversing warfarin effect, the INR may not be a true reflection of the whole coagulation system; in particular, a normal INR may not reflect 100% activity of all the vitamin K-dependent factors.

Other inhibitors of coagulation

A relatively uncommon cause of acute bleeding is the development of inhibitors against specific coagulation factors. These conditions are more common in the elderly and have a range of clinical presentations, from asymptomatic patients with abnormal coagulation tests, to patients with severe, life-threatening haemorrhage. Inhibitors are most commonly directed against factor VIII or vWF, but have been described to most other coagulation factors.

Lupus anticoagulant is most commonly associated with a prothrombotic state, but in rare cases it can have haemorrhagic manifestations owing to acquired inhibitors of coagulation factors.

No specific inhibitor identified

Unfortunately, with unpleasant frequency, cases are found in critical care in which pathological bleeding continues in the face of strenuous diagnostic and therapeutic efforts. There is abundant evidence that clinical outcomes are improved in such patients if haemorrhage is arrested early, by whatever means, before the patient acquires a dilutional coagulopathy and concomitant activation of the protective inflammatory cascades. In such a situation, the patient may enter a coagulopathic spiral from which it may become extremely difficult to 'catch up.'

Abnormal blood results

Thrombocytopenia

Some of the commonest causes of thrombocytopenia are those due to incorrect sampling or artifact. If the sample starts to clot before mixing with anticoagulants in the collection tube, the platelet count

Table 33.2 Causes of thrombocytopenia

Category		Example
Artefactual (false reading)	Clot in sample platelets clumped	
Congenital	Rare inherited disorders	May-Hegglin anomaly Bernard Soulier syndrome
Defective production	Bone marrow aplasia	Aplastic anaemia, drugs
	Metabolic disorders	B_{12}, folate deficiency Renal failure Alcohol abuse
	Abnormal bone marrow	Myelodysplasia, leukaemia, lymphoma, myeloma, osteopetrosis, myelofibrosis, cytotoxics, radiation, viruses, drugs
Loss from circulation	Massive transfusion	Dilutional effect
	Enlarged spleen	Platelet pooling
Diminished survival	Immune mediated	
	Disseminated intravascular coagulation	Trauma, burns, malignancy, infection
	Thrombotic thrombocytopenic purpura	
	Damage during circulation	Leaking artificial valves Cardiopulmonary bypass

may be extremely low owing to platelet clumping. Although the laboratory staff checks for visible clots in the sample, these are not always apparent; therefore, unexpectedly low results should be repeated.

As a general rule a platelet count higher than 100 $\times 10^9$/L is adequate to maintain haemostasis, and a count $>50 \times 10^9$/L should be adequate if no recent haemostatic insult has taken place.

Thrombocytopenia may be due to either increased platelet consumption or decreased platelet production. This distinction is important because appropriate treatment differs and the wrong treatment may aggravate the situation. In critical care, the majority of such cases are due to dilution or consumption.

DECREASED PLATELET PRODUCTION

Thrombocytopenia owing to reduced platelet production by the marrow is less common in critical care. Causes include pharmacological agents (cyclosporine, quinine, chloramphenicol) and malignant marrow infiltration. This is usually associated with evidence of failure of other marrow constituents: falling haemoglobin, low reticulocyte count and neutropenia. If doubt exists, diagnosis may be made on marrow biopsy showing absent or reduced megakaryocytes. Treatment is supportive by way of platelet transfusion aimed at maintaining a platelet count above 20×10^9/L in the absence of bleeding, and above 50×10^9/L if haemorrhage is present.

DECREASED PLATELET FUNCTION

Inherited platelet function defects are rare and are usually known before admission. A much more frequent occurrence is pharmacological impairment of platelet function. Ultimately, if pathological bleeding is present and suspicion of a platelet defect has arisen then platelets should be transfused.

Table 33.3 Examples of drugs causing platelet dysfunction

Mechanism of action	Drug examples
Inhibition of the thromboxane pathway	Aspirin, NSAIDs, losartan, furosemide
Inhibition of serotonin uptake	Tricyclic antidepressants, fluoxetine
Inhibition of ADP receptor	Clopidogrel, ticlopidine
Inhibition of phosphodiesterase	Dipyridamole, aminophylline, sildenafil, caffeine
Group IIb/IIIa fibrinogen interaction	Abciximab, eptifibatide, tirofiban, fibrinolytic agents
Unknown mechanism of action	Acetazolamide, cimetidine, hydroxychloroquine, penicillins, dextran, procaine, phenothiazines, cyclosporin, clofibrate, chlorpheniramine

Abbreviations: ADP, adenosine diphosphate; NSAIDs, nonsteroidal anti-inflammatory drugs.

INCREASED PLATELET DESTRUCTION

Increased platelet destruction is common:

- after surgery or trauma;
- in DIC and sepsis;
- heparin-induced thrombocytopenia;
- idiopathic (or immune) thrombocytopenic purpura;
- drugs (e.g. Gp IIb/IIIa blockers);
- post-transfusional purpura; and
- hypersplenism.

The presentation of all of the above conditions, with the exception of heparin-induced thrombocytopenia (Chapter 31) is identical. Bleeding secondary to thrombocytopenia tends to be predominantly in skin and mucosa but may of course be at any site and, in particular, may aggravate surgical bleeding. Platelet count is obviously low, and TEG may indicate reduced platelet function.

IMMUNE THROMBOCYTOPENIC PURPURA

Immune thrombocytopenic purpura is caused by circulating antiplatelet auto-antibodies, which cause peripheral destruction of platelets in the reticuloendothelial system. The diagnosis is based on the exclusion of other causes of thrombocytopenia. In general, the condition is not associated with severe bleeding, even when the platelet count is very low. Immune thrombocytopenic purpura may be idiopathic, but can be associated with a number of underlying conditions, such as lymphoproliferative disorders (e.g. chronic lymphocytic leukaemia), autoimmune diseases (e.g. systemic lupus erythematosus) and infections (such as HIV).

No treatment is recommended if the patient is asymptomatic and the platelet count is greater than 30×10^9/L. First-line treatment is based on steroids with concomitant administration of intravenous immunoglobulin in the presence of bleeding.

THROMBOTIC THROMBOCYTOPENIC PURPURA

Thrombotic thrombocytopenic purpura is a rare condition characterized by thrombocytopenia, microangiopathic haemolytic anaemia, fluctuating neurological symptoms, renal impairment and fever. The neurological symptoms can include headache, bizarre behaviour, transient ischaemic attacks and coma. However, up to 35% of patients have no neurological symptoms at presentation.

There are currently no diagnostic tests available for this condition, but features include characteristic schistocytes (fragments) on the blood film, elevated lactate dehydrogenase levels, reflecting intravascular haemolysis, and normal coagulation tests. The underlying pathogenesis has recently become clearer with the identification of a vWF-cleaving protease (ADAMTS-13), which breaks down the ultralarge vWF multimers known to accumulate. The action of this protease is blocked by an inhibitor in thrombotic thrombocytopenic purpura. It is important to have a high index of suspicion in a patient with thrombocytopenia and any of these symptoms. Management is by plasma exchange. Platelet transfusion is contraindicated because it exacerbates the syndrome.

POST-TRANSFUSION PURPURA

Post-transfusion purpura is an increasingly rare complication of blood transfusion. It results in severe thrombocytopenia, which typically occurs 2 to 14 days after transfusion. This is due to antibodies directed against the human platelet antigen in the recipient, and therefore directed against donor platelets within the transfusion. Post-transfusion purpura can be identified by testing the donor for anti-human platelet antigen antibodies. Treatment is with intravenous immunoglobulin with or without steroids, and appropriate antigen-negative cellular components should be given for any future transfusions. The incidence of post-transfusion purpura has been dramatically reduced by the introduction of leukodepleted blood products. This is thought to be due to a reduction in exposure to sensitizing antigens.

HYPERSPLENISM

Patients with splenomegaly and portal hypertension frequently present with chronic, stable thrombocytopenia owing to sequestration of platelets in the portal circulation. In simple cases, the total circulating platelet mass is within normal limits and bleeding problems are not conspicuous. However, such patients may bleed heavily perioperatively and require platelet transfusions.

Table 33.4 Examples of drugs causing neutropenia

Analgesics and NSAIDs	Indomethacin, phenacetin, paracetamol, phenyl-butazone, aminopyrine
Anticonvulsants	Phenytoin, carbamazepine
Antithyroid drugs	Thiouracil, methimazole
Phenothiazines	Chlorpromazine
Antiarrhythmic	Quinidine

Abbreviation: NSAIDs, nonsteroidal anti-inflammatory drugs.

Neutropenia

Neutropenia in critical care may be due to severe sepsis, malignant infiltration of the marrow or, most commonly, secondary to drugs. Bone marrow biopsy may be necessary in cases of diagnostic difficulty. The severity and duration of neutropenia may be ameliorated by the administration of colony-stimulating factor.

Anaemia

Reduced haemoglobin concentrations in critical care patients are nearly always due to blood loss and consequently fairly obvious. Other causes may be obscure, but the inherited anaemias have usually been diagnosed before admission. Checking the appearance of the blood smear, the mean corpuscular volume and reticulocyte count usually allows diagnosis of the problem. Anaemias may be divided into those due to failure of production and those due to reduced survival in the circulation. There are only two broad groups of causes of the latter: blood loss from the circulation or haemolysis. In both, the reticulocyte count should be raised, and in haemolysis the bilirubin climbs.

Haemolytic anaemias

Haemolysis may be immune or mechanical. In all haemolytic anaemias, the Coomb's test is positive.

In this clinical setting, the commonest is an isoimmune problem (allergic to own species) and thus a problem for the blood transfusion laboratory. Less commonly, the cause is autoimmune – due to connective tissue disorders, lymphoproliferative disorders or, rarely, infections or drugs.

The mechanical causes of haemolysis, in addition to raised reticulocyte count and rising bilirubin, are likely to display red cell abnormalities on the blood film, with red cell fragments seen.

Sickle cell anaemia

The main problems associated with sickle cell disease in critical care situations are vaso-occlusive phenomena and haemolysis. The former can lead to acute painful crises and end-organ failure. Therapy is aimed at preventing crises or treating them. The mainstays of treatment are optimal hydration, oxygenation and exclusion of other problems such as infection. It is recommended that such patients receive aggressive analgesia, folic acid supplementation and thromboprophylaxis.

Red cell transfusion lowers the percentage of haemoglobin S by both simple dilution and suppression of erythropoietin and thus production by the marrow. Reduction of haemoglobin S levels to less than 25% should minimize the short-term risk of new crises.

Haematological malignancy

In very general terms, haematological malignancies, as seen in critical care, may be divided into three broad groups:

1. acute leukaemias, high-grade lymphomas and bone marrow transplant patients;
2. the myeloproliferative disorders; and
3. myelodysplastic disorders and low-grade lymphoproliferative disorders.

Acute leukaemia

The predominant clinical problem with cases of acute leukaemia or high-grade lymphoma (especially after chemotherapy) is that of marrow failure. Red cell and platelet support is required, as well as extreme care with haemostasis. However, by far the major clinical challenge is likely to be profound neutropenia and the risk of overwhelming sepsis. Absolute barrier nursing should be imposed if possible, energetic investigation for potential sites of infection (which may be by atypical organisms and fungi) and very aggressive treatment once an infection is suspected. Filgastrim (colony-stimulating factor) may be useful in stimulating neutrophil production if the neutropenia is due to recent chemotherapy.

Myeloproliferative disorders

The myeloproliferative disorders (chronic granulocytic leukaemia, polycythaemia rubra vera, essential thrombocythaemia and myelofibrosis) constitute a group of diseases in which one or more marrow cell lines proliferate. The clinical presentation is highly variable; the proliferating cells may have normal, increased or decreased function. Thus, for example, a patient with essential thrombocythaemia and a high platelet count may present problems with bleeding if platelet function is impaired, or thrombosis if platelet function is normal or increased. The distinction is usually obvious clinically. This group of disorders generally do not cause problems in critical care, with the exception of postoperative bleeding, which should be treated with platelet transfusions regardless of the platelet count.

Myelodysplastic disorders and low-grade lymphoproliferative disorders

Low-grade lymphoproliferative disorders such as chronic lymphocytic leukaemia and smouldering myeloma and the myelodysplastic syndromes such as chronic myelomonocytic leukaemia and sideroblastic leukaemia are generally considered to be relatively benign by haematologists. They are all common and occur predominantly in the elderly.

Perhaps because they usually present little problem to haematologists, often requiring no treatment at all, they are deemed as 'normal' in the context of surgery. However, they frequently cause serious, usually chronic, and extremely difficult-to-treat problems with haemostasis or sepsis.

It is well known that cardiac surgery produces an altered activation of the inflammatory response, owing to the combination of surgical trauma, cardiopulmonary bypass (CPB) and ischaemia–reperfusion injury. Patients with chronic lymphoproliferative disease may therefore progress to the acute phase of leukaemia as a result of surgery, a complex and poorly understood response by the bone marrow to stress. A dramatic myelomonocytic leukaemoid reaction may be produced, with a clinical picture of systemic inflammatory response to sepsis and multiorgan dysfunction; this may be very difficult to diagnose. The pathways responsible for this response are unknown. Patients with chronic haematological disease may therefore benefit from a strategy aimed at decreasing their exposure to inflammatory stimuli. Off-pump coronary artery bypass surgery avoids the need for CPB, but still causes significant surgical trauma; it may precipitate disease acceleration less commonly.

Key points

- Elevated aPTT may be due to congenital or acquired haematological disease, although prolonged heparin effect is most common.
- Thrombocytopenia owing to excessive platelet destruction or decreased production is common. Drugs used in critical care may also affect platelet function or numbers.
- Cardiothoracic surgery or critical illness can lead to acceleration of haematological malignancy.

FURTHER READING

Crowther M, McDonald E, Johnston M, *et al.* Vitamin K deficiency and D-dimer levels in the intensive care unit: a prospective cohort study. *Blood Coagul Fibrinolysis* 2002;13:49–52.

Geerts W, Selby R. Prevention of venous thromboembolism in the ICU. *Chest* 2003; 124(Suppl):S357–363.

Lee LY, DeBois W, Krieger KH, *et al.* The effects of platelet inhibitors on blood use in cardiac surgery. *Perfusion* 2002;17:33–37.

Raivio P, Suojaranta-Ylinen R, Kuitunen A. Recombinant factor VIIa in the treatment of postoperative hemorrhage after cardiac surgery. *Ann Thorac Surg* 2005;80:66–71.

Chapter 34

Heparin-induced thrombocytopenia

T. STRANG AND A. KOSTER

Introduction

Heparin-induced thrombocytopenia (HIT) is a potentially catastrophic side effect of heparin therapy. Paradoxically, HIT is associated with a high risk of thrombosis despite heparin treatment and a low platelet count.

Pathophysiology

Heparin administration may often trigger an immunogenic reaction, and up to 50% of patients develop heparin-dependent antibodies after cardiac surgery and cardiopulmonary bypass (CPB), usually within 5 to 10 days of exposure.

An immune disorder, HIT is characterized by the binding of immunoglobulin G antibodies to the heparin molecule, building a complex of heparin and platelet factor 4. In a proportion of these patients, this immune complex will bind to the platelet Fc receptor, activate platelets and trigger thrombin generation.

In contrast with many immunological disorders, there is convincing evidence that in HIT the antibodies are transient and typically disappear 40 to 100 days after cessation of heparin therapy. Reintroduction of heparin within that time period reinitiates the reaction instantly, but it is accepted that heparin can be used again after 100 days (if a patient requires heparinization for CPB, for example).

Incidence

The true incidence of HIT in cardiothoracic critical care patients is unknown. It is estimated that it affects about 1% of cardiac surgical patients treated postoperatively with unfractionated bovine heparin. The incidence is lower when low-molecular-weight heparins are used (0.1%). About 50% of patients have suffered a thrombotic event by the time of diagnosis, and 50% of the those remaining progress to a clinically significant thrombotic event.

Diagnosis

The clinical diagnosis of HIT is challenging and requires integration of clinical presumption and laboratory tests.

Clinical presumption

Clinical presumption is based on the rules of the four Ts.

TIMING

Typical onset (60% of cases)

Typically, HIT presents between the 4th and 10th day of heparin treatment. Platelet count falls in most patients in the aftermath of cardiac surgery, but this is usually transient and recovers quickly. A secondary drop in platelet count to below half of the baseline count is highly suggestive of HIT, and any decrease by 50% of the peak platelet count should be considered as HIT until proven otherwise.

Table 34.1 Probability scoring for the clinical diagnosis of heparin-induced thrombocytopenia

	2 points	1 point	0 point
Thrombocytopenia	>50% fall or nadir 20–100	30–50% fall or nadir 10–20	≤30% fall or nadir ≤ 10
Timing	Day 5 to day 10 or rapid if recent exposure	After day 10	Before day 4
Thrombosis	Yes	Possible	No
Other	No	Possible	Likely

6–8 points: high probability
4–5 points: intermediate probability
0–3 points: low probability

Rapid onset (30% of cases)

Heparin-induced thrombocytopenia can happen immediately on heparin exposure or rapidly after initiation of therapy. It is usually associated with re-exposure to heparin within 100 days of a first episode. It can also lead to an anaphylactoid-type reaction, mediated by immunoglobulin E antibodies.

Delayed onset (10% of cases)

The onset of HIT can occur several days after the last dose of heparin.

THROMBOSIS

Any of these can occur as a presentation of HIT:

- Localized venous thrombosis (e.g. deep venous thrombosis, adrenaline infarction).
- Pulmonary embolism.
- Arterial thrombosis (particularly lower limbs in cardiac patients).
- Graft thrombosis, thrombi associated with central venous lines.
- Heparin-induced skin lesions at subcutaneous injection sites (i.e., indurated nodules or necrotizing lesions [20%]).

PLATELET COUNT

The median nadir for thrombocytopenia is above 50×10^9/L and severe thrombocytopenia is not typical.

OTHER CAUSES

Other causes of thrombocytopenia are unlikely. Thrombocytopenia is not uncommon on critical care units. One of the commonest causes is ethylenediamine tetra-acetic acid-induced thrombocytopenia, a laboratory artefact. Therefore, a second analysis of blood using a citrated sample should be performed to rule this out.

Patients with sepsis or those undergoing renal replacement therapy or mechanical heart support (including intra-aortic balloon pumping) often have low platelets in the absence of HIT.

Because of the difficulty in defining the cause of thrombocytopenia, a pretest probability score has been devised. This may be useful in helping the clinician decide to instigate often relatively unfamiliar therapy that may have its own hazards.

Laboratory confirmation of diagnosis

Several types of test are available. Platelet activation assays (using washed platelets) have the highest sensitivity but are technically demanding. Enzyme-linked immunosorbent assays are easier to conduct and are very sensitive, but lack specificity. These tests have a high negative predictive value with negative results allowing discontinuation of alternative anticoagulants.

Positive results are more open to interpretation; the positive predictive value is only moderate. The clinician should therefore discuss the clinical history and pretest probability with an immunologist or specialist haematologist. In the light of these factors, a clinical opinion of the significance of a positive test can be judged.

It must be emphasized that HIT is principally a clinical diagnosis, supported by laboratory findings. Testing in the absence of clinical suspicion is not recommended (and screening is of no value). If the test is performed on a large number of patients, antibodies will be frequently detected without the presence of the syndrome, and this is of no clinical or therapeutic significance.

Delays in obtaining laboratory results confirming the diagnosis of HIT are common. A result typically takes 3 days to produce, depending on the test in use and the clinical expertise of the laboratory. Therefore, consideration must be given before receipt of test results to changing anticoagulation, as below.

Treatment

Once HIT is suspected, it is essential to stop all heparin (including heparin given in line flushes). It is also essential to assess the lower limbs for signs of deep venous thrombosis, and look for signs of thrombosis in other organs (gut, arms, etc.).

An alternative anticoagulant must be started if the pretest probability of HIT is high (>6), unless there are significant contraindications. Of untreated patients, 50% progress to a thrombotic event even after cessation of heparin.

Warfarin must be avoided because it induces an acquired protein C deficiency (even if the International Normalized Ratio is high), leading in turn to thrombosis. Warfarin should only be reinstituted later, when the acute phase of the HIT has passed; until then, anticoagulation should be maintained by other means. Prophylactic platelet transfusion may also contribute to thrombosis and should be avoided – it is worth noting that bleeding is rare in HIT, despite the low platelet count.

Low-molecular-weight heparins may also trigger the formation of HIT antibodies, and are therefore also contraindicated.

Various alternatives to heparin are available, but they may be difficult to administer and monitor. The most popular are danaparoid (a factor Xa inhibitor) and lepirudin (recombinant hirudin – a direct thrombin inhibitor). Neither offers the ideal solution; they may both increase the risk of haemorrhage and dosing can be difficult in renal failure. Both are probably equally effective and selection of drug usually reflects local guidance and availability of suitable monitoring.

Monitoring is not required for routine danaparoid use, unless renal impairment is present or there is a significant risk of haemorrhage (i.e., surgical patient) or thrombosis (i.e., patient on extracorporeal membrane oxygenation). In these cases, factor Xa levels can be measured and these reflect anticoagulation effect satisfactorily.

The activated partial thromboplastin time is used to monitor the effect of lepirudin, unless low levels of prothrombin are present, in which case the Ecarin clotting time must be used. This requires specific handling and calibration, and is best performed in specialized laboratories.

Once the platelet count has recovered, and if continued anticoagulation is required, warfarin can be started; alternative anticoagulation should be continued for at least 3 days, guided by local expertise.

Haemofiltration and haemodialysis

The incidence of HIT in chronic haemodialysis patients mirrors that of surgery. The disease tends

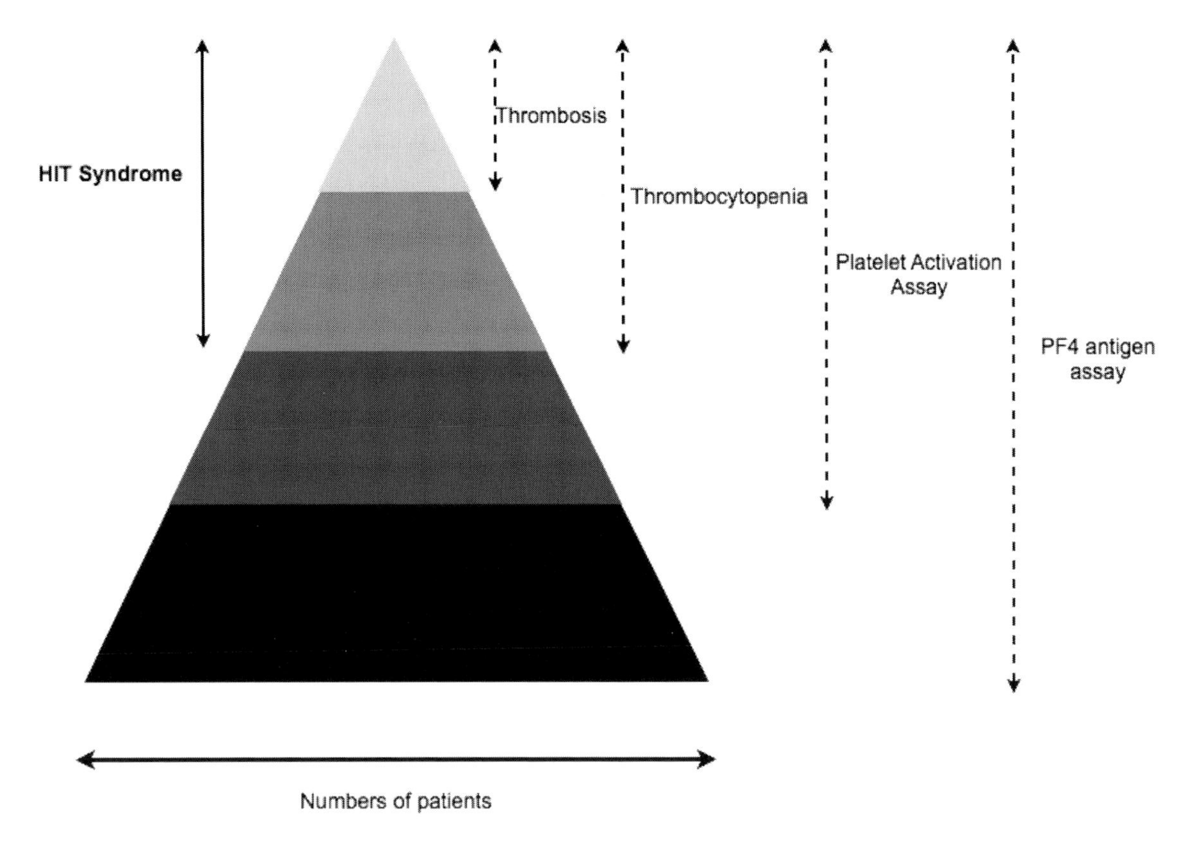

Figure 34.1 The proportion of patients suffering from HIT among those presenting with antibodies. Note that some patients present with a decrease in platelets but do not develop thrombosis.

to present as a fall in platelets or clots in the circuit rather than patient thrombosis, and should be suspected if the filter requires very frequent changing. As above, all administration of heparin must cease while diagnosis is confirmed. The use of low-molecular-weight heparin, aspirin, regional heparinization or filtration without anticoagulant is not recommended. Danaparoid or lepirudin may be administered (both will have a prolonged half-life). Other alternatives include anticoagulation of the circuit with prostacyclin or citrates.

Anticoagulation during cardiac surgery

Anticoagulation during cardiac surgery in patients with a diagnosis of HIT poses a special problem; to date, no alternative anticoagulants have been approved for this indication. The fact that cardiac surgery is usually associated with major surgical trauma and requires high degrees of anticoagulation for CPB, means that certain 'safety features' are necessary for an anticoagulation strategy in this instance, to provide adequate anticoagulation and avoid excessive bleeding. A safe anticoagulation strategy during cardiac surgery should have an immediate effect, a short half-life or be reversible by the use of an antidote. Reliable monitoring by a point-of-care assay should also be available. Therefore, the choice of strategy should be guided by local knowledge and experience; laboratory and specialist support are essential.

Key points

- Heparin-induced thrombocytopenia is an underrecognized complication of heparin administration.
- Heparin-induced thrombocytopenia must be treated promptly because its consequences can be devastating.
- Diagnosis should be clinical, supported by the laboratory tests. These tests taken alone have a very low predictive value.
- Warfarin is contraindicated in the acute phase of HIT.

FURTHER READING

Koster A, Kukucka M. Anticoagulation of patients with heparin-induced thrombocytopenia in cardiac surgery. *Curr Opin Anaesthesiol* 2004;17:71–74.

Warkentin TE, Greinacher A. *Heparin induced thrombocytopenia*. New York: Marcel Dekker; 2003.

Warkentin TE, Greinacher A. Heparin-induced thrombocytopenia: recognition, treatment, and prevention: the Seventh ACCP Conference on Antithrombotic and Thrombolytic Therapy. *Chest* 2004;126(3 Suppl):311S–337S.

3.5 *Gastrointestinal System in Cardiothoracic Critical Care*

Chapter 35

Nutrition

D.V. COLLINS AND T. RYAN

Nutrition in health and critical illness

In health, the hormonal response to nutrition is substrate-controlled. During the fed state, glucose and amino acids stimulate insulin secretion, thereby decreasing glucagon secretion. The net effect is that glycogen reserves and protein synthesis increase, with excess carbohydrate, amino acids and fats converted to lipids. During the fasted state, plasma levels of glucose and amino acids decline, reducing insulin secretion and increasing glucagon secretion, stimulating gluconeogenesis and glycogenolysis.

During critical illness, the nutritional hormones are no longer substrate-controlled. There is an increase in sympathetic tone and catecholamine secretion. In the septic state, in addition to the hormonal stress response, tumour necrosis factor-α and interleukin-1 are produced, causing an increase in glucose intolerance and in skeletal muscle protein catabolism. Glucocorticoids regulate muscle proteolysis and increase the utilization of the resulting amino acids in the liver.

Optimal nutritional support in the critically ill patient can only be achieved when the patient is in the convalescent phase of injury; nutritional supplementation will not reverse the factors causing proteolysis, gluconeogenesis or lipolysis. Appropriate nutritional provision lessens the negative effects of stress and injury associated with critical illness, particularly protein depletion.

In the elective or uncomplicated cardiac surgery context, short periods of fasting of 24 to 48 hours are of no consequence, especially if the patient is assessed to be well nourished before surgery. In the cardiac patient who has a complicated perioperative course, the early, appropriate institution of nutrition is very important.

Nutritional assessment

A patient's nutritional status may be assessed by anthropometry, biochemistry and dietary evaluation.

Anthropometry

Anthropometry is the measurement of size, weight and proportions of the body.

WEIGHT

Weight is a very useful indicator if the patient does not have oedema or ascites. Patients should be weighed and have their height measured on admission. Initial weight should be compared with the patient's normal/usual weight. The per cent weight loss can be calculated (Figure 35.1) and serial measurements taken to record any change.

BODY COMPOSITION

Assessing body composition is useful because estimates of fat and muscle stores are normally distributed. Triceps and subscapular skin-fold thickness allows calculation of fat stores, and mid-arm

$$\text{\% weight loss from normal weight} = \frac{\text{usual weight - actual weight}}{\text{usual weight}} \times 100$$

Figure 35.1 Equation.

muscle circumference measures muscles stores. Ideally, patients should have serial examinations performed to monitor change.

BIOCHEMISTRY

Hydration status, liver function, renal function and anaemia are all relevant in the assessment of a patient's nutritional status. Albumin is a poor correlator, but is indicative of the degree of catabolism.

DIETARY ASSESSMENT

The patient's intake is established by taking a dietary history whenever possible. Actual calorie and protein can be calculated from the dietary history. This can then be compared to estimated nutritional requirements.

Nutritional requirements

Nutritional requirements may be divided into four areas: energy; nitrogen; fluid and electrolyte; and micronutrients.

Table 35.1 Criteria used to assess nutritional risk

Weight
Involuntary weight loss of >10% of usual body weight within 6 months;
Involuntary weight loss of 5% of usual body weight in 1 month;
Weight of 20% over or under ideal body weight.
Triceps skin-fold thickness/mid-arm muscle circumference
Measurements ≤25th percentile are indicative of mild malnutrition
Measurements ≤10th percentile are indicative of moderate malnutrition
Measurements ≤5th percentile are indicative of severe malnutrition

Energy requirements

Energy requirements are expressed in kilocalories and can be estimated as follows:

- Calculate the approximate basal metabolic rate (in kcal/24 hours) using the modified Schofield's equation (weight measured in kilograms).
- Adjust for stress using Elia's nomogram.
- Add a combined factor for activity and diet-induced thermogenesis.
- If an increase in energy stores is required, add 400 to 1000 kcal/day.

Recommendations for energy provision are:

- 20 to 25 kcal/kg body weight (BW) per day during the acute and initial phase of critical illness – energy provision in excess of this may be associated with a less favourable outcome;
- 25 to 30 kcal/kg BW per day during the anabolic recovery phase; and
- up to 25 to 30 kcal/kg BW per day for patients with severe undernutrition.

In clinical practice, most critically ill patients are given 22 to 25 kcal/kg to avoid the metabolic complications of overfeeding. Feeding should be commenced slowly in the severely malnourished.

Nitrogen requirements

Nitrogen requirements are anything from 0.16 to 0.30 g nitrogen/kg in 24 hours (1–2 g protein/kg in 24 hours) depending on the degree of catabolism.

For patients on total parenteral nutrition, the maximum amount of nitrogen that can be administered is 18 to 20 g/24 hours because the liver cannot metabolize more than this.

Fluid and electrolyte requirements

Fluid and electrolyte requirements will be influenced by the patient's clinical condition. Fluid

Table 35.2 Modified Schofield equation

Age (y)	Male	Female
10–17	BMR = 17.7 × weight + 657	BMR = 13.4 × weight + 692
18–29	BMR = 15.1 × weight + 692	BMR = 14.8 × weight + 487
30–59	BMR = 11.5 × weight + 875	BMR = 8.3 × weight + 846
60–74	BMR = 11.9 × weight + 700	BMR = 9.2 × weight + 687
Over 75	BMR = 8.4 × weight + 821	BMR = 9.8 × weight + 624

Abbreviation: BMR, basal metabolic rate.

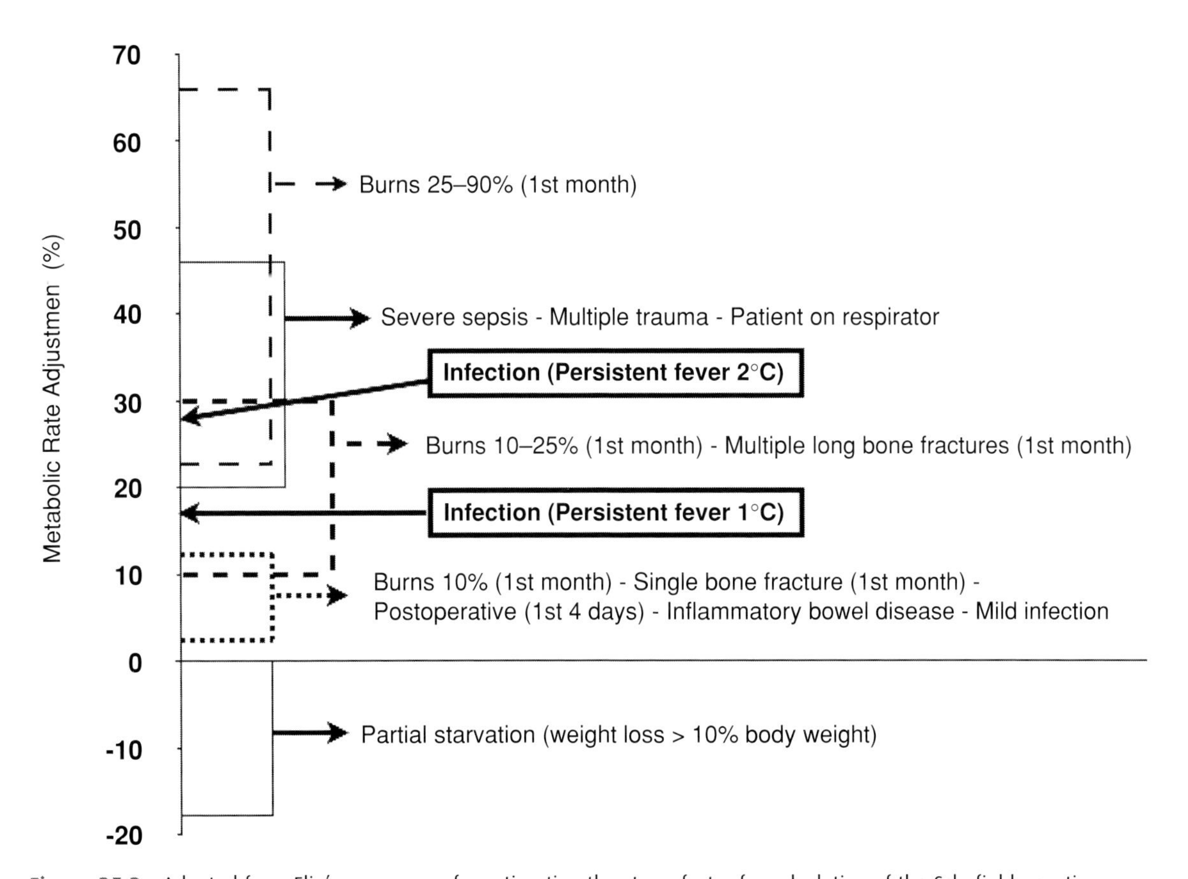

Figure 35.2 Adapted from Elia's nomogram for estimating the stress factor for calculation of the Schofield equation.

Table 35.3 Combined factor to be added

Bed-bound, immobile	+10%
Bed-bound, mobile/sitting	+15%–20%
Mobile on ward	+25%

requirement can be calculated by 30 to 35 mL/kg over 24 hours plus 500 mL/24 hours per degree of pyrexia. Electrolyte requirements need to be balanced against losses.

Micronutrient requirements

Vitamins are dietary compounds that act as cofactors for intermediary metabolism. Vitamin K and the other water-soluble vitamins should be administered routinely, especially in patients receiving parenteral nutrition; deficiency may develop within 4 weeks without intake. The body stores of vitamins A, D and E are usually sufficient for at least 3 months. Thiamine requirements may increase to 250 mg/d, folic acid requirements to 5 mg/d and vitamin C may need to be increased to 500 mg/d.

With the exception of zinc, the body stores of other essential trace elements such as copper, iodine, iron, manganese, cobalt, selenium, chromium, fluoride and molybdenum are usually sufficient for up to 3 months. Zinc at a dose of 2.5 mg/d is required in critically ill patients; when diarrhoea persists, up to five times the daily requirement may need to be administered. If a patient requires feeding via the parenteral route for more than 3 months, trace elements should also be administered.

Impact of hypocaloric feeding

Because critically ill patients are catabolic, and hypermetabolic, the risk of underfeeding is real. In cardiac patients, a negative energy balance (calculated as energy delivery minus target), and hypocaloric feeding is correlated with an increasing number of complications, particularly infections.

Refeeding syndrome

Patients at less than 75% of ideal body weight and who have lost a large amount of weight rapidly are at risk of the refeeding syndrome during the 2 to 3 weeks of restarting feeding.

Malnourished patients can have depleted intracellular phosphate stores. Refeeding and a shift from fat to carbohydrate metabolism leads to hypophosphataemia, resulting in impaired energy stores owing to depletion of intracellular adenosine triphosphate, and tissue hypoxia owing to reduced levels of erythrocyte 2,3 diphosphoglycerate. Hypophosphataemia can therefore cause severe impairment of myocardial contractility.

If a patient is deemed at risk of refeeding syndrome, feeding should start slowly (e.g. 20 kcal/kg) and increase by 100 to 200 kcal/d. Potassium and phosphate levels should be closely monitored.

Table 35.4 Nitrogen requirement according to catabolism

Level of catabolism	Protein requirement (g/kg per day)	Equivalent nitrogen (g/kg per day)
Normometabolic	1	0.16
Intermediate catabolic	1.25–1.5	0.2–0.25
Hypermetabolic	1.5	0.25–0.32

Table 35.5 Adult requirements for electrolytes

Sodium	60–100 mmol/d or 1 mmol/kg
Potassium	50–100 mmol/d or 1 mmol/kg
Calcium	20 mmol/d or 0.2 mmol/kg
Magnesium	12–14 mmol/d or 0.2 mmol/kg
Phosphate	25 mmol/d or 0.3 mmol/kg
Chloride	60–100 mmol/d or 1 mmol/kg

Meeting nutritional requirements

Balanced nutritional support should provide 50% of energy from carbohydrate, 30% from lipid and 20% from protein.

Parenteral nutrition

Total parenteral nutrition requires the use of a compounded solution containing amino acids, glucose, fat, electrolytes, trace elements and vitamins. Protein is given as mixtures of essential and nonessential synthetic L-amino acids. Energy is provided in a ratio of 150 to 250 kcal per gram of protein nitrogen. Energy requirements must be met if amino acids are to be utilized for tissue maintenance and this is usually provided by a mixture of carbohydrate and fat (usually 30%–50% as lipid) to give better utilization of amino acids than glucose alone.

Some centres give parenteral nutrition as an amino acid-dextrose mixture while giving, on a once weekly basis, 500 mL of 20% intralipid to avoid the development of essential fatty acid deficiency.

The sole use of glucose as an energy source may lead to hyperinsulinaemia that prevents the mobilization of endogenous lipid. The physiological maximum for glucose oxidation is estimated to be approximately 4 mg/kg per minute. Exceeding this limit leads to hepatic steatosis, with an increased respiratory quotient, which may pose problems when patients are being weaned from mechanical ventilation. Consequently, there is a limit to the amount of energy that can be safely provided with glucose alone and it is preferable that energy is always given as a combination of glucose and lipid. The

Table 35.6 Estimated daily allowance of micronutrients depending on nutritional route

Trace element	Enteral route (μmol/24 h)	Parenteral route (μmol/24 h)
Chromium	1–2	0.2–0.4
Cobalt	Given as B_{12}	Given as B_{12}
Copper	16–32	8–16
Fluoride	0.05–0.16	0.05–0.08
Iodine	0.6–1.2	0.6–1.2
Iron	180–270	18–45
Manganese	27–94	1.3–2.7
Molybdenum	1–2	0.1–0.2
Selenium	0.5–1.0	0.5–1.0
Zinc	62–184	31–92

simultaneous infusion of fat has other advantages: there is reduced water and electrolyte retention (high energy to fluid volume ratio) and reduced propensity to reactive hypoglycaemia after the infusion has been discontinued. Fat should not be administered at a rate greater than 50 mg/kg per hour (1.2 g fat/kg per day). Phosphate should be added to allow phosphorylation of glucose: between 20 and 30 mmol/L of enteral nutrition is required.

Enteral nutrition

Tube feeding is indicated when oral intake is inadequate and the gastrointestinal tract is otherwise functional. Enteral feeding may be delivered via a large-bore nasogastric tube initially, resorting as soon as possible to a fine-bore feeding tube to reduce the likelihood of sinusitis. Prepared formula feeds provide a mixture of nutrients equivalent to a normal diet. The composition of commonly used enteral feeds is well known and readily available from manufacturers.

If absorption is impaired, an enteral feeding tube may need to be placed duodenally or jejunally. There is no evidence from any studies performed to date that a reduction in residual volume in the stomach reduces the incidence of pulmonary infection, mortality or critical care length of stay. If enteral feeding is required for more than 1 month, a gastrostomy, duodenostomy or jejunostomy may be required.

INSTITUTION OF ENTERAL FEEDING

Canadian and European guidelines recommend early initiation of enteral nutrition (≤48 hours) in all patients. This is especially important in patients with obvious undernutrition at the time of surgery. It is also indicated in patients who have not maintained their oral intake above 60% of the recommended target for 10 days. Enteral feeding should be commenced at a low rate of 10 to 20 mL/h increasing in a stepwise fashion every 12 to 24 hours according to tolerance up to the target rate. Early enteral feeding (≤36 hours) is associated with a significantly lower incidence of infections and a reduced length of hospital stay, but does not affect mortality or noninfectious complications. High-dose dopamine and noradrenaline are correlated with poor tolerance of enteral feeding.

Undernutrition after transplantation is a major factor influencing outcome, and it is important to initiate normal diet or enteral nutrition as early as possible after heart or lung transplantation.

Table 35.7 Various options by which enteral feeding may be administered

Route	Placement method
Nasogastric	Via nasopharynx
Nasoduodenal/nasojejunal	Manually by tube rotation method Endoscopically with snare/guide wire method Fluoroscopically At laparotomy
Percutaneous endoscopic gastrotomy	Endoscopically
Percutaneous gastrotomy	Radiologically
Percutaneous jejunostomy	Radiologically
Jejunostomy	Surgical placement

GASTRIC VERSUS JEJUNAL FEEDING

The European guidelines suggest that jejunal feeding should only be attempted if intolerance to gastric feeding persists. There is some evidence that earlier initiation of nasojejunal feeding in patients at high risk of gastric intolerance (inotropic support, high doses of sedatives, high nasogastric drainage) is beneficial, especially in patients at increased risk of regurgitation and aspiration (e.g. nursed in the supine position). However, there is no evidence that nasojejunal feeding reduces the incidence of pneumonia, length of stay or mortality.

MOTILITY AGENTS

As a class, motility agents have a beneficial effect on gastrointestinal motility, but their routine use is not recommended. There are no studies demonstrating a beneficial effect of prokinetics on outcome. Administration of metoclopramide increases gastrointestinal transit and feed tolerance; a single dose of erythromycin may facilitate small bowel feeding tube placement. Both drugs should be considered as a strategy to optimize nutritional intake in instances of gastrointestinal intolerance.

Enteral versus parenteral nutrition

Systemic analysis examining randomized controlled trials comparing enteral with parenteral nutrition in critically ill patients concluded that enteral feeding resulted in a significant decrease in the incidence of infectious complications in the critically ill and may be less costly. But there is no proven impact on mortality, length of critical care stay or number of ventilator days when compared with parenteral nutrition. Current guidelines strongly recommend enteral over parenteral feeding in patients with a functional gastrointestinal tract.

Parenteral nutrition should be given to those patients who cannot reach their nutritional targets with enteral nutrition alone (≤60% of caloric requirement) or when enteral nutrition is contraindicated or not tolerated.

Insulin therapy

A landmark study of 1,548 patients, published in 2001 by Van den Berghe and colleagues, compared intensive insulin therapy with a conventional therapy regime in critically ill surgical patients. The critical care case mix was predominantly elective cardiovascular surgery. The target glucose range was 4.4 to 6.1 mmol/L in the intensive insulin therapy group, versus 10 to 11.1 mmol/L in the conventional group. Intensive insulin therapy was associated with reduced critical care and hospital mortality and significant reductions in prolonged ventilatory support and renal replacement therapy. Interestingly in this study, the early provision of nutrition after admission was a feature with intravenous glucose being administered at a dose of 200 to 300 g per 24 hours for the first day. Total enteral nutrition was then attempted as early as possible.

Table 35.8 Contraindications to enteral feeding

Contraindications
Intestinal obstructions or ileus
Severe shock
Intestinal ischaemia
High output enterocutaneous fistula (>500 mL/d)
Significant radiation enteritis
Significant chemotherapeutic mucositis
Severe inflammatory bowel disease
Colovaginal fistula
Short bowel syndrome (≤200 cm viable small intestine)
Severe intra-abdominal sepsis

Antioxidants, trace elements and vitamins

Oxygen-derived free radicals or reactive oxygen species play an important role in the development of organ dysfunction in critically ill patients. Reactive oxygen species cause cellular damage and death by attacking cellular proteins, polysaccharides, nucleic acids and polyunsaturated fatty acids. Antioxidants counter the effects of reactive oxygen species by a process of reduction or by delaying or inhibiting the oxidation of molecules.

In critical illness, there are reduced stores of antioxidants, reduced plasma or intracellular concentrations of free electron scavengers or cofactors, and decreased activity of enzymatic systems involved in the detoxification of reactive oxygen species. Supplementation with vitamins and trace elements (selenium or zinc) has been shown to improve antioxidant capacity in critically ill patients. There is, however, insufficient evidence routinely to recommend administration of selenium or others above the recommended daily allowance. Further studies are required before definitive recommendations can be made.

Key points

- Enteral nutrition is recommended over parenteral nutrition in critically ill patients with an intact gastrointestinal tract.
- There is no significant difference in efficacy in feeding jejunally versus the gastric route.
- A trial of a prokinetic agent is recommended for patients who do not tolerate sufficient enteral feeding.
- If target values cannot be met by enteral feeding alone, supplementation with parenteral nutrition should be considered.
- If enteral feeding is not tolerated, total parenteral nutrition should be given to meet the nutritional targets of the patient.
- In critically ill surgical patients receiving nutritional support, intensive insulin therapy to maintain blood glucose levels between 4.4 and 6.1 mmol/L should be considered.

FURTHER READING

Heyland DK, Dhaliwal R, Drover JW, *et al.* Canadian clinical practice guidelines for nutrition support in mechanically ventilated, critically ill adult patients. *J Parenter Enteral Nutr* 2003;27:355–373.

Kreymann KG, Berger MM, Deutz NEP, *et al.* ESPEN guidelines on enteral nutrition: intensive care. *Clin Nutr* 2006;25:210–223.

Van den Berghe G, Wouters P, Weekers F, *et al.* Intensive insulin therapy in the critically ill patients. *N Engl J Med* 2001;345:359–366.

Chapter 36

Gastrointestinal catastrophe

E. CAMERON AND P.J. ROBERTS

Introduction

A range of different gastrointestinal (GI) complications can occur following cardiac surgery. Gastrointestinal haemorrhage is the most common, but mesenteric ischaemia has the highest mortality. Gastrointestinal complications occur in between 0.5% and 5.5% of patients and are associated with a significant excess mortality. Off-pump coronary artery bypass surgery does not appear to protect against such complications.

Gastrointestinal haemorrhage

Upper gastrointestinal haemorrhage

Clinically significant upper GI haemorrhage occurs in up to 4% of patients after cardiac surgery and has a high mortality.

Patients commonly present with haematemesis, melaena or drop in haemoglobin, but unexplained hypotension may occur before blood loss becomes apparent. Some of these patients are on antiplatelet drugs or anticoagulants and approximately 20% to 30% of cases require surgical treatment. Stress ulcer prophylaxis is controversial and under investigation currently. Endoscopy of the upper GI tract is mandatory once resuscitation has been performed. It aids diagnosis, allows endoscopic therapy and appears to be safe. However, the high rate of surgical intervention suggests that therapeutic endoscopy is less effective or bleeding more severe than in other patient groups.

Patients with liver disease tend to have a worse prognosis which is directly related to the degree of liver dysfunction or failure. Evidence of *Helicobacter pylori* infection should be sought, but it is important to remember that acid suppression reduces the sensitivity of biopsy-based tests and breath tests.

ENDOSCOPIC THERAPY

Endoscopic therapy is indicated when active ulcer bleeding, fresh adherent clot or visible vessels are observed. Options include adrenaline injection, use of a heater probe, electrocoagulation and clips; combination treatment appears to be most effective. After such treatment, high-dose intravenous proton pump inhibitors may reduce the risk of rebleeding and surgical intervention (80 mg omeprazole IV bolus followed by infusion at 8 mg/h for 72 hours).

SURGICAL INTERVENTION

Surgery is more commonly required for rebleeding if a duodenal ulcer is situated posteriorly (may erode through the gastroduodenal artery) or a gastric ulcer is situated high on the lesser curve of the stomach (may erode a branch of the left gastric artery).

Oral proton pump inhibitors should be continued for at least 3 months in peptic ulcer disease. In patients with gastric ulceration, the possibility of neoplastic disease should be considered and these patients should undergo follow-up endoscopy to ensure ulcer healing and allow biopsy. Decisions

Table 36.1 Predisposing conditions for gastrointestinal complications
Valve surgery (in part due to use of anticoagulation)
Preoperative renal failure
Poor left ventricular ejection fraction
Age >80 years
Prolonged mechanical ventilation (with effects on splanchnic vasoconstriction)
Hypoperfusion (including prolonged aortic cross clamp time)
Intra-aortic balloon pump

on whether to continue, stop in the short term or reverse anticoagulation need to be individualized, but must balance the risk of thrombosis against the high mortality from bleeding in this patient group. Aspirin, clopidogrel and nonsteroidal anti-inflammatory drugs should be stopped whenever possible.

Lower gastrointestinal tract haemorrhage

Bleeding from the lower GI tract most commonly presents with large amounts of fresh or altered blood per rectum. As with upper GI haemorrhage, this is probably exacerbated by anticoagulation and antiplatelet treatments. Common causes include

- diverticular disease;
- angiodysplasia;
- colitis, which may be ischaemic, infective or indeed idiopathic (ulcerative colitis and Crohn's disease);
- colonic polyps and cancer; and
- anorectal lesions.

It is often difficult from the history alone to determine the cause of the bleeding, although sudden onset with associated pain is more suggestive of

Table 36.2 Causes of upper gastrointestinal haemorrhage
Peptic ulceration
Oesophagitis
Erosions (gastric or duodenal)
Varices
Mallory-Weiss tear
Upper gastrointestinal tract neoplasm
Vascular lesions (angiodysplasia)
Aortoenteric fistulae (previous aortic graft surgery)

Table 36.3 Endoscopic findings and risk of rebleeding

Finding	Risk (%)
Clean ulcer base	3
Oozing ulcer	10
Adherent clot	30
Visible vessel	50
Actively bleeding vessel	90

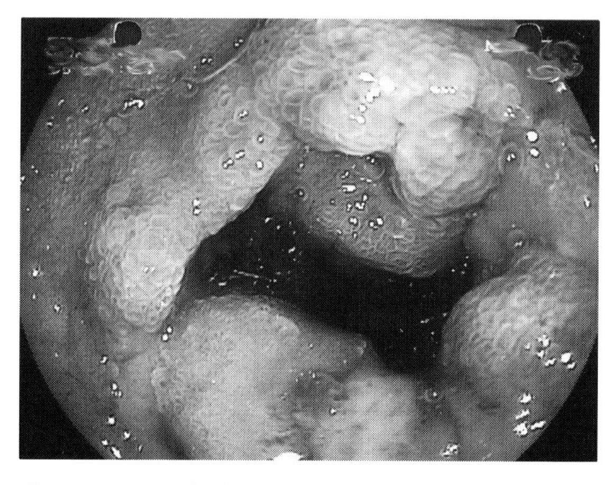

Figure 36.1 Multiple ulcers in the first part of the duodenum with marked oedema. This patient presented 6 days after bypass surgery with haematemesis and melaena. The patient settled with cessation of antiplatelet drugs and the use of omeprazole orally.

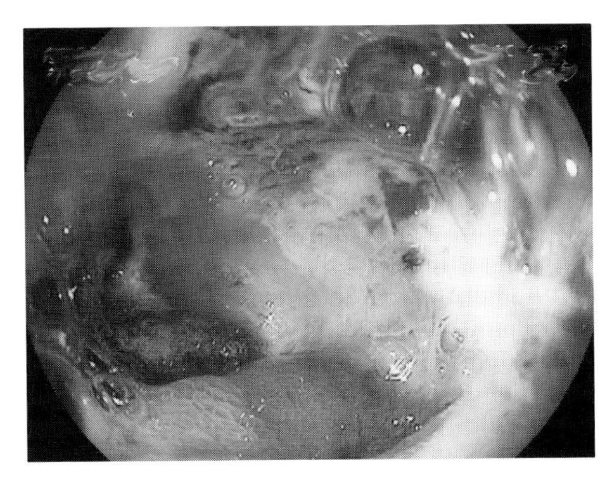

Figure 36.2 Large posterior duodenal ulcer in a patient after valve surgery and treated with anticoagulants. Although no definite visible vessel is seen, there is fresh blood and he had adrenaline injection into the ulcer and high-dose omeprazole infusion. He, however, bled again, was taken to theatre and did well after surgery to the ulcer.

ischaemic colitis. Occasionally there may be prior symptoms to suggest underlying colonic disease such as diarrhoea, mucus and bleeding per rectum. *Clostridium difficile* is increasingly common,

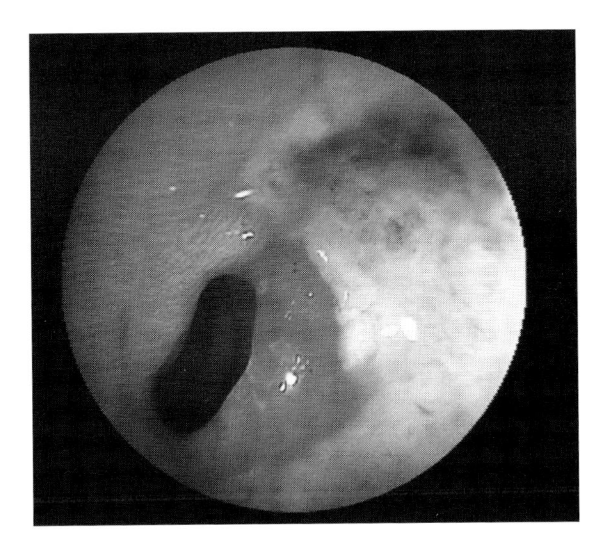

Figure 36.3 Prepyloric ulcer in post-bypass patient who had also been on diclofenac (a nonsteroidal anti-inflammatory) and presented with melaena. The patient settled with conservative treatment and cessation of offending drugs.

and the associated diarrhoea can lead to severe pseudomembranous colitis. Risk factors include multiple broad-spectrum antibiotic usage, readmission to hospital and age greater than 80 years.

Attempts should be made to localize the source of the bleeding; flexible sigmoidoscopy is safe in this group of patients, but colonoscopy may be required. Luminal blood is the main endoscopic finding, but colitis, pseudomembranous colitis, bleeding diverticulae and ischaemic changes may be identified, which may alter treatment.

In severe bleeding, an upper GI source should be sought initially and then lower GI tract evaluation carried out. Mesenteric angiography and surgical intervention are other treatment options if endoscopic and medical treatments fail.

Mesenteric ischaemia

Although less common than haemorrhage (0.1%–0.5%), mesenteric ischaemia has a particularly high mortality rate (67%–85%). After cardiac surgery, most cases are related to nonocclusive mesenteric ischaemia, although this patient group also tends to have risk factors for mesenteric arterial thrombosis and embolism. Nonocclusive ischaemia tends to be caused by low-flow states exacerbated by the use of vasoconstrictors. Risk factors include prolonged cardiopulmonary bypass, use of an intra-aortic balloon pump, emergency surgery and advanced age.

Diagnosis can be challenging in the critical care setting owing to the diversity of presentation and the compounding effects of analgesia and sedation. Symptoms include constipation, nausea or vomiting, diarrhoea (possibly bloody), melaena and most commonly abdominal pain. Abdominal signs may be subtle but peritonitis is more apparent if frank gangrenous bowel has developed. Investigations commonly undertaken include:

- blood tests: for rising markers of inflammation (C reactive protein, white cell count);
- arterial blood gases for metabolic acidosis, often with a raised lactate;

- abdominal radiographs/ultrasound scan, which are often normal, and may exclude other causes;
- computed tomography, which may demonstrate occlusive mesenteric ischaemia, bowel wall thickening or pneumatosis (air in the bowel wall);
- angiography, which may demonstrate obstructive causes; and
- endoscopy, which may be performed if melaena or falling haemoglobin are present and may occasionally demonstrate ischaemic mucosa with almost confluent ulceration of the first and second parts of the duodenum.

Laparotomy may be the only method to provide a true and accurate diagnosis, and should not be delayed if signs and symptoms are highly suggestive, particularly in the setting of a rapidly worsening metabolic acidosis with no other explanation. Surgery may include bowel resection and reanastomosis or stoma formation, but in extensive cases may be futile. It is not unusual to discover that most if not all of the bowel is dead or not viable on opening the abdomen, and open-and-shut surgery is then the best option. Experience may allow avoidance of surgery if prognosis is terrible. Palliative care should then be instituted promptly.

Hepatobiliary complications

Acalculous cholecystitis may occur in 0.1% to 0.2% of patients and is probably caused by a combination of factors including increased viscosity of bile, reduced cholecystokinin-induced gallbladder contraction (as a result of lack of enteral nutrition) and gallbladder ischaemia. Mortality is much higher than in calculous cholecystitis. Diagnosis is based on clinical suspicion and the findings on imaging (ultrasound or computed tomography). Broad-spectrum antibiotics are required and either cholecystectomy or cholecystotomy (if not fit for surgery) may be necessary if medical treatment is unsuccessful.

Pancreatitis occurs in 0.02% to 0.40% of critical care patients, and is often secondary to reduced tissue perfusion, but gallstone pancreatitis must be excluded. If severe gallstone disease or cholangitis is diagnosed, early endoscopic bile duct sphincterotomy should be considered.

Ischaemic hepatitis may occur in up to 3.3% of patients and is usually due to decreased hepatic perfusion, contributed to by hepatic congestion. Typically patients develop jaundice with a large rise in transaminases and a coagulopathy; this often resolves rapidly with an improvement in hepatic perfusion. It is clearly important to exclude other causes of hepatic dysfunction, such as drug-related and viral. Patients with preexisting chronic liver disease are at significant risk of decompensation, and a high rate of complications is seen in this group after cardiac surgery, including sepsis, renal failure, variceal haemorrhage and death.

Pseudo-obstruction

Postoperative ileus is a relatively common occurrence in critical care and the diagnosis of acute colonic pseudo-obstruction may be made.

Definition

Acute colonic pseudo-obstruction is defined as the presence of massive colonic dilatation in the

Table 36.4 Predisposing factors associated with acute colonic pseudo-obstruction
Age
Sepsis
Electrolyte imbalance (hypokalaemia, hypocalcaemia, hypomagnesaemia)
Drugs (particularly opiates, tricyclic antidepressants, anti-parkinsonian drugs)
Renal failure
Untreated hypothyroidism

absence of mechanical obstruction. Ischaemia and perforation are severe and life-threatening complications of this condition, which become more likely if the caecal diameter is measured as greater than 10 to 12 cm on plain abdominal radiographs and when distension lasts longer than 5 days.

Management

Mechanical obstruction must be excluded. Water-soluble contrast enema should be considered to exclude distal colonic obstruction, even when computed tomography of the abdomen appears normal; the enema itself may help to relieve the acute colonic pseudo-obstruction. Initial conservative management includes stopping oral feeding, intravenous fluids, nasogastric suction and, if possible, frequent position changes in bed. Predisposing factors should be sought and corrected. Sepsis should be considered, including intra-abdominal sepsis, and treated accordingly. Regular abdominal radiographs (every 12 hours) should be performed to monitor the caecal diameter. A trial of conservative treatment is appropriate in patients with little abdominal pain, who do not have features suggestive of peritonitis or ischaemia. A period of up to 48 hours of conservative management appears to be safe before endoscopic or surgical intervention.

Pharmacological therapy

There are anecdotal reports of success with prokinetics such as erythromycin and metoclopramide. Neostigmine, an anticholinesterase parasympathomimetic agent, should be considered, but may cause tachycardia and is therefore often contraindicated in cardiac critical care.

Endoscopic treatment

Colonoscopic decompression of the colon is preferred over radiological attempts. However, perforation has been described in up to 3% of patients when using colonoscopy.

Surgical intervention

Caecostomy and colectomy carry a significant risk and should be reserved for those patients who have either failed colonoscopic treatment or demonstrate signs of ischaemia, peritonitis or perforation.

Key points

- Acute upper and lower GI haemorrhage are relatively common conditions with an appreciable morbidity and mortality; it may necessitate stopping antiplatelet/anticoagulant medication.
- Early diagnostic and therapeutic upper GI endoscopy is required in significant haemorrhage and negative findings should prompt lower GI endoscopy.
- Mesenteric ischaemia should always be considered if metabolic acidosis is unexplained, even in the absence of abdominal signs and symptoms.
- Laparotomy carries significant added risk but should not be delayed if haemorrhage persists or acidosis worsens. It may also be required to decompress a grossly distended caecum.

FURTHER READING

Andersson B, Nilsson J, Brandt J, *et al.* Gastrointestinal complications after cardiac surgery. *Br J Surg* 2005;92:326–333.

Bolcal C, Iyem H, Sargin M, *et al.* Gastrointestinal complications after cardiopulmonary bypass: sixteen years of experience. *Can J Gastroenterol* 2005;19:613–617

Geller A, Petersen BT, Gostout CJ. Endoscopic decompression for acute colonic pseudo-obstruction. *Gastrointest Endosc* 1996;44: 44–150.

Rockall TA, Logan RF, Devlin HB, *et al.* Risk assessment after acute upper gastrointestinal haemorrhage. *Gut* 1996;38:316–321.

Chapter 37

Liver failure

A. ROSCOE AND J.M. WILLIAMS

Introduction

After cardiothoracic surgery, a mild elevation in the serum concentration of liver enzymes is not uncommon. It is usually transient with little or no clinical sequelae. In contrast, acute hepatic failure is a rare but serious complication. It is associated with multiorgan dysfunction syndrome and carries a poor prognosis.

Functions of the liver

The liver is the largest solid organ in the body. It receives oxygenated blood via the hepatic artery and nutrient-rich blood from the portal vein. The liver performs a variety of important functions.

Carbohydrates in the diet are converted to hexoses and transported to the liver via the portal veins. Glucose enters hepatocytes passively, where it is converted to glycogen. Maintenance of blood glucose concentrations within narrow limits is regulated by insulin and glucagon. Amino acids removed from the blood are utilized for protein synthesis and gluconeogenesis. Approximately 10 to 20 g of albumin is synthesized per day, depending on nutritional status and endocrine balance. The degradation of amino acids leads to nitrogenous waste, in the form of ammonia, which is then converted to urea.

The vitamin K-dependent clotting factors (II, VII, IX and X) are formed in the liver. Other important synthesized proteins include α- and β-globulins, fibrinogen, antithrombin III, α_1 acid glycoprotein, haptoglobin and C-reactive protein.

Short-chain fatty acids undergo oxidation in the liver, with the production of ketones and acetoacetate. Kupffer cells lining the hepatic sinusoids phagocytose infective and inflammatory mediators, which are then degraded by lysosomal enzymes.

One of the principal roles of the liver is xenobiotic metabolism. Lipophilic substances are made more hydrophilic by phase I reactions (oxidation, reduction and hydrolysis). Phase II biotransformations (glucuronidation, sulphation, acetylation) usually inactivate substances by conjugation. These processes allow elimination via bile and urine.

The liver acts as a reservoir of blood, containing 400 to 500 mL. During hypovolaemia, half of this may be mobilized to increase effective circulatory volume.

Definition of liver failure

Acute hepatic failure

Acute hepatic failure is a potentially reversible and progressive liver dysfunction in the absence of preexisting liver disease. It can be temporally classified into hyperacute (encephalopathy within 10 days of symptoms) and fulminant (10–30 days).

Subacute hepatic failure

Subacute hepatic failure is progressive liver dysfunction, in the absence of preexisting liver disease,

Table 37.1 Functions of the liver

1. Carbohydrate metabolism
2. Protein metabolism
3. Synthesis of coagulation factors
4. Urea production
5. Lipid metabolism
6. Bile synthesis
7. Hormone metabolism
8. Defence against infection
9. Drug metabolism
10. Blood reservoir
11. Storage of vitamins and minerals
12. Heat production

characterized by the occurrence of ascites and/or encephalopathy.

'Acute-on-chronic' hepatic failure

This is the development of liver failure in the presence of preexisting liver disease. This classification has important prognostic implications.

Table 37.2 Causes of postoperative jaundice

Bilirubin overload
Congenital
Secondary to drug administration
Prosthetic valves and extracorporeal circulation
Sepsis
Resorption of haematoma
Haemolysis of transfused blood
Hepatocellular dysfunction
Hepatitis-like pattern
Anaesthesia-induced hepatitis
Secondary to drug administration
Ischaemia-induced hepatitis
Viral hepatitis
Preexisting chronic liver disease
Cholestatic pattern
Benign postoperative intrahepatic cholestasis
Secondary to drug administration
Sepsis
Ischaemia-induced cholestasis
Gilbert's syndrome
Extrahepatic biliary obstruction
Gallstone obstruction
Postoperative cholecystitis or pancreatitis

From Salmeron and Rodes.

Causes of liver failure

It is important to distinguish between postoperative jaundice and acute liver failure. Jaundice after cardiac surgery and cardiopulmonary bypass is not uncommon and is often of no clinical significance. It may be characterized as a benign postoperative cholestatic jaundice, often in a patient who has been bleeding, received a blood transfusion or suffered a period of hypotension. It is not associated with signs of hepatocellular failure. Clinical examination and investigations are essentially normal other than the presence of jaundice and a mixed hyperbilirubinaemia and elevated alkaline phosphatase. The condition resolves spontaneously.

In contrast, acute liver failure after cardiac surgery is rare and is often related to multiple organ failure and sepsis. It is associated with an extremely poor prognosis. It is characterized by a marked rise in serum transaminases, often only moderate elevation in bilirubin levels and the systemic effects associated with acute liver failure. The stigmata of chronic liver disease are absent.

The commonest cause by far in the United Kingdom is paracetamol overdose. However, after cardiac surgery, the development of acute liver failure is most likely to be as part of a pattern of multiple

Table 37.3 Causes of acute liver failure

Infective
Hepatitis A, B, C
Hepatitis non-A, -B, -C, -D, -E
Yellow fever
Leptospirosis
Sepsis
Drug-induced
Paracetamol
Halothane
Nonsteroidal anti-inflammatory drugs
Rifampicin
Isoniazid
Ecstasy
Sodium valproate
Monoamine oxidase inhibitors
Toxins
Alcohol
Mushroom poisoning (*Amanita phalloides*)
Phosphorus
Carbon tetrachloride
Ischaemic
Hepatic vein occlusion
Shock
Cardiac surgery
Ischaemic hepatitis
Metabolic
Wilson's disease
Reye's syndrome
Fatty liver of pregnancy
Galactosaemia

organ failure secondary to sepsis or as the result of an ischaemic injury resulting in organ hypoperfusion and hypoxia. In severe sepsis and septic shock the presence of hypotension, hypoxaemia, arteriovenous shunting, microcirculatory dysfunction, impaired ability of the cell to utilize oxygen as well as the direct cellular effects mediated by the inflammatory response all contribute to hepatocellular injury. The resultant organ damage further contributes to systemic circulatory dysfunction, which in turn leads to worsening hepatic injury.

In the cardiac surgical population, acute liver failure may occasionally result from an ischaemic injury (e.g. cardiogenic shock or biventricular failure). Perioperative factors that may contribute to a reduction in hepatocellular oxygenation as a result of decreased hepatic blood flow or increased splanchnic vascular resistance, include hypotension, shock, haemorrhage, hypoxaemia, vasopressor drugs and positive-pressure ventilation. Ischaemic hepatic injury is characterized by centrilobular necrosis, the severity of which is related to the degree of cellular hypoperfusion and hypoxia. Massive centrilobular necrosis leads to acute liver failure and has a poor prognosis. Cardiopulmonary bypass, and the associated inflammatory response, is not by itself implicated in the development of acute liver failure.

System involvement

The liver plays a central role in homeostasis. As a consequence of the liver's role in many synthetic, metabolic and excretory processes, acute severe hepatic dysfunction results in profound pathophysiological derangements throughout the body's organ systems.

Central nervous system

Hepatic encephalopathy invariably develops in patients with acute liver failure. It is characterized by behavioural and personality changes, altered levels of consciousness and ultimately coma. The pathogenesis of hepatic encephalopathy is complex and poorly understood, but many factors have been implicated. Portosystemic shunting and the inability of the liver to detoxify circulating metabolites leads to an increase in plasma levels of neurotoxic substances, including ammonia, mercaptans, fatty acids and amines. This may be combined with altered blood–brain barrier function, altered cerebral metabolism and levels of neurotransmitters. The development of cerebral oedema may also reduce cerebral perfusion pressure leading to

Table 37.4 Systemic effects of acute liver failure

System	Effects
Central nervous system	Hepatic encephalopathy
	Cerebral oedema
	Respiratory alkalosis
Cardiovascular system	Reduced systemic vascular resistance
	Increased cardiac output
	Portosystemic and arteriovenous shunting
	Increased intravascular volume
Respiratory system	Pleural effusions
	Pulmonary oedema
	Atelectasis, ventilation/perfusion mismatch shunting
Renal system	Hepatorenal syndrome
	Acute renal failure
Immune system	Impaired humoral and cell-mediated immunity
	Increased susceptibility to bacterial, fungal and viral infections
Coagulation system	Impaired clotting factor production
	Platelet dysfunction
	Disseminated intravascular coagulation
Metabolic effects	Impaired protein synthesis and hypoalbuminaemia
	Hypoglycaemia
Hypokalaemia, hyponatraemia, hypomagnesaemia, hypophosphataemia	
Metabolic acidosis and impaired lactate metabolism	Altered drug handling
	Hepatoadrenal syndrome

cellular ischaemia. Cerebral oedema occurs in 40% to 70% of patients with grade III or IV encephalopathy. It is the single greatest cause of death in acute liver failure. It presents clinically with tachycardia, tachypnoea, abnormal pupillary reflexes, muscle rigidity and decerebrate posturing. Papilloedema is an uncommon finding.

Cardiovascular system

Cardiovascular effects include a fall in systemic vascular resistance, increased circulating volume, sodium and fluid retention and an increased cardiac output (CO). However, in patients with pre-existing cardiac disease or severe sepsis, myocardial impairment may result in a significantly reduced CO and subsequent tissue hypoperfusion. Portosystemic and arteriovenous shunting may be extensive. There may also be impaired responsiveness to vasoactive drugs.

Respiratory system

Respiratory function may be compromised by several mechanisms.

- Critical-illness-related muscle dysfunction affects spontaneous ventilation.
- Airway control may be compromised by the onset of cerebral oedema and reduced level of consciousness.
- Respiratory alkalosis is typical in hepatic encephalopathy with hyperventilation in the nonventilated patient.
- Ventilation/perfusion mismatching (hepatopulmonary syndrome), shunting, atelectasis and increased susceptibility to infection occur frequently.
- Pleural effusions, alveolar capillary endothelial dysfunction and pulmonary oedema occur as do reductions in tidal volume, functional residual capacity and vital capacity.
- Long-standing portal hypertension can give rise to pulmonary hypertension (portopulmonary hypertension).

Renal system

Renal dysfunction may occur as a direct result of acute liver failure or, more commonly, as a result of the underlying cause of the acute liver failure. Causes include sepsis, hypotension and hypoperfusion, haemorrhage and massive transfusion. The renal injury is commonly acute tubular necrosis. Acute renal failure causes volume overload, metabolic acidosis and hyperkalaemia, and exacerbates existing metabolic derangement caused by acute liver failure.

Hepatorenal syndrome is a progressive increase in plasma creatinine, oliguria and low urinary sodium concentrations with normal renal histology. It often resolves if the underlying liver dysfunction recovers. With normally functioning kidneys, acute liver failure results in sodium and water retention, which may contribute to the development of ascites, peripheral oedema and pleural effusions. Hypokalaemia may result from diuretic use, renal tubular defects, diarrhoea and vomiting, alkalosis and secondary hyperaldosteronism. The development of hyper- or hyponatraemia depends on the relative amounts of water and sodium retained.

Coagulation system

Coagulopathy is commonly seen in acute liver failure. Significant reduction in the production of clotting factors, all of which are produced in the liver, other than factor VIII, with an elevated prothrombin time and International Normalized Ratio, reduced platelet counts with platelet dysfunction and low-grade disseminated intravascular coagulation lead to an increased tendency to bleed, although major haemorrhage is uncommon.

Immune system

Immune function is compromised in acute liver failure with the result that bacterial and fungal infections are common. Up to 90% of patients have systemic bacterial infection, with 30% acquiring a systemic fungal infection. Translocation of organisms from the gut, impaired neutrophil and Kupffer cell function and the presence of multiple invasive lines make these patients highly susceptible to infection.

Metabolism

Metabolic derangement is a key feature of acute liver failure. Hypoglycaemia is common and results from impaired hepatic gluconeogenesis, glycogenolysis and increased levels of circulating insulin. Electrolyte abnormalities include hyponatraemia, hypokalaemia, hypomagnesaemia and hypophosphataemia. Reduced production of protein, especially albumin, contributes to the development of ascites, peripheral oedema and increased capillary leak. The ability to bind to and carry drugs is impaired. Alkalosis is the commonest acid–base disturbance in primary acute liver failure, but in the presence of hypotension and tissue hypoperfusion, metabolic acidosis is more common and indicates a poor prognosis. Hyperlactataemia may result from anaerobic metabolism in hypoxic tissue, as a result of the liver's inability to metabolize lactate or a combination of both. In severe hepatic hypoperfusion, the liver may produce lactate secondary to anaerobic glycolysis.

Reduced hepatic blood flow, altered enzyme function, reduced plasma protein concentrations, increased circulating levels of endogenous compounds, acid–base disturbance and renal dysfunction all contribute to abnormal drug metabolism and excretion.

Hepatoadrenal syndrome is not uncommon in the liver failure patient and may be related to sepsis and multiorgan dysfunction.

Management

Treatment of postoperative acute liver failure involves appropriate monitoring, supportive care, potential artificial liver support and possible transplantation.

In addition to routine postoperative critical care monitoring, a pulmonary artery catheter, or other means of measuring CO, is recommended. Patients may benefit from intracranial pressure (ICP) monitoring to allow early detection of intracranial hypertension. A jugular bulb catheter may be inserted to assess cerebral oxygenation.

Encephalopathy grades III and IV are associated with an increased risk of cerebral oedema. Initial

Table 37.5 Basic management strategies for acute hepatic failure

Correct aggravating factors of encephalopathy
Maintain cerebral perfusion pressure
Control serum glucose levels
Avoid hypoxaemia, hypercapnea and high levels of positive end-expiratory pressure
Use fluid resuscitation, inotropes and vasopressors to support cardiovascular system
Institute renal replacement therapy (continuous venovenous haemofiltration)
Give antimicrobial therapy
Prescribe prophylaxis for gastrointestinal bleeding

relief of aggravating factors is important. This includes the correction of electrolyte imbalances, diagnosis and treatment of gastrointestinal haemorrhage, appropriate antimicrobial therapy for infection, and control of serum glucose levels. Intracranial pressure monitoring is recommended if the facilities and expertise are available, but the placement of such a monitoring device is not without risk in a coagulopathic patient. A 30-degree head up tilt is employed to aid venous drainage from the head. Boluses of mannitol are given if the serum osmolality is less than 320 mosm/L or with rises in ICP. Ventilation parameters are set to correct any hypoxaemia and achieve normocapnea. High levels of positive-end expiratory pressure should be avoided as they may increase hepatic venous pressure and ICP.

Patients are typically hyperdynamic with a low systemic vascular resistance, high CO and increased stroke volume. Fluid resuscitation is combined with vasopressor therapy to achieve a mean arterial pressure sufficient to provide a cerebral perfusion pressure greater than 50 mmHg. Inotropic and vasoconstrictive therapy is directed by pulmonary artery catheter measurements or other CO monitor.

Early renal support with continuous venovenous haemofiltration is advised. Bicarbonate-buffered (lactate-free) replacement fluid is required because the failing liver is often unable to metabolize lactate to bicarbonate, resulting in a severe lactic acidosis. A serum sodium concentration of 140 to 150 mmol/L is the aim.

Early enteral nutrition should be established. Prophylactic H_2 blockers or proton pump inhibitors are given to prevent upper gastrointestinal haemorrhage. The use of lactulose and neomycin therapy is no longer recommended.

Red blood cells and platelet transfusions are often required to maintain adequate haemoglobin and platelet levels. Prothrombin time is a good marker of hepatic function and should only be corrected with fresh frozen plasma if the patient is actively bleeding.

Sepsis is a major cause of mortality in acute hepatic failure. Antimicrobial agents are given prophylactically. They should be broad-spectrum and cover both Gram-positive and Gram-negative organisms. Additional antifungal therapy is also recommended.

There is growing interest and research into the use of artificial and bioartificial liver support systems. However, there are no clinical data that have shown an improvement in mortality in the cardiac surgical patient.

Key points

- Postoperative hepatic failure carries a poor prognosis.
- Acute liver failure results in systemic dysfunction.
- In the cardiothoracic critical care setting, it is usually the result of severe sepsis or hepatic ischaemia.
- Treatment is supportive.

FURTHER READING

Tandon BN, Bernauau J, O'Grady J, *et al.* Recommendations of the International Association for the Study of the Liver Subcommittee on the nomenclature of acute and subacute liver failure. *J Gastroenterol Hepatol* 1999;14:403–4.

Marik PE, Gayowski T, Starzl TE; Hepatic Cortisol Research and Adrenal Pathophysiology Study Group. The hepatoadrenal syndrome: a common yet unrecognized clinical condition. *Crit Care Med* 2005;33:1254–59.

Chapter 38

Abdominal hypertension and abdominal compartment syndrome

M.L.N.G. MALBRAIN AND M.L. CHEATHAM

Introduction

A compartment syndrome exists when the increased pressure in a closed space threatens the viability of surrounding tissue. When this occurs in the abdomen, the rise of intra-abdominal pressure (IAP) may have a marked impact on end-organ function within and outside the abdominal cavity. The development of intra-abdominal hypertension (IAH) and abdominal compartment syndrome (ACS) are of importance in the care of critically ill patients. Intra-abdominal hypertension is a graded phenomenon that can be acute or chronic, primary or secondary and localized or generalized. Abdominal compartment syndrome is considered to be an 'all-or-nothing' phenomenon.

Definitions

Intra-abdominal pressure is the steady-state pressure within the abdominal cavity. It is expressed in mmHg and measured at end-expiration in the complete supine position after confirming the absence of abdominal muscle contractions and with the transducer zeroed at the level of the midaxillary line. Normal IAP is approximately 5 to 7 mmHg in critically ill adults. Intra-abdominal hypertension is defined as a sustained or repeated elevation of IAP to 12 mmHg or higher.

Abdominal compartment syndrome is defined as a sustained IAP above 20 mmHg associated with new organ dysfunction. Abdominal perfusion pressure (APP), where APP = MAP − IAP

Recognition of intra-abdominal hypertension and abdominal compartment syndrome

Clinical awareness

There still appears to be underrecognition of the syndrome and one must be aware of its existence to recognize it. Some clinicians dispute its existence.

Aetiology

Abdominal compartment syndrome can develop both in nonsurgical and surgical patients. Conditions associated with IAH/ACS can be classified into four categories:

- decrease in abdominal wall compliance;
- increase in intraluminal contents;
- intra-abdominal collection of fluid, air or blood; or
- capillary leak and fluid resuscitation.

Massive volume resuscitation after a first insult can lead to increased IAP, particularly postoperatively or in a septic patient. This is as a result of capillary leak, shock with ischaemia–reperfusion injury and the release of cytokines combined with the increase in total extracellular volume.

Diagnosis

CLINICAL AND RADIOLOGICAL EXAMINATION

Neither clinical examination (abdominal perimeter or girth) nor radiology (plain radiography of the

Table 38.1 Consensus definitions of abdominal compartment syndrome

Definition 1	IAP is the steady-state pressure concealed within the abdominal cavity.
Definition 2	APP = MAP − IAP
Definition 3	FG = GFP − PTP = MAP − (2 × IAP)
Definition 4	IAP should be expressed in mmHg and measured at end-expiration in the complete supine position after ensuring that abdominal muscle contractions are absent and with the transducer zeroed at the level of the midaxillary line.
Definition 5	The reference standard for intermittent IAP measurement is via the bladder with a maximal instillation volume of 25 mL of sterile saline.
Definition 6	Normal IAP is approximately 5–7 mmHg in critically ill adults.
Definition 7	IAH is defined by a sustained or repeated pathologic elevation of IAP ≥12 mmHg.
Definition 8	IAH is graded as follows: Grade I: IAP 12–15 mmHg Grade II: IAP 16–20 mmHg Grade III: IAP 21–25 mmHg Grade IV: IAP > 25 mmHg
Definition 9	ACS is defined as a sustained IAP >20 mmHg (with or without an APP ≤60 mmHg) that is associated with new organ dysfunction/failure.
Definition 10	Primary ACS is a condition associated with injury or disease in the abdominopelvic region that frequently requires early surgical or radiological intervention.
Definition 11	Secondary ACS refers to conditions that do not originate from the abdominopelvic region.
Definition 12	Recurrent ACS refers to the condition in which ACS redevelops following previous surgical or medical treatment of primary or secondary ACS.

Abbreviations: ACS, abdominal compartment syndrome; APP, abdominal perfusion pressure; FG, filtration gradient; GFP, glomerular filtration pressure; IAH, intra-abdominal hypertension; IAP, intra-abdominal pressure; MAP, mean arterial pressure; PTP, proximal tubular pressure.

chest or abdomen, abdominal ultrasound or computed tomography) can assess IAP accurately. The key to recognizing ACS in a critically ill patient is the demonstration of an elevated IAP: 'measuring is knowing!'

INTERMITTENT MEASUREMENT OF INTRA-ABDOMINAL PRESSURE

The abdomen and its contents are relatively noncompressive and compliant, so that pressure within the abdomen behaves in accordance with Pascal's law. The IAP measured at one point may be assumed to represent the IAP throughout the abdomen. Intra-abdominal pressure can be measured directly (invasive method) or indirectly (noninvasive method).

- Direct measurement relies on the insertion of an intraperitoneal catheter attached to a pressure transducer.
- Indirect measurement relies on conduction of the pressure to easily accessible cavities (rectal, uretal, vesical, gastric). Intra-abdominal pressure measured in the bladder is emerging as the gold standard.

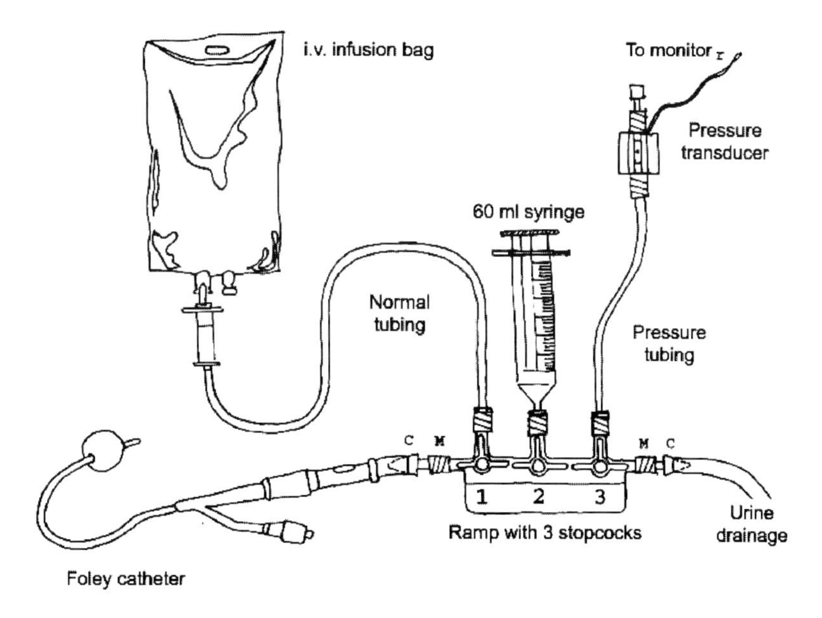

Figure 38.1 Using a patent Foley catheter with clamped drainage tube, 10 to 25 mL of sterile water is infused into the bladder via 3 three-way stopcocks placed in series between the Foley catheter and the urine drainage tubing. By turning, the stopcocks 'open' and 'close' to either the saline infusion bag or the pressure transducer, the bladder can be primed and the bladder pressure as estimate for IAP can be measured afterwards. The bladder pressure measured with a transducer correlates well with directly measured IAP.

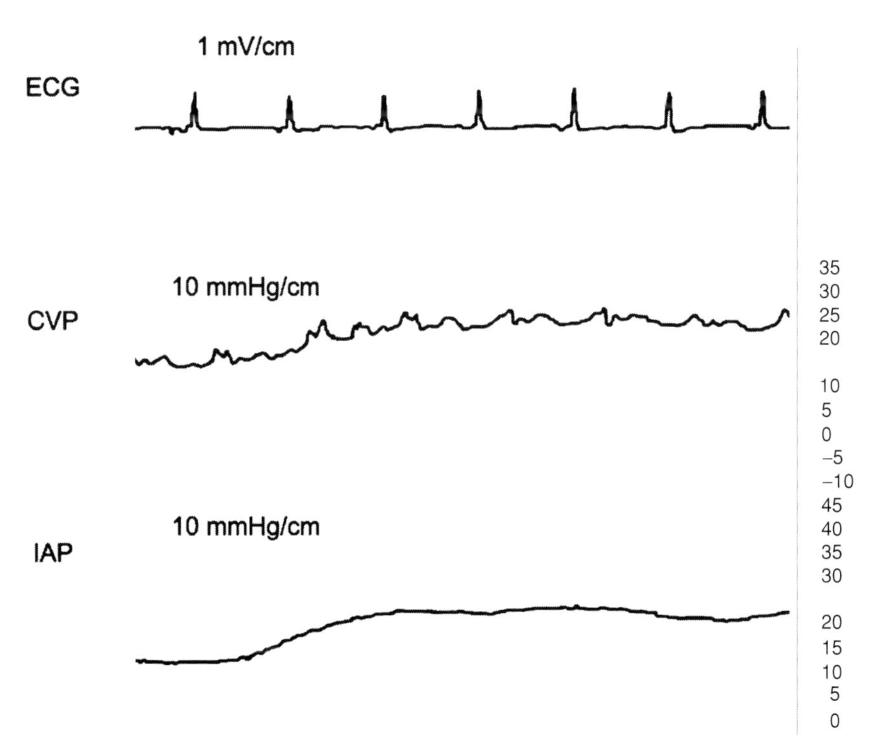

Figure 38.2 Simultaneous electrocardiography, CVP and IAP tracing before and during abdominal compression. The abdominothoracic transmission can be calculated as follows: The change in end-expiratory IAP: $\Delta IAP = 20 - 12.5 = 7.5$ mmHg. The change in end-expiratory CVP: $\Delta CVP = 25 - 12.5 = 12.5$ mmHg. The index of abdominothoracic transmission $= \Delta IAP/\Delta CVP = 7.5/12.5 = 60\%$.

CONTINUOUS MEASUREMENT OF INTRA-ABDOMINAL PRESSURE

Methods to measure IAP continuously have been developed and include measurement via the stomach (using air-chamber membranes), peritoneal cavity (using air-chamber or piezo-resistive membranes) and bladder (using a continuous irrigation).

ABDOMINAL PERFUSION PRESSURE

Abdominal perfusion pressure (APP = MAP – IAP) has been proposed as a more accurate predictor of visceral perfusion and a potential endpoint for resuscitation. A target APP of at least 60 mmHg has been demonstrated to correlate with improved survival from IAH and ACS.

RENAL PERFUSION PRESSURE AND FILTRATION GRADIENT

Elevated IAP significantly decreases renal artery blood flow and compresses the renal vein, leading to renal dysfunction and failure. Oliguria often develops at an IAP of 15 mmHg and anuria at 25 mmHg in the normovolaemic patient. Renal perfusion pressure (RPP = MAP – IAP) and renal filtration gradient (FG = GFP – PTP = [MAP – IAP] – IAP = MAP – [2 × IAP], where GFP is glomerular filtration pressure and PTP is proximal tubular pressure) have been proposed as key factors in the development of IAP-induced renal failure.

Pathophysiological implications

Neurological function

Increased IAP causes cephalad displacement of the diaphragm. Cerebral perfusion pressure decreases owing to a functional obstruction of cerebral venous outflow caused by the increased intrathoracic pressure in combination with the reduced systemic blood pressure (owing to decreased preload and cardiac output [CO]). Cerebral blood flow and therefore jugular bulb saturation decrease.

Table 38.2 Neurological effects related to intra-abdominal pressure

Intracranial pressure	↑↑
Cerebral perfusion pressure	↓↓
Cerebral blood flow	↓↓
Jugular bulb saturation	↓↓

Key: ↓↓, decreased; ↑↑, increased.

Cardiovascular function

Because of the cephalad movement of the diaphragm, intrapleural and intrathoracic pressures increase. Filling pressures (central venous pressure [CVP], pulmonary artery wedge pressure) seem to be elevated, but intravascular volume may remain low.

When IAP rises above 10 mmHg, CO drops owing to an increase in afterload and a decrease in preload and left ventricular compliance. Systemic vascular resistance increases owing to mechanical compression of vascular beds. Preload is reduced because of the reduction in stroke volume and venous return. Mean arterial blood pressure may initially rise owing to shunting of blood away from the abdominal cavity, but thereafter decreases.

Transmural filling pressure, calculated at end-expiration is a more accurate estimation of preload: transmural CVP = CVP – intrathoracic pressure.

A quick estimate of transmural filling pressures can also be obtained by subtracting half of the IAP: transmural CVP = CVP – IAP/2.

Pulmonary function

The abdominal and the thoracic compartment are linked across the diaphragm and on average a 50% (range, 25%–80%) transmission of IAP to the thorax has been noted. Intra-abdominal hypertension causes a reduction of the functional residual

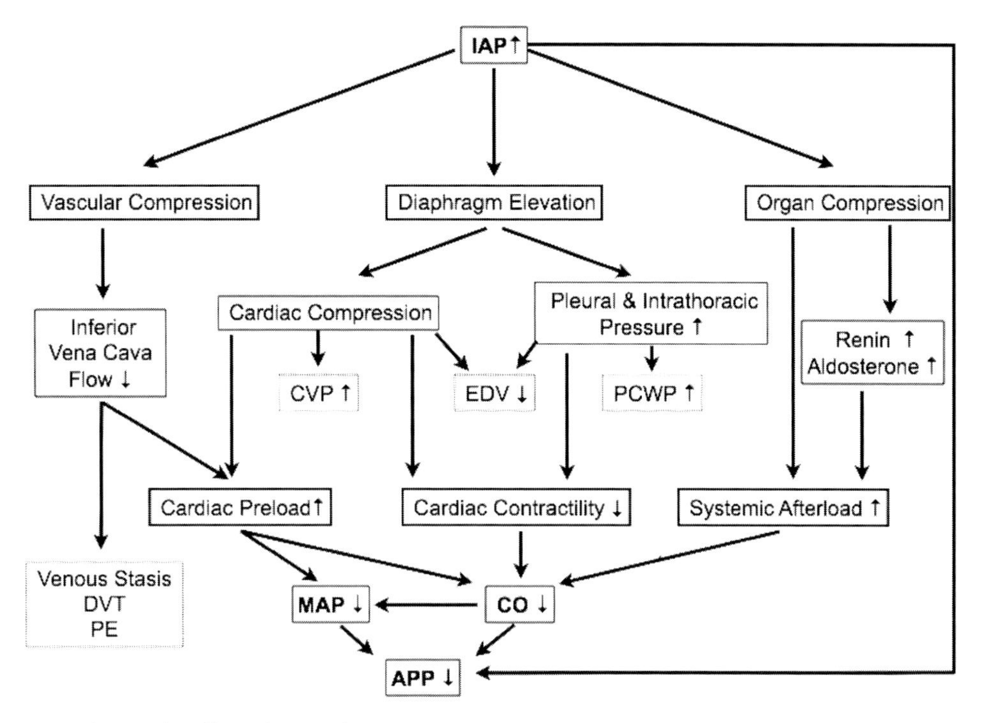

Figure 38.3 Cardiovascular effect of IAH and ACS.

capacity. Intra-abdominal pressure increases with inspiration as the diaphragm contracts and decreases with expiration and diaphragmatic relaxation.

Hepatic function

Animal and human studies have shown impairment of hepatic cell function and liver perfusion even with only moderately elevated IAP. Increased IAP is associated with decreased hepatic arterial flow, decreased venous portal flow and increased portal collateral flow.

Renal function

Intra-abdominal hypertension ($\geq$15 mmHg) is independently associated with renal impairment and increased mortality.

The mechanisms behind these changes are not entirely understood, but include reduced renal perfusion, reduced CO, increased systemic vascular resistance and humoral and neurogenic factors. Prompt reduction of IAP may have dramatic beneficial effect on urine output in patients with primary and secondary ACS.

Gastrointestinal function

Increasing IAP may reduce visceral perfusion and lead to local intracellular acidosis. This may be a precursor of multiple organ failure. Intra-abdominal hypertension therefore triggers a vicious cycle leading to intestinal oedema, ischaemia and bacterial translocation.

Abdominal wall

Increased IAP has been shown to reduce abdominal wall blood flow by direct compression, leading to local ischaemia and oedema. This can decrease abdominal wall compliance and further exacerbate IAH, setting up a vicious circle. Abdominal

Table 38.3 Cardiovascular effects related to intra-abdominal pressure

Pleural and intrathoracic pressure	↑↑
Pulmonary artery wedge pressure	↑↑
Central venous pressure	↑↑
Transmural filling pressure	↓
Right ventricular end-diastolic volume	↓
Right, global and left ventricular ejection fraction	↓
Stroke volume variation	↑
Inferior vena caval flow	↓↓
Venous return	↓↓
Left ventricular compliance and contractility	↓↓
Cardiac output	↓↓
Systemic vascular resistance	↑↑
Mean arterial pressure	↓↑
Pulmonary artery pressure	↑↑
Pulmonary vascular resistance	↑↑
Heart rate	↓↑
Mixed venous oxygen saturation	↓↓

Key: ↑↑, increased; ↑, slightly increased; ↓↓, decreased; ↓, slightly decreased; ↓↑, increased or decreased.

wall muscle and fascial ischaemia may contribute to infective and noninfective wound complications (e.g. dehiscence, herniation, necrotizing fasciitis) often seen in this patient population.

Clinical management

The management is based on three principles:

- specific procedures to reduce IAP and the consequences of ACS;
- general support (intensive care) of the critically ill patient; and
- optimization, including surgical decompression, to counteract some of the specific adverse effects.

Table 38.4 Pulmonary effects related to intra-abdominal pressure

Diaphragm elevation	↑↑
Intrathoracic pressure	↑↑
Pleural pressure	↑↑
Functional residual capacity	↓↓
All lung volumes (total lung capacity, tidal volume, etc.) (~restrictive disease)	↓↓
Auto-positive end-expiratory pressure	↑↑
Compression atelectasis	↑↑
Peak airway pressure (volume-controlled minute ventilation)	↑↑
Mean airway pressure	↑↑
Plateau airway pressure	↑↑
Pulmonary vascular resistance	↑↑
Static chest wall compliance	↓↓
Static lung compliance	↓
Hypercarbia – P_{CO_2} retention	↑↑
Pa_{O_2} and Pa_{O_2}/Fi_{O_2}	↓↓
Dead-space ventilation	↑↑
Ventilation–perfusion mismatch	↑↑
Oxygen consumption	↑↑
Metabolic cost and work of breathing	↑↑
Alveolar oedema	↑↑

Key: ↑↑, increased; ↑, slightly increased; ↓↓, decreased; ↓, slightly decreased.

Medical treatment

IMPROVEMENT OF ABDOMINAL WALL COMPLIANCE

The relationship between abdominal contents and IAP is exponential. Sedation and even muscle

Table 38.5 Hepatic effects related to intra-abdominal pressure

Effect	
Hepatic arterial flow	↓↓
Portal venous blood flow	↓↓
Lactate clearance	↓↓
Glucose metabolism	↓↓
Mitochondrial function	↓↓
Cytochrome p450 function	↓↓

Key: ↓↓, decreased.

paralysis can help to control IAH by increasing abdominal wall compliance. Body positioning also affects IAP.

EVACUATION OF INTRALUMINAL CONTENTS

Ileus is common in most critically ill patients. Non-invasive evacuation of abdominal contents may be considered in severe cases by means of nasogastric suction, rectal tube and enemas, and possibly even endoscopic decompression. This can be done in conjunction with prokinetics such as metoclopramide, neostigmine or erythromycin.

Table 38.6 Renal effects related to intra-abdominal pressure

Effect	
Renal perfusion pressure	↓↓
Filtration gradient	↓↓
Renal arterial blood flow	↓↓
Renal venous blood flow	↓↓
Glomerular filtration rate	↓↓
Antidiuretic hormone	↑↑
Sympathetic nervous system stimulation	↑↑

Key: ↑↑, increased; ↓↓, decreased.

Table 38.7 Gastrointestinal effects related to intra-abdominal pressure

Effect	
Abdominal perfusion pressure	↓↓
Superior mesenteric artery blood flow	↓↓
Coeliac blood flow	↓↓
Mucosal blood flow	↓↓
Intestinal mucosal perfusion	↓↓
Intramucosal pH (gastric tonometry)	↓↓
Intestinal oedema	↑↑
Bacterial translocation	↑↑
Bowel ischaemia	↑↑

Key: ↑↑, increased; ↓↓, decreased.

EVACUATION OF ABDOMINAL FLUID COLLECTION

Drainage of ascites if present may result in a decrease in IAP and in patients with liver cirrhosis and oesophageal varices, paracentesis helps to decrease variceal wall tension and the risk of rupture and bleeding. In cardiac critical care, draining ascites is controversial because of the concern about introduction of infection.

CORRECTION OF CAPILLARY LEAK AND POSITIVE FLUID BALANCE

Fluid loss should be replaced to prevent splanchnic hypoperfusion. Low-dose infusion of an inotrope that increases CO without causing excessive vasoconstriction may also reduce the intestinal mucosal perfusion impairment induced by moderate increases in IAP. Dobutamine or enoximone may be the most suitable inotropic agents. In the early stages, diuretic therapy in combination with albumin can be considered to mobilize the oedema, but only if the patient is haemodynamically stable. The institution of renal replacement therapy with fluid removal should be considered early.

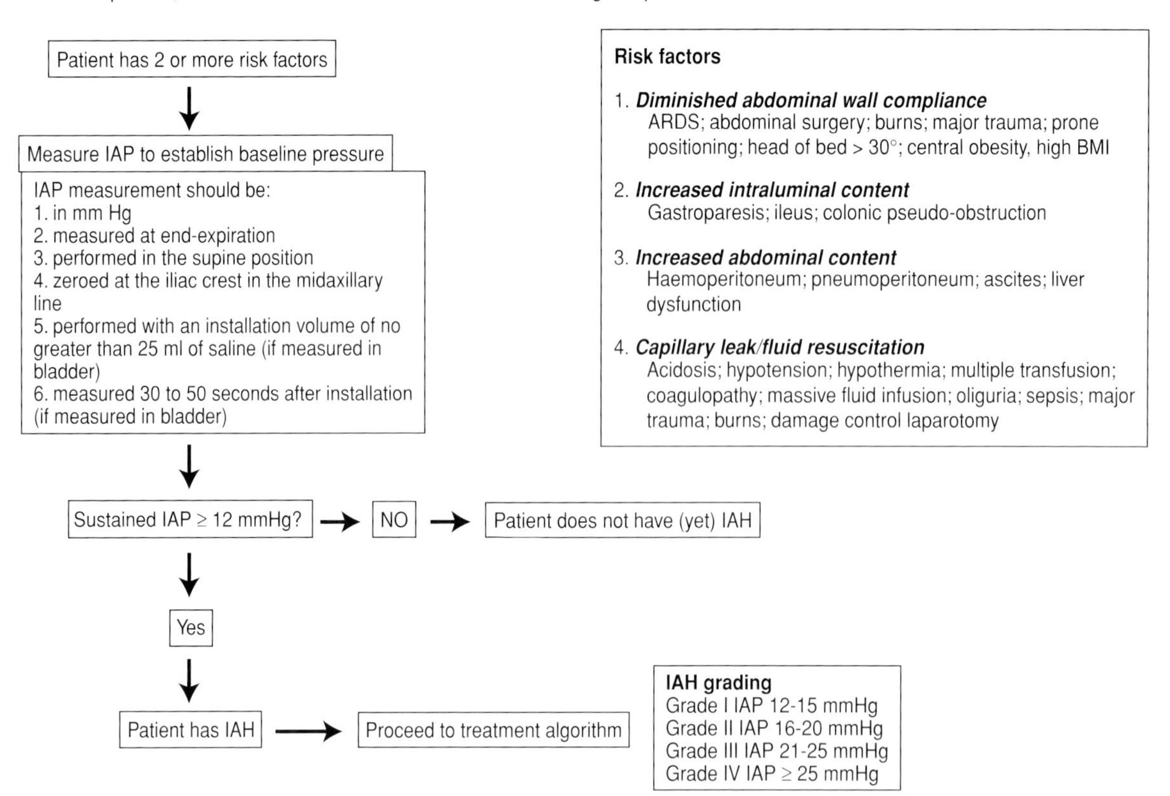

Figure 38.4 Algorithm for the clinical assessment of IAH and ACS.

SPECIFIC TREATMENTS

The application of continuous negative abdominal pressure by means of a cuirass has been studied in animals and humans. This may lead to a decrease in IAP and increase end-expiratory lung volumes. It may be appropriate to target APP, where APP = MAP − IAP, to a level that reduces the risk of impaired splanchnic perfusion and subsequent organ dysfunction. Octreotide, a long-acting somatostatin analogue, has been shown to affect neutrophil infiltration and improve the reperfusion-induced oxidative damage after decompression of secondary IAH.

Surgical decompression

Although decompression remains the only definitive management for ACS, the timing of this procedure is controversial. After decompression, the patient is at risk of ischaemia–reperfusion injury, venous stasis and fatal pulmonary embolism. Leaving the abdomen open was originally intended for patients with diffuse intra-abdominal infections, and often used in combination with a planned 'second-look' approach. Because of the increased awareness of the deleterious effects of IAH, such treatment, either prophylactic or therapeutic, is becoming more common in critical care. Several

INTRA-ABDOMINAL HYPERTENSION (IAH) / ABDOMINAL COMPARTMENT SYNDROME (ACS) MANAGEMENT ALGORITHM

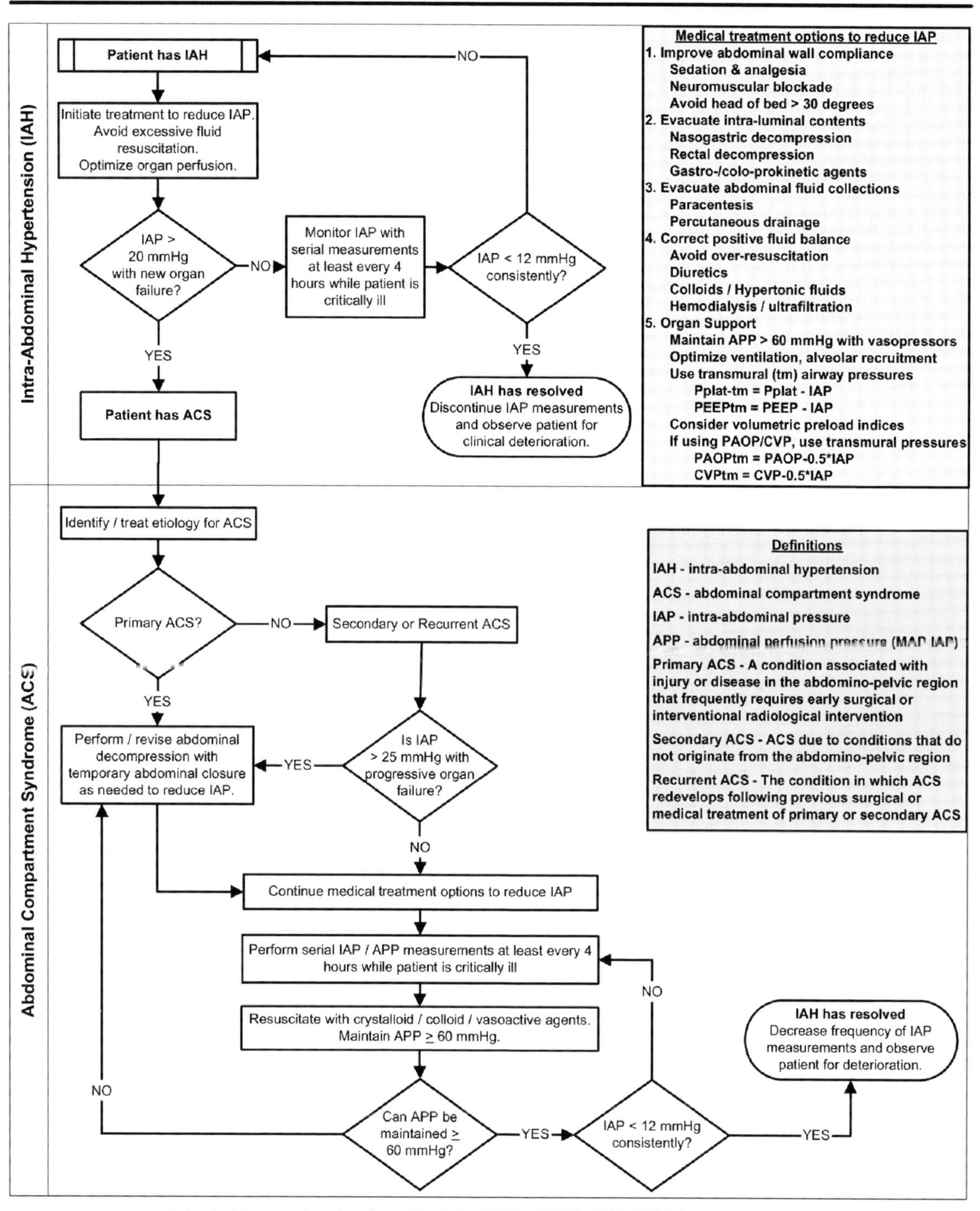

Adapted from *Intensive Care Medicine* 2006; 32(11):1722-1732 & 2007; 33(6):951-962.

Figure 38.5 Algorithm for the clinical management of IAH and ACS.

Table 38.8 Medical treatment options for intra-abdominal hypertension and abdominal compartment syndrome

1. Improvement of abdominal wall compliance
- Sedation
- Pain relief (not fentanyl!)
- Neuromuscular blockade
- Body positioning
- Negative fluid balance
- Skin pressure decreasing interfaces
- Weight loss
- Percutaneous abdominal wall component separation

2. Evacuation of intraluminal contents
- Gastric tube and suctioning
- Gastroprokinetics (erythromycin, cisapride, metoclopramide)
- Rectal tube and enemas
- Colonoprokinetics (neostigmine, prostigmine bolus or infusion)
- Endoscopic decompression of large bowel
- Colostomy
- Ileostomy

3. Evacuation of peri-intestinal and abdominal fluids
- Ascites evacuation
- CT- or US-guided aspiration of abscess
- CT- or US-guided aspiration of haematoma
- Percutaneous drainage of (blood) collections

4. Correction of capillary leak and positive fluid balance
- Albumin in combination with diuretics (furosemide)
- Correction of capillary leak (antibiotics, source control, . . .)
- Colloids instead of crystalloids
- Dobutamine (not dopamine!)
- Dialysis or CVVH with ultrafiltration
- Ascorbinic acid in burn patients

5. Specific therapeutic interventions
- Continuous negative abdominal pressure
- Negative external abdominal pressure
- Targeted abdominal perfusion pressure
- Experimental: Octreotide and melatonin

Abbreviations: CT, computed tomography; CVVH, continuous venovenous haemofiltration; US, ultrasound.

methods for temporary abdominal closure are available.

Key points

- Recognition of the role of IAP and the development of ACS is increasing.
- Increasing abdominal pressure may splint the diaphragm and makes filling pressures appear high.
- Measurement of IAP may be advantageous, and this may be undertaken easily via the bladder or stomach.
- Abdominal compartment syndrome may be associated with multiorgan failure, and is specifically implicated in renal and gastrointestinal dysfunction.
- Surgical decompression by laparotomy may be necessary if abdominal pressure continues to rise despite conservative measures.

FURTHER READING

Balogh Z, Jones F, D'Amours S, *et al.* Continuous intra-abdominal pressure measurement technique. *Am J Surg* 2004;188;679–684.

Cheatham ML, Malbrain ML, Kirkpatrick A, *et al.* Results from the International Conference of Experts on Intra-abdominal Hypertension and Abdominal Compartment Syndrome. II. Recommendations. *Intensive Care Med* 2007;33:951–962.

Malbrain ML. Abdominal pressure in the critically ill. *Curr Opin Crit Care* 2000;6:17–29.

Malbrain ML, Cheatham ML, Kirkpatrick A, *et al.* Results from the International Conference of Experts on Intra-abdominal Hypertension and Abdominal Compartment Syndrome. I. Definitions. *Intensive Care Med* 2006;32:1722–1732.

World Society on Abdominal Compartment Syndrome [homepage on the Internet]. Available at: www.wsacs.org.

3.6 *Immune System and Infection in Cardiothoracic Critical Care*

Chapter 39

The role of the immune system in critical illness

H.F. GALLEY

Introduction

The immune system has evolved to provide protection against invading pathogenic organisms, foreign cells and cancer cells. This chapter describes basic mechanisms involved in innate and acquired immune responses and describes the particular relevance for critical illness, notably sepsis and multiple organ dysfunction syndromes.

Innate immunity

Immunity is the state of protection from infectious disease or our own altered cells, and comprises both specific and nonspecific components. Nonspecific, or innate immunity, is the basic in-built resistance to disease and consists of four defensive barriers that offer protection through anatomical, physiological, phagocytic and inflammatory strategies.

Anatomical barriers

THE SKIN

Intact skin prevents the penetration of most pathogens. The thinner outer epidermis is renewed every 2 to 4 weeks and does not contain blood vessels. The thicker dermis is composed of connective tissue and contains blood vessels, hair follicles, sebaceous glands and sweat glands. The sebaceous glands produce the oily substance sebum, made up of lactic acid and fatty acids, which keeps the pH of the skin at around 4 to inhibit bacterial growth. Breaks in the skin such as small cuts and insect bites are obvious routes of infection.

MUCOUS MEMBRANES

Many pathogens can enter the body by penetrating mucous membranes, although they are protected by saliva, tears and mucus, which wash away organisms and also contain antiviral and antibacterial substances.

In the lower respiratory and gastrointestinal tracts, organisms trapped in mucus are propelled out of the body by ciliary action. Some organisms have evolved such that they can evade this defence mechanism. For example, the influenza virus has a surface molecule that enables it to attach to cells in the mucus membrane, preventing it being washed away through the action of cilia. The adherence of bacteria to mucous membranes depends on the interaction of protrusions on the bacteria and specific glycoproteins on some mucous membrane or epithelial cells, which explains why certain tissues are more susceptible to bacterial invasion.

Physiological barriers

If an organism manages to breach the anatomical barriers, there are several physiological protection mechanisms. Physiological barriers include temperature, pH (gastric acidity prevents the growth of many organisms) and a variety of soluble factors. Lysozyme, found in mucus, is an enzyme that cleaves the peptidoglycan layer of bacterial cell

Table 39.1 The four components of the innate immune response

Anatomical barriers	Skin, mucous membranes	Sebum, mucous, ciliary action
Physiological barriers	pH, temperature, soluble factors	Complement, lysozyme, interferons
Endocytosis/phagocytosis	Neutrophils, macrophages, natural killer cells	Phagosome, lysozyme
Inflammatory response	Vasodilatation, increased capillary permeability, leukocyte margination, chemical mediators	Cytokines, acute phase proteins, histamine, kinins, complement, phagocytosis

walls. Interferons (IFNs) are produced by virus-infected cells and bind to nearby cells causing a generalized antiviral state.

COMPLEMENT

Complement is a group of serum proteins that circulate in an inactive state. Activation converts the inactive proenzymes to active enzymes through an enzyme cascade, which results in membrane-damaging reactions, destroying pathogenic organisms and facilitating their clearance. There are two pathways of complement activation. The classical pathway involves activation by specific immunoglobulin molecules, and the alternative pathway is activated by a variety of micro-organisms and immune complexes. Each pathway results in the generation of a membrane attack complex that

- displaces phospholipids within cell membranes,
- makes large holes in and disrupts the membrane, and
- results in bacterial cell lysis.

Complement components also amplify reactions between antigens and antibodies, attract phagocytic cells to sites of infection and activate B lymphocytes. The complement system is nonspecific and will, in theory, attack its own body cells as well as foreign cells. To prevent host cell damage, there are regulatory mechanisms that restrict complement reactions to specific targets.

Endocytosis and phagocytosis

Another important innate defence mechanism is the ingestion of extracellular macromolecules and particles by endocytosis and phagocytosis respectively. In endocytosis, macromolecules in extracellular fluid are internalized by invagination of the plasma membrane to form endocytic vesicles. Enzymes then degrade the ingested material. Phagocytosis involves ingestion of particles, including whole micro-organisms, via expansion of the plasma membrane to form phagosomes. Virtually all cells are capable of endocytosis, but phagocytosis occurs in only a few specialized cells. Professional phagocytes are the polymorphonuclear neutrophils, mast cells and macrophages.

Cells infected with viruses and parasites are killed by large granular lymphocytes, termed natural killer (NK) cells, and eosinophils. Once particles are ingested into phagosomes, they fuse with lysosomes and the contents are digested.

The inflammatory response

The inflammatory response to tissue damage or invasion by pathogenic organisms results in vasodilatation, increased capillary permeability and influx of phagocytic cells.

- Vasodilatation results in engorgement of the capillary network, causing tissue redness or erythema and increased tissue temperature.
- Increased capillary permeability enables an influx of fluid and cells from the capillaries into the tissue.
- Migration of leukocytes into the tissues, particularly phagocytes, involves a complex series of events, including margination or adherence of cells to the endothelial cell wall, extravasation or movement of the cells between the capillary cell walls into the tissue, and chemotaxis, the migration of the cells through the tissue to the site of inflammation.

The inflammatory response is initiated by chemical mediators, produced from the invading organisms, damaged cells and cells of the immune system. These include the acute-phase proteins:

- C-reactive protein is produced by the liver and binds to the C polysaccharide component found on many bacteria and fungi. This binding activates the complement system, resulting in both complement-mediated lysis and increased phagocytosis.
- Histamine is released from mast cells, basophils and platelets and binds to receptors on capillaries and venules, leading to increased vascular permeability and vasodilatation.
- Kinins cause vasodilatation and increased capillary permeability and bradykinin also stimulates pain receptors in the skin.

REGULATION OF THE INFLAMMATORY RESPONSE

Severe infection with Gram-negative organisms leads to the appearance of endotoxin or lipopolysaccharide (LPS) in the bloodstream, activating the transcription factor nuclear factor kappa B (NF-κB). Toll-like receptors (TLRs) are pathogen-associated molecular pattern receptors for a variety of molecules from bacteria, viruses and fungi. The TLRs are important for both innate and acquired immunity because interaction of TLRs with pathogen-associated molecular patterns on cells such as neutrophils and macrophages drives innate immune responses, whereas activation of TLRs expressed on antigen-presenting cells leads to the initiation of adaptive immunity via T cells.

Nuclear factor-κB is involved in the regulation of gene expression of a huge number of cytokines, growth factors, adhesion molecules and enzymes involved in the inflammatory response. It is maintained in a nonactivated state in the cytoplasm by association with an inhibitor subunit, IκB. Proteolysis of IκB in response to activation by LPS and cytokines reveals a previously hidden nuclear recognition site. This then prompts the NF-κB to move into the nucleus where it binds onto target DNA and results in mRNA expression.

Activation of NF-κB leads to increased gene expression of several important mediators involved in the inflammatory response, including chemokines, cytokines and adhesion molecules. Activation of NF-κB has been shown to be increased in critically ill patients – and associated with nonsurvival – in several studies.

Interferons are the body's first line of antiviral defence. By inducing the expression of hundreds of IFN-stimulated genes, IFNs can block virus replication. Viruses are able to counteract the antiviral response through mechanisms that control IFN signalling and block the actions of IFN-stimulated gene products. Studies of influenza, hepatitis C, herpes simplex and vaccinia viruses have revealed the importance of IFNs for the control of virus replication and pathogenesis. Various viral proteins are able to either activate TLRs or to block TLR function. Some viruses may even need cellular activation via TLRs to enable entry into the cell or replication.

Another receptor important for host responses to infection is the triggering receptor expressed on myeloid cells (TREM-1). It is expressed on neutrophils and a subset of monocytes. In vitro studies

Table 39.2 Toll-like receptor ligands

Toll-like receptor	Ligand (s)	Other points
TLR-1	Triacyl lipoproteins	Activates nuclear factor-κB
TLR-2	Lipoproteins, Gram-positive peptidoglycan, lipoteichoic acids, fungi, viral glycoproteins, zymosan	Promotes apoptosis
TLR-3	Double stranded viral RNA	Stimulates IFNs which activate anti-inflammatory pathways
TLR-4	LPS, viral glycoproteins	LPS binds to CD14 via LPS binding protein, and activator protein-1
TLR-5	Flagellin	Feeds into TLR-4 pathway
TLR-6	Diacyl lipoproteins	Promotes apoptosis
TLR-7	Antiviral compounds, single stranded RNA	Feeds into TLR-4 pathway
TLR-8	Small synthetic compounds, single stranded RNA	
TLR-9	Unmethylated CpG DNA	Feeds into TLR-4 pathway
TLR-10	Unknown	

Abbreviations: IFN, interferon; LPS, lipopolysaccharide; TLR, toll-like receptor.

have shown that TREM-1 is upregulated in response to Gram-positive and Gram-negative bacteria, mycobacteria and bacterial cell wall components, including both LPS and lipoteichoic acid. Triggering of the TREM-1 receptor induces the secretion of IL-8, tumour necrosis factor (TNF)-α, IL-1β and monocyte chemotactic protein-1 and release of the enzyme myeloperoxidase. One of several pathways with a role in signalling in the innate immune response, TREM-1 has been shown to have a role in critically ill patients with sepsis.

Acquired immunity

Specificity, diversity, memory and the ability to discriminate 'self' from 'non-self' are key features of the acquired or specific immune system. It has four distinct phases: the recognition of antigen, the activation of lymphocytes, the effector phase of antigen elimination and the return to homeostasis and antigenic memory.

The acquired immune response is further classified into humoral and cell-mediated immunity. The humoral component involves interaction of B lymphocytes with antigen and their proliferation and differentiation into antibody-secreting plasma cells. Antibody is the effector of the humoral response via binding to the antigen, neutralizing and facilitating its removal. This process also activates the complement system. Binding of micro-organisms to antibodies on the cell surface of B cells leads to preferential selection of these antibody-producing cells. This is termed 'priming,' and subsequent responses are faster and amplified, and provide the basis of vaccination.

T-lymphocytes can only recognize antigen in the presence of cell membrane proteins called

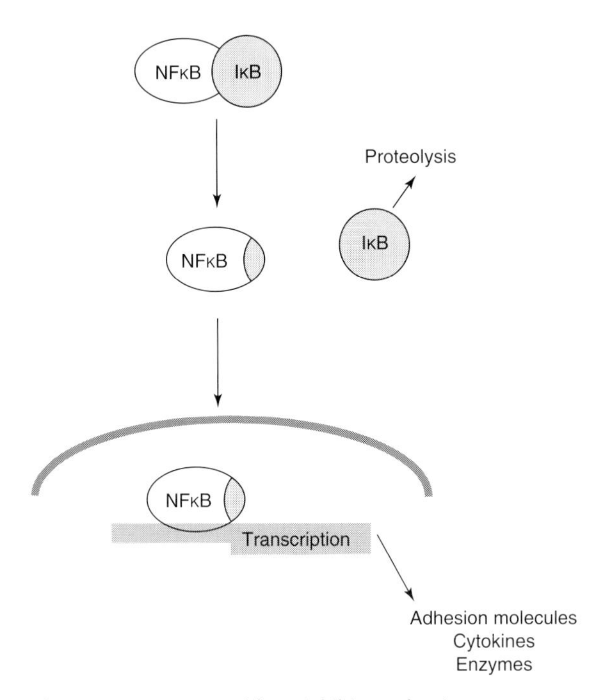

Figure 39.1 NF-κB with an inhibitor subunit, IκB. Proteolysis of IκB in response to activation by LPS and cytokines reveals a previously hidden nuclear recognition site. NF-κB moves into the nucleus where it binds onto target DNA and results in mRNA expression.

the major histocompatibility complex (MHC) molecules. Effector T cells generated in response to antigen associated with MHC are responsible for cell-mediated immunity. There are two main types of T cells: T helper cells and T cytotoxic cells.

- T helper cells secrete cytokines, which are low-molecular-weight proteins, that activate various phagocytic cells, B cells and T cytotoxic cells.
- Circulating T helper cells are capable of unrestricted cytokine expression and are prompted into a more restricted and focused pattern of cytokine production depending on signals received at the outset of infection.
- T cytotoxic cells recognize antigen–MHC molecule complex and are able to eliminate altered self cells, virus-infected cells, foreign tissue grafts and tumour cells.

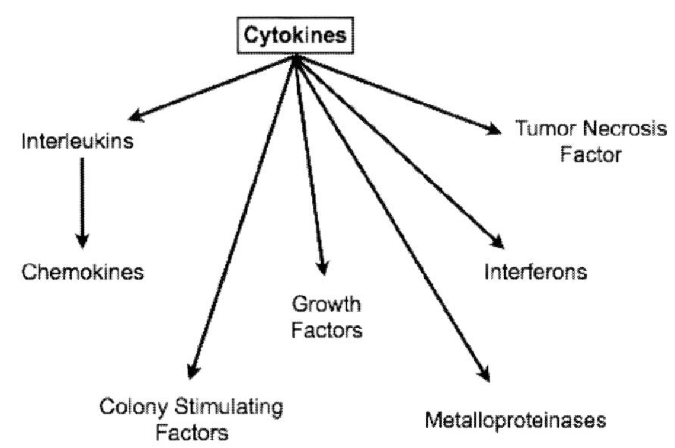

Figure 39.2 Cytokines released signals.

Antigens are any substance capable of interacting with the products of a specific immune response. Antigens capable of eliciting a specific immune response are called 'immunogens.' Foreign protein antigens must be degraded into small peptides and complexed with MHC molecules to be recognized by a T cell, a process called 'antigen processing.'

Mature immunocompetent animals possess large numbers of antigen reactive T and B cells. Before any contact with an antigen, each T and B lymphocyte already possesses specificity to antigens. This is achieved by random gene rearrangements in the bone marrow during maturation of lymphocytes. The initial encounter of antigen-specific lymphocytes with an antigen induces a primary response, and later encounters or secondary responses are more rapid and heightened.

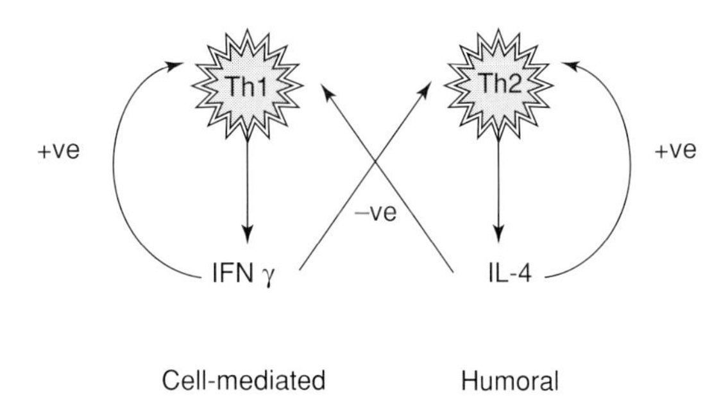

Figure 39.3 Cellular interactions mediated by cytokines. -ve denotes inhibition and +ve activation.

Cell-mediated immunity

Leukocytes develop from a common pluripotent stem cell during haematopoiesis, and proliferate and differentiate into the different cells in response to haematopoietic growth factors.

- The lymphocyte is the only cell to possess specificity, diversity, memory and recognition of self/non-self.
- Monocytes, macrophages and neutrophils are accessory immune cells responsible for phagocytosis.
- Macrophages are important in antigen processing and presentation in association with MHC molecules, and secretion of cytokines.
- Different maturational stages of lymphocytes can be distinguished by their expression of specific molecules on the cell membranes, which are called 'cluster of differentiation' or CD antigens.

Antibodies

The protein molecules that combine specifically with antigens are called 'antibodies' or 'immunoglobulins.' Antibody molecules consist of two identical light chains and two identical heavy chains joined by disulphide bonds. Each heavy and light chain has a variable amino acid sequence region and a constant region. The unique heavy chain constant region sequences determine the five classes or isotypes of antibody.

Cytokines

Orchestration of immune response depends on communication between cells by soluble molecules given the generic term 'cytokines.' They are involved in both innate and acquired immune responses and have a transient and tightly regulated action. They regulate both the amplitude and duration of the response. Cytokines are highly active at very low concentrations, combining with small numbers of high-affinity cell-surface receptors and producing changes in the patterns of RNA and protein synthesis. They have multiple effects on growth and differentiation in a variety of cell types with considerable overlap and redundancy between them. Specific mode of action depends on the stimulus, the cell type and the presence of other mediators and receptors.

Interferons (IFN-α, -β and -γ) are a family of broad-spectrum antiviral agents that also modulate the activity of other cells, particularly IL-8 and platelet-activating factor (PAF) production, antibody production by B cells and activation of cytotoxic macrophages.

Growth factors regulate the differentiation, proliferation, activity and function of specific cell types. The best known are colony-stimulating factors, which cause colony formation by haematogenic progenitor cells.

A labile alkyl phospholipid, PAF is released from a variety of cells in the presence of antigen and leukocytes in response to immune complexes. In addition to its actions on platelets, the effects of PAF include the priming of macrophages to other inflammatory mediators and alterations of microvascular permeability.

Arachidonic acid metabolites include the prostaglandins and leukotrienes, which have profound inflammatory and vascular actions, and may regulate, and be regulated by, other cytokines. The biological activities of cytokines are regulated by specific cellular receptors. Often, these receptors comprise multiple subunits providing phased stages of activation and biological action. Binding of a cytokine to one type of receptor may result in interactions with another receptor.

Soluble cytokine receptors have been identified that compete with membrane-bound receptors, thus regulating cytokine signals. Such soluble receptors may be membrane-bound receptors that are shed into the circulation either intact or as truncated forms (e.g. soluble TNF receptors), or may begin as related precursor molecules that are enzymatically

Table 39.3 Characteristics of immunoglobulin isotypes

Antibody isotype	Half-life in serum (d)	Specific effector function	Other information
IgG	23	• Neutralization of bacteria • Facilitation of phagocytosis • Complement activation (classical pathway) • Antibody-dependent cellular toxicity mediated by NK cells • Inhibits B-cell activation	• Crosses placenta; provides neonatal passive immunity. • Most common.
IgM	5	• Antigen receptor for naïve B cells • Complement activation (classical pathway)	• Viral neutralization • Bacterial agglutination • Complement activation
IgD	3	• Antigen receptor for naïve B cells	• Membrane bound, no secreted form
IgA	6	• Provides mucosal immunity	• Secreted into gut lumen, respiratory tract and breast milk
IgE	2	• Antibody-dependent cellular toxicity mediated by eosinophils • Mast cell degranulation	• Provides immunity against helminths • Involved in hypersensitivity reactions

Abbreviations: IG, immunoglobulin; NK, natural killer.

cleaved (e.g. IL-1R). Soluble cytokine receptors not only mediate biological activity, but control desensitization to ligands by reduced availability, decreased signalling and stimulating cellular mechanisms, which can result in lack of activity.

Cancer immunology

Tumour cells display surface structures that are recognized as antigenic and promote an immune response. Macrophages mediate tumour destruction by lytic enzymes and production of TNF-α; NK cells recognize tumour cells and either bind to antibody-coated tumour or secrete a cytotoxic factor active only against tumour cells. Tumour cell antigens can often elicit the generation of specific serum antibodies, which activate the complement system. However, some tumours are able to endocytose the hole in the cell membrane produced by the membrane attack and repair the cell membrane before lysis occurs. Complement products can also induce chemotaxis of macrophages and neutrophils and release of toxic mediators. Ironically, antibodies to tumour cells may also enhance tumour growth, possibly by masking tumour antigens and preventing recognition by NK cells.

Immune responses in the critically ill: Sepsis, systemic inflammatory response syndrome and multiple organ dysfunction syndrome

Severe infection leads to triggering of the innate immune response, including activation of phagocytic cells and activation of the alternative complement cascade, leading to the production of TNF-α and IL-1β. Secondary mediators, including other cytokines, prostaglandins and PAF, are then released, with further activation of complement and the acute phase response, expression of adhesion molecules, T-cell selection, antibody production and release of oxygen-derived free radicals. Other toxins and cellular debris must also trigger such a systemic inflammatory response; this process also occurs in the absence of infection, resulting in the term 'systemic inflammatory response syndrome.'

Local effects of the inflammatory response are essential for the control of infection. Prolonged systemic exposure to high concentrations of cytokines and other components of the immunoinflammatory cascade may contribute to the development of multiorgan dysfunction syndrome. The endothelium, which plays a pivotal role in the regulation of haemostasis, vascular tone and fibrinolysis, may be damaged, and this has profound consequences. The endothelium produces several substances that regulate inflammation and regional perfusion, including nitric oxide, vasoactive arachidonic acid metabolites and cytokines. Phagocytic cells are in constant contact with the endothelium and disturbance of the relationship between these two cell types may result in direct tissue damage as a result of local production of oxygen-derived free radicals, hypochlorous acid and proteolytic enzymes. Another hypothesis to explain the observed tissue damage and organ dysfunction is that of local tissue ischaemia and hypoxia as a result of microthrombi formed by a coagulopathy or platelet or white cell aggregates.

Immunotherapy in sepsis

Mortality from sepsis associated with metabolic acidosis, oliguria, hypoxaemia or shock has remained high, despite treatment of the source of infection, intravenous fluids, nutrition and mechanical ventilation for respiratory failure. During the initial response to infection, tissue macrophages generate inflammatory cytokines, including TNF-α, IL-1 and IL-8 in response to bacterial cell wall products. Although cytokines play an important part in host defence by attracting activated neutrophils to the site of infection, inappropriate and excessive release into the systemic circulation may lead to widespread microvascular injury and multiorgan failure. Clinical trials that tested immunotherapies aimed at modulating the excessive expression of key cytokines, such as ILs and TNF-α, designed to reduce the mortality rate associated with sepsis, have overall been either equivalent or inferior to placebo. Both soluble receptors and monoclonal antibodies directed against receptors can be used to block the interaction of a cytokine with its receptor. This then prevents transduction of the appropriate biological signal in the target cell. The cloning of genes encoding cytokine receptor chains and the characterization of their soluble forms has resulted in new approaches to anticytokine therapy. Injection of a recombinant soluble receptor might prevent the deleterious effect of excessive cytokine production. In addition to soluble receptors, monoclonal antibodies that block cellular cytokine receptors can be used as anticytokine therapy. However, these small molecules have short half-lives and therefore derived molecules with longer half-lives and higher affinity have now been developed. However, it has been shown that cytokines in complex with such binding proteins are still available for receptor binding. It is possible that these complexes can still act as agonists in vivo depending on concentrations of other mediators and relative receptor expression. Another approach to minimizing the deleterious effects of the uncontrolled inflammatory process is to blunt the final common pathways of damage (i.e., using either agents which decrease free radical production or antioxidants that inactivate free radicals as they are produced).

Blockade of any single or combined immune/inflammatory mediator may not be successful for a number of reasons. First, the inflammatory process is a normal response to infection and is essential not only for the resolution of infection but also for the initiation of other adaptive stress responses required for host survival. Second, the profound redundancy of action of many cytokines means that there are many overlapping pathways for cellular activation and further mediator release. In addition, the synergism of actions and effects of cytokines suggests that imbalance in the process of the immune response may be adversely affected by inhibition of a single agent. Exogenously administered anticytokine therapy may have unrecognized effects owing to interaction with naturally occurring immunomodulators or their receptors. Finally, the timing of any potential anticytokine therapy is clearly crucial.

Activated protein C

In vitro data indicate that activated protein C exerts an anti-inflammatory effect by inhibiting the production of TNF-α, IL-1β and IL-6 by monocytes and limiting monocyte and neutrophil adhesion to the endothelium. Reduced levels of protein C are found in the majority of patients with sepsis and are associated with an increased risk of death, which is the rationale for the administration of human recombinant activated protein C (Chapter 40).

Key points

- The human immune system consists of both innate (nonspecific) and acquired (specific) immune responses.
- Innate immune responses comprise anatomical and physiological barriers, endocytosis and phagocytosis and the inflammatory response.
- Acquired immune responses comprise humoral responses (mainly via B cells) and cell-mediated responses (mainly via T cells).
- Low-molecular-weight mediator proteins called cytokines are the orchestrators of inflammation.
- There is profound redundancy in the immune system, which goes some way towards explaining the lack of success of various immunotherapies in critical illness.

FURTHER READING

Aderem A, Ulevitch RJ. Toll-like receptors in the induction of the innate immune response. *Nature* 2000;406:782–787.

Galley HF. *Critical care focus 10: Inflammation and immunity*. London: BMJ Books; 2003.

Nasraway SA. The problems and challenges of immunotherapy in sepsis. *Chest* 2003;123 (Suppl):451S–459S.

Vincent JL. Management of sepsis in the critically ill patient: key aspects. *Expert Opin Pharmacother* 2006;7:2037–2045.

Chapter 40

Sepsis and the systemic inflammatory response syndrome

H. GERLACH AND S. TOUSSAINT

Introduction

Despite recent advances, 'the systemic inflammatory response syndrome' (SIRS), severe sepsis and septic shock still have an increasing incidence and unchanged mortality. The development of organ failure determines the course and prognosis of the septic patient. Progress has been made, particularly in areas such as pathophysiology, diagnosis, standard and adjunctive therapy, as well as experimental approaches. This includes genomic information for stratifying subgroups of patients, and a broader field of laboratory diagnostics from clinical studies and basic research on the cellular mechanisms of inflammation and organ dysfunction.

Systemic inflammatory response syndrome

The term SIRS was introduced in 1992 to denote the constellation of findings that result from systemic activation of the innate immune response, irrespective of the cause. The concept was that SIRS could be triggered by localized or generalized infections, trauma, thermal injury or sterile inflammatory processes, such as acute pancreatitis. From an operational standpoint, SIRS was considered to be present when patients had prespecified criteria.

The inflammatory events responsible for clinical derangements such as severe infection, sepsis, or septic shock are thought to be similar. These events lead to circulatory instability with respiratory distress according to the extent of infection and/or the intensity of the host response, culminating in single or multiple organ dysfunction syndromes. A major factor contributing to the belief that mediation of septic shock proceeds via well-defined molecular and cellular pathways irrespective of microbial taxonomy is the extensive database concerning bacterial septic shock syndromes. For Gram-negative bacteraemia or endotoxinaemia, data are especially compelling to causally link excessive production or prolonged activity of host-derived proinflammatory cytokine mediators with the intravascular inflammation, cardiopulmonary dysfunction and organ injury characteristic of septic shock.

Sepsis, severe sepsis and septic shock

Sepsis is defined as the combination of a SIRS with a localized and/or systemic infection that is responsible for the inflammatory response. It is a major cause of death worldwide, with a large impact on mortality in the critical care unit. Sepsis is an aggressive and multifactorial disease state resulting from the host response to infection. Although a localized and controlled inflammatory reaction helps to control infection, a dysregulated response may lead to multiple organ failure and determines the course and prognosis of the septic patient. Patients usually die of sepsis owing to severe organ dysfunction, and deaths are often attributed to these conditions rather than to sepsis. Despite intensive care, mortality remains as high as 54% for severe sepsis

Table 40.1 Criteria of the systemic inflammatory response syndrome: present when at least two of the four criteria are diagnosed

Body temperature: >38°C or ≤36°C
Heart rate: >90 min^{-1}
Respiratory rate: >20 min^{-1} or $Paco_2$ ≤32 mmHg or mechanical ventilation
White blood cell count: >12,000 cells μL^{-1} or ≤4,000 μL^{-1} or >10% immature forms

and septic shock. The combination of sepsis and a concomitant organ dysfunction is called 'severe sepsis'; if volume-refractory hypotension is present, the criteria for 'septic shock' are fulfilled.

The PIRO concept

Despite the definitions for sepsis, severe sepsis and septic shock, these terms do not allow for precise characterization and staging of patients with this condition.

A classification scheme for sepsis has been proposed – called PIRO – that stratifies patients on the basis of their *p*redisposing conditions, the nature and extent of the *i*nsult (or in the case of sepsis, *i*nfection), the nature and magnitude of the host *r*esponse, and the degree of concomitant *o*rgan dysfunction. It is important to emphasize that the PIRO concept presented herein is rudimentary; extensive testing and further refinement are needed before it can be considered ready for routine application in clinical practice.

Predisposition

Premorbid factors have a substantial impact on outcome in sepsis, modifying both the disease process and the approach taken to therapy. This point is emphasized by recent data showing that genetic factors play a greater role in determining the risk of premature mortality owing to sepsis than they do in influencing the risk of premature death from other common conditions, such as cancer or cardiovascular diseases. Beyond genetic variability, however, the management of patients with sepsis, and hence the outcome of the disease, is clearly influenced by factors such as the premorbid health status of the patient and the reversibility of concomitant diseases.

Infection

The site, type and extent of infection have a significant impact on prognosis. A bilateral bronchopneumonia is a more extensive process than a localized pneumonia, and a generalized faecal peritonitis is a more extensive process than appendicitis. Patients with secondary nosocomial bacteraemia experience a higher mortality than those with catheter-related or primary bacteraemia. Similarly, there is evidence that the endogenous host response to Gram-positive organisms differs from that evoked by Gram-negative organisms.

Response

In general, novel therapies for sepsis target the host response, rather than the infecting organism. The host response has proven to be difficult to characterize. Putative biologic markers of response severity include circulating levels of procalcitonin, interleukin-6 and many others.

Organ dysfunction

The severity of organ dysfunction is an important determinant of prognosis in sepsis. Whether the severity of organ dysfunction can aid in therapeutic stratification is less clear. Nevertheless, there is some evidence that neutralization of tumour necrosis factor, an early mediator in the inflammatory cascade, is more effective in patients without significant organ dysfunction, whereas activated protein C (APC) may provide more benefit to patients with greater as compared with lesser disease burden.

The potential utility of the proposed PIRO model lies in being able to discriminate morbidity arising from infection from morbidity arising from the response to infection. Interventions that modulate the response may impact adversely on the ability to contain an infection; conversely, interventions that target the infection are unlikely to be beneficial if the morbidity impact is being driven by the host response. Premorbid conditions establish a baseline risk, independent of the infectious process, whereas acquired organ dysfunction is an outcome to be prevented.

Pathophysiology

The inflammatory processes, which play a role in pathogenesis of diseases like severe infections, sepsis and septic shock, have certain similarities. They represent a physiologic host response by the immune system against endogenous (e.g. tissue necrosis) or exogenous (e.g. micro-organisms, trauma) stimuli to protect the organism and restore homeostasis. Hence, inflammation is an essential part of the innate as well as the adaptive immune system. In the initial phase, the inflammation is often a predominantly local syndrome with a more or less pronounced, transient systemic response. On the other hand, this SIRS is potentially harmful when it is part of a generally overwhelming process. This may lead to circulatory instability by vasodilatation owing to production of nitric oxide and ongoing microcirculatory failure ending with a single or combined organ dysfunction or failure.

The control of these local and systemic proinflammatory mechanisms by anti-inflammatory counterbalance is therefore an important protective process against further enhancement of inflammation. If, however, the anti-inflammatory reaction gets too strong, this may lead to decreased immune competency with so-called second-hit infections, for example, after major surgery. This is especially important for patients with sepsis after cardiothoracic surgery, who are often in an immunosuppressive phase.

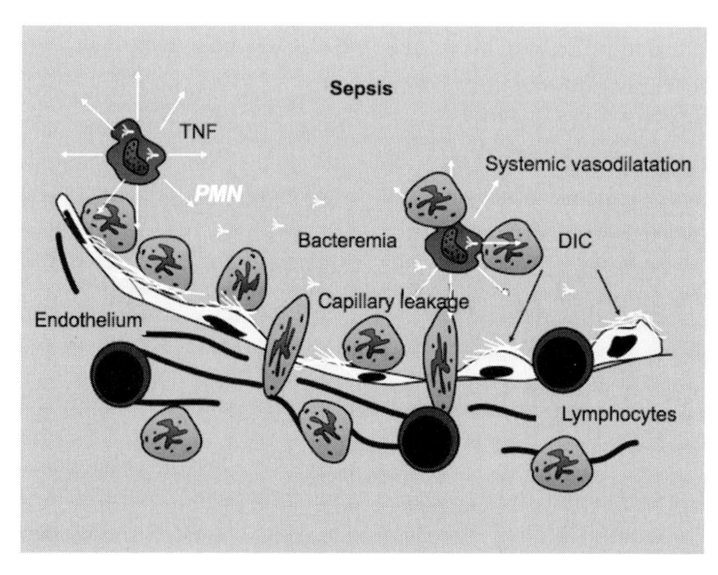

Figure 40.1 Systemic inflammation and microvascular failure. In case of systemic inflammation, the vascular endothelium is stimulated by cytokines like tumour necrosis factor (TNF), which stimulates a procoagulatory response with disseminated intravascular coagulation (DIC), a capillary leakage syndrome, adherence and transmigration of white blood cells and systemic vasodilatation with loss of peripheral vascular resistance followed by hypotension. PMN is polymorphonuclear cells.

Components of these pro- and anti-inflammatory processes are found in the innate immune system, mainly as endothelial cells, polymorphonuclear cells, macrophages, and so on, as well as in the adaptive immune system, represented by specific humoral B-cell and cellular T-cell immunity. Additional components are the coagulation as well as the complement system, eicosanoid metabolism and the endocrine system.

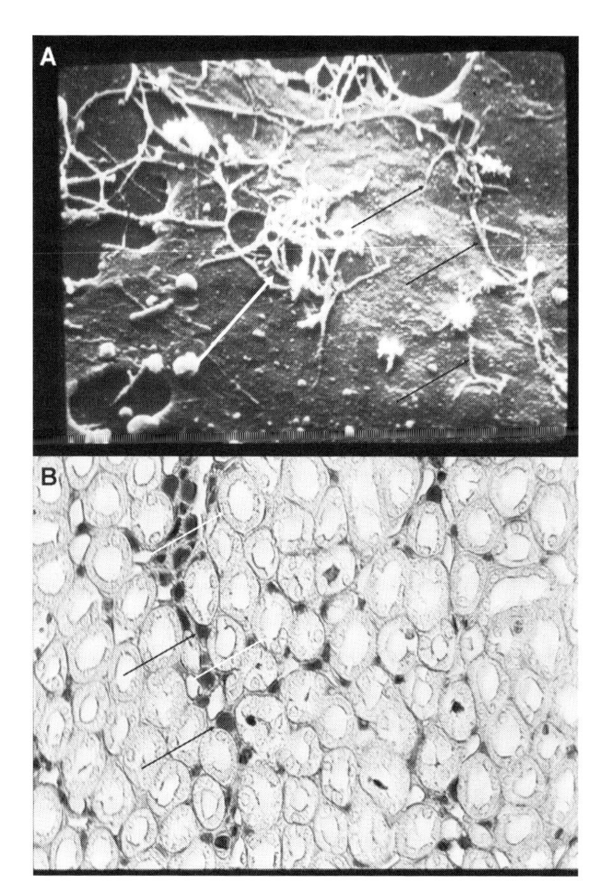

Figure 40.2 Microvascular clot formation and hypoperfusion. (*A*) After stimulation, the vascular endothelium starts to produce fibrin on the cellular surface (*black arrows*). The initial fibrin strings are combined, thus forming fibrin clots (*white arrow*). (*B*) Induction of acute renal failure in sepsis. Around the tubuli in the kidney (*white arrows*), the peritubular capillaries are filled with fibrin clots (*black arrows*), which induces acute renal failure.

Management of sepsis

The management of sepsis is significantly better today than it was 30 years ago, with the advent of a number of successful strategies. However, new strategies must be embraced to improve patient outcomes still further. Moreover, sepsis is an acute condition that kills rapidly and requires a combination of therapeutic approaches, because no single therapy is available that is capable of targeting the multiple pathophysiological components of either condition.

Initial resuscitation of septic patients

HAEMODYNAMIC SUPPORT

Fluid resuscitation should be commenced early to reverse hypotension, hypovolaemia and organ dysfunction and restore effective tissue perfusion and cellular metabolism. This may consist of natural or artificial colloids or crystalloids; there is no evidence-based support for one type of fluid over another. If fluid resuscitation fails to restore adequate arterial pressure and organ perfusion, vasopressors, and potentially inotropes, should be administered. Either noradrenaline or dopamine (through a central line as soon as available) is the first-choice vasopressor agent to correct hypotension in septic shock. Care must be taken when commencing patients on vasopressor or inotropic therapy because studies have indicated that their administration causes detrimental effects, including adverse vasoconstrictive effects, impaired splanchnic blood flow and oxygenation, reduced pH and negative effects on growth and thyroid hormones.

During the first 6 hours of treatment, the goals of initial resuscitation of sepsis-induced hypoperfusion (associated with hypotension or lactic acidosis) should be categorized.

SOURCE CONTROL

Every patient presenting with severe sepsis should be evaluated for the presence of a focus of

Table 40.2 Early goal-directed therapy of sepsis

The following goals should be achieved:
Central venous pressure: 8–12 mmHg (12–15 mmHg in mechanically ventilated patients)
Mean arterial pressure ≥65 mmHg
Urine output >0.5 mL/kg per hour
Central venous saturation ≥70%, or mixed venous O_2 [SvO_2] saturation ≥65%

potentially treatable infection. This may include the drainage of an abscess, the debridement of infected necrotic tissue, the removal of a potentially infected device or the definitive control of a source of ongoing microbial contamination. If surgical treatment is required, this should take place as soon as possible after initial resuscitation.

ANTIBIOTIC THERAPY

Initiating aggressive fluid resuscitation is the first priority when managing patients with severe sepsis or septic shock. However, prompt administration of antimicrobial agents is also required. Intravenous antibiotic therapy should be started within the first hour of recognition of severe sepsis after appropriate cultures have been obtained. This should include one or more drugs that have activity against the likely pathogens (bacterial or fungal) and penetrate into the presumed source of sepsis. The choice of drugs should be guided by the susceptibility patterns of micro-organisms in the community and in the hospital, and also depends on complex issues related to the patient's history (including drug intolerance) and the underlying disease.

Supportive measures

RENAL REPLACEMENT THERAPY

The incidence of renal failure requiring dialysis is low in sepsis patients (≤5%); however, the risk of mortality in sepsis patients with acute renal failure exceeds 50%.

LOW-PRESSURE VENTILATION

An estimated 25% to 42% of sepsis patients develop acute lung injury. The use of low tidal volumes (6 mL/kg ideal body weight) may reduce the risk of mortality in acute lung injury patients by up to 22% and increase the number of ventilator-free days in the first 28 days compared to conventional treatment.

MAINTENANCE OF NORMOGLYCAEMIA

In patients in critical care after surgery, intensive insulin therapy reduces in-hospital mortality and morbidity, and strict adherence to protocols is required.

Adjunctive therapies

LOW-DOSE CORTICOSTEROIDS

Corticosteroids are known to exert anti-inflammatory effects by inhibition of cellular signal transduction pathways, which are responsible for synthesis and expression of proinflammatory mediators. In low doses, steroids have been shown to reduce morbidity and mortality in septic shock patients. Infusion of hydrocortisone has been shown to lead to an increase in mean arterial pressure, systemic vascular resistance and a decline of heart rate, cardiac index and noradrenaline requirement. Hydrocortisone withdrawal has been shown to induce haemodynamic and immunological rebound effects.

Current evidence suggests that administration of individualized low-dose corticosteroids restores haemodynamic stability and differentially modulates the immunological response to stress by way of anti-inflammation rather than immunosuppression, which may play a major role in the management of septic shock patients, in conjunction with other therapeutic strategies.

ACTIVATED PROTEIN C

Physiologically, three main inhibitors are involved in the host defence against an overwhelming activation of coagulation during sepsis: the tissue factor pathway inhibitor, antithrombin and the protein C system. They are involved in controlling or decreasing the considerable amount of generated thrombin induced by the activation and release of tissue factor from monocytes and endothelium. Protein C is a serine protease, which is activated by endothelium-bound thrombomodulin, and – together with its cofactor protein S – inhibits the procoagulant factors Va and VIIIa. Activated protein C also acts as anti-inflammatory protein, by modulating intracellular signalling, cytokine secretion, cellular or lymphocyte apoptosis, and leukocyte–endothelial interactions.

Drotrecogin alpha (activated) is a recombinant human version of APC that represents the first therapy against sepsis to show efficacy in a Phase III clinical trial. This treatment exerts its effects by multiple modes of action: inhibition of coagulation, reduced inflammation and promotion of fibrinolysis. In addition to the significant mortality reductions, treatment with drotrecogin alpha (activated) has

Table 40.3 Sequential Organ Failure Assessment (SOFA) score

	0	1	2	3	4
Respiratory Pao_2/Fio_2 (mmHg)	>400	≤400	≤300	≤200	≤100
Coagulation Platelets ($10^3/mm^3$)	>150	≤150	≤100	≤50	≤20
Liver Bilirubin (μmol/L)	≤20	20–32	33–101	102–204	≥204 or support
Cardiovascular Hypotension	No hypotension	MAP ≤70 mmHg	Dopamine ≤5 μg/kg/min or dobutamine or phosphodiesterase inhibitor	Dopamine >5 μg/kg/min or adrenaline or noradrenaline ≤0.1 μg/kg/min	Dopamine >15 μg/kg/min or adrenaline or noradrenaline >0.1 μg/kg/min or circulatory assistance
Central nervous system Glasgow Coma Scale	15	13–14	10–12	6–9 or intracranial pressure	≤6
Renal Creatinine, μmol/L (or urine output)	≤110	110–170	171–299	300–440 (or ≤500 mL/d)	>440 or (≤200 mL/d) or renal replacement therapy

Abbreviation: MAP, mean arterial pressure.

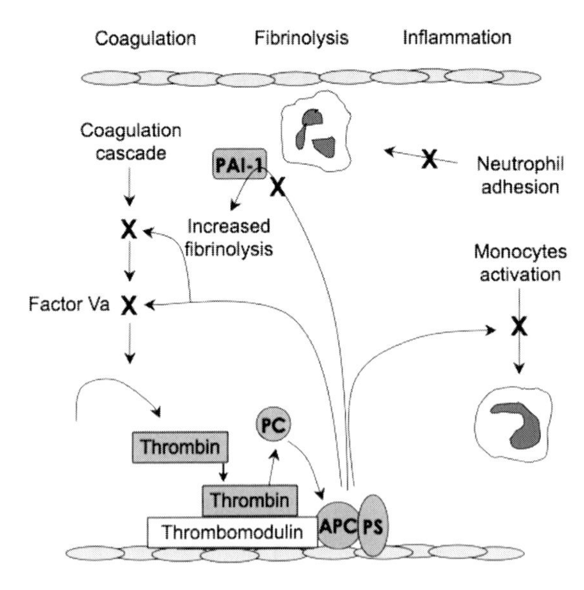

Figure 40.3 Effect of APC on the response to sepsis.

been shown to reduce cardiovascular and respiratory organ dysfunction in the first 7 days; mortality reductions were achieved at the expense of a modest 1.4% increase in the risk of serious bleeding.

To assess morbidity in these patients, Sequential Organ Failure Assessment (SOFA) scores for cardiovascular, respiratory, renal, haematologic and hepatic organ systems were measured for 28 days. Mean cardiovascular SOFA scores were significantly lower for patients treated with drotrecogin alpha (activated) compared with placebo patients over this time period.

Table 40.4 The surviving sepsis resuscitation bundle

Goals to be achieved within the first 6 hours after diagnosis of sepsis:
Serum lactate measured
Blood cultures obtained prior to antibiotic administration
Broad-spectrum antibiotics administered within 1 hour
Initial minimum volume of 20 mL/kg of crystalloid (or colloid equivalent)
Apply vasopressors for hypotension
Achieve central venous pressure of >8 mmHg
Achieve central venous oxygen saturation of >70%

Table 40.5 The surviving sepsis management bundle

Goals to be achieved within the first 24 hours after diagnosis of sepsis:
Administration of low-dose steroids in case of refractory septic shock
Administration of drotrecogin alpha (activated) according to standardized critical care policy
Glucose maintained ≤8.3 mmol/L
Inspiratory plateau pressure maintained ≤30 cmH_2O in ventilated patients

'BUNDLES'

Recently published research has shown that reductions in mortality are achievable, and that an incremental, combination therapy-based approach is the key to diminishing sepsis-associated mortality. The Surviving Sepsis Campaign is targeted to implement a core set of management protocols in hospital environments where change in behaviour and clinical impact can be measured. The first step in this next phase will be to deploy a 'change bundle.' Recent data reveal that the implementation of bundles in critical care is able to reduce mortality.

Key points

- Severe sepsis and septic shock have an increasing incidence, and the mortality rate of more than 50% is unacceptably high.
- The balance between pro- and anti-inflammatory mechanisms is crucial for adequate host response.
- Fast haemodynamic stabilization and immediate antibiotic therapy are the key points for initial resuscitation of the septic patient.
- Implementing bundle strategies improves process quality and is probably reducing mortality.

FURTHER READING

Cohen J. The immunopathogenesis of sepsis. *Nature* 2002;420:885–891.

Dellinger RP, Carlet J, Masur H, *et al*. Surviving Sepsis Campaign guidelines for management of severe sepsis and septic shock. *Intensive Care Med* 2004;30:536–555.

Kortgen A, Niederprum P, Bauer M. Implementation of an evidence-based "standard operating procedure" and outcome in septic shock. *Crit Care Med* 2006;34:943–949.

Levy M, Fink MP, Marshall JC, *et al*. 2001 SCCM/ESICM/ACCP/ATS/SIS International Sepsis Definitions Conference. *Intensive Care Med* 2003;29:530–538.

Chapter 41

Infection control

G.M. JOYNT AND C.D. GOMERSALL

Introduction

Infection is a major cause of death and morbidity in hospitals. A large proportion of these infections are acquired in the hospital and the term 'nosocomial infection' refers to infection that was neither present nor incubating at the time of hospital admission, but acquired by the patient during his or her hospital stay. The risk of nosocomial infection in the critical care unit is particularly high, and the attributable morbidity, mortality and financial costs are substantial. It is often forgotten that critical care unit staff are also at risk of exposure to cross-infection and its negative consequences.

The goal of infection control is to identify, prevent and control nosocomial infections of patients and staff by implementing strategies based on sound scientific principles and epidemiologic techniques.

There is now good evidence supporting positive outcomes after implementation of several individual infection control procedures, and the implementation of a comprehensive infection control programme that systematically incorporates individual components remains the best method for achieving positive outcomes.

Infection control programme

An infection control team should be responsible for determining policies and procedures, and ensuring disciplined implementation. To achieve this, the membership of the team must include senior management, medical and nursing staff with sufficient authority to approve and implement policy.

The essential components of an infection control programme are:

- Development and implementation of measures to prevent transmission of infectious agents and to reduce risks for device- and procedure-related infections.
- Surveillance to monitor patients and health care personnel for acquisition of infection and/or colonization.
- Investigation of infection problems identified by surveillance or relevant individual observations.
- Effective management of identified infection problems and outbreaks.

The programme should have mechanisms to ensure that all personnel working inside a patient setting must receive documented training and updates on infection control procedures. There should also be regular audit of compliance with policies, as well as review of surveillance of infection patterns to assess program performance. Audit and surveillance data should be benchmarked against relevant local and external sources.

Measures to prevent transmission of infectious agents

The approach to minimizing or eliminating cross-infection is based on strategies that interrupt recognized methods of transmission.

Table 41.1 Methods of transmission of infection

Direct contact transmits organisms from body surfaces, surgical wound or secretions to staff hands and then to a second patient's body surface.
Indirect contact occurs when the transmission from body surfaces secretions or hands to the next patient occurs via a contaminated object.
Droplet transmission of exhaled particles (>5 μm in diameter) is promoted by speaking, coughing, sneezing or interventions such as suction, but droplets are usually spread only a short distance as they do not remain suspended in air very long.
Airborne transmission of droplet nuclei ($\leq$5 μm in diameter) is promoted by coughing in particular and particles remain suspended in air for long periods increasing potential transmission distance.
Common vehicle transmission describes spread through inanimate objects, nonsterile fluids, and instruments such as laryngoscopes, bronchoscopes and stethoscopes.

Isolation measures

Based on the method of transmission, specific infection isolation methods to protect patients and health care staff from cross-infection have been devised.

High-risk procedures

Certain high-risk procedures increase the risk of infectious disease transmission, both to health care staff and other patients.

These procedures should be performed in isolation rooms with appropriate ventilation (8–12 air changes per hour), with staff protected by high-grade personal protective equipment (PPE) as for airborne precautions.

The transport of potentially infectious patients should be for essential purposes only and suitable precautions should be taken to reduce transmission risks. These may include a mask (or bacterial/viral filter if intubated) of the appropriate efficiency for the patient while in transit as well as provision of all transporting staff, including assisting staff, with appropriate PPE. Ensure the removal of unnecessary personnel, patients or public from transport routes and elevators.

Environmental infection control

There should be adequate procedures for the routine care, cleaning and disinfection of environmental surfaces. Often forgotten surfaces in this category include keyboards and telephones. Frequent cleansing and disinfection of high-use objects in patient areas can be achieved with hypochlorite-based solutions or other hospital-use approved detergent/disinfectant. For large blood or body fluid spills, use a 1:100 dilution (500–615 ppm available chlorine) to decontaminate nonporous surfaces after cleaning. Disposable barrier coverings for keyboards and similar objects should be considered.

Personal equipment such as pagers, mobile phones and pens may also become contaminated and should never be handled in the clinical area without prior handwashing. Also avoid unnecessary touching of beds, bedrails and bedside equipment such as stethoscopes, measuring tapes and torches.

Hand cleansing

There is good epidemiologic evidence to suggest that organisms are carried from one patient to another via the hands of health care personnel.

Table 41.2 Methods to prevent transmission of infection

Standard precautions – should be practiced at all times in critical care
- Hands must be cleansed before and after every patient contact.
- Gloves, gowns and eye protection must be used in situations where exposure to body secretions or blood is considered possible.
- Sharp instruments and needles must be disposed of safely in special containers.
- Soiled linens must be disposed of in impervious bags.
- Blood, faeces, urine and substances significantly contaminated with them must be disposed of in proper sanitary facilities.

Droplet precautions – for all severe community-acquired respiratory infections, until the organism is identified (e.g. influenza, *Neisseria meningitides*)
- Patients should be isolated in single rooms.
- Wear a good-quality surgical face-mask when within 1–2 m of the patient.
- Eye protection such as visors or goggles are optional and depend on specific circumstances (e.g. excessive patient coughing, closeness of contact and need for performing high-risk procedures).

Airborne precautions – suspected or confirmed infections known to be airborne, or newly recognized infections before methods of spread are known (e.g. tuberculosis, measles, varicella)
- Patients require single isolation rooms with negative air pressure and a minimum of 8–12 air changes per hour
- When entering the room, wear a mask respirator with a particle filtering capacity of ≥95% that allows a tight seal over the nose and mouth. Individuals should have been 'fit tested' to establish which make of mask is most suitable. Correct mask placement technique is important.
- Eye protection such as full-face shields or goggles are optional and depend on specific circumstances (e.g. excessive patient coughing, closeness of contact, need for high-risk procedures).

Contact precautions – infections that can be spread by direct patient contact or by indirect contact with inanimate objects and/or environmental surfaces (e.g. respiratory viruses, enteric viruses, *Clostridium difficile*), multiple drug resistant organisms, including methicillin-resistant *Staphylococcus aureus*.
- Patients should be isolated or cohorted with patients who have the same infection.
- Wear gloves and an apron for all patient contact.
- Wear gowns if there is likely to be prolonged direct contact with the patient (daily clinical examination) or any infective material.
- All protective equipment must be removed before exiting infected areas.

Table 41.3 High-risk procedures for transmission of infection

High-risk procedures
- Nebulization
- Bag-mask ventilation
- Endotracheal intubation
- Bronchoscopy
- Endoscopy
- Cardiopulmonary resuscitation

Hand cleansing is possibly the single most important infection control measure when managing critically ill patients. It is important to note that gloves do not replace hand cleansing. Washing gloves, spraying gloves with antiseptic or double gloving to allow continual use is not recommended. When wearing gloves, to avoid cross-infecting other patients and contaminating environmental surfaces, health care workers must change gloves after

Table 41.4 Key aspects of hand cleansing

Regular educational campaigns should stress and audit good hand-cleansing technique.
Cleanse hands after touching blood, body fluids, secretions, excretions, and contaminated items, whether or not gloves are worn.
Wash hands before and immediately after every patient contact.
Use antimicrobial soap for routine hand washing, especially if hands are visibly dirty.
Use a waterless, alcohol-based antiseptic hand rub such as chlorhexidine in alcohol if hands are not visibly dirty.
Wash hands or use hand rub before putting on a pair of new gloves and immediately after gloves are removed.
Cleanse hands between touching different body sites in the same patient when indicated.

all procedures and in between patients. The technique of hand cleansing is simple to learn, but is often not properly performed and rules about when to wash are inconsistently followed.

To be able to achieve high hand cleansing compliance, regular, repeated educational campaigns are needed and cleansing facilities must be immediately and conveniently available. In this regard the liberal distribution of waterless antiseptic dispensers throughout the critical care unit is easily achieved and cost effective.

Personal protective equipment

When using specialized PPE, staff must always carefully follow manufacturer's instructions on proper use and always seek advice in case of doubt. The following general principles are crucial:

- Remove gloves and other PPE promptly after use, before touching noncontaminated items and environmental surfaces in the critical care unit – never walk around, answer phones or write notes with gloves on.
- Used PPE should be treated as contaminated and should not be taken out of the workplace into nonclinical areas except during patient transport.
- Remove a soiled PPE as promptly as possible, and wash hands or shower to avoid micro-organism spread to yourself or others.
- Implement protocols to ensure that reusable equipment is not used for the care of another patient until it has been cleaned and reprocessed appropriately. Ensure that single-use items are discarded immediately and properly.

Measures to reduce risks for device- and procedure-related infections

Common device- and procedure-related infections in critically ill patients include:

- nosocomial and ventilator-associated pneumonia;
- surgical site infections;
- catheter-related infections;
- urinary tract infections in catheterized patients; and
- sinusitis.

There are well-established infection control procedures that minimize the important device- and procedure-related infections.

Antibiotic prophylaxis is particularly important for the reduction of surgical site and other postoperative infections in patients who have undergone cardiopulmonary bypass surgery, which is associated with a substantial systemic inflammatory response.

Table 41.5 Infection control interventions that have been shown to reduce the incidence of nosocomial pneumonia

Established interventions

The institution of an educational and infection control program targeting nosocomial pneumonia.
Hand washing before and after patient contact.
Avoid intubation where possible (use of noninvasive ventilation in appropriate patient groups).
Use orotracheal instead of nasotracheal intubation.
Avoid reintubation.
Weekly ventilator circuit changes (not more frequently).
Nursing patients in semirecumbent position (30–45 degrees), particularly when receiving enteral feed to prevent aspiration.
Minimizing blood transfusion.
Avoiding paralysis and deep sedation in intubated, mechanically ventilated patients.
Encourage deep breaths, movement about the bed, and early ambulation.
Incentive spirometry for patients at high-risk of pneumonia.

Controversial methods with some evidence-based support

Selective decontamination of the digestive tract may be useful in units where the incidence of multi-drug-resistant pathogens is low.
Continuous aspiration of subglottic secretions via special endotracheal tube.
Isolation of patients with multi-drug-resistant pathogens.
Rotation of empirical antibiotic choices.
Immunonutrition.

Medical devices such as catheters and drains must be removed as soon as they are no longer required.

Sterility and asepsis

Procedures and equipment should always be kept as clean as possible. Certain emergency procedures in critically ill patients require the need for sterile technique in addition to general antisepsis and cleanliness. Sterile technique is required for central venous catheter placement, urinary catheter placement, percutaneous chest drain placement and blood cultures. Aseptic technique is sufficient for

Table 41.6 Infection control interventions that have been shown to reduce the incidence of surgical site infections

Appropriate use of prophylactic antibiotics. Antibiotics must be circulating at the start of the operation and must be maintained in an adequate concentration during the entire operation and the immediate postoperative period. Antibiotics should be continued for no longer than 24–48 hours.

Perform proper skin preparation using appropriate antiseptic agents.

When necessary, use appropriate hair removal techniques – clipping rather than shaving.

Monitor and maintain normoglycaemia.

Maintain normothermia.

Strict adherence to standard precautions, and if indicated, contact precautions when undertaking wound care.

Table 41.7 Infection control interventions that have been shown to influence the incidence of catheter-related infections

The unnecessary use of central venous catheters must be avoided.

The strict implementation of systems for educating nurses and doctors about infection control, standardization of catheter insertion and the care process reduces infection.

Specific preventive measures include

Use a central venous catheter with the minimum number of ports or lumens essential for the management of the patient.

Use a sterile insertion technique including the use of a mask, sterile gown, sterile gloves and a large sterile sheet for both new site insertion or guidewire exchange. Chlorhexidine 0.5% (1:200) in 70% alcohol is recommended to clean the skin.

Consider the risk/benefit ratio of the site in individual cases.

Reduced infectious complications occur at the subclavian site (rather than a jugular or femoral site) in adult patients, but the risk for mechanical complications may be higher (e.g. pneumothorax, arterial puncture, vein laceration, subclavian vein stenosis, haemothorax, air embolism or catheter misplacement)

Use of antibiotic impregnated catheters. Routine use is not recommended, but may be cost effective when the catheter is expected to remain in place >5 days, in patients at high risk of catheter-related infections and in whom treatment may be complicated (e.g. severely immunocompromised patients)

Despite infection control disadvantages, catheters used for haemodialysis should be placed in a jugular or femoral vein rather than a subclavian vein to avoid subclavian vein stenosis.

Catheter replacement

It is not advantageous to routinely replace central venous catheters solely for the purpose of reducing the incidence of infection.

It is not advantageous to remove central venous catheters on the basis of fever alone. Clinical judgment should determine the appropriateness of removing the catheter if infection is present elsewhere or if a noninfectious cause of fever is suspected.

Replacement of catheters by guidewire exchange techniques with appropriate catheter and blood specimen surveillance is acceptable. In patients strongly suspected of having catheter-related infection, or if specimens return positive, a new catheter must be placed at a different site.

Catheter care

Do not unnecessarily interfere with catheter hubs and three-way taps. Multiple catheter manipulations increase the risk of catheter-related infections.

Use transparent dressings as a routine and do not routinely use topical antibiotic ointment or creams on insertion sites.

Replace dressing when the catheter is removed or replaced, the dressing becomes damp, loosened or soiled or inspection of the site is necessary.

Replace gauze dressing every 2 days and transparent dressings every 7 days on short-term catheters.

Infusate care

Unless clinically indicated, replace administration sets at 72-hour intervals

Replace blood product or lipid emulsion administration tubing within 24 hours.

Table 41.8 Infection control interventions that have been shown to reduce the incidence of catheter-associated urinary tract infections

Avoid unnecessary catheterization.
Minimize duration of catheterization (consider using condom catheter).
Use sterile technique on insertion.
Minimize manipulations and if the catheter or drainage system is manipulated, maintain strict sterility.
Bladder irrigation with antibiotic solutions, application of local antibiotics or other antimicrobial agents do not reduce catheter-associated urinary tract infections.
There is some evidence supporting not routinely changing catheters at regular intervals.
Note: Treatment of asymptomatic bacteria does not reduce the incidence of febrile episodes and increases the risk of colonization with multi-drug-resistant bacteria.

peripheral venous cannula placement and arterial catheter placement.

Antibiotic use and infection control

Early, appropriate administration of antibiotics in critical illness is associated with improved outcomes. However, exposure of bacteria to antibiotics leads to antibiotic resistance. Antibiotic resistance is rapidly becoming a major infection control problem in critically ill patients. To avoid multi-antibiotic resistance, it is essential to try to avoid unnecessary and broad-spectrum antibiotic use. This can be done by rigorously applying the following important principles.

- Only use antibacterial antibiotics if bacterial infection is suspected.
- Use antibiotics in sufficient dosage.
- Use the narrowest spectrum antibiotic appropriate for the clinical setting.
- Adjust antibiotics on the basis of culture results – usually to less broad-spectrum combinations or single agents.
- Stop antibiotics as soon as possible.

Prevention of specific infections and staff protection

Staff immunization is sometimes required to protect against microbial threats such as influenza or hepatitis B. Postexposure prophylaxis and follow-up (e.g. after HIV or hepatitis B exposure) should be available if required. Postexposure follow-up

Table 41.9 Important components of sterile and aseptic techniques in the critical care unit

Sterile technique
All articles used in the procedure have been sterilized.
Only persons who are sterile may touch sterile articles.
Wear a surgical mask.
Wash hands thoroughly for one minute using an antimicrobial hand wash and apply sterile gown and gloves.
Note that once worn, gowns are considered sterile only from the waist to shoulder level in front, and to 2 inches above the elbows.
Cleanse skin (large field) with chlorhexidine.
Chlorhexidine 0.5% (1:200) in 70% alcohol is the agent of choice to clean the working surface/skin.
After cleansing, create a large sterile area with the use of sterile drapes.
The equipment tray is sterile and should only be touched by sterile persons.
Aseptic technique
Gloves, but usually not a gown are worn.
The surface is cleaned in the same way as for the sterile technique, but sterile drapes are used to protect only the immediate working area.

programmes after exposure to hepatitis C should also be available. Health care staff potentially exposed to tuberculosis should also undergo appropriate evaluation, follow-up and treatment if required. Institutional guidelines and procedures should be followed when exposures such as these have potentially occurred.

Surveillance

Surveillance programmes are designed to establish baseline rates and susceptibility patterns of microorganisms, evaluate the impact of specific control measures, identify possible outbreaks and high-risk patient groups, with the objective of reducing the morbidity, mortality and costs associated with infection. It is also becoming increasingly necessary to perform surveillance to meet compliance requirements with accrediting and regulatory agencies that use surveillance data to assess unit performance. There are established surveillance programmes such as the National Nosocomial Infections Surveillance System (NNIS) managed by the Centers for Disease Control and Prevention (CDC) and the Health Protection Agency that offer standardized definitions and freely available benchmarking data. Some data specifically generated for cardiothoracic units are reported by NNIS.

At a practical level, efficient surveillance requires that individual critical care units have sufficient infection control personnel to collect the data, standardized protocols and definitions of infections and sufficient numbers of beds to yield enough cases of hospital-acquired infection for reliable estimation of the incidence and trends over time.

Investigation and management of infection control problems

Surveillance data should identify potential infection problems in the critical care unit and may necessitate a review of the existing infection control programme. If the problem is sufficiently severe, directed intervention may be necessary. A description of the detailed management of infectious disease outbreaks is beyond the scope of this chapter; however, this type of intervention commonly takes the form of the introduction of a short-term eradication programme involving the use of combinations of one or more of selective decontamination of the digestive tract or other methods of reducing colonization, high-grade antibiotic prophylaxis and high-grade infection control precautions. Specialist assistance for outbreak management is available from many governmental organizations such as the Health Protection Agency in the United Kingdom, and the CDC in the United States.

Key points

- Handwashing is the single most important infection control measure and all staff should wash hands or use alcoholic hand rub before and after every patient contact.
- Antibiotic prophylaxis is important for the reduction of surgical site and other postoperative infections.
- Antibiotic treatment should focus on narrow-spectrum drugs, selected on the basis of culture results and stopped as soon as possible, based on microbiological advice.
- Medical devices such as catheters and drains should be removed as soon as they are no longer required.

FURTHER READING

Department of Health and Human Services, The Centers for Disease Control and Prevention (CDC) [homepage on the Internet]. Infection Control in Healthcare Settings. Available at: www.cdc.gov/ncidod/dhqp/index.html; www.cdc.gov/ncidod/dhqp/nnis_pubs.html.

Health Protection Agency (HPA) [homepage on the Internet]. Centre for Infections, Epidemiology and Surveillance. Available at: www.hpa.org.uk/cfi/about/epidem_surveil.htm.

Chapter 42

Infective endocarditis

J.M. BYGOTT AND J.E. FOWERAKER

Definition

Infective endocarditis (IE) is an endovascular microbial infection of cardiovascular structures (such as native valves and atrial or ventricular endocardium) and/or intracardiac foreign bodies (such as prosthetic valves, pacemaker or intracardiac defibrillator leads and surgically created conduits). It most commonly affects sites where turbulent blood flow or endothelial damage encourages formation of platelet thrombi, offering a protected area where micro-organisms can adhere and replicate. Lesions may be friable, producing systemic emboli. Complications related to IE may necessitate critical care admission. Difficult to diagnose, IE often requires prolonged medical therapy; surgical intervention may be necessary. It is uniformly fatal if untreated.

Epidemiology

Despite modern antibiotic and surgical therapy, mortality rates remain around 25%, with death resulting primarily from congestive heart failure, sepsis and central nervous system embolic events. Historically, IE was closely linked to rheumatic heart disease, with bacteraemia of oral or dental origin the usual source of infection. But owing to a dramatic decrease in rheumatic fever in developed countries and the use of antibiotics with the emergence of antibiotic-resistant organisms, the organisms causing the disease and the sites of infection have changed.

The proportion of patients with no known pre-existing cardiac lesion has risen to over 50%. The advent of high-dependency care, transplant surgery and the wide range of intravascular devices have created a new population at risk of nosocomial IE.

Pathogenesis

Normal vascular endothelium is resistant to microbial infection, but damage to the endothelial surface of the heart or blood vessels induces platelet and thrombin deposition, producing thrombotic vegetations to which micro-organisms can bind. Endocarditis is classically associated with 'jet lesions' where blood flowing from a high-pressure area through an orifice to an area of lower pressure produces a high-velocity jet. Vegetations are usually found in the lower pressure area, for example, on the atrial surface of the mitral valve.

Low-grade pathogens can bind to damaged valves (e.g. viridans streptococci), whereas high-grade pathogens such as *Staphylococcus aureus* may affect normal valves.

Clinical features

Bacteraemia

Infective endocarditis is characterized by a constant bacteraemia, which may present as pyrexia, rigors, malaise, anorexia, headache, confusion and arthralgia. However, in the elderly, fever may be absent.

Table 42.1 Predisposing conditions

Congenital heart disease
Septal defects (usually ventricular)
Degenerative valve disease
Rheumatic heart disease
Mural thrombus
Intravenous drug abuse (right-sided infections)
Cardiac surgery, including mechanical and bioprosthetic valves

Tissue destruction

Endocarditis classically affects valve cusps, leaflets or chordae tendinae. Tissue destruction results in valvular incompetence, cusp perforation or rupture of the chordae producing a cardiac murmur that may change in character with time. Infection may progress and extend beyond the valve into the paravalvular structures. Aortic root abscess is a serious complication. When the abscess extends through the aortic wall into other tissues or cavities, a fistula or pseudoaneurysm may be formed. Involvement of the conducting tissue leads to heart block.

Infection of a mechanical valve often involves the sewing ring and may produce annular abscess, paravalvular leak and prosthetic dehiscence. Infection of a bioprosthetic valve may also involve the valve leaflets, resulting in destruction or perforation and consequent valvular incompetence. Large vegetations may obstruct a prosthetic valve, but rarely a native valve.

Embolization

Emboli are reported in 20% to 40% of cases and may present as a cerebrovascular accident, arterial occlusion of a limb, myocardial infarction, sudden unilateral blindness or infarction of the spleen or kidney. In right-sided endocarditis, recurrent septic pulmonary emboli may be misinterpreted as pneumonia. Emboli usually occur before or within a few days of starting antimicrobial therapy. Mycotic aneurysms may occur in the cerebral circulation and have been reported in 3% of clinical cases but found in 15% of cases at autopsy. They may produce subarachnoid haemorrhage.

Circulating immune complexes

Immune complex deposition may cause many of the extracardiac manifestations of IE. However, these classic signs are relatively uncommon. They include splinter haemorrhages, Osler nodes, Roth spots and vasculitic rash. Splenomegaly is noted on computed tomography in at least 50% of patients. Immune complex deposition can cause glomerulonephritis, and proteinuria; haematuria and cellular urinary casts are common.

Aggressive endocarditis

Damaging and rapidly progressive IE may be caused by certain highly pathogenic organisms, including *S. aureus*. In contrast with less aggressive infections, there is high fever, large vegetations develop quickly, significant valve failure occurs early and septic emboli are more common, with a resultant higher case fatality rate.

Nosocomial endocarditis

This is a complication of nosocomial bacteraemia. The probability of IE increases if bacteraemia persists for more than 36 to 48 hours. The importance of early removal of infected intravascular lines and prompt treatment of other infections is paramount in reducing the risk of bacteraemia. Transplant patients are at particular risk of nosocomial endocarditis because of the atrial and large-vessel suture lines. Repeated biopsy of the right ventricle may add risk by injury to the tricuspid valve and ventricular endocardium.

Prosthetic valve endocarditis

Prosthetic valve endocarditis occurs in 1% to 5% of patients with valvular prostheses. Prosthetic valve

Table 42.2 Causative organisms, native versus prosthetic valve endocarditis

Organism	Native and late prosthetic valve (%)	Early prosthetic valve (≤60 d) (%)
Streptococcus spp.	52	3
Enterococcus spp.	11	8
Staphylococcus aureus	11–35	22
Coagulase-negative staphylococci	8	32
Coxiella burnetii	2	≤1
Gram-negative bacteria, HACEK	1–3	11
Fungi	≤1	1–7

endocarditis is five times more common with aortic than mitral prostheses. Early prosthetic valve endocarditis (within 60 days of surgery) accounts for 30% of cases. This is caused by either contamination of the prosthetic valve at implantation or early postoperative bacteraemia. The commonest organisms are usually coagulase-negative staphylococci, such as *S. epidermidis*.

Factors associated with poor outcome include *S. aureus* infection, early prosthetic valve endocarditis, heart failure and neurological complications. Septic shock and mediastinitis are predictive of increased mortality.

Endocarditis in the critical care setting

For the subset of patients with complications of IE requiring critical care admission, there is high morbidity and mortality. Overall in-hospital mortality may be as high as 45%. Congestive heart failure during the course of IE is a well-known reason for critical care admission. Neurological complications such as cerebral emboli or brain haemorrhage are found in up to 60% of cases of IE admitted to critical care. *S aureus* is likely to be the predominant organism causing IE in patients admitted to critical care (>50% in some studies) because of its high rate of complications.

Any patient with a persistent fever after surgery, especially after valve or transplant surgery, must be investigated for IE. These investigations may need to be repeated at regular intervals; diagnosis in critically ill patients is often difficult.

Diagnosis

Laboratory

BLOOD CULTURES

Blood cultures are integral to IE diagnosis. Isolation of the organism enables an effective antibiotic treatment regimen to be devised. Bacteraemia in IE is usually constant; when blood cultures are taken they are usually all positive. Three sets of blood cultures are recommended (a total of 30–60 mL of blood), ideally a minimum of 1 hour apart, from different venepuncture sites. Taking multiple sets can help to assess the relevance of bacteria such as coagulase-negative staphylococci, which can cause endocarditis but are also common skin contaminants. The frequency of blood culture-negative endocarditis is around 5%. This is usually due to prior administration of antibiotics. Stopping antibiotics and reculturing may help to isolate an organism; it may take up to 4 days after stopping antibiotics before bacteraemia can be detected.

BLOOD TESTS

An elevated C-reactive protein and erythrocyte sedimentation rate are almost invariable and can be useful in monitoring response to therapy. A polymorphonuclear leukocytosis is found in the majority of cases and normocytic normochromic anaemia is often present. Serum antibodies to atypical organisms should also be sought.

OTHER

Culture of emboli from skin lesions may be important in making a diagnosis where blood cultures are negative (e.g. in fungal infections). After cardiac surgery, tissue specimens become available for culture and microscopy; it is important that specimens are sent to microbiology and not all sent to histopathology in formalin. Cardiac tissue from culture-negative endocarditis can also be tested by polymerase chain reaction.

Echocardiography

Echocardiography can demonstrate vegetations as small as 1 to 2 mm; it may also demonstrate abnormal blood flow patterns and detect intracardiac abscesses. Visualization is more difficult with prosthetic valves, especially echodense mechanical valves. A negative result does not exclude endocarditis. Echocardiography should be performed as soon as possible in suspected cases of endocarditis. This is normally done with transthoracic echocardiography. Transoesophageal echocardiography has improved the rate of diagnosis, especially in the presence of a prosthetic valve. Transoesophageal echocardiography reveals vegetations in 25% or more of cases with negative transthoracic echocardiography and also has much better specificity. It also makes it easier to visualize complications such as abscess, fistula and paravalvular leak.

Criteria for diagnosis

The 'Duke Criteria' are diagnostic and investigational criteria that are used in suspected cases of IE. Major diagnostic criteria include positive blood cultures or positive echocardiogram.

Table 42.3 The Duke Criteria

Major

- Positive blood culture either with an organism recognized to cause endocarditis or >1 positive culture >12 hours apart, or 3 positives from 3 cultures drawn ≥1 hour apart.
- Evidence of endocardial damage: Echocardiographic evidence of vegetations on valves or supporting structures, on an implant or in the turbulent path of a high-flow jet; or new valvular regurgitation.

Minor

- Known predisposition to endocarditis.
- Temperature ≥38°C.
- Evidence of focal vasculitis or emboli.
- Immunological features.
- Single positive blood culture or blood culture of uncertain significance.
- Serological evidence of infection known to cause endocarditis.
- Echocardiographic finding of uncertain significance.

Clinical criteria: 2 major criteria; 1 major and 3 minor; or 5 minor criteria.

Microbiology

Although almost any micro-organism can cause IE, certain species are more likely to be implicated. Overall, viridans streptococci and staphylococci account for about two thirds of all cases.

STREPTOCOCCI

Viridans-type streptococci are the commonest cause of community-acquired IE and late-onset prosthetic valve endocarditis. These streptococci are part of the normal oropharyngeal flora. They are organisms of low virulence and thus usually only infect previously abnormal heart valves. Lower rates of microbiological relapse and mortality have traditionally been associated with viridans streptococci. Common species include *S sanguis*, *S mutans* and *S oralis*.

Pyogenic streptococci (haemolytic streptococci) are more aggressive and may affect a previously normal valve. Group B streptococcus (*S. agalactiae*) is the commonest cause. This organism is found in normal flora in the genital and gastrointestinal tracts.

Streptococcus pneumoniae endocarditis is rarely seen, although it is sometimes diagnosed at autopsy of patients with overwhelming pneumococcal infection.

ENTEROCOCCI

Enterococci form part of the normal gastrointestinal flora. They are more virulent but still of low pathogenicity, and more resistant to antibiotics. Most cases of enterococcal IE are community acquired, although they may occasionally follow urinary tract instrumentation or line-related infection.

STAPHYLOCOCCI

S. aureus is an important and aggressive pathogen in community-acquired IE and is also the commonest cause of hospital-acquired disease. Methicillin-resistant strains (MRSA) are now commonly encountered. Prosthetic valve infection may be associated with sternal wound sepsis. *S. aureus* is the commonest pathogen causing endocarditis in intravenous drug users.

Coagulase-negative staphylococci, such as *S. epidermidis*, are mostly pathogens of prosthetic valves. These organisms are usually of low pathogenicity; however, due to their prolific growth in biofilms, they may be difficult to eradicate from prosthetic material.

OTHER ORGANISMS

The species of the HACEK group are fastidious slow-growing organisms that are oropharyngeal commensals and have a predilection for heart valves, such that their presence in blood cultures is virtually synonymous with IE. The group consists of *Haemophilus spp. (aphrophilus/paraphrophilus)*, *Actinobacillus actinomycetemcomitans*, *Cardiobacterium hominis*, *Eikenella corrodens* and *Kingella kingae*. Vegetations with these organisms are classically large, usually the result of diagnostic delay and prolonged illness.

ORGANISMS THAT CANNOT BE ROUTINELY CULTURED

Coxiella burnetii (Q-fever), *Bartonella* spp., *Chlamydia* spp. and *Brucella* spp. infection usually affects patient with preexisting valve lesions. Diagnosis usually relies on serology.

Fungal endocarditis is very rare and more likely to occur on prosthetic than native valves, or in intravenous drug users. Most infections are nosocomially acquired: broad-spectrum antibiotic treatment predisposes to *Candida* infection. Blood cultures are only intermittently positive with *Candida*. For other fungi (e.g. *Aspergillus*) diagnosis is usually made by culture of the fungus from the excised valve or detection on valve histology.

Treatment

Close liaison between clinicians and microbiologists is recommended in devising an appropriate antibiotic regimen. Careful susceptibility testing should be done on isolates by testing the mean inhibitory concentration of the antibiotic.

High antibiotic doses are required, usually given intravenously for the duration of treatment. Dose of antibiotic and course duration depends on the isolate, degree of antibiotic susceptibility and whether a native or prosthetic valve is involved. Frequently, antibiotic combinations are given for synergy.

Because of the difficulty in reaching a diagnosis, empiric treatment may occasionally be necessary. In patients who have been chronically unwell for many weeks, antibiotic treatment can often be deferred until blood cultures are positive and the pathogen is known.

Resolving fever and stabilization of cardiac function are signs that infection is resolving. The C-reactive protein is a useful monitor of progress.

Table 42.4 Summary of recommendations for the treatment of infective endocarditis

Empirical treatment

Clinical course	Recommended	Alternatives
Aggressive IE	Flucloxacillin 8–12 g IV daily in 4–6 divided doses plus gentamicin 1 mg/kg IV 8-hourly	If penicillin allergy, intracardiac prosthesis or suspected MRSA: vancomycin 1 g IV 12-hourly plus gentamicin 1 mg/kg 8-hourly plus rifampicin orally 300–600 mg 12-hourly
Indolent IE	Penicillin 7.2 g IV daily in 6 divided doses or amoxicillin/ampicillin 2 g IV 6-hourly plus gentamicin 1 mg/kg IV 8-hourly	

Definitive treatment

Organism	Recommended	Alternatives
Viridans streptococci	Penicillin 1.2–2.4 g IV 4-hourly plus gentamicin 1 mg/kg IV 8-hourly Duration 2–6 weeks: depends on penicillin susceptibility and complications Prosthetic valve endocarditis: treatment duration 6 weeks	If risk of gentamicin toxicity is high: penicillin 1.2–2.4 g IV 4-hourly for 4–6 weeks If penicillin allergy: substitute vancomycin 1 g IV 12-hourly for penicillin
Enterococci	Penicillin 2.4 g IV 4-hourly or ampicillin/amoxicillin 2 g IV 4-hourly plus gentamicin 1 mg/kg IV 8-hourly for ≥4 weeks (depending on susceptibility) Prosthetic valve endocarditis: treatment duration ≥6 weeks	If penicillin allergy: substitute vancomycin 1 g IV 12-hourly for penicillin or ampicillin
Staphylococcal endocarditis Native valve	MSSA: flucloxacillin 2 g IV 6-hourly (4-hourly in patients >85 kg) for 4 weeks	If penicillin allergy: use 2 agents: vancomycin 1 g IV 12-hourly plus rifampicin 300–600 mg orally 12-hourly or gentamicin 1 mg/kg 8-hourly or sodium fusidate 500 mg 8-hourly orally for 4 weeks
S. aureus and coagulase-negative Staphylococci	MRSA: use 2 agents: vancomycin 1 g IV 12-hourly plus rifampicin 300–600 mg orally 12-hourly or gentamicin 1 mg/kg 8-hourly or sodium fusidate 500 mg 8-hourly orally for 4 weeks	
Staphylococcal endocarditis Prosthetic valve *S. aureus* and coagulase-negative Staphylococci	Use 3 agents: flucloxacillin 2 g IV 4–6 hourly (for MSSA) or vancomycin 1 g IV 12-hourly (MRSA) plus rifampicin 300–600 mg orally 12-hourly and/or gentamicin 1 mg/kg IV 8-hourly and/or sodium fusidate 500 mg orally 8-hourly	If penicillin allergy: use 3 agents: vancomycin 1 g IV 12-hourly plus rifampicin 300–600 mg orally 12-hourly and/or gentamicin 1 mg/kg IV 8-hourly and/or sodium fusidate 500 mg orally 8-hourly

(*continued*)

Table 42.4 *(continued)*

Definitive treatment

Organism	Recommended	Alternatives
HACEK organisms	Ceftriaxone 2 g IV daily for 4 weeks	Ampicillin-sensitive organisms: ampicillin/amoxicillin 2 g IV 4–6 hourly for 4 weeks plus gentamicin 1 mg/kg IV 8-hourly for first 2 weeks

Note. Gentamicin dose should be modified according to renal function and drug levels. Penicillin and vancomycin doses also need to be adjusted in renal impairment.
Abbreviations: IV, intravenous; MRSA, methicillin-resistant Staphylococcus aureus; MSSA, methicillin-sensitive Staphylococcus aureus.

Fever on treatment

Continuing fever is rarely due to inappropriate antibiotic treatment. The usual cause is abscess formation of the valve ring or the cardiac septum. Large vegetations or the presence of necrotic tissue may also inhibit clearance of infection. In these circumstances surgery is indicated. A coexisting focus of infection such as lung, soft tissue, liver or cerebral abscess may have arisen from nosocomial bacteraemia and cause continuing fever. Other concomitant infections, such as from the urinary tract, respiratory tract and intravascular lines, should be sought and excluded. Drug allergy may cause fever that is likely to subside once antibiotics have been stopped.

Surgical management

Several studies suggest that combined medical and surgical therapy can reduce both early and late mortality in patients with a complicated course.

Congestive heart failure has remained the strongest indication for surgery in IE. Medically treated patients with moderate-to-severe heart failure owing to endocarditis-related valvular dysfunction have a mortality rate of 56% to 86% compared with 11% to 35% among patients treated with combined medical and surgical therapy. The beneficial effect of surgery persists even in the presence of comorbidity; therefore, the occurrence of other complications such as acute renal failure is not a contraindication for valve replacement. Close clinical monitoring and serial echocardiography aid

Table 42.5 Complications where surgery should be considered during active infective endocarditis

Haemodynamically significant valve malfunction
Refractory congestive heart failure
Early prosthetic valve endocarditis
Evidence of perivalvular extension
Persistent infection after 7–10 days of adequate antibiotic therapy
Infection due to organisms with poor inherent response to therapy (fungi, *Brucella* spp., *Coxiella* spp., *Staphylococcus lugdenensis*, *Enterococcus* spp. with high-level gentamicin resistance, Gram-negative organisms)
Mobile vegetation >10 mm size before or during first week of antibiotic treatment
Recurrent emboli despite appropriate antibiotic therapy
Obstructive vegetations

timing of surgical intervention, which should be early rather than late.

Antibiotic therapy must be continued postoperatively unless the patient has already completed a successful course of treatment preoperatively. Valve tissue should be sent to microbiology at the time of surgery and duration of postoperative antibiotic therapy discussed with microbiologists.

Prophylaxis

Although antibiotic prophylaxis has an important place in endocarditis prevention, the importance of early treatment of infections and removal of intravascular and other devices (e.g. urinary catheters, endotracheal tubes) cannot be overemphasized.

Various recommendations for the prophylaxis of IE have been published around the world and are based on similar principles. Procedures involving noninfected skin incisions and no mucosal breach, such as cardiac catheterization, do not require prophylaxis. High-risk procedures include surgical procedures on the upper respiratory tract, nasal packing, nasal intubation, cystoscopy, urethral dilatation and hepatic and biliary operations. Prophylaxis for other procedures such as upper endoscopy, sigmoidoscopy, colonoscopy and barium enema may be recommended in high-risk patients. Performing a risk assessment and discussion with a microbiologist may be required.

Table 42.6 Cardiac conditions for which antibiotic prophylaxis is indicated for high-risk procedures

History of previous endocarditis
Prosthetic cardiac valves
Surgically constructed shunt/conduit
Complex congenital heart disease
Complex left ventricular outflow abnormalities, including aortic stenosis and bicuspid aortic valves
Acquired valvulopathy*
Mitral valve prolapse*

**With echocardiographic documentation of substantial leaflet pathology and regurgitation.*

Key points

- Infective endocarditis is difficult to diagnose, but should be suspected whenever fever persists and especially after cardiothoracic surgery.
- Blood cultures should always be taken before starting treatment, which may need to continue for a considerable time via the intravenous route.
- Surgery should be considered if there is a clinical deterioration or infection persists.
- Streptococci and staphylococci are the most commonly implicated organisms, but virtually any other organism may also cause infective endocarditis, especially if prosthetic material is present.

FURTHER READING

Baddour LM, Wilson, WR, Bayer AS, *et al.* Infective endocarditis: diagnosis, antimicrobial therapy, and management of complications: a statement for healthcare professionals from the Committee on Rheumatic Fever, Endocarditis, and Kawasaki Disease, Council on Cardiovascular Disease in the Young, and the Councils on Clinical Cardiology, Stroke, and Cardiovascular Surgery and Anesthesia, American Heart Association: endorsed by the Infectious Diseases Society of America. *Circulation* 2005;111:e394–e434.

British Society of Antimicrobial Chemotherapy [homepage on the Internet]. Recommendations. Available at: www.bsac.org.uk.

Elliott TS, Foweraker J, Gould FK, *et al*. Guidelines for the antibiotic treatment of endocarditis in adults: report of the Working Party of the British Society for Antimicrobial Chemotherapy. *J Antimicrob Chemother* 2004;54:971–981.

Gould FK, Elliott TS, Foweraker J, *et al*. Guidelines for the prevention of endocarditis: report of the Working Party of the British Society for Antimicrobial Chemotherapy. *J Antimicrob Chemother* 2006;57:1035–1042.

Horstkotte D, Follath F, Gutschik E, *et al*. Guidelines on prevention, diagnosis and treatment of infective endocarditis executive summary; the task force on infective endocarditis of the European society of cardiology. *Eur Heart J* 2004;25:267–276.

3.7 *Endocrine System in Cardiothoracic Critical Care*

Chapter 43

Endocrine function

F.M. GIBSON AND A.A. KLEIN

Introduction

'The constancy of the internal environment is the condition that life should be free and independent. . . . So far from the higher animal being indifferent to the external world, it is on the contrary in a precise and informed relation with it, in such a way that its equilibrium results from a continuous and delicate compensation, established as by the most sensitive of balances.'

— Claude Bernard 1813–1878

The 'internal milieu' is a complex system influenced and controlled by the combined effects of the endocrine, nervous and immune systems. The actions of these systems are further complicated by their differing responses to acute and chronic stressors, features that are readily identifiable in the post cardiac surgical patient. At the time of writing, the catalogue of hormones recognized as active in the maintenance of this human equilibrium consists of 55 compounds, and doubtless the number will continue to grow.

The state of knowledge in relation to these issues is advancing day by day, and management strategies of patients in the cardiac surgical critical care area are similarly in a state of flux; we are indeed in the era of 'known knowns, known unknowns and unknown unknowns.'

The pituitary

Chronic pituitary insufficiency

Common causes of chronic pituitary insufficiency include pituitary adenomas (the most common), inflammatory destruction, surgical removal, radiation-induced destruction of pituitary tissue, subarachnoid hemorrhage and postpartum pituitary necrosis (Sheehan syndrome). Presentation is frequently slow and insidious, with or without headaches, neuro-ophthalmologic symptoms and focal neurological deficits. Most commonly, generalized fatigue and weakness may be the predominant complaints. The findings on laboratory evaluation may be consistent with hypogonadism, growth hormone deficiency, central hypothyroidism and adrenal insufficiency – all controlled through the hypothalamic–pituitary axis. Cardiac surgery in patients with chronic panhypopituitarism has been demonstrated to be well tolerated, with maintenance therapy targeted on those hormones known to be deficient. Thyroid hormones should be used with caution, in the knowledge that symptoms of angina and potential myocardial ischaemia and acute infarction may be precipitated.

Acute hypopituitarism

Acute hypopituitarism may occur after cardiac surgery with cardiopulmonary bypass, by a process known as 'pituitary apoplexy,' a rarely reported complication. It is characterized by a catastrophic degeneration of the pituitary gland, the origin of which may be by bleeding into or necrosis within a pituitary gland adenoma. This may then compress nearby structures. This syndrome may be indicated by unexplained hyponatraemia, headache, ptosis, nausea and vomiting, altered level of consciousness,

Table 43.1 Molecular basis of hormones

Amines	Catecholamines, thyroxine
Peptides	Adrenocorticotrophic hormone, vasopressin, insulin
Lipid/phospholipid	Cortisol

change in mental state and fever. In the case of blindness as a result of pituitary apoplexy, early surgical intervention may lead to complete recovery.

Growth hormone

Growth hormone homeostasis may become abnormal in critical illness, and growth hormone levels are certainly much lower than would be expected. This contributes to the 'wasting syndrome' commonly seen after a period of critical illness, with fat deposition and protein degradation. This may persist until some time after recovery, even when additional nutrition is provided. Growth hormone supplementation, however, has been demonstrated to be associated with increased mortality. This may be because of increased catabolism (significant insulin resistance may occur) along with increased metabolic rate and the inadequate nutrition that is likely despite best efforts.

The thyroid

Thyroid hormones are key regulators of metabolism and are known to exert effects on many different organs. Cardiac surgery in patients with known thyroid disease rarely upsets the established hormone equilibrium, provided treatment is continued during the critical care admission. There is evidence, however, that mortality among female patients on thyroid replacement therapy is higher than might be expected. In prolonged critical illness, the multiple and complex alterations in the hypothalamic–pituitary–thyroid axis result in what is commonly referred to as the euthyroid sick syndrome or nonthyroid illness syndrome. Thyroid hormone levels are reduced in nonthyroid illness syndrome in proportion to the severity and probably the length of the illness. Serum levels of thyroid hormone below 4 μg/dL are associated with an increased risk of mortality up to 50%.

Iatrogenic causes

The inotrope, dopamine, is known to inhibit thyroid-stimulating hormone secretion, and it is postulated that dopamine may precipitate hypothyroidism in nonthyroid illness syndrome. Amiodarone may induce both hypo- and hyperthyroidism. It is very rich in iodine, with a 100-mg tablet containing 250 times the recommended daily iodine intake. Thyroid dysfunction with prolonged administration occurs because of both the iodine content and direct toxicity of the drug on the parenchyma of the thyroid gland; this is made more pronounced by rifampicin treatment.

The adrenals

Adrenal insufficiency can be subdivided into three broad categories:

1. Chronic primary adrenal insufficiency, known as Addison's disease, is the result of destruction of the adrenal cortex. The most common causes include autoimmune disease (about 70%–80%), tuberculosis (about 20%), adrenal haemorrhage, adrenal metastases, and acquired immunodeficiency syndrome in association with cytomegalovirus or other pathogens.
2. Chronic secondary adrenal insufficiency occurs when insufficient adrenocorticotrophic hormone is available to stimulate the adrenal cortex. Most commonly it is due to exogenous glucocorticoid therapy, but it can also be the result of generalized hypopituitarism.
3. Acute adrenal crisis may result from inadequate steroid replacement during periods of high stress (such as major surgery or critical illness) in patients with chronic adrenal insufficiency. It also occurs in patients with acute adrenal

haemorrhage or as part of the syndrome of pituitary apoplexy.

Chronic adrenal insufficiency leads to glucocorticoid deficiency, with clinical features including hypotension, weakness, fatigue, anorexia, weight loss, nausea and vomiting. Eosinophilia and normocytic anaemia are common, along with hypocalcaemia and hypoglycaemia on occasion.

An addisonian crisis may occur in the setting of acute adrenal insufficiency; this is characterized by nonspecific symptoms of shock, with rapid deterioration in the patient's haemodynamic state. Hyponatraemia and hyperkalaemia, along with dehydration, are common features. The lack of cortisol causes failure of maintenance of vascular tone, causing vasodilatation and hypotension, which is often resistant to vasopressors. This may, however, respond to steroid replacement and fluid resuscitation.

Steroid supplementation

Patients receiving long-term corticosteroid therapy fall into two different categories. The majority have chronic autoimmune or inflammatory diseases such as asthma, ulcerative colitis or rheumatoid arthritis. The remainder require steroid treatment because of chronic adrenal insufficiency. Whichever category patients fall into, additional steroids in the form of intravenous hydrocortisone should be administered perioperatively, for up to 3 days and certainly until oral treatment has been reestablished. This may be by regular bolus (50 mg 4–6 times a day) or infusion (150–300 mg over 24 hours). Patients who received steroid treatment in the months before surgery may also require steroid supplementation in this manner.

Acute adrenal failure

Although adrenal insufficiency is thought to occur in 0.1% or less of the population, postoperative patients in the critical care unit are acknowledged to be at risk of acute adrenal failure, with an incidence of up to 28% in some series. There is some evidence that administration of hydrocortisone to all patients with hypotension and a high vasopressor requirement may be beneficial in terms of reduction of vasopressor dose and improved survival.

Adrenal function may be assessed by means of the short synacthen test. This may help to identify those patients who will benefit from corticosteroid therapy. Its interpretation in critical care practice in patients suffering from septic shock can be difficult. In fact, the test is a measure of reserve, not adrenal function, and interpretation of the result should take into account the baseline cortisol level. No consensus exists as to what constitutes the lowest safe limit of cortisol in critically ill patients.

Hypoadrenalism in critical illness

This may be due to a number of factors, including specific damage to the adrenals or the pituitary, previously undiagnosed chronic disease or acute destruction of the adrenal gland from haemorrhage or infection. Probably more commonly, hypoperfusion or cytokine-induced inhibition of the adrenal or the hypothalamic–pituitary area leads to functional impairment of different components of the axis. Some drugs used in critical care may also lead to an exaggeration of hypoadrenalism, such as rifampicin (increased metabolism of cortisol) and ketoconazole and etomidate (interference with steroid-manufacturing enzymes). The clinical presentation is usually a cathecholamine-dependent hyperdynamic shock, which is difficult to distinguish from other conditions, such as sepsis syndrome. Such patients are often responsive to steroid treatment, despite the absence of biochemical or histological adrenal insufficiency; this may be explained by desensitization of glucocorticoid responsiveness at the cellular level. Glucocorticoid treatment may result in recoupling of the desensitized adrenergic receptors and thus restore responsiveness in blood pressure.

Diabetes and insulin therapy

Diabetes may be defined as an abnormality of insulin production or effect that results in elevated blood sugar. It is managed by dietary control, with or without oral medication or parenteral (subcutaneous) insulin administration.

Routine cardiac surgery

Many diabetic patients present for cardiac surgery because diabetes is a significant risk factor for coronary artery disease. The majority of these have insulin infusions started during surgery, which should be continued in critical care and through to the ward, until a normal diet and the normal diabetic regime is resumed. A number of patients may exhibit elevated blood glucose levels during surgery, despite no previous history of diabetes. Insulin infusion may be commenced in these patients also, although blood glucose may rapidly return to normal after admission to critical care and insulin may then be stopped.

Critical illness

Hyperglycaemia and insulin resistance are common in critically ill patients, even when glucose homeostasis has previously been normal. Patients undergo a variety of metabolic changes in response to the stress from surgery, trauma or sepsis. Increased secretion of stress hormones (cortisol and catecholamines), growth hormone and glucagon leads to an increase in gluconeogenesis, glycogenolysis, lipolysis and proteolysis. This can result in hyperglycaemia and insulin resistance, even in patients with no history of diabetes mellitus. The frequency of uncontrolled blood glucose in diabetics is even higher, because diabetic patients cannot increase insulin production to counteract the effect of the increase in catabolic hormones; in some patients, the insulin requirements may increase 10-fold or more. High-carbohydrate feeding in the form of hyperalimentation or enteral feeding can also contribute to increased glucose levels. Therefore, providing adequate amounts of insulin to promote euglycaemia and enough nutrition to avoid hypoglycaemia, proteolysis and lipolysis is a challenge in critically ill patients.

Insulin regime

There is a body of evidence that strict glycaemic control in critical care substantially reduces morbidity and mortality. Overall mortality has been shown to decrease from 8% to 4.6%, and serious morbidity from 20.2% to 10.6% among patients admitted for longer than 5 days. Intensive glucose control also decreased the number of bloodstream infections by 46%, the frequency of acute renal failure requiring dialysis or haemofiltration by 41%, the frequency of critical illness and polyneuropathy by 44%, and the median number of blood transfusions by 50%. There is also evidence that tight blood sugar control may considerably improve postoperative recovery of myocardial contractile function and reduce the incidence of atrial arrhythmias after cardiac surgery.

Use of insulin protocols in critically ill patients improves blood glucose control and reduces morbidity and mortality in critically ill populations. Glucose levels in critically ill patients should be controlled through implementation of insulin protocols with the goal to achieve normoglycaemia, regardless of a history of diabetes. Frequent monitoring is very important to avoid hypoglycaemia, using point-of-care whole-blood or capillary blood analysis. Protocols use a sliding scale of insulin infusion, titrated against regular blood glucose measurements. These should be at least hourly during the first 24 hours of the infusion, and such frequent monitoring may need to continue during the acute phase of the illness. Once blood glucose levels are stable, monitoring may become less frequent, although this should be reviewed regularly. The exact glucose concentration to be aimed for is controversial, as a target of between 4.4 and 5.6 mmol/L may be associated with an increased incidence of hypoglycaemia. In the majority of cases, blood glucose levels below 6.5 mmol/L are adequate. Computerized sliding scale protocols have been developed, with some success.

Key points

- Hypothyroidism accompanying critical illness is common, and may be exacerbated by dopamine or amiodarone treatment; thyroid function tests should be considered.
- Glucocorticoid deficiency is also common, and systemic steroid supplementation should be considered if shock is refractory to inotropic support or in cases of sepsis/systemic inflammatory response to sepsis.
- Maintenance of normoglycaemia is of crucial importance; sliding scale parenteral insulin therapy is mandatory to manage elevated blood glucose, although threshold for treatment is the subject of debate.

FURTHER READING

Burman KD, Wartofsky L. Thyroid function in the intensive care unit setting. *Crit Care Clin* 2001;17: 43–57.

Ligtenberg JJ, Zijlstra JG. Hormones in the critically ill patient: to intervene or not to intervene? *Intensive Care Med* 2001;27:1567–1577.

Pittas AG, Siegel RD, Lau J. Insulin therapy for critically ill hospitalized patients: a meta-analysis of randomized controlled trials. *Arch Intern Med* 2004;164:2005–2011.

Van den Berghe G, Wouters PJ, Bouillon R, *et al.* Outcome benefit of intensive insulin therapy in the critically ill: insulin dose versus glycemic control. *Crit Care Med* 2003;31:359–366.

3.8 *Neurological System in Cardiothoracic Critical Care*

Chapter 44

Sedation and analgesia

M. DURAND AND C.C. ARVIEUX

Introduction

To provide adequate sedation and analgesia is integral to the care and management of the patient in critical care.

Indications

The postoperative patient

In contrast to most other types of surgery, patients after cardiac surgery are usually sedated and ventilated in the immediate postoperative period, until normothermia and haemodynamic stability are achieved and lack of bleeding is confirmed.

NORMOTHERMIA

Sedation allows a reduction of oxygen consumption during rewarming; it inhibits shivering. Shivering is associated with a three- to four-fold increase in O_2 consumption and leads to an increase in CO_2 production with respiratory acidosis. Intraoperative hypothermia should be avoided where possible and active warming employed. Increasing sedation or adding clonidine may be beneficial if shivering persists.

HAEMODYNAMIC STABILITY

Early postoperative haemodynamic instability can have many causes, and might necessitate reexploration or further investigation. Deep levels of sedation were advocated in the past to reduce the stress response of cardiac surgery and the incidence of myocardial ischaemia, but this is no longer thought to be beneficial. Moreover, heavy sedation has itself been associated with increased myocardial ischaemia.

The non postoperative patient

The most common reason for sedation in critical care is to permit mechanical ventilation and tolerance of the artificial airway (endotracheal tube). Low levels of sedation should be used and patients should ideally be easy to rouse and remain calm and cooperative.

Sedation

Sedation is most effective if a balanced combination of drugs is used. Most commonly, a sedative is administered concurrently with an opioid, but on occasion single agents may be sufficient. Daily sedation breaks lead to improved weaning and reduce length of stay in critical care. Sedation is discontinued after full clinical assessment, usually in the morning. The patient is then allowed to wake up so that neurological status may be assessed. If the patient is comfortable and tolerates the tube and ventilation, then resedation is not necessary. Most often sedatives are restarted, but at a lower dose. Sedation breaks may lead to precipitous extubation or cardiovascular deterioration if not carefully monitored.

When starting sedation, a loading dose should be administered and followed by continuous infusion.

If more sedation is required, another bolus should be prescribed and the infusion rate increased. Sedative agents accumulate when administered for long periods of time. This may delay weaning and prolong critical care stay. Many agents have deleterious effects on haemodynamics, including pulmonary vasculature, and this needs to be considered. Tolerance to sedatives is often seen, as is withdrawal after discontinuation. Unfortunately, no sedative produces rapid eye movement sleep, and deprivation may be associated with psychological disturbance after recovery. Therefore, sedatives should be used with care and for no longer than necessary.

Principles of sedation

SEDATION SCORES

These should be frequently assessed and reviewed to allow titration of sedatives. There are many in clinical use, but none can be employed when muscle paralysis is required. Monitors for sedation levels are currently being investigated, and the Bispectral Index Monitor (BIS) has been studied the most; a BIS score of 60 is approximately equivalent to a Ramsay score of 6. This may be particularly useful when paralysis is used, but the amount of paralysis itself may have an effect on the BIS score.

PROPOFOL

This intravenous anaesthetic agent has a hypnotic and sedative effect at subanaesthetic dose (usually 2–4 mg/kg per hour). Its main advantages are that a steady level of sedation can be easily achieved with a fast recovery when interrupted even after prolonged infusion. Its disadvantages are high lipid content and a vasodilatory effect that may contribute to haemodynamic instability. Rarely, 'propofol infusion syndrome' occurs in patients receiving propofol for longer than 5 hours. This can lead to progressive cardiac failure, arrhythmia associated with rhabdomyolysis, metabolic acidosis and hyperkalaemia. At high doses, muscle necrosis and profound lactic acidosis are possible, and are related to the inhibition of both fatty acid oxidation and oxidation–phosphorylation in mitochondria. Propofol acts as a trigger substrate in the presence of priming factors such as high levels of catecholamines or cortisol. Renal replacement therapy may be needed to eliminate propofol and its toxic metabolites. For long-term sedation, the clinical impact of propofol-induced hypertriglyceridaemia is not known. Rare infection outbreaks related to the contamination of large vials of propofol and substandard handling techniques have been reported.

Table 44.1 Basic principles of sedation

Patients should be comfortable and pain free.
Anxiety should be minimized.
Patients should be calm and cooperative.
Patients should be able to tolerate the ventilator and artificial airway, plus any other forms of organ support necessary such as the need to lie flat with an intra-aortic balloon pump in situ).
Patients must not be paralysed and awake.

Table 44.2 Ramsay Sedation Scale

1	Patient is anxious and agitated or restless, or both.
2	Patient is cooperative, oriented, and tranquil.
3	Patient responds to commands only.
4	Patient exhibits brisk response to light glabellar tap or loud auditory stimulus.
5	Patient exhibits a sluggish response to light glabellar tap or loud auditory stimulus.
6	Patient exhibits no response.

MIDAZOLAM

This sedative agent with hypnotic and anxiolytic properties is usually administered as an infusion (1–5 mg/h), but can be administered by intermittent bolus (1 or 2 mg). Despite its short half-life, accumulation may occur, especially in the elderly or in renal and hepatic failure. Metabolized by cytochrome P450, it competes with other drugs such as fentanyl for its breakdown. Practically, most studies have found no major difference between midazolam and propofol in relation to mechanical ventilation duration, quality of sedation or haemodynamic stability. Recovery time is usually shorter with propofol, but this seems to have little impact on time spent in critical care. The most important difference is in the feasibility of a daily sedation break for assessment. Propofol is best suited for short-term sedation and midazolam for sedation longer than 36 to 48 hours.

CLONIDINE AND DEXMEDETOMIDINE

Clonidine and dexmedetomidine are α_2-receptor agonists. They inhibit sympathetic activity and reduce plasma adrenaline and noradrenaline levels. They decrease heart rate, blood pressure and reduce the haemodynamic and neuroendocrine response to stimulus. Both are sedative and analgesic, but do not cause respiratory depression. Experience is limited and there is no clear advantage over propofol for short-term sedation. Clonidine can be administered as an adjunct to reduce the dose of other sedatives if patients are resistant. It also has an additive effect to the analgesia provided by opioids. During weaning from sedation, clonidine seems particularly useful in managing confusion or agitation, especially if the patient is at risk of self-harm.

REMIFENTANIL AND SUFENTANIL

Both remifentanil and sufentanil seem clinically to have anxiolytic properties, in addition to being very potent analgesics. Remifentanil has a very short, context-sensitive half-life, and when administered by infusion may provide sufficient sedation to enable tolerance of mechanical ventilation when used as a sole agent. However, agitation, distress and acute pain on withdrawal are commonly seen, especially if the infusion is stopped precipitously. This has limited the widespread use of remifentanil. Withdrawal of remifentanil may be best managed by substituting a small dose of another opioid such as morphine for a short period. Sufentanil has a longer half-life and does not induce the same state of clinical dependence.

Analgesia

Pain

Pain after cardiac surgery is not limited to the wound itself. It also encompasses procedural pains such as line insertions and drain removal. Intense post-operative pain may induce a stress response with increased myocardial oxygen consumption, which can lead to myocardial ischaemia. If pain is not managed appropriately, a reduction of mobility and difficulty in coughing or breathing deeply may lead to increased morbidity and mortality. Pain contributes to agitation as well as psychosis and interferes with sleep. It is probably for these reasons that a strong relationship exists between level of pain and length of stay in critical care and in hospital.

The dose of morphine required is lower after sternotomy than thoracotomy, but there is wide variation between patients. The intensity of pain diminishes during the first week after surgery, and its anatomical localization varies (at day 7, the pain is mainly located in the back of the shoulders). After sternotomy, pain intensity is greatest on days 1 and 2 with only 10% of patients being pain free (this increases to 20% at day 7). Chest drains contribute to pain and should be removed as soon as it is safe to do so, but it must be remembered that their removal is itself particularly painful. Administration of opiates or entonox (nitrous oxide and oxygen premixed 50:50) is indicated.

Pain assessment

Accurate assessment of pain during the postoperative period is an essential component of pain management. A standard method must be used to document patients' postoperative pain, with a visual analogue scale being the most widely used. Patients rate their pain between 0 (no pain) and 10 (the worst imaginable pain).

Well-informed patients cope better with post-operative pain and have less anxiety; therefore, good preoperative education is essential. Anaesthetic technique may influence postoperative pain. Perioperative administration of large doses of opioid can induce delayed hyperalgesia and acute tolerance to the analgesic effect of morphine. This is observed with several opioids like remifentanil or fentanyl. This may be prevented by an intraoperative infusion of a small-dose of NMDA-receptor antagonist (ketamine, 0.5 mg/kg).

Analgesic administration

Opiates in critical care may be administered either by nurse-delivered boluses (intravenously or subcutaneously) or by continuous infusion, with the rate adjusted according to pain. Patient-controlled analgesia may be used when the patient is awake, and may lead to lower pain scores and reduced side effects.

Perioperative thoracic epidural analgesia reduces postoperative pain scores and cardiac complications. Its use is usually limited to thoracic surgery or trauma, where the excellent analgesia provided allows earlier extubation and reduces the incidence of reintubation. Some centres use epidural analgesia for cardiac surgery, but this is controversial because of the perceived increased risk of epidural haematoma associated with systemic heparinization. If an epidural is used, it should be sited at the appropriate level (high thoracic), and an infusion is commenced after a loading dose. The infusion usually consists of a standard mixture of local anaesthetic (often bupivacaine) and opioid (commonly fentanyl), according to local protocol. Such a mixture is designed to ensure adequate analgesia without excessive muscle weakness. Sympathetic block is a common disadvantage of the thoracic epidural, with the resulting vasodilatation possibly contributing to postoperative hypotension. Additional inotropes or vasoconstrictors may be necessary if hypotension persists after judicious intravascular volume expansion. Epidural infusion is often reserved for patients only lightly or not at all sedated so that unexpected, rare, but important neurological complications (such as epidural abscess or haematoma) can be recognized immediately. The epidural catheter should be removed by day 5 to reduce the risk of infection, and the use of anticoagulants should be taken into account when planning catheter insertion or removal. Morphine may also be given intrathecally. Doses vary widely, and ventilatory depression or delayed extubation may be a problem although analgesia is excellent.

Morphine

Morphine is the most commonly used opioid, and also the least expensive. It acts on central μ_1 and μ_2 opioid receptors, and has a rapid onset of action of less than 5 minutes and a maximum effect within 20 minutes. It is usually well tolerated, and major side effects include sedation, respiratory depression, cognitive dysfunction, constipation, nausea and vomiting. The main limitation of morphine use is the accumulation of active metabolites associated with renal dysfunction that leads to prolonged sedation and ventilatory depression. It is metabolized in the liver to morphine-3-glucuronide (a potent antanalgesic) and morphine-6-glucuronide (an analgesic excreted by the kidney).

Fentanyl

Fentanyl is approximately 100 times more potent than morphine, and has a more rapid onset of action (3 minutes). In low doses, its duration of action (20 minutes) is limited by redistribution. Tissues may become saturated and duration of effect prolonged at higher doses. In renal failure, the metabolite norfentanyl may accumulate, and may cause toxic delirium. Fentanyl also accumulates in hepatic failure. For these reasons, fentanyl infusion

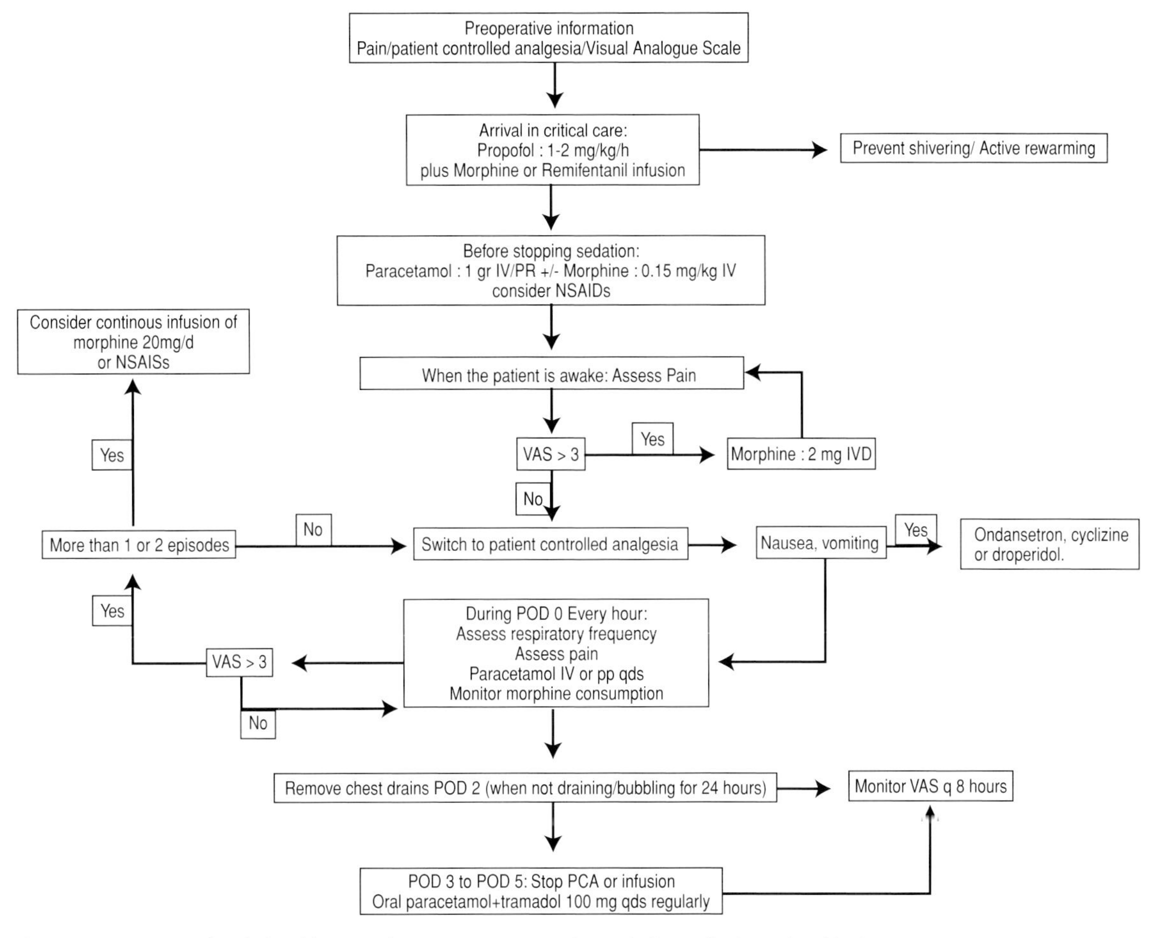

Figure 44.1 Example of algorithm used to treat postoperative pain in cardiothoracic critical care.

is not commonly used in critical care. Conversely, it is usually reserved for patients in renal failure.

Nonopioid analgesics

TRAMADOL

Tramadol is a synthetic, centrally acting analgesic agent with two distinct, synergistic mechanisms of action, acting as both a weak opioid agonist and an inhibitor of monoamine neurotransmitter reuptake. Oral and parenteral tramadol effectively relieve moderate to severe postoperative pain in most patients. The most common adverse events (incidence of up to 6%) are nausea, dizziness, drowsiness, sweating, vomiting and dry mouth. Importantly, unlike other opioids, tramadol has no clinically relevant effects on respiratory or cardiovascular parameters. Tramadol is often administered regularly after cardiothoracic surgery, usually after discontinuation of morphine or epidural infusion. Parenteral or oral tramadol has proved to be an effective and well-tolerated analgesic agent. Tramadol seems to have no analgesic property in a minority of patients, for whom an alternative treatment is required.

PARACETAMOL

Although its exact mechanism of action is not fully understood, the blockade of prostaglandin E2 production by central cyclo-oxygenase 3 inhibition is likely to account for the analgesic properties of paracetamol. It has a weak anti-inflammatory effect, probably by slight inhibition of peripheral cyclo-oxygenase 1 inhibitors. It can be given intravenously, rectally, orally or via the nasogastric tube. It is most effective when administered regularly four times a day.

Nonsteroidal anti-inflammatory drugs

Nonsteroidal anti-inflammatory drugs (NSAIDs) are very effective analgesics, but their use is limited by nephrotoxicity, especially in preexisting renal failure or when cardiac failure is present. Their use is also associated with an increased risk of gastrointestinal haemorrhage. Diclofenac, ibuprofen and naproxen are used after cardiothoracic surgery, but should be avoided in patients with renal failure or a history of gastrointestinal haemorrhage.

CYCLO-OXYGENASE-2 INHIBITORS

Cyclo-oxygenase-2 (COX-2) inhibitors are powerful analgesics that were thought initially not to induce gastrointestinal or bleeding complications. Unfortunately, COX-2 inhibitors increase thrombotic events, particularly cardiac. They also reduce renal blood flow and increase the risk of renal failure; therefore, their use has declined.

NEFOPAM

Nefopam is a non-narcotic analgesic not structurally related to other analgesic drugs. It provides analgesia comparable with a moderate dose of parenteral morphine, but is more powerful than paracetamol. It is usually well tolerated. The commonest side effects are sweating, nausea and sedation. Nefopam prevents shivering, but is less efficient than clonidine.

Neuromuscular blockade

Neuromuscular blockers have no sedative or analgesic properties. Except in the setting of tracheal intubation, the use of neuromuscular blockers to effect muscle paralysis has declined substantially over the last 20 years. Most clinicians now employ them as a last resort, and they are very rarely administered by infusion. Their association with

Table 44.3 Specific complications of neuromuscular blockade

Vecuronium
Vecuronium has been reported to be more commonly associated with prolonged blockade once discontinued, compared with other neuromuscular blocking agents.
Patients receiving vecuronium and corticosteroids were at increased risk of prolonged weakness once the drug was discontinued.
Atracurium
Atracurium has minimal cardiovascular adverse effects and is associated with histamine release at higher doses.
Laudanosine is a breakdown product of Hofmann elimination of atracurium and has been associated with central nervous system excitation. This has led to concern about the possibility of precipitating seizures in patients who have received extremely high doses of atracurium or who are in hepatic failure. Long-term infusions have been associated with the development of tolerance, necessitating significant dose increases or conversion to other neuromuscular blocking agents. Atracurium has been associated with persistent neuromuscular weakness as have other neuromuscular blocking agents.
Cisatracurium
Prolonged weakness has been reported following the use of cisatracurium.
Pancuronium
The two adverse effects of pancuronium that are commented on frequently are vagolysis and an increase in heart rate

prolonged weakness has been the biggest factor in the decline in their popularity. This prolonged weakness may be more common when aminoglycoside antibiotics or corticosteroids are administered concurrently because of their interaction at the neuromuscular junction. Spontaneous muscle breakdown during total muscle inactivity has also been postulated.

Muscle relaxants are indicated only in the following conditions:

- Facilitation of invasive modes of ventilation, when they are not tolerated by an adequately sedated patient, especially when hypoxia is an issue;
- Open chest – surgical bleeding or indwelling vascular cannulae may necessitate the patient's chest being left open for a short time and the patient being kept completely still; and
- To allow invasive procedures such as bronchoscopy and transoesophageal echocardiography.

Atracurium is the most commonly used drug. It is metabolized by Hoffman degradation so its effect is not prolonged in renal failure. Vecuronium, pancuronium and cisatracurium are also used.

Table 44.4 General complications of the use of neuromuscular blocking drugs in critically ill patients

Risk of prolonged muscle weakness
Anxiety and panic if patient is awake yet paralysed
Autonomic and cardiovascular effects (i.e. vagolytic)
Decreased lymphatic flow
Risk of generalized loss of muscle conditioning
Peripheral nerve injury
Corneal abrasion, conjunctivitis
Myositis ossificans
Potential central nervous system toxicity

Key points

- Sedation is common postoperatively and during mechanical ventilation.
- A combination of sedatives and opioids by infusion is still the most used method of sedation and analgesia.
- Monitoring of sedation by regular scoring with sedation breaks is necessary to avoid prolonging critical care stay.
- Multimodal analgesia should be employed, commonly regular paracetamol, tramadol with or without NSAIDs. Opioids may also be required if pain is severe.
- Neuromuscular blockade is rarely used because it is associated with prolonged muscle weakness.

FURTHER READING

Bainbridge D, Martin JE, Cheng DC. Patient-controlled versus nurse-controlled analgesia after cardiac surgery – a meta-analysis. *Can J Anaesth* 2006;53:492–499.

Chaney MA. Intrathecal and epidural anesthesia and analgesia for cardiac surgery. *Anesth Analg* 2006;102:45–64.

Elia N, Lysakowski C, Tramer MR. Does multimodal analgesia with acetaminophen, nonsteroidal antiinflammatory drugs, or selective cyclooxygenase-2 inhibitors and patient-controlled analgesia morphine offer advantages over morphine alone? Meta-analyses of randomized trials. *Anesthesiology* 2005;103:1296–1304.

Kehlet H, Jensen TS, Woolf CJ. Persistent postsurgical pain: risk factors and prevention. *Lancet* 2006;367:1618–1625.

Mueller XM, Tinguely F, Tevaearai HT, *et al.* Pain location, distribution, and intensity after cardiac surgery. *Chest* 2000;118:391–396.

Chapter 45

Neurological complications

J.D. STEARNS AND C.W. HOGUE

Introduction

General advances in perioperative care now allow for the benefits of cardiac surgery to be extended to older and higher risk patients with low operative mortality. High survival in this at-risk surgical population places increased emphasis on complications as determinants of patient outcomes. Neurological complications are a particular concern owing to their relationship with older age and their association with other morbidity.

Clinical spectrum

Neurological complications after cardiac surgery manifest as a myriad of presentations.

Stroke is the most clinically obvious complication with an incidence rate that depends on the type of surgery, the characteristics of the patients and the method of diagnosis (e.g. clinical examination vs brain imaging). The period of vulnerability to brain injury extends beyond the immediate perioperative period and, in many series, the highest incidence is in the postoperative period.

Disorders of consciousness and cognition are a more frequent type of neurological complication than stroke. These complications include encephalopathy, delirium and more subtle disturbances of cognition. In fact, impaired memory, visual disturbances, difficulty with fine motor movements and attention are the commonest types of neurological complications. The frequency of such neurocognitive dysfunction varies depending on the patients studied, the psychometric battery employed, the methods of data analysis and the timing of testing. The rates are much higher the first week after surgery, but many such deficits are reversible and due to pain, electrolyte disturbances, hypoxaemia and the residual effects of anaesthetics, sedatives and analgesic drugs. Nonetheless, neurocognitive dysfunction at hospital discharge and 1 month later is an important determinant of long-term decline in cognitive capabilities.

Brain imaging performed immediately after surgery suggests an even higher prevalence of cerebral infarction, as high as 45% in some centres. Many of these infarcts are not accompanied by motor or sensory deficits and their impact on higher cerebral function, including cognition, cannot always be demonstrated immediately after surgery. The long-term consequences of clinically 'silent' postoperative strokes are yet to be defined, but they may be associated with slow deterioration in cognitive ability in elderly patients.

Impact on patient outcome

Stroke after cardiac surgery is associated with up to a 10-fold higher operative mortality rate, and a higher risk for death at 1, 5 and 10 years after surgery compared with patients not suffering stroke. Both encephalopathy and neurocognitive dysfunction are associated with higher mortality rates compared with patients not experiencing these deficits. For survivors, all forms of perioperative

Table 45.1 Types and range of frequency of neurological complications reported after cardiac surgery

Type of injury	Range of incidence (%)
Stroke	1.5–5.5
Encephalopathy	6–32
Neurocognitive dysfunction	
At hospital discharge	50–80
1 month after surgery	20–40
6 months after surgery	10–30
Upper extremity neuropathy	
Brachial plexus/ulnar nerve	7–37.7
Other nerves	6
Phrenic nerve injury	
Ice slush during surgery	32–34
No ice slush	2–6
Optic neuropathy	0.06–0.11
Reduced visual acuity	4.5
Dysphagia	
TOE during surgery	7.9
No TOE	1.8

Abbreviation: TOE, transoesophageal echocardiography.

neurological complications are associated with prolonged hospitalization, higher hospital costs, greater likelihood of discharge to a secondary care facility, impaired functional capacity and impaired quality of life after surgery.

Peripheral nerve injury may also occur after cardiac surgery. The long-term outcome of such injury is less well documented, but in many instances recovery occurs over a period of months, provided nerve sheath continuity is not disrupted.

Proposed mechanisms

Cerebral embolism and cerebral hypoperfusion are the two basic mechanisms for brain injury during cardiac surgery. Macroembolism is demonstrated at autopsy and on brain imaging studies. Microembolism is more common and results from a variety of sources including air, atherosclerotic debris, cellular aggregates, thrombi, lipids and other particulate matter. Cerebral hypoperfusion may be global or regional. The latter can occur from localized cerebral arterial stenosis. Cerebral embolism and hypoperfusion are likely to be interrelated in many instances. Cerebral hypoperfusion might impair clearance of microemboli, for example, increasing the duration of tissue anoxia or increasing the dwell time of emboli and thus aggravating endothelial injury.

Excitatory neurotransmitters accumulate at the site of neuronal injury. This 'excitotoxicity' and the inflammatory processes (resulting from surgery or developing locally at the site of brain injury) are believed to exacerbate neuronal injury. Ischaemic brain injury is necrotic and apoptotic. The ultimate manifestation depends on whether the injury is regional or global, permanent or transient, and the location and extent of neuronal ischaemic damage. Brain infarction affecting the motor cortex results in a clinical stroke, whereas the same extent of injury affecting less dominant brain areas might only manifest as neurocognitive dysfunction.

Many candidates for cardiac surgery have widespread atherosclerotic disease affecting the cerebral vasculature. Separating underlying neuropathology from acute brain injury is often difficult. Brain imaging of patients before cardiac surgery demonstrates a high prevalence of preexisting cerebral infarction, white matter changes and hippocampal sclerosis. Autopsy studies of patients who died shortly after cardiac surgery have identified evidence of Alzheimer's disease in a high number of patients (~10%–14%). It is not surprising that candidates for cardiac surgery have a high prevalence of often clinically silent brain injury; since cerebrovascular disease, and its consequences, is common in elderly individuals, particularly in those with diabetes and hypertension. Poor performance on preoperative

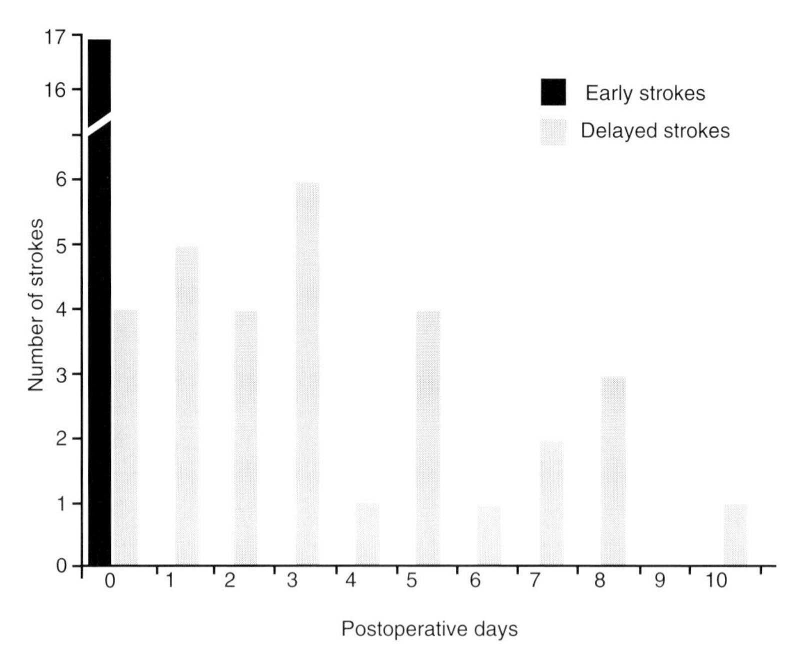

Figure 45.1 Time course of new clinical strokes in a cohort of nearly 3,000 patients. The majority of strokes in this series occurred after emergence from general anaesthesia. (From Hogue CW, *et al.* Reprinted with permission from the American Heart Association).

neuropsychological testing may be a surrogate marker for preexisting cerebrovascular disease.

Risk factors

Many preoperative risk factors are associated with the risk for neurological complications. Both intraoperative and postoperative variables may further influence risk for adverse neurological events.

Atherosclerosis of the aorta

Atheromatous plaques of the ascending aorta are vulnerable to dislodgement during aortic manipulations (e.g. cannulation for cardiopulmonary bypass [CPB], cross-clamping, proximal coronary artery bypass grafting [CABG] anastomosis). Atheroembolism is increasingly recognized as an important risk factor for perioperative stroke. Also, severe atherosclerosis of the ascending aorta is likely to identify patients with extensive cerebrovascular disease. Epiaortic ultrasound at the time of surgery is more sensitive than transoesophageal echocardiography, and much more sensitive than direct palpation, for detecting atherosclerosis of the ascending aorta.

Age

Age is consistently reported as a risk factor for neurological complications. This implies that the frequency of such complications increases with the rising prevalence of older surgical patients. The risk for neurological complications imparted by age, however, is probably related to age-associated vascular disease rather than age per se.

Prior stroke

Previous stroke is one of the strongest indicators of risk for a new neurological deficit after surgery. A history of stroke identifies patients with atherosclerosis of the aorta and the cerebral vasculature who are prone to subsequent stroke even in the absence

Table 45.2 Preoperative risk factors for stroke, encephalopathy, and neurocognitive dysfunction

Stroke	Encephalopathy	Neurocognitive dysfunction
Age >65 years	Age >65 years	Age
Aortic atherosclerosis	Prior stroke	Prior stroke
Diabetes	Diabetes	Aortic atherosclerosis
Hypertension	Hypertension	Poor left ventricular function
Female gender	Carotid bruit	Elevated creatinine
Prior stroke	Peripheral vascular disease	Level of education
Peripheral vascular disease		Smoking
Renal failure		Alcohol abuse
Pulmonary disease		
Intra-aortic balloon pump		
Unstable angina		
Smoking		
Aortic stenosis		
Mitral insufficiency		
First reoperation		

of surgery. Clinical history of stroke identifies only a small portion of patients with prior brain infarctions. Preoperative brain magnetic resonance imaging may identify brain infarction in 40% to 60% of patients. These brain infarcts are usually not associated with a clinical history of stroke.

Gender

Female gender has been found in single and multicentre studies to be associated with increased risk for neurological complications after cardiac surgery. A higher prevalence of risk factors for stroke in women compared with men is one explanation for this observation. The fact that female gender remained an independent predictor of stroke, even after statistically adjusting for other stroke risk factors, implicates unknown variables as a cause of this higher risk.

Medical conditions

Diabetics are at higher risk for neurological complications independent of other risk factors. The mechanism for this risk is not known, but it might be due to a higher prevalence of other stroke risk factors or the propensity for hyperglycaemia.

Hypertension predisposes to stroke in the general population. It is not surprising that even patients with controlled hypertension are at risk for perioperative neurological complications. This risk might be due to altered cerebral autoregulation predisposing to cerebral hypoperfusion during CPB or during periods of haemodynamic instability.

Genetic factors

Several genotypes have been identified to predispose to perioperative neurological complications including the apolipoprotein $\varepsilon 4$ allele, C-reactive protein (3′UTR 1846C/T), interleukin-6 (-174G/C) polymorphisms, as well as polymorphisms associated with platelet glycoprotein receptors. Active investigation continues and the list of candidate polymorphisms is growing. Verification of genetic variants that increase susceptibility to brain injury in larger, multinational patient populations is needed. Identifying risk based on genotype holds promise for more accurate risk stratification and, possibly, an enhanced understanding of the mechanisms of neurological complications.

Cerebral microembolic counts

Cerebral microembolisms composed of either particulate or gaseous material are detected during CPB with transcranial Doppler monitoring in virtually all patients. A relationship between the number of transcranial Doppler high-intensity signals ('HITS') during CPB and neurocognitive dysfunction after CABG surgery has been demonstrated. This relationship, however, has not been shown for patients undergoing open-chamber cardiac valve surgery where HIT counts are higher. The composition of the embolic material, rather than simply the number of HITS, may play a bigger role in the aetiology of brain injury. Fatty material has been found on autopsy in dogs and in humans in small cerebral arterioles after surgery with CPB. The lipid emboli are believed to arise from epicardial adipose tissue that is returned to the CPB circuit via pericardial suction. These fatty emboli are difficult to filter, leading some researchers to advocate first processing pericardial suction blood with a cell saver before reinfusion, but this remains unproven.

Anaemia

Low haematocrit ($\leq$21%) on CPB is suggested, based on observational studies, to be independently associated with stroke and mortality after cardiac surgery. Increases in cerebral blood flow and increased oxygen extraction are the primary compensatory responses to reduced tissue oxygen content. Thus, anaemia might lead to brain injury not only by reducing tissue oxygen delivery, but by also increasing the cerebral blood flow and, hence, the embolic load. Whether transfusion of packed red blood cells reduces the risk for neurological complications after cardiac surgery has not been proven. Prospective randomized trials in nonsurgical critically ill patients found that mortality was actually less in patients 55 years of age or younger with a conservative versus liberal transfusion trigger (haematocrit 21% vs 30%). Post hoc analysis of this trial suggested that more critically ill patients with cardiovascular disease might benefit from maintaining a 'higher' haematocrit. Further investigations are needed to guide transfusion practices during and after CPB.

Acid–base management

Alpha-stat pH management is the most widely used approach for acid–base management during CPB in adults. Although there are conflicting data, this management approach is based on studies suggesting better neurocognitive outcomes compared with pH stat management during CPB. In children, pH stat management is believed to lead to better neurobehavioural development after hypothermic circulatory arrest.

Pulsatile versus nonpulsatile flow

Nonpulsatile flow is the de facto standard for CPB, mostly because prior difficulties with ensuring delivery of pulsatility during CPB. Newer technologies are capable of easily generating pulsatile flow; some data suggest lower systemic vascular resistances, less sympathetic activation, attenuation of the systemic inflammatory response to CPB and better renal function after surgery when pulsatile CPB is used rather than nonpulsatile flow. One prospective randomized study found no differences in neurocognitive dysfunction after CABG surgery with pulsatile compared with nonpulsatile CPB. The patients studied tended to be younger and had fewer stroke risk factors than contemporary cardiac surgical patients.

Hyperglycaemia

Hyperglycaemia extends the size of cerebral infarctions in laboratory experiments. A relation between hyperglycaemia (>140 mg/dL) and worse neurological outcome after stroke or cardiac arrest has been demonstrated in humans. There are few clinical data establishing that prevention of hyperglycaemia with aggressive infusion of insulin during or after CPB leads to improved neurological outcome. Data from trials in critical care patients show that maintaining glucose levels below 130 mg/dL with insulin infusion leads to improved outcomes. Those studies did not focus on neurological complications, included mostly noncardiac surgical patients and the benefits were apparent when patients were in critical care for longer than 3 days. These same data suggested worse outcomes with this strategy in less ill patients requiring shorter critical care stays.

Duration of cardiopulmonary bypass

Long CPB increases the time the brain is exposed to embolism and possible hypoperfusion. This exposure may have a cumulative effect on the brain or it may merely increase the chance for a critical embolic event. On the other hand, long CPB duration tends to be associated with complex cardiac disease requiring extensive surgery. Such patients are prone to multiple adverse events that may be independent of CPB duration.

Inadvertent cerebral hyperthermia

Excessive rewarming of patients after hypothermic CPB is associated with jugular bulb O_2 desaturation indicative of cerebral O_2 supply/demand mismatch. These events have been found to be associated with postoperative neurocognitive dysfunction. Maintaining arterial blood temperature of the CPB perfusate no higher than 37°C during rewarming and avoiding nasopharyngeal temperature higher than 36°C are advocated by some clinicians.

Atrial fibrillation

Atrial fibrillation occurs in 20% to 45% of patients after CABG surgery and at even higher rates after valve surgery. Many studies have found atrial fibrillation to be a predictor of neurological complications, but most studies do not document the fact that the atrial arrhythmias actually occurred before the onset of the cerebral event; that is, stroke itself may precede the atrial fibrillation rather than vice versa. Clinical investigations have shown that anticoagulation reduces the incidence of stroke in nonsurgical and often ambulatory populations with atrial fibrillation. Most clinicians consider anticoagulation for patients with postoperative atrial fibrillation lasting longer than 48 hours or when it is present at the time of hospital discharge. The balance of risks and benefits of this approach specifically in patients after cardiac surgery has not been adequately investigated.

Improving neurological outcomes

Approaches for improving neurological outcomes after cardiac surgery can be physical, such as changing the conduct or circuit of CPB, or pharmacological.

Early studies showed better neurological outcomes when a 20- to 40-micron in-line filter and a membrane oxygenator were used. The evidence to date does not support the widespread, routine use of any pharmacological therapy for limiting the extent of brain injury during or after CPB.

Further neuroprotective manoeuvres can be targeted at patients identified as being at particular risk by epiaortic ultrasound in patients over 65 years of age or for those at risk for neurological

Table 45.3 Summary of results of clinical trials evaluating neuroprotective drugs during cardiac surgery

Drug	Primary mechanism	General findings
Thiopental	↓ $CMRO_2$	Early results showing improved neurocognitive function compared with placebo early after surgery were not confirmed in later studies. The contradictory findings can be explained by types of CPB apparatus (e.g. bubble oxygenator), approach to rewarming and limited long-term patient follow-up in the earlier work.
Propofol	↓ $CMRO_2$	Multicentre study showed no difference in cognitive complications 5–7 or 50–70 days after surgery propofol vs controls.
Nimodipine	Ca^{++} channel blocker	Large, single-centre study stopped early by data and safety monitoring committee owing to higher mortality in nimodipine treated vs control group without evidence of neuroprotective benefit.
Prostacyclin	↓ platelet aggregation, ↓ inflammation	Small, single-centre study showed no difference in cognitive outcomes 2 weeks after surgery compared with controls.
GM1 ganglioside	↓ EAA signalling	No evidence of efficacy in small, preliminary, placebo-controlled trial.
Remacemide	NMDA receptor antagonist	Encouraging results showing better performance on psychometric measures and better global cognitive function in remacemide treated patients compared with placebo. Further confirmatory investigations are needed.
Pegorgotein	Antioxidant	Early study showed no benefit of the drug for reducing the frequency of neurocognitive dysfunction.
Aprotinin	Mechanism(s) unknown; maybe due to ↓ inflammation/↓ pericardial aspirate	Post hoc analysis of prospectively randomized studies that were primarily designed to test the blood-sparing effects of the drug showed lower stroke rates in aprotinin treated patients compared with control patients. Inconclusive data regarding benefit for improving neurocognitive outcomes. Meta-analysis that included larger patient sample size showed aprotinin had a neutral effect on stroke rates compared with placebo.
Lidocaine	Na^+ channel blockade; membrane stabilization/↓ EAA release	Two single-centre, small studies showed neurocognitive outcome slightly improved with lidocaine. Limitations of these investigations included small sample sizes, limited psychometric battery and only short-term patient follow-up. The findings have not been confirmed in more rigorous investigations.
Clomethiazole	GABA receptor agonist	No difference in the frequency of neurocognitive dysfunction was demonstrated compared with placebo in pilot study.
Pexelizumab	↓ C5a and C5b-9	Multicentre study demonstrated that, compared with placebo, pexelizumab led to improvement in visuospatial performance, but no effect on global cognition compared with placebo.
Magnesium	Multiple mechanisms including ↓ Ca^{++} entry and ↓ EAA signalling	Contradictory findings regarding benefit for perioperative neuroprotection. Recent single-centre study suggested some benefit on neurocognitive function compared with placebo.

Abbreviations: CABG, coronary artery bypass grafts; $CMRO_2$, cerebral metabolic rate for oxygen; EAA, excitatory amino acid; GABA, γ-aminobutyric acid; NMDA, N-methyl D-aspartate.

complications. Techniques that can be considered when aortic atherosclerosis is identified include:

- Use of a modified aortic cannula that limits the 'sandblasting' effect of CPB perfusion.
- Use of an aortic cannula with a 'net' to capture embolic material (these are available, but there is no conclusive evidence of their benefit for improving neurological complications).
- Use of the single-cross clamp technique for all CABG anastomoses, distal and proximal.
- Avoidance of proximal CABG anastomosis by using all arterial conduits.
- Considering alternative arterial cannulation sites (axillary or femoral arteries).
- Aiming for relatively high mean arterial pressure during CPB ($\geq$70–80 mmHg) in elderly and high-risk patients (although data on the most appropriate blood pressure for CPB are not conclusive).
- Avoiding 'low' haematocrit. Optimal haematocrit during and after CPB has not been defined, particularly in patients at high risk for neurological complications. A haematocrit of 21% or lower is associated with high risk for stroke and mortality in retrospective studies.
- Processing pericardial suction aspirate with a cell saver before return to the CPB circuit. Although some centres have adopted this practice, evidence supporting its safety and efficacy awaits rigorous evaluation.
- Avoiding cerebral hyperthermia during rewarming patients after hypothermic CPB. The temperature of the blood returning to the arterial circulation should be kept no higher than 37°C.
- Avoiding hyperglycaemia (blood glucose $>$140 mg/dL). A caveat with this recommendation is that there are no data to date showing that 'tight' glucose control during CPB markedly improves neurological outcomes after cardiac surgery.

Other considerations

'Off-pump' coronary artery bypass grafting

The data thus far have shown neither benefit nor increased risk for neurological complications by avoiding CPB. Approach to surgery should be individualized and must consider the experience and skill of the surgical team for providing good surgical outcomes with 'off-pump' surgery.

Neurobiochemical markers of brain injury

Markers have been proposed as an adjunct to other modalities to assess and even predict neurological injury after cardiac surgery. The presence of proteins that are brain specific, such as protein S-100B and neuron-specific enolase, has been well correlated with adverse neurological outcome in patients after stroke, traumatic brain injury and brain damage caused by circulatory arrest. Likewise, these markers have been shown to correlate with adverse neurological events in patients after cardiac surgery. Some of the enthusiasm for these markers has been dampened by data suggesting that they may be falsely elevated by non-brain-specific proteins that resemble proteins such as S-100B or by impaired clearance rather than production during CPB.

Neuromonitoring

Several monitors have been proposed for the detection of brain injury during cardiac surgery including the raw or processed electroencephalogram and monitors of brain oxygenation such as jugular venous blood saturation. Each monitor has limitations precluding widespread clinical acceptance. Noninvasive monitoring of frontal lobe brain oxygenation with near-infrared spectroscopy (NIRS) has received most recent attention. Light in the 680 to 800 nm range penetrates bone at a depth of 1.3 to 2.0 cm from the scalp. Algorithms for subtracting light absorption from the superficial scalp and muscle layers are required. Unlike pulse oximetry, NIRS does not distinguish between arterial, brain tissue or venous oxygen saturation. Near-infrared spectroscopy provides a highly regional, venous-weighted oxyhaemoglobin saturation measurement that is related to brain oxygen and metabolic state. Interindividual precision is in the $\pm$ 10% range and intraindividual precision in the $\pm$3% range. The benefits of NIRS monitoring during cardiac surgery might thus be for identifying trends of compromised brain oxygenation. Current data involving the most widely used NIRS device suggests that values less than 40% to 45%, or a change of 20% from baseline, represent risk for neurological injury. Criticisms of NIRS monitoring include the limited spatial resolution that excludes important brain areas such as the motor and sensory cortex, occipital cortex, brain stem and brain areas supporting cognition and memory (e.g. hippocampus and medial temporal cortex). Although studies have demonstrated that low NIRS values identify individuals at risk for neurological complications, investigations have been limited by retrospective study design, failure to perform broad psychometric measurements or brain imaging studies and the inclusion of mostly short-term outcomes. More important, rigorous investigations are needed to assess whether interventions based on real-time NIRS monitoring during CPB result in improved patient outcomes. Such interventions for low NIRS values include raising the blood pressure, ensuring optimal CPB flow, red blood cell transfusion and possibly allowing blood pH to rise to increase cerebral blood flow.

Assessing early neurological function after cardiac surgery

The manner in which neurological function is assessed after cardiac surgery varies from institution to institution and there is no evidence to suggest which approach is best for evaluating a patient with 'slow' awakening. A cursory neurological examination is performed as soon as feasible, assessing the ability of the patient to follow commands and to move all extremities. In the event that a patient demonstrates focal deficits, an appropriate next step is to perform an immediate computed tomography (CT) scan of the patient's head. In patients who are slow to awaken or who demonstrate encephalopathy or delirium a differential diagnosis should include the following:

- hypoxia;
- hypercarbia;
- residual anaesthetics (e.g. opioids, benzodiazepines, hypnotics, or muscle relaxants);
- prior alcohol or drug abuse or withdrawal;
- hypoglycaemia or hyperglycaemia;
- electrolyte abnormalities (e.g. sodium, calcium);
- hypothermia; and
- hypothyroidism.

Rare diagnoses such as neurological or systemic infection, uraemia, liver failure, seizures (perhaps masked by the effects of anaesthetics or sedatives) and cerebral tumours should also be considered. If a patient has not demonstrated return of neurological function 12 hours after the cessation of sedatives and narcotics, a CT scan of the head is also indicated. The CT scan can reveal evidence of central neurological injury such as intraventricular haemorrhage, embolic or thrombotic cerebral vascular accidents, normal pressure hydrocephalus or pathology consistent with dementia or cognitive impairment syndromes. Although rare after cardiac surgery, any evidence of subarachnoid haemorrhage may warrant the use of transcranial Doppler to evaluate cerebral perfusion and to assess for cerebral vasospasm.

Ultimately, a comprehensive neurological examination should be performed, including the assessment of cranial nerves, cerebellar function, motor and sensory function, mini-mental status examinations and tests of cognition. Further diagnostic testing is dictated by the results of this examination.

Key points

- Diagnosis of neurological complications depends on the extent of patient examination. Subtle deficits of cognition and memory can be found in 20% to 40% of patients 1 month after surgery using psychometric testing. Evidence of brain embolism can be demonstrated in a similar percentage of patients using brain magnetic resonance imaging, although the latter are not always associated with clinical stroke or neurocognitive dysfunction.
- Neurological complications are associated with increased mortality, longer hospitalization, higher health care costs and diminished quality of life after surgery.
- Patients at high risk for neurological complications include the elderly, patients with prior stroke, diabetics, hypertensives and females.
- Aetiology of neurological complications is believed to be cerebral macro- or microembolism and cerebral hypoperfusion exacerbated by inflammatory processes induced by surgical trauma and CPB.
- There are no drugs that have conclusively been found to lead to improved neurological outcomes after cardiac surgery.

FURTHER READING

Herrmann M, Ebert AD, Galazky I, *et al.* Neurobehavioral outcome prediction after cardiac surgery: role of neurobiochemical markers of damage to neuronal and glial brain tissue. *Stroke* 2000;31:645–650.

Hogue CW Jr, Murphy SF, Schechtman KB, *et al.* Risk factors for early or delayed stroke after cardiac surgery. *Circulation* 1999;100:642–647.

Hogue CW Jr, Palin CA, Arrowsmith JEA. Management of cardiopulmonary bypass and neurologic complications: a critical appraisal of current practices. *Anesth Analg* 2006;103:21–37.

McKhann GM, Grega MA, Borowicz LM Jr, *et al.* Stroke and encephalopathy after cardiac surgery. *Stroke* 2006;37:562–571.

Roach GW, Kanchuger M, Mora-Mangano C, *et al.* Adverse cerebral outcomes after coronary bypass surgery. Multicenter Study of Perioperative Ischemia Research Group and the Ischemia Research and Education Foundation Investigators. *N Engl J Med* 1996;335:1857–1863.

Chapter 46

Psychiatric illness during and after discharge from critical care

C.R. WEINERT

Introduction

The physical consequences of critical illness are relatively easily recognized by clinicians, families and patients. Less apparent are psychological symptoms that appear during critical illness and afterwards and that can combine to create symptom clusters of sufficient severity that a specific psychiatric disorder results. Recognizing the psychological symptoms that are expected after major illness and knowing the usual severity and duration of symptoms is an important skill for clinicians caring for patients during and after critical care. Almost all psychiatric research on the epidemiology and treatment of depression, anxiety or post-traumatic stress disorder (PTSD) has been conducted with patients not in critical care units, so that translating research from ambulatory patients with little medical comorbidity to critically ill patients is difficult.

No clinical recommendations can be made that are supported by multiple trials performed in critical care patients.

Defining psychiatric illness

Psychiatrists in Europe and the United States generally use categorical schema to define disorders based on counting symptoms and behaviours, although there is substantial evidence that psychiatric symptoms and conditions occur on a continuum.

For instance, by DSM-IV criteria, the basis for defining depression-related mood disorders is the presence of a Major Depressive Episode (MDE), which requires 2 weeks or more of either daily depressed mood or anhedonia (inability to gain pleasure from enjoyable experiences). In addition, four other concurrent somatic or psychological cardinal symptoms should be present, such as low energy, feeling of worthlessness, suicidal ideation, anorexia or psychomotor agitation or retardation. The episode has to be of sufficient severity to cause impairment in social or occupational function or symptomatic distress for the patient, such that, for instance, they seek relief of symptoms from health care providers.

The aetiology of the MDE is further categorized by the clinician into 'disorders' such as those due to the direct physiological effect of substances (both illicit and prescribed), medical conditions (mood disorder due to a general medical condition) or other conditions such as bereavement or bipolar illness. If these conditions do not completely account for the mood symptoms then Major Depressive Disorder is diagnosed.

In research studies, these symptoms are elicited by structured interviews, often complemented by a patient-completed severity score. In clinical practice, interviews and chart reviews are less formal, but a cursory examination and psychiatric interview of patients with serious medical illnesses could lead to an incorrect diagnosis and prescription of ineffective or harmful therapies.

The difficulty in determining the cause(s) of depressive symptoms in acutely ill or rehabilitating medical and surgical patients is clear. What is likely more predictive of a 'true' depressive episode is the severity and persistence of depressive symptoms in the face of improving physical status.

Depression

Large studies in patients with and without medical illnesses have clearly demonstrated that depression increases patient suffering, decreases quality of life and is consistently associated with increased mortality. Depression severity affects the prognosis more than disorder classification. This is important because it suggests that depression is a spectrum disorder and using 'diagnostic' breakpoints underestimates the total depression symptom burden that resides in the large group with 'subthreshold' diagnoses.

In hospitalized patients, depression is associated with readmission and higher acute care and rehabilitation costs, even after adjusting for comorbidity.

Although there is substantial evidence that treating established major depression associated with medical illness is effective, medical comorbidity remains a risk factor for nonresponse to antidepressants.

Difficulties in assessing depression after critical illness

Because of the acute nature of critical illness, all studies lack a detailed baseline evaluation such that it is impossible to determine the extent to which the medical illness, surgical procedure, anaesthetic treatment or postoperative course contributes to the patients' outcome several weeks or months later. Even the quasi-experimental designs used in studies to evaluate changes in cognition after cardiac surgery have highlighted the challenges in defining the cause(s) of changes in brain function from a precritical care baseline. Moreover, compared with neuropsychological testing, measurement of psychiatric illness is performed with less reliable instruments and psychopathological severity is estimated with fewer normative data than in the noncritical care population. Therefore, determining cause and effect in postcritical care psychiatric illness is very difficult.

Patients expressing symptoms of low mood or anhedonia may have conditions other than major depressive disorder. Transient (not most of the day or nearly every day) or mild symptoms that improve with increasing functional status in the hospital, discharge to home or at a postoperative clinic visit, are more indicative of an adjustment disorder with depressed mood. This can be managed with general supportive interactions and by informing the patient and family of the good prognosis for symptom resolution.

Realistically, only experience can determine when a postcritical care patient is expressing more than the expected amount of psychological distress relative to the severity of their medical illness and the speed and completeness of physical recovery. This clinical wisdom can be more quickly gained if clinicians routinely ask all their patients about a limited number of mood symptoms (e.g. low mood, energy, sleep, hopelessness) during recovery in the hospital and at follow-up clinic visits.

Delirium

An important condition to distinguish from depression is delirium. Delirium affects up to 80% of intubated medical critical care patients and is associated with increased length of hospital stay and 6-month mortality. Delirium usually presents as a hypoactive, withdrawn patient; the agitated form occurs in a minority of critical care patients. Delirium in the hospital leads to increased risk for cognitive dysfunction after discharge; however, in critical care patients, the extent to which delirium is a risk factor for postcritical care depression is unknown. Ongoing studies of medicines to prevent or treat critical

Table 46.1 Differential diagnosis of medical patients exhibiting signs and symptoms of depression

Diagnosis	Defining characteristics	Treatment
Adjustment disorder with depressed mood	Transient and nonsevere symptoms that respond to supportive comments. Symptoms diminish with improved physical function.	Create supportive atmosphere.
Delirium	Fluctuating level of consciousness, inattention and confusion.	Treat underlying cause – usually the systemic inflammatory response syndrome or drug effects. Antipsychotics may control behavioural manifestations but, in critical care patients, there is little evidence that it changes the natural course of the disease.
Brain ischaemia	Focal neurological signs, abnormal brain imaging.	Prevent further brain insults.
Drug effects	Currently receiving daily doses of opiates, benzodiazepines or other neurologically active medication.	Wean drugs as tolerated without creating acute abstinence syndromes.
Drug withdrawal	Recent and prolonged sedation (>5 days) with high-dose opiates or benzodiazepines or precritical care substance or alcohol abuse. Patients have increased autonomic activity and are usually more anxious appearing than depressed. It is difficult to distinguish withdrawal symptoms from numerous other causes in adult patients.	Increase dose until symptoms resolve and then taper with longer acting medications.
'Sickness behaviour' associated with systemic inflammation	Fever, leukocytosis, elevated C-reactive protein.	Clinical judgment is required to determine whether the medical condition accounts for all of the depressive symptoms (mood disorder owing to a general medical condition). If not, then the patient may have both a medical and psychiatric diagnosis.

care delirium give clinicians greater evidence about the efficacy and adverse effects of using first- and second-generation antipsychotics in delirious critical care patients.

Depression after acute coronary syndromes

Depression after myocardial infarction, unstable angina or coronary revascularization procedure doubles the odds of having another cardiac event or dying from any cause. However, no trial has shown that antidepressant therapy improves cardiovascular outcomes in depressed patients. However, treating depressed patients with coronary artery disease is safe and effective in alleviating depressive symptoms. Unlike tricyclic antidepressants, selective serotonin reuptake inhibitors (SSRIs) do not cause orthostatic hypotension and do not decrease cardiac conduction or heart rate variability, although the safety and efficacy of SSRI therapy in critical care patients has not been established. Reports of SSRI-associated bleeding and platelet dysfunction as well as electrolyte disorders and the serotonin syndrome suggest caution.

Nonpharmacological interventions to prevent or treat postmyocardial infarction depression have been tested, but the results have been disappointing. Postmyocardial infarction psychological therapy, counselling and stress management do not reduce depression, anxiety or cardiac events.

There are no large studies specifically aimed at treating depressed patients with antidepressants or psychotherapy while they are in the critical care unit. Small, uncontrolled series using 'psychostimulants' to improve ventilator weaning in depressed critical care patients do not provide sufficient data to draw conclusions regarding the safety and efficacy of these medications. Yet antidepressants are probably widely used in patients recovering from respiratory failure (although usually after they leave the critical care unit).

It is important that delirium is not misdiagnosed as a mood disorder. Depression in patients recovering from critical care in all but its most severe, suicidal form is not a medical emergency.

The ingrained practice of intensivists to rapidly intervene and reassess for treatment response is probably counterproductive when dealing with depressed, medically ill patients. It is good practice to observe patients for several days after a possible diagnosis of depression is raised by the patient, family or caregivers. The persistence and severity of mood symptoms should be carefully documented, and the absence of delirious behaviour confirmed. Practitioners should also remain objective and critically examine their own or other caregivers' feelings that they too would 'feel depressed' if they were in the patient's situation. One consistent finding from studies of postcritical care psychiatric illness is that the majority (approximately 75%) of patients surviving prolonged acute respiratory failure recover without significant psychological injury.

Table 46.2 Interventions to improve the psychological outcome of critical care patients

Tracheostomy allowing more mobilization, oral feeding, verbal communication and reduction in sedative exposure.
Wean as many neurologically active medications as possible while treating pain adequately.
Physical therapy and health psychology consultation, if available.
Structure regular sleep–wake cycles using behavioural and medication-based interventions.
Present clear goals for rehabilitation and return to home.
Enlist family support in presenting a positive attitude.
Review course of illness and acknowledge common symptoms of flashbacks, fear and amnesia that the patient may believe indicates brain injury.
If patient was taking an antidepressant before critical care admission, consider restarting it or initiate a short-acting SSRI antidepressant with the fewest drug–drug interactions. For persistent or severe symptoms or before starting more than low doses of tricyclic medications or any monoamine oxidase inhibitor, consult with a psychiatrist with experience in treating medically ill patients.

Abbreviation: SSRI, selective serotonin reuptake inhibitor.

Pathogenesis of depression in critically ill patients

It is now recognized that afferent and efferent neural pathways can control the inflammatory state by allowing communication between the brain and periphery. 'Sickness behaviours,' such as fatigue, anorexia, psychomotor slowing, sleep alteration and anhedonia, overlap cardinal symptoms of MDE, and are at least partially mediated by inflammatory cytokines. Although antidepressants are not typically considered immunomodulatory medications, they may abrogate some of the deleterious effects of systemic inflammation on mood symptoms.

On a more basic neuroscience level, it is known that animals exposed to environmental stress have impaired neuronal growth and development in the hippocampus and demonstrate stereotypical behaviours analogous to some human mood behaviours. This neuronal atrophy can be prevented by antidepressant drugs administered during the stress interval. Proof that the observed neuronal changes directly mediate the observed behaviours during stress is lacking and the molecular events that link stress to neuronal or glial dysfunction and the actions of antidepressants remain obscure.

However, these observations have led to the hypothesis that the brain structures responsible for depressive symptoms and behaviours are adversely affected during critical illness and that specific areas of the central nervous system can be 'psycho-protected' by prophylactic administration of antidepressants during the medical stress period. This hypothesis has not yet been tested in human critical illness. Although the ultimate cause of any mood symptom or behaviour is brain neuronal activity, it is also useful to consider psychodynamic explanations for critical care depression, such as loss of function and independence, inability to communicate and fear of dying or having unrelieved suffering.

Post-traumatic stress symptoms after critical illness

Acute respiratory failure is a life-threatening condition and psychological and behavioural responses can be expected owing to intolerable symptoms or a threat to life similar to that experienced by victims of military or civilian trauma. However, caregivers are often concerned that the unpleasant memories of fear and anxiety associated with acute severe illness and/or life-support therapies could be recalled later by patients, resulting in a variable amount of psychological distress that persists after patients physically recover.

At follow-up several years after severe acute lung injury, nearly one third (28%) of patients score above the threshold value on the Post-Traumatic Stress Syndrome Inventory, which is highly predictive of a formal post-PTSD diagnosis. There is a positive relationship between PTSD symptoms and the number of distressing symptoms (e.g. pain, anxiety, dyspnoea, nightmares) that patients experienced during their critical care treatment years earlier. Patients with PTSD have little mood psychopathology, but high levels of anxiety symptoms and somatoform symptoms. The critical care length of stay is longer for those who later develop PTSD compared to those with subthreshold or no PTSD. Animal models suggest that 'fight-or-flight' chemicals such as adrenaline and cortisol enhance memory consolidation for stressful events, yet humans with established PTSD have lower cortisol levels than normal people. Endogenous substances released during severe medical stress may affect the emotional response to recall of unpleasant memories. The content of the critical care memory may be more important than the number of memories, and delusional memories (e.g. nightmares, hallucination, persecutory delusions) cause persistent emotional distress more than factual, albeit unpleasant, memories (e.g. pain, anxiety).

Studies have opposing clinical implications for sedation of patients in critical care units. Some suggest that complete amnesia for the critical care experience would prevent PTSD symptoms and that the critical interval for PTSD pathogenesis is during weaning when sedatives are reduced. However, complete amnesia is difficult to achieve and delirious memories (possibly promoted by sedative medications) may lead to worse psychological outcomes. This hypothesis is, however, supported by good evidence that daily sedation interruption (sedation breaks) leads to improved psychological recovery after prolonged respiratory failure.

Anxiety

Anxiety and autonomic arousal are inevitable responses to life-threatening illness. Combined with impaired level of consciousness and ventilator dyssynchrony, this can lead to distressing and dangerous behaviours often characterized under the catch-all term 'anxious.' However, mechanical ventilation itself (unless poorly set up relative to the patient's ventilatory needs) is usually not a primary cause of an intubated patient's agitated or anxious behaviour. Even in very anxious patients cared for by psychiatrists, oral benzodiazepines sometimes combined with SSRI medications are usually sufficient to alleviate symptoms without decreasing alertness. Behaviours in the critical care unit requiring frequent doses of intravenous benzodiazepines or potent hypnotics such as propofol are more likely the result of delirium, untreated pain, severe dyspnoea or drug intoxication rather than simple anxiety. Similarly, postcritical care anxious complaints of restlessness, generalized discomfort, insomnia, distressing rumination about death or disability (especially at night) and constant need for reassurance may indicate a withdrawal syndrome from opiates or benzodiazepines administered during critical care stay. Symptoms should respond to reassurance, education about the common nature of the complaints and tapering doses of a regularly scheduled medium-duration oral benzodiazepine, with possibly a larger dose at bedtime.

Key points

- Patients recovering from critical illness have survived tremendous stress to their physical and psychological health.
- There are few interventions that are safe and effective in preventing or treating psychiatric illness for patients in the critical care unit.
- Clinicians should proactively ask their patients about mood, anxiety and PTSD symptoms.
- If complaints or behaviours are persistent or severe, careful evaluation and treatment involving both medications and nonpharmacological interventions may be useful.

FURTHER READING

Chevrolet JC, Jolliet P. Clinical review: Agitation and delirium in the critically ill – significance and management. *Crit Care* 2007;11;214.

Griffiths RD, Jones C. Delirium, cognitive dysfunction and posttraumatic stress disorder. *Curr Opin Anaesthesiol* 2007;20:124–129.

Miller RR 3rd, Ely EW. Delirium and cognitive dysfunction in the intensive care unit. *Curr Psychiatry Rep* 2007;9:26–34.

SECTION 4 Procedure-Specific Care in Cardiothoracic Critical Care

Chapter 47

Routine management after cardiac surgery

N.E. DRURY AND S.A.M. NASHEF

Introduction

Early postoperative management after cardiac surgery takes place in the critical care unit, enabling the provision of advanced respiratory, cardiovascular and renal support. The patient usually remains intubated and ventilated, with close monitoring of haemodynamic variables, cardiac rhythm and chest drain output. The aim is to achieve metabolic stability through the control of cardiovascular and respiratory parameters.

However, this is threatened even before arrival in the critical care area. Transfer of the patient from the operating table to the critical care unit has the potential for displacement or disconnection of tubes, lines, drains and pacing wires. The risk can be minimized by careful handling, portable monitoring and accompaniment by both anaesthetic and surgical staff.

On arrival, the patient is received by the critical care team to whom relevant information is communicated. Baseline routine tests including arterial blood gas analysis are carried out. In some units, a portable plain chest radiograph is also taken on admission.

Assessment of the adult cardiac surgical patient

Evaluation requires review of the case notes, the patient, the observation charts recording haemodynamic and other parameters, laboratory and radiological tests and an electrocardiogram.

The case notes provide the patient's background information including operative and preoperative data. The admission clerking gives details of the diagnosis, demographics, status (routine, urgent, emergent), preoperative ventricular function and comorbidity, particularly respiratory, renal and neurological dysfunction. The operation note should describe what was done, what was not done, any problems encountered and details of the placement and numbers of drains and pacing wires.

Examination of the patient is an important part of the assessment and should not be lost in the large quantity of data generated by monitors. On arrival in critical care, the patient should be warm, well-perfused and adequately sedated. Physical examination, notably of the heart, lungs and peripheral circulation, should be performed and documented so that any future change in status that may require intervention can be appreciated.

Observation charts provide a detailed and easily interpretable record of a patient's stay on the critical care unit. Many units currently record physiological data on a single sheet of paper every day, providing an overview of recent progress. The main variables are ventilatory parameters, arterial blood gases, basic and advanced cardiovascular variables, neurological status and fluid balance, including infusions, nutrition, urine output and drains. Several units have recently replaced paper and pen recording with an electronic clinical information system (Chapter 66). All clinical variables are recorded and presented on a visual display unit, allowing rapid and flexible manipulation of both real-time and historical patient data, as well as a reliable detailed digital record of the patient's stay.

Although analysis of actual values is important, the plotting of trends and responses to therapy provides a more dynamic perspective. Think about applied cardiovascular physiology: What is the gradient of this patient's Starling curve and where is the patient in relation to it now? The response of mean arterial and right atrial pressure to a judicious fluid challenge is a useful guide to a patient's cardiovascular status in the absence of more invasive monitoring, such as a pulmonary artery catheter.

The reliability of data should also be considered: a 'failure of intelligence' may result in inappropriate action as much in critical care as in politics! For example, pressures from a nonzeroed transducer may be misleading; 'anuria' may be due to a blocked urinary catheter; and pulmonary artery catheter data are only reliable if the catheter is in the right place and correctly calibrated.

Laboratory and radiological investigations are the principal adjuncts to clinical monitoring. Blood samples are routinely sent to haematology and biochemistry for a full blood count, coagulation studies, serum electrolytes and liver function tests, with further tests requested as appropriate. Arterial blood sampling is used to provide a bedside assessment of gas exchange and metabolic state; many analysers also provide data on haematocrit, haemoglobin, potassium, glucose and lactate concentrations. A portable plain chest radiograph enables the diagnosis of a number of postoperative problems.

Assessment of the cardiac silhouette and mediastinum is also useful for comparison with future films. An electrocardiogram should also be obtained, although interpretation of ventricular complex morphology is difficult in the initial period after cardiac surgery and is not the most specific tool for the diagnosis of postoperative ischaemia.

The team-based approach

The care of the surgical patient on cardiothoracic critical care is explicitly multidisciplinary. The core membership comprises the intensivist, cardiac surgeon and critical care nurse, with regular input from the physiotherapist, pharmacist and dietician. This team of professionals frequently reviews the patient throughout the day on regular ward rounds and as required in the intervening periods. As complications arise, other specialists may be consulted for advice including the cardiologist, haematologist, renal physician, general or vascular surgeon, radiologist, psychologist or even speech and language therapist.

The operating surgeon should play a pivotal role in this team, having met the patient preoperatively, discussed the risks and benefits of the intervention, obtained informed consent and taken knife to skin and beyond. The surgeon has had an unrivalled view of the patient's anatomy and response to physiological stimuli. It is therefore important implicitly to trust the surgeon's opinion on his or her patient. On the other hand, few surgeons express their self-doubts, uncertainties or reservations in the immediate aftermath of a tricky case. It is in their nature to be optimistic about their cases, ability and judgment; else they would not operate on sick hearts. It is therefore important implicitly to doubt the surgeon's opinion. Needless to say, there is a balance to be sought in the objective assessment of every patient.

Key points

- Transfer from the operating theatre to critical care is a potentially hazardous journey.
- Assessment of the postoperative cardiac surgical patient should include the notes, the charts, the investigations and the patient.
- The surgeon has a pivotal role on the multidisciplinary team.

Chapter **48**

Management after coronary artery bypass grafting surgery

N.E. DRURY, S.A.M. NASHEF
AND N. BREITENFELDT

Introduction

Coronary artery bypass grafting (CABG) is the commonest cardiac operation performed. Its purpose is to relieve angina and help prevent myocardial infarction by bypassing narrowed or occluded coronary arteries. This is done by suturing a pedicled arterial graft (such as a left internal mammary artery [LIMA]) or a free graft (such as a segment of saphenous vein or a radial artery) to the affected coronary artery downstream from the lesion. A pedicled LIMA brings its blood supply with it from the subclavian artery. A free graft needs to be joined to a nearby source of oxygenated arterial blood, usually the ascending aorta.

Most CABG is done on cardiopulmonary bypass with cardioplegic cardiac arrest, but it is possible to achieve good results without cardiopulmonary bypass on the beating heart. This chapter deals with specific problems that may be encountered after CABG.

Myocardial ischaemia

The heart should not be ischaemic after CABG. If the electrocardiograph shows ischaemic changes, this may indicate:

- myocardial damage owing to
  - poor protection during surgery or
  - compromise of a coronary artery;
- incomplete revascularization, leaving a segment of myocardium still ischaemic;
- a technical graft problem (such as thrombosis, occlusion or kink); or
- spasm of a coronary artery.

Although myocardial protection is an important issue in all cardiac surgery, it can be more problematic in CABG because of the native coronary disease. Incomplete revascularization renders the ungrafted coronary territory unprotected and is more common in off-pump (beating heart) surgery.

After CABG, coronary or graft vasospasm may affect normal, diseased or bypassed vessels as well as the bypasses themselves, especially arterial conduits. The aetiology remains unclear and the diagnosis is often difficult. Typically, it can occur during a catecholamine surge, such as on waking up or extubation, and may follow the administration of vasopressor drugs. Spasm should be considered in the differential diagnosis of any patient with electrocardiographic evidence of ischaemia, dysrhythmias or low cardiac output, especially if the surgeon is confident about the quality of graft. Initial management is supportive with optimization of the cardiac indices: preload, heart rate, contractility and afterload. Nitrates or calcium channel antagonists are often started, but are negatively inotropic and may precipitate a further fall in mean arterial pressure by decreasing systemic vascular resistance. If inotropic support is required, a phosphodiesterase inhibitor is the agent of choice because it also produces coronary vasodilatation. The diagnosis may be confirmed on contrast coronary angiography but a lack of haemodynamic improvement should prompt a return to the operating room to exclude a technical graft problem.

Postoperative ischaemia may also be due to early graft failure. Low conduit flow detected intraoperatively may be due to poor surgical technique and should lead to immediate reconstruction of the anastomosis. Intracoronary air embolism produces ischaemic changes that usually resolve spontaneously, usually within minutes. In patients receiving a radial artery graft, the calcium channel blocker diltiazem is often used for the first few months to prevent spasm and graft occlusion. Vein graft patency is improved by the early administration of antiplatelet therapy (aspirin or clopidogrel) and these conduits may be preferable in patients with poor left ventricular function owing to an increased requirement for vasoactive drugs in the early postoperative period.

Minimally invasive coronary surgery

Minimally invasive direct coronary artery bypass surgery involves the (usually off-pump) anastomosis of the LIMA to the left anterior descending artery via an anterior thoracotomy with excision of the rib. Epicardial pacing wires are not routinely placed and symptomatic bradycardia may occasionally require temporary transvenous pacing. In addition, minimally invasive direct coronary artery bypass can be performed as part of a staged hybrid procedure with subsequent percutaneous coronary intervention to other diseased vessels; it should be remembered that in the interim, these patients are incompletely revascularized.

Donor harvest site

The major free graft conduit harvest sites are the leg (long and short saphenous vein) and the forearm (radial artery), usually on the nondominant side. In some patients, the harvest site is more painful than the sternotomy incision (heart surgery is often a pain in the leg!). Complications include pain, paraesthesia, bleeding, dehiscence and infection; the incidence is increased by patient factors (obesity, diabetes, peripheral vascular disease) and operative factors (poor technique with excessive soft tissue trauma, nerve injury, formation of tissue flaps and haematoma). Wound infection requires prompt treatment, including antibiotic therapy, debridement and negative pressure dressings.

Case study

A 68-year-old woman is admitted to the critical care unit following in-house urgent CABG using LIMA and saphenous vein conduits. She has three-vessel ischaemic heart disease with moderate left ventricular function after a recent myocardial infarction. The procedure was uneventful and she was weaned off cardiopulmonary bypass without inotropic support. Two mediastinal and a left pleural drain were placed and closure was routine. Her observations on transfer from the operating room are: heart rate, 80 bpm; sinus rhythm; BP, 112/58 mmHg (mean, 73); right atrial pressure (RAP), 8 mmHg; and drainage, 200 mL/h.

Over the next 3 hours, her blood pressure drifts downwards: heart rate, 110 bpm; sinus rhythm; BP, 86/44 mmHg (mean, 58); RAP, 4 mmHg; and drainage, 150 mL/h.

She is felt to be underfilled and, after two boluses of 250 mL of colloid, her blood pressure rallies to a mean of 68 with a RAP of 9. However, over the subsequent 2 hours, her blood pressure slides again and does not respond to a further fluid challenge. At least the bleeding seems to have stopped as the last 3 hours are recorded as 150 mL, 50 mL and 0 mL: heart rate, 124 bpm; sinus rhythm; BP, 73/43 mmHg (mean, 53); RAP, 16 mmHg; and drainage, 0 mL/h.

An infusion of noradrenaline (norepinephrine) is commenced at 2 μg/min in an attempt to improve her blood pressure but with little effect. Her peripheries are now cool and arterial blood gases reveal a worsening metabolic acidosis with a base deficit of 6. A pulmonary artery catheter is floated to assess her low cardiac output state and provides the following data: cardiac index, 1.9 L/min/m^2; pulmonary artery pressure (PAP), 28/15 mmHg (mean, 21); and pulmonary artery occlusion pressure, 19 mmHg.

Cardiac tamponade is suspected and a transoesophageal echocardiogram demonstrates a large pericardial collection with compression of the right atrium and right ventricle. She is transferred to the operating room for exploration and an arterial bleeding point is found at the LIMA harvest site on the anterior chest wall. After cessation of bleeding, she is returned to the critical care unit and remains stable overnight. She is extubated on the following morning and discharged home on the postoperative day 7.

Learning points

- In clinical practice, the signs of postoperative cardiac tamponade can be subtle. Although drain output naturally declines in the nonbleeding patient, an abrupt decrease following a period of significant drainage may paradoxically be bad news: the drains may be blocked. Another clue for tamponade in this patient is the combination of hypotension, elevated filling pressures and compensatory tachycardia; note that the right atrial pressure rise was late, as the open left pleural cavity can accommodate a substantial amount of haemorrhage before the heart is compressed.
- Any cardiac surgical patient with increasing inotrope requirements and rising filling pressures without a clear reason for worse cardiac function should be presumed to have tamponade until proven otherwise.
- In many units, routine plain chest radiography is not carried out immediately after surgery. In this patient, a radiograph would have demonstrated a wide mediastinum and a fluid-filled left chest. There are indications for chest radiography beyond problems with ventilation.
- In this scenario, the institution of an infusion of noradrenaline (norepinephrine) was inappropriate. It is a powerful catecholamine that increases systemic vascular resistance (alpha effect), contractility and heart rate ($beta_1$ effects) with a secondary rise in myocardial oxygen demand and a fall in organ perfusion. Noradrenaline is useful in patients whose hypotension is due to low systemic vascular resistance as in septic shock. In this case, hypotension was due to low cardiac output; systemic vascular resistance was elevated and would have risen further with noradrenaline. This is likely to have worsened to the low cardiac output state and the acidosis. If the diagnosis is uncertain, it is preferable to float a pulmonary artery catheter early and institute evidence-based inotropic therapy.
- The indications for reopening in the early postoperative period are bleeding, low cardiac output state with suspected tamponade or cardiac arrest. Reexploration is associated with increased morbidity, mortality and length of stay in hospital, and is a risk factor for sternal wound infection.

FURTHER READING

Hirsch WS, Ledley GS, Kotler MN. Acute ischemic syndromes following coronary artery bypass graft surgery. *Clin Cardiol* 1998;21:625–632.

Chapter 49

Management after valve surgery

N.E. DRURY, S.A.M. NASHEF
AND N. BREITENFELDT

Care after a heart valve operation is determined by both the operative intervention and the pathophysiological status of the patient, with particular regard to ventricular function and the presence of pulmonary hypertension. In adults, operations on the aortic or mitral valve form the vast majority of such cases. This chapter deals primarily with the anatomical and physiological issues specific to surgery for heart valve disease.

Aortic valve surgery

Anatomical concerns

The leading cause of aortic stenosis in the elderly is a calcific degenerative process that often extends beyond the annulus into the wall of the aorta with calcified, atheromatous plaques. Aortic cannulation, aortotomy, excision of the valve and annular decalcification are all potential sources of particulate debris that increase the risk of perioperative stroke in this group. Cardiac structures that lie close to the aortic annulus are at risk during removal of the native valve, decalcification of the annulus or valve suture placement. The atrioventricular node lies near the base of the right coronary cusp and may be injured to produce complete heart block; if persistent, a permanent pacemaker may be needed. The anterior leaflet of the mitral valve may also be accidentally hitched up, producing new mitral regurgitation. The ostia of the coronary arteries are very close to the aortic annulus and may be compromised by the valve sutures or by an implanted valve that is too large or badly seated. If the implanted valve is not adequately sutured to the aortic annulus, a large paravalvular leak may cause haemodynamically important aortic regurgitation and a small one may cause haemolysis. Nowadays, intraoperative transoesophageal echocardiography is routinely used at the end of the procedure to screen for problems.

Physiological considerations

In aortic stenosis, the left ventricle (LV) gradually develops concentric hypertrophy to eject blood through the shrinking valve orifice and this increases myocardial oxygen demand. The ventricle also becomes stiff with reduced wall compliance (diastolic dysfunction). Cardiac output (CO) is therefore more dependent on ventricular filling (preload): left-sided filling pressure needs to be adequate following surgery. Left ventricular end-diastolic pressure is best estimated by the pulmonary capillary wedge pressure obtained from a pulmonary artery catheter. Coordinated atrial contraction may contribute up to 30% of ventricular filling in the presence of diastolic dysfunction and therefore new postoperative atrial fibrillation has a detrimental effect on both stroke volume and CO.

The operative relief of the stenosis in the presence of a dynamic LV tends to result in hypertension. This response is usually delayed by several hours and may only become apparent after admission to the critical care unit. Antihypertensive medication is then required to protect suture lines and reduce myocardial oxygen demand. Vasodilators, such as nitroglycerin and sodium nitroprusside, are the mainstay of treatment in the immediate postoperative period. On the other hand, if presentation for surgery is late, the LV may have become dilated, producing systolic dysfunction and dictating the need for inotropic drugs in the early postoperative period.

Aortic regurgitation produces volume loading of the LV leading to a dilated, compliant chamber. Systolic dysfunction is common with compensatory eccentric hypertrophy. After surgery, most patients remain vasodilated and may require vasoconstrictors to maintain blood pressure. The LV is less dependent on filling pressures, but more sensitive to any excessive increase in afterload. If hypertension develops, β-blockade is more effective than further vasodilatation.

Mitral valve surgery

Anatomical concerns

When possible, repair of the mitral apparatus is preferable to valve replacement. Mitral valve repair involves a combination of procedures to the valve leaflets, chordae tendinae and annulus. If the valve must be replaced, this should ideally be done with as much preservation of the subvalvular apparatus as possible: these structures play a crucial role in the maintenance of LV morphology; if their integrity is lost, the ventricle becomes more globular and less efficient. Decalcification or suturing of the mitral annulus may result in complete heart block by damage to the atrioventricular node and conduction system. The circumflex coronary artery runs in the atrioventricular groove and injury or compression may produce inferobasal ischaemia. The coronary sinus and aortic valve are also in close proximity and may be at risk. The most feared complication of mitral surgery is rupture of the LV. Overly aggressive debridement or traction on the mitral annulus may lead to disruption of the atrioventricular groove. Excessive removal of chordae and papillary muscle may lead to free wall rupture. This is now rare owing to routine preservation of the posterior chordal apparatus. Although most commonly detected during surgery, ventricular rupture may occur in the early postoperative period owing to LV overdistension or hypertension, and is often fatal. Treatment can be either conservative (intra-aortic balloon, surgical glue to the exit site, packing the chest and hoping for the best) to dealing directly with the problem (return to theatre, removal of the valve, patch repair of the ventricle from within, replacing the valve and hoping for the best). Intermediate methods (trying to suture the exit point of the haemorrhage) are useless because the blood simply tracks through to a new exit point.

Physiological considerations

In pure mitral stenosis, the LV cavity is small and most patients are diuretic dependent before surgery. Postoperatively, stroke volume depends on the maintenance of adequate filling pressures, largely determined by the degree of pulmonary hypertension and its reversibility. In severe disease, pulmonary hypertension and right ventricular dysfunction are common. Right ventricular dysfunction usually responds better to inotropic support rather than further filling. Ventilatory failure is commonly due to pulmonary hypertension and fluid overload, requiring aggressive diuresis.

Chronic mitral regurgitation causes volume loading of the LV with increased preload and decreased afterload and wall stress owing to offloading through the regurgitant valve. In chronic regurgitation, the LV becomes dilated and compliant, with little or no elevation in pulmonary vascular resistance. After restoration of mitral function, the rise in LV wall stress may reveal underlying LV dysfunction, compromising CO and requiring inotropic support, particularly in ischaemic mitral regurgitation. Improved results with early mitral repair have meant that surgery is now usually performed before the onset of significant LV impairment or pulmonary hypertension.

Acute mitral regurgitation can be due to papillary muscle rupture after myocardial infarction. Adaptive mechanisms are limited and the rapid rise in pulmonary pressures causes pulmonary oedema. Postoperatively, ventricular dysfunction is common, reflecting the recent acute myocardial insult.

Valve implant considerations

All implanted valves, whether bioprosthetic or mechanical, have an increased risk of infection compared with a native valve. In these patients, there should be a lower threshold for starting empirical antimicrobial therapy if there is evidence of systemic or local infection likely to lead to bacteraemia. In addition, procedures performed on the critical care unit that may cause a bacteraemia should be covered with prophylactic antibiotics.

Prosthetic heart valves are susceptible to thrombotic complications, particularly during the first 3 months after implantation. The risk is significantly greater in mechanical valves or in the mitral position. In high-risk patients (atrial fibrillation, large left atrium, history of thromboembolic events or known thrombotic tendency), anticoagulation with intravenous heparin should be considered once the risk of pericardial bleeding has declined, usually after postoperative day 2. This should be continued until oral anticoagulation with warfarin is therapeutic.

Case study

An 83-year-old man has had elective aortic valve replacement with a 21-mm bovine pericardial valve for severe aortic regurgitation. The procedure was uneventful and he was weaned off cardiopulmonary bypass with ease but required atrioventricular pacing for bradycardia. Two mediastinal drains were placed and closure was routine. On arrival in the critical care unit, he appears stable: heart rate, 90 bpm; paced rhythm; blood pressure (BP), 96/54 mmHg (mean, 68); right atrial pressure (RAP), 9 mmHg; O_2 saturation (sat), 98%; and drainage, 50 mL/h.

Routine blood tests including a coagulation screen are normal. A chest radiograph has not yet been obtained; however, 3 hours later, he rapidly deteriorates: heart rate, 110 bpm; sinus, rhythm; BP, 56/43 mmHg (mean, 47); RAP, 22 mmHg; O_2 sat, 77%; drainage, 50 mL/h.

The acute respiratory compromise does not respond to manual ventilation with 100% oxygen. His mean BP is falling and a bolus of adrenaline (epinephrine) is given. On examining his chest, the right side is hyper-resonant with absent breath sounds. A tension pneumothorax is diagnosed and needle thoracocentesis produces a characteristic hiss of air. A lateral chest drain is rapidly inserted. However, after decompression, his mean arterial pressure soars: heart rate, 140 bpm; paced rhythm; BP, 192/115 mmHg (mean, 141); O_2 sat, 99%; drainage bubbling+++.

While watching the BP, the chest drain bottle suddenly fills with blood and the patient suffers a cardiac arrest. An emergency resternotomy is performed, the mediastinum is suctioned and open cardiac massage initiated. With volume resuscitation and further adrenaline, spontaneous circulation returns after 4 minutes and the bleeding is found to be originating from a rupture at or near to the aortotomy site. Digital control is obtained as a senior surgeon scrubs to repair the aorta. Four units of packed cells are given and inotropic support commenced.

The patient remains haemodynamically stable for the next 48 hours and the inotropes and sedation are being weaned. However, he is slow to wake and appears neurologically inappropriate. Brain computed tomography shows a new watershed infarct of the left cerebral hemisphere and a small, old, right-sided infarct. His critical care stay is further complicated by pneumonia with sputum retention and lobar collapse. He is eventually weaned from the ventilator with the aid of a tracheostomy. There is some recovery of neurological function such that he can move his right leg, open his eyes to speech and breathe spontaneously. Thirty-four days after surgery, he is transferred to his local hospital for rehabilitation.

This dramatic case illustrates a number of valuable points.

Learning points

- Even a seemingly routine and stable patient has the potential to deteriorate rapidly on the cardiothoracic critical care unit. In this case, it is likely that an inadvertent and unnoticed injury to the lung was incurred, perhaps during sternotomy or chest closure. Positive-pressure ventilation led to the development of a tension pneumothorax and started a chain of events with serious long-term sequelae.
- The hypertensive rebound after decompression of the tension pneumothorax was exacerbated by adrenaline (epinephrine). Rapid fluxes in BP, even for short periods, can be dangerous in the postoperative period. Increased stress on a fragile, sutured elderly aortic wall can lead to dehiscence, rupture and rapid exsanguination.
- When haemodynamic deterioration occurs, it is important wherever possible to identify the cause before giving treatment. This case also highlights the value of examining the patient: even cursory assessment of the chest may have picked up the pneumothorax and directed treatment appropriately.
- A period of 'downtime' (loss of CO), albeit brief, can cause cerebral damage with serious consequences for neurological function and subsequent recovery. This is especially true in the elderly.

FURTHER READING

Mackay JH, Arrowsmith JE. Aortic valve disease. In: Mackay JH, Arrowsmith JE, eds. *Core topics in cardiac anaesthesia*. Cambridge: Cambridge University Press; 2004:169–173.

Mackay JH, Wells FC. Mitral valve disease. In: Mackay JH, Arrowsmith JE, eds. *Core topics in cardiac anaesthesia*. Cambridge: Cambridge University Press; 2004:175–182.

Chapter 50

Management after aortic surgery

N.E. DRURY, S.A.M. NASHEF
AND N. BREITENFELDT

Surgery of the thoracic aorta can be divided into elective and emergency interventions. Emergency operations are usually for acute aortic dissection, but may also be for rupture of an atherosclerotic aneurysm. Occasionally, patients with traumatic transection survive to hospital and may be treated surgically. They often have associated injuries – particularly to the head, spine and abdomen – that may require prompt intervention. A thorough evaluation and multidisciplinary approach is therefore essential.

Preoperative management

Emergency aortic surgery patients are often received by the cardiothoracic critical care unit from the referring hospital before operation, so some preoperative critical care may be needed. Although there should not be any unnecessary delay in definitive therapy, those who reach a tertiary centre have already self-selected for immediate survival. A period of focused assessment and stabilization is beneficial as theatre staff and resources are coordinated. It is worthwhile to remember that every organ in the body derives its blood supply from the aorta, so that the injured aorta can place any organ at risk. This is especially true of acute aortic dissection where any organ system can be compromised at any time in the evolution of the condition.

A brief history should be obtained including symptoms, time since onset, past medical history, medication and allergies, if not previously documented. Recurrence or worsening of pain in a patient with dissection is suggestive of extension and potential rupture. Sensory or motor impairment may indicate that the brain is at risk. Abdominal pain may point to visceral ischaemia and there may be blatant evidence of limb underperfusion.

On examination, the presence and strength of all pulses should be recorded, in particular at the carotid, radial and femoral. Differential upper limb pulses are suggestive of compromise to the great vessels arising from the aortic arch. Absent or weak femoral pulses may indicate obstruction to the descending aorta. Muffled heart sounds may indicate a pericardial collection; the diastolic murmur of aortic regurgitation is heard if the integrity of aortic valve has been affected. Neurological examination is important to document any preoperative deficit. If possible, informed consent should be obtained, explaining the risks and benefits of this high-risk but life-saving surgery. Hypertension is exacerbated by the catecholamine surge associated with severe pain and by injury to the baroreceptors of the aortic arch. The aim should be a systolic pressure of less than 100 mmHg, adequate to maintain tissue perfusion while decreasing shear stress on the aortic wall. The pharmacological agent of choice is an intravenous β-blocker such as esmolol (short acting, cardioselective) or labetalol (α and β effects, direct vasodilator). If a further reduction in blood pressure (BP) is required, a vasodilator such as nitroprusside may be added; this should not be commenced until β-blockade is effective to prevent a reflex tachycardia.

Operative features relevant to postoperative care

The wise intensivist obtains as much information as possible about what was done in the operating theatre, because this information is invaluable for postoperative management.

The disease process can affect either a localized portion of the aorta or be more widespread, determining the surgical approach and circulatory strategy. The aorta is divided into five anatomical sections from the sinuses of Valsalva to the bifurcation: aortic root, ascending aorta, aortic arch, descending thoracic aorta and abdominal aorta. The procedure involves resection of the diseased aortic segment and replacement by a vascular graft. Depending on the segment, associated procedures may include repair or replacement of the aortic valve and reimplantation of various arteries into the graft, such as the coronary arteries or the great vessels.

Intervention to the root and ascending aorta is performed on cardiopulmonary bypass. If the aortic arch is affected, a period of deep hypothermic circulatory arrest (DHCA) with systemic cooling to 20°C or below may be required. Neurological complications can occur especially if the period of DHCA exceeds 45 minutes; older patients are at greatest risk. Cerebral protection can be improved with intermittent or continuous low-flow via selective antegrade or retrograde perfusion. Other adjuncts include high-dose steroids, phenobarbitone and packing the head in ice. Long bypass times and DHCA predispose to coagulopathy and, as a result of this, aortic operations are often bloody affairs. Aprotinin reduces intraoperative bleeding after DHCA but may be associated with an increase in postoperative neurological and renal dysfunction.

In surgery of the descending thoracic or thoracoabdominal aorta, the spinal cord and kidneys are at particular risk of ischaemia. An arterial shunt or partial femorofemoral bypass improves perfusion distal to the cross-clamp and decreases the incidence of paraplegia and renal injury. Other measures include cerebrospinal fluid drainage and pharmacological agents.

Postoperative care

Hypertension must be closely controlled because it threatens both suture lines and what is left of the native aorta; this can be aided by adequate analgesia. Antihypertensive medication should be continued indefinitely to decrease the risk of long-term complications such as recurrent dissection or aneurysm formation.

Branch vessels that have been reimplanted into a vascular graft may have compromised flow. Compromise of a reimplanted coronary artery after aortic root surgery leads to myocardial ischaemia, ventricular dysfunction and arrhythmias. Spinal cord ischaemia may result from hypotension or the inability to identify or successfully reimplant the posterior intercostal or lumbar artery (usually between T8 and L1) that feeds the artery of Adamkiewicz, the main supply of the spinal cord. It is a major cause of postoperative paraplegia after thoracoabdominal aortic surgery due to anterior spinal cord syndrome.

Once stability has been achieved and the sedation can be lightened, the patient's neurological status can be fully assessed. Any new disability should be carefully elicited and documented including tone, power, sensation, reflexes and continence. Comparison should be made with both the contralateral side and documented preoperative status where possible.

Vascular grafts are also prone to infective complications, particularly during the early postoperative period. Few catastrophes in medicine are as disheartening as an infected aortic prosthesis. Any sepsis should be treated aggressively and invasive procedures covered with appropriate antibiotic prophylaxis.

Case study

A 56-year-old man presented to his local emergency department at midday with severe chest and back pain of 2 hours duration. His femoral pulses were weak and his BP was 45 mean on the left arm but unrecordable at the right brachial. Computed tomography (CT) demonstrated an aortic dissection extending from the aortic root to the bifurcation with no contrast to the right kidney and reduced enhancement of the left. He was referred to a specialist centre for further management of his type A dissection; en route, he became hypertensive, requiring infusions of labetalol and nitroglycerin. On arrival at 15:10 hours, his observations are: heart rate, 76 bpm; sinus rhythm; BP, 112/54 mmHg (mean, 73); urine output, 5 mL/h (dark); neurological, alert, anxious

He is intubated via rapid sequence induction and taken to theatre expeditiously. Transoesophageal echocardiography demonstrates a dissection flap in the ascending aorta and central aortic regurgitation. Cannulation is performed via the right atrium and left femoral artery. After aortic cross-clamping, the ascending aorta is replaced with resuspension of the aortic valve and hemi-arch replacement with the distal anastomosis performed on DHCA. On rewarming, his urine output remains minimal and there is a moderate acidosis requiring the administration of bicarbonate. He is transferred back to the critical care unit at around 20:00 hours. heart rate, 90 bpm; paced rhythm; BP, 108/64 mmHg (mean, 78); urine output, 8 mL/h; central venous pressure, 8 mmHg; cardiac output, 5.6 L/min; femoral pulses, barely palpable.

Over the next 6 hours, he appears to be doing well with good haemodynamics and minimal chest drain bleeding. The only cause for concern is that he remains anuric. Renal replacement therapy (continuous venovenous haemofiltration) is started but this fails to control his acidosis, which slowly worsens despite frequent additional doses of bicarbonate. By the morning, it is noted that his legs are mottled and his abdomen is distended. An exploratory laparotomy is performed. This reveals extensive established intestinal infarction; the abdomen is closed without resection. After discussion with his family, treatment is withdrawn and he rapidly succumbs from multiorgan failure.

Learning points

- Aortic dissections typically occur spontaneously in individuals with an underlying condition such as hypertension, Marfan's syndrome or bicuspid aortic valve, but may be iatrogenic (e.g. a cardiac catheterization laboratory disaster). The dissection can originate anywhere in the aorta, but wherever the original tear happens, the false lumen of the dissection may extend in either direction and compromise any arterial branches in its path. Most patients are diagnosed on the basis of a CT scan with intravenous contrast from the referring institution. Transoesophageal echocardiography can identify an intimal flap in the thoracic aorta, although this should not be performed in a conscious, unsedated patient because it may precipitate a hypertensive surge with catastrophic sequelae.
- Emergent surgery is indicated for all patients with acute type A dissection (defined as involving the ascending aorta) who are deemed salvageable. Without intervention, this condition has a mortality of around 1% per hour over the first 48 hours; it is one of the few true cardiac surgical emergencies. Surgery improves survival to over 80%. The aim is to preserve life by averting three major causes of death: catastrophic heart failure (owing to free aortic regurgitation), myocardial infarction (owing to coronary compromise) and tamponade (owing to intrapericardial rupture). Peripheral malperfusion syndrome occurs in up to one third of patients with acute type A dissection and is an important cause of postoperative death. Branch vessels are compromised by bulging of the

false lumen or extension of the dissection into the artery, leading to distal ischaemia. In most cases, perfusion improves with ascending aortic repair and restoration of flow through the true lumen. Persistent inadequate organ perfusion can be difficult to diagnose but should be considered in patients with an unexplained acidosis, abdominal distension, absent femoral pulse or neurological deficit.

- This patient probably had occlusion of the abdominal aorta with impact on the renal, celiac, mesenteric and femoral circulation. Renal dysfunction preoperatively should have raised the alert, and persistent acidosis with anuria postoperatively was a strong indicator of a major perfusion defect. Treatment options to restore blood flow include radiograph-guided or open abdominal aortic fenestration, stenting or additional surgical procedures such as axillofemoral bypass. The ideal set-up is a hybrid theatre suite enabling a combined open and endovascular approach to aortic dissection, although this is not commonplace.

FURTHER READING

Knowles AC, Kneeshaw JD. Aortic dissection. In: Mackay JH, Arrowsmith JE, eds. *Core topics in cardiac anaesthesia*. Cambridge: Cambridge University Press; 2004:187–190.

Misso SL, Knowles AC. Deep hypothermic circulatory arrest. In: Mackay JH, Arrowsmith JE, eds. *Core topics in cardiac anaesthesia*. Cambridge: Cambridge University Press; 2004:279–282.

Taylor EJS, Mackay JH. Descending thoracic aorta surgery. In: Mackay JH, Arrowsmith JE, eds. *Core topics in cardiac anaesthesia*. Cambridge: Cambridge University Press; 2004: 195–200.

Chapter 51

Management after thoracic surgery

K. VALCHANOV AND S. GHOSH

Introduction

Lung resection varies in the amount of lung resected and the approach, and ranges from segmentectomy or wedge resection to lobectomy or pneumonectomy. It may be performed using a minimally invasive technique (video-assisted thoracoscopic surgery [VATS]) or via a thoracotomy. Irrespective of the type of resection undertaken or approach chosen, the aim is to have the patient extubated, breathing spontaneously and able to cough and expectorate secretions with minimal discomfort as soon as possible after the procedure.

Thoracic surgical patients often have significant comorbid conditions. The association between smoking, emphysema, lung cancer and cardiovascular disease is widely accepted. The preponderance of comorbid disease, together with the extent of surgery and the surgical approach, predispose to numerous potentially serious complications.

The aim of preoperative assessment and optimization is to identify patients at risk of complications and to take measures to prevent such complications from arising. Good postoperative care aims not only to recognize and treat complications that have already occurred, but also to prevent the progression from minor to major complication.

Mortality

Mortality after lung resection has generally improved over the years with improved diagnostic and treatment strategies. The 30-day mortality rate for lung resection is between 4% and 5% and is inversely proportional to the experience of the surgical centre. Pneumonectomy carries a higher mortality risk compared with lobectomy, which in turn carries a higher mortality rate than wedge lung resections.

The most frequent cause of death is acute lung injury (ALI) and acute respiratory distress syndrome (ARDS), followed by bronchopleural fistula and empyema, cerebrovascular accidents and cardiac events.

Cardiac dysfunction

Arrhythmias

The commonest arrhythmia after lung resection is atrial fibrillation (AF). The incidence of AF ranges from 10% to 20% after lobectomy, to 40% after pneumonectomy. It is most prevalent on the second postoperative day, and the predisposing factors include male gender, older age, preexisting cardiac disease, extent of surgery and fluid overload. In one third of patients who develop AF, onset is associated with chest infection or sepsis. Patients who develop AF are more likely to develop other complications and it is associated with a longer hospital stay and higher mortality.

There is no evidence that prophylactic digitalization is of benefit, but there is some evidence that metoprolol, magnesium, flecainide or amiodarone may reduce the incidence of postoperative AF if

Table 51.1 Common complications post lung resection (in order of frequency of occurrence)

Air leak and pneumothorax
Bleeding
Pain
Sputum retention and atelectasis
Arrhythmias
Cardiac dysfunction
Pulmonary oedema and acute respiratory distress syndrome
Pulmonary embolism
Death

administered prophylactically. The treatment of AF, once it has occurred, can be pharmacological or by synchronized direct current cardioversion. Pharmacological treatment strategies vary, but generally include optimization of electrolyte status (magnesium, potassium and acid–base balance), followed by administration of a therapeutic agent such as digoxin, β-blockers, amiodarone or flecainide. Prophylactic anticoagulation with low-molecular-weight heparin is recommended as an early measure during the acute phase postoperatively to prevent the development of thrombus in the atrial appendage.

Myocardial ischaemia

The incidence of electrocardiographic changes indicative of myocardial ischaemia has been reported as 3.8% after thoracic surgery, and the mortality may be up to 32% to 70%. The perioperative factors most strongly predictive of ischaemic events are poor preoperative exercise tolerance and intraoperative hypotension. The incidence of myocardial infarction has been found to be 0.13% for patients with no prior cardiac history and 2.8% to 17% for patients with previous infarction. Rigorous preoperative assessment and selection can limit the incidence of postoperative morbidity and mortality ascribable to myocardial ischaemia. Patients who are considered at risk of myocardial ischaemia

Table 51.2 Mortality after lung resection: Peer-reviewed publications

Author	Year	Years analysed	No. cases	30-day mortality, %	30-day mortality, % pneumonectomy	30-day mortality, % lobectomy	30-day mortality, % wedge resection
Fryjordet	1971	1949–1976	277	13.5	—	—	—
Weiss	1974	1963–1965	364	14	17	10	0
Ginsberg	1983	1979–1981	2200	3.7	6.2	2.9	1.4
Romano	1992	1983–1986	12439	4.1	11.6	4.2	3.8
Deslauriers	1994	1988–1989	783	3.8	—	—	—
Wada	1998	1994	7099	1.3	3.2	1.2	0.8
Harpole	1999	1991–1995	3516	5.2	11.5	4	—
Watanabe	2004	1987–2002	3270	0.6	3.1	0.3	0.3

should ideally be invasively monitored intra- and postoperatively. Appropriate measures should be taken to maintain cardiac filling pressures and arterial blood pressure at optimum levels and consideration given to the use of inotropes, vasopressors or vasodilators to prevent or limit the sequelae of ischaemic myocardial dysfunction.

Heart failure

Theoretically, the strain on the right ventricle (RV) should increase with the increase in afterload after lung and pulmonary artery resection. However, the RV end-diastolic pressure in fact remains stable in the first few hours postoperatively, and only increases significantly on the first and second days.

As concomitant cardiac disease is not uncommon in patients undergoing lung resection, postoperative cardiac failure is a distinct probability and preventative measures such as careful monitoring of fluid balance need to be taken.

Pulmonary embolism and heart herniation are rare causes of RV decompensation but carry very high mortality after lung resection. Heart herniation may occur if the pericardium is opened intraoperatively and not adequately closed.

Table 51.3 Predisposing factors for acute lung injury/acute respiratory distress syndrome after lung resection

Preoperative	Postoperative
Age >60	Extent and duration of surgery
Male gender	Pneumonectomy (right > left, carinal > noncarinal)
Chronic alcohol/ tobacco abuse	High inflation pressure during ventilation
Chronic suppurative disease	Intra- and postoperative fluid load
Concurrent cardiac disease	Volume of blood loss
Prior radiation or chemotherapy	Administration of blood products
Residual lung function ≤55%	Nonbalanced hemithorax drainage after pneumonectomy

Acute lung injury and acute respiratory distress syndrome

Pulmonary oedema is a feared complication as it may progress to fulminant ALI or ARDS (see Chapter 27). The incidence of ALI/ARDS ranges from 0.1% to 0.2% post VATS, 1% post lobectomy, and to 2% to 4% post pneumonectomy, but carries a 53% to 74% mortality. The onset is usually on postoperative days 1 to 4. The aetiological factors are not well understood, but at a biochemical level altered cellular metabolism, lactic acidosis and altered enzyme kinetics have been noted, predisposing to interstitial oedema and cell destruction. Hyperoxia, generation of reactive oxygen species and endothelial-derived cytokines have been implicated in the pathophysiological process, but the relative contributions of perioperative fluid balance, barotrauma from positive-pressure ventilation, the effect of lung handling and surgery and the underlying disease state remain unclear.

The treatment strategies for this condition are similar to the strategies for ALI in general and are summarized below:

- ventilatory support (avoid barotrauma, consider noninvasive ventilation);
- permissive hypercapnoea;
- rigorous blood gas monitoring and limitation of FiO_2 to minimum required for target PaO_2;
- conservative fluid management (monitor right atrial pressure, pulmonary capillary wedge pressure, and urine output); and
- avoid blood products owing to risk of transfusion-related lung injury.

The utilization of nitric oxide (NO) in low concentrations (5–40 ppm) may initially improve oxygenation by vasodilating pulmonary capillaries in better ventilated regions of lung and so improve ventilation/perfusion matching, but the effect is often short lived. Current opinion is that the use of NO in ALI/ARDS is of limited value and does not reduce the risk of mortality significantly.

BALANCED PLEURAL DRAINAGE

After pneumonectomy, the space within the pneumonectomized hemithorax gradually fills with fluid over a period of weeks. In the immediate postoperative period, close clinical and radiological monitoring is required for signs of accumulation of blood or air and for mediastinal shift (movement of the mediastinal contents from their midline position as a result of changes in intrathoracic pressure). This cavity can be managed with:

- no drainage;
- underwater seal drain clamped and released intermittently to allow assessment of blood loss and release any trapped air; or
- balanced pleural drainage (injection/aspiration of air to limit mediastinal shift)

The use of balanced pleural drainage has been associated with a lower incidence of postoperative ALI/ARDS. This may be because limitation of movement of the heart and pulmonary vessels from their usual position reduces changes in transpulmonary vascular pressures in the remaining lung and so decreases the propensity for the development of pulmonary oedema; or it may be that maintenance of the mediastinal contents in their midline position reduces the mechanical stresses on the residual lung caused by overdistension or compression.

Air leak and pneumothorax

The residual lung tissue after lung resection usually expands and fills the pleural space. However, if there are damaged areas on the lung surface these can communicate with the pleura causing air leak from the drains or a pneumothorax in the absence of an effective patent drain. The air leak can be either an alveolar–pleural fistula, when there is open communication with lung parenchyma, or a bronchopleural fistula, when the communicating segment is a larger bronchus.

Management is usually conservative. The alveolar–pleural fistulae often seal over the first few days. This is aided by spontaneous ventilation and application of negative pressure suction to chest drains. If, however, suction is too vigorously applied, it may perpetuate the air leak and in some cases cause respiratory compromise as a result of loss of tidal volume. Prolonged air leak after lung resection can occur in up to 16% of cases.

Bronchopleural fistula

Bronchopleural fistula is a persistent communication between the bronchial stump and the pleura, resulting in persistent air leak. The fluid-filled pleural space may become infected leading to sepsis. The incidence is approximately 2% after pneumonectomy, and is more common after right pneumonectomy. It is most often diagnosed at days 7 to 10 postoperatively. Onset of breathlessness, exacerbated in the supine position, a low-grade pyrexia and blood-stained expectoration are the classical presentation. The typical radiological finding is an air–fluid level within the pneumonectomized hemithorax, with repeat radiographs showing a falling fluid level. Emergency surgical treatment is often required, and repair of the stump with an omental or muscle patch is required. More recently, the use of tissue glue applied bronchoscopically to seal the defect has been advocated. Thoracoplasty to occlude the pneumonectomy space may also be considered.

Anaesthetic induction and intubation in this situation can be challenging, because the patients can be very anxious, hypoxic and unstable. In the absence of a chest drain, there is a risk of tension pneumothorax during positive-pressure ventilation; furthermore, the application of positive pressure may fail to produce adequate ventilation if large volumes of inspired gas are lost through the fistula. Positive-pressure ventilation may also exacerbate spillover of the infected pleural fluid into the bronchial tree as gas is forced under positive pressure into the pleural cavity via the fistula, displacing fluid. Intubation and positive-pressure ventilation may be required to manage respiratory distress accompanying sepsis or for surgical closure of the fistula.

Inhalational induction and subsequent lung isolation with a double-lumen endobronchial tube in the semi-erect position offers good protection against lung soiling with infected fluid and avoids positive-pressure ventilation to the bronchial stump. However, inhalational induction to the depth of anaesthesia required for passage of an endobronchial tube can be accompanied by cardiovascular compromise, particularly in septic, unstable patients, and can be difficult to safely achieve in practice. The use of rapid sequence induction and intubation has been advocated as offering a more rapid means of securing the airway, with superior intubating conditions if suxamethonium is used. Awake fibreoptic endobronchial intubation has also been described in this situation.

Bleeding

Bleeding is a relatively common complication after thoracic procedures, and rethoracotomy for haemostasis is needed in approximately 2% of cases. Bleeding is usually from the lung parenchyma, bronchial vessels or intercostal arteries. It is usually detected from the effluent chest drainage, but chest drains may be blocked and in the presence of hypotension and tachycardia a chest radiograph may be informative. The indications for rethoracotomy are rapid blood loss, a large intrathoracic collection, which may be infected, or persistent hypoxia owing to compression of the lung or pulmonary veins.

Pain

Thoracotomy ranks among the most painful of surgical procedures. The constant motion of respiration and coughing compounds the pain from muscles that have been transected or overstretched and torn, and ribs that have been partially excised or fractured during thoracotomy.

Pain relief after thoracic procedures has been offered via many modalities, including systemic analgesics, epidural analgesia, paravertebral or intercostal blocks, intrapleural regional anaesthesia or cryoanalgesia. Ineffective analgesia often results in poor chest expansion and expectoration leading to atelectasis and chest infection. The surgical technique can be modified to reduce the severity of pain – VATS is significantly less painful than thoracotomy.

Epidural analgesia is the gold standard. There is variability in the analgesic regimens used, as well as whether the epidural is placed in the thoracic or lumbar spine. Although epidural infusions have been shown to reduce the incidence of chest infection and improve the results of respiratory function tests after thoracotomy, there is no evidence that they have changed the surgical outcome. On the other hand, large numbers of complications have been attributed to the epidural insertion and to the management of epidural infusions postoperatively.

A safer regional analgesic technique in the form of paravertebral blockade of the thoracic nerve roots has been advocated by some. However, the analgesia may often not be as effective as that provided by an epidural infusion, and failure of the technique is unfortunately relatively common. Complications are certainly reduced, however, and placement of the paravertebral catheter may be performed either percutaneously or under direct vision by the surgeon from within the thoracic cavity during the operation.

Sputum retention, atelectasis and chest infection

Poor respiratory reserve, combined with inadequate analgesia and infrequent physiotherapy often leads to atelectasis and respiratory tract infection.

The incidence of pneumonia after thoracic surgery is 5% to 25%, and carries a mortality of around 20%. Preoperative predictors include old age, chronic obstructive pulmonary disease, significantly reduced forced expiratory volume and prolonged/extensive surgery. Common pathogens are *Haemophilus*, *Streptococcus* and *Pseudomonas*. The best treatment is probably prevention, but once established the infective complications should be promptly treated with appropriate antibiotics, commenced after acquisition of sputum samples for microbiological analysis, ample analgesia and physiotherapy.

Key points

- Acute lung injury is the most common cause of death after lung surgery; pulmonary oedema is strongly associated with ALI and care with fluid balance is very important.
- Atrial fibrillation is a frequent complication, and may be the first indicator of impending sepsis or pneumonia.
- Continuing air leak after thoracic surgery necessitates prolonged pleural drainage and leads to increased hospital length of stay.
- Good analgesia is a priority and reduces the incidence of atelectasis and pneumonia.

FURTHER READING

De Decker K, Jorens PG, Van Schil P. Cardiac complications after noncardiac thoracic surgery: an evidence-based current review. *Ann Thorac Surg* 2003;75:1340–1348.

Grinchnik KP, D'AmicoTA. Acute lung injury and acute respiratory distress syndrome after pulmonary resection. *Semin Cardiothorac Vasc Anesth* 2004;8:317–334.

Van Schil P, Van Meerbeeck J, Kramer G, *et al.* Morbidity and mortality in the surgery arm of EORTC 08941 trial. *Eur Resp J* 2005;26:192–197.

Watanabe S, Asamura H, Suzuki K, *et al.* Recent results of postoperative mortality for surgical resections in lung cancer. *Ann Thorac Surg* 2004;78:999–1003.

Chapter 52

Lung volume reduction surgery

R.A. SAYEED AND T.K. WADDELL

Pathophysiology of emphysema

Emphysema is characterized by the loss of lung parenchyma elasticity and alveolar wall destruction with dilatation of the lung unit distal to the terminal bronchiole. In severe emphysema, symptoms of breathlessness and exercise limitation result from the combined effects of several factors that reduce the efficiency of breathing. Loss of elastic recoil of the lung and progressive destruction of normal lung parenchyma lead to dynamic small airways collapse, increased airways resistance, and reduced expiratory driving force. The resulting reduction in expiratory flow produces hyperinflation and gas trapping. Chest wall and diaphragmatic contraction become less efficient owing to suboptimal chest wall mechanics, and the increased work of breathing and hyperinflation produce the sensation of breathlessness.

In addition to these mechanical factors, the reduction in the available alveolar capillary surface area impairs gas exchange and may affect pulmonary haemodynamics. Emphysema may coexist with poor nutritional status, general deconditioning and other comorbidities, particularly related to smoking, that also contribute to poor exercise tolerance.

Lung volume reduction surgery

The rationale for lung volume reduction surgery (LVRS) is to improve the mismatch between the size of the lungs and the thoracic cavity by removing space-occupying, hyperinflated, emphysematous areas of lung that contribute little to gas exchange; LVRS relieves hyperinflation, improves elastic recoil and decreases small airways resistance, leading to improved chest wall and diaphragmatic mechanics and reduced work of breathing. Ventilation–perfusion mismatch is improved and the reduction in intrathoracic pressure is beneficial for the cardiac output. Following the National Emphysema Treatment Trial in the United States and earlier smaller series, there is now clear evidence of the benefits of LVRS in selected patients.

Patient assessment and selection criteria

In addition to a routine history and physical examination to confirm the severity of emphysema and to identify any comorbidities, patients undergo extensive preoperative investigation to identify suitable operative candidates. Patients suitable for LVRS must have appropriate motivation for preoperative pulmonary rehabilitation and surgery.

As well as a detailed pulmonary assessment, operative candidates undergo detailed cardiac assessment and further invasive assessment by right heart catheterization; coronary angiography may then be indicated.

The ideal candidate has severe emphysema with dyspnoea at rest or on minimal exertion and impaired quality of life, despite optimal medical management. Disease distribution should be heterogeneous on computed tomography of the

Table 52.1 Patient selection criteria for lung volume reduction surgery

Emphysema
Disabling dyspnoea
$FEV_1 \leq 40\%$ predicted
Residual volume >180% predicted
Total lung capacity >120% predicted
Hyperinflation on chest radiograph
Heterogeneous disease on computed tomography

chest and quantitative ventilation–perfusion scan, with accessible 'target areas' of severe destruction and minimal or absent perfusion, and other areas of more well-preserved lung parenchyma. Criteria have been identified to exclude patients at high surgical risk or in whom surgery is unlikely to be beneficial.

The preservation of satisfactory respiratory muscle function is indicated by a normal or minimally elevated $Paco_2$; an elevated $Paco_2$ (>7 kPa) is considered a risk factor. However, even patients with $Paco_2$ at 8 kPa may be considered for surgery in absence of other risk factors, but at a higher risk of postoperative respiratory failure. The functional adequacy of the lung parenchyma that would remain after LVRS may be assessed by the Pao_2 at rest and the transfer coefficient for carbon monoxide (DL_{CO}): a Pao_2 of 6 kPa or less on air and DL_{CO} of 30% or less have been shown to be predictors of poor outcome. Other factors predictive of poor outcome are a history of chronic sputum production (i.e., bronchiectasis or chronic bronchitis rather than emphysematous obstructive pulmonary disease), age greater than 70 years, pulmonary hypertension (peak systolic pulmonary artery pressure >50 mmHg), poor exercise tolerance and previous thoracic surgery.

Table 52.2 Contraindications to lung volume reduction surgery

$FEV_1 \leq 20\%$ predicted *and* $DL_{CO} \leq 20\%$ predicted
$FEV_1 \leq 20\%$ predicted *and* homogeneous disease distribution on CT scan
Pulmonary hypertension (peak systolic PA pressure >50 mmHg)
$Paco_2$ >7 kPa
$Pao_2 \leq 6$ kPa on air
6-minute walk ≤120 m
Non-upper lobe disease predominance
Previous thoracic surgery

Abbreviations: CT, computed tomography; DL_{CO}, transfer coefficient for carbon monoxide; PA, pulmonary artery.

Preoperative management

The patient should have stopped smoking for at least 6 months. Oral steroids should be weaned or reduced to the lowest dose tolerated, ideally less than 5 mg prednisone daily, and the patient's nutritional status should be optimized. Operative candidates undergo a course of pulmonary rehabilitation over 6 to 10 weeks to improve exercise tolerance and pulmonary hygiene; patients with active bacterial respiratory tract infections should be excluded.

Surgical procedure

A thoracic epidural catheter is placed before surgery if there are no contraindications, for optimal postoperative analgesia. Surgery is performed under general anaesthesia with double-lumen endotracheal intubation to allow single-lung ventilation. The surgical approach may be through median sternotomy or by bilateral video-assisted thoracoscopic surgery; no clear differences in outcome between these approaches have been shown. Regardless of the approach, lung volume reduction is achieved by resecting 20% to 30% of each lung as one to three stapled wedge resections of the target areas. The staple lines are often buttressed with bovine pericardial or polytetrafluoroethylene strips to reduce air leaks. Bilateral chest drains are placed at the end of surgery, usually two drains to each pleural space. Unilateral procedures are rarely performed – only in case of unilateral disease, previous contralateral pleurodesis, previous thoracotomy, or extensive air leak on the first operated side.

Postoperative management

GENERAL MEASURES

A multidisciplinary approach is needed to minimize postoperative morbidity by meticulous attention to the prevention and aggressive treatment of complications. The main features of the postoperative management are excellent pain control, early mobilization, and aggressive chest physiotherapy. These patients are most often looked after in critical care or a high-dependency setting

The $Paco_2$ often rises to 10 to 13 kPa after periods of single-lung ventilation and so the patient is extubated as early as possible after surgery once the baseline $Paco_2$ has been attained. Early extubation is beneficial to avoid coughing or gagging and to minimize the duration of positive-pressure ventilation of the fragile, operated lungs. The Pao_2 is maintained close to baseline because a high Pao_2 may be deleterious in a patient with preoperative CO_2 retention.

Thoracic epidural analgesia is maintained for 4 to 5 days to avoid or reduce the requirement for opioid analgesia with the associated risks of oversedation and respiratory depression. If parenteral opioids are required, these should be given as small doses of short-acting drugs or as low-dose, patient-controlled analgesia with careful monitoring to avoid respiratory depression; oral opioids are avoided until the epidural catheter is removed.

Early mobilization, incentive spirometry and regular chest physiotherapy are very important. Regular nebulized bronchodilators should be administered for at least 48 hours before resuming usual bronchodilator therapy. Retained secretions may require nasotracheal suctioning; fibreoptic bronchoscopy may be needed up to twice daily for retained secretions, and a minitracheostomy (a 5.4-F tracheostomy tube inserted through the cricothyroid membrane) can be inserted if more frequent suctioning is necessary.

The chest tubes are connected to underwater-seal drainage without suction, because this is believed to reduce the size and duration of any air leak; the indications for suction are described elsewhere in this chapter. Chest drains are removed in stages 24 to 48 hours after cessation of any air leak.

COMPLICATIONS

With complication rates up to 85% to 100% in some series, and up to 60% excluding air leaks, LVRS carries a high morbidity. Postoperative complications are tolerated poorly in patients with end-stage respiratory disease and any complication has the potential to be life threatening. Early recognition and prompt, aggressive management of complications are vital to prevent further deterioration. Readmission to critical care is advocated early if severe complications are detected.

Table 52.3 Common postoperative complications

Respiratory
- Prolonged air leak
- Large pleural space
- Respiratory failure
- Pneumonia

Cardiovascular
- Atrial fibrillation
- Myocardial ischaemia

Gastrointestinal
- Bleeding
- Ileus
- Bowel perforation

PROLONGED AIR LEAK

Prolonged air leaks are a major source of morbidity and prolonged hospital stay; nearly half of patients have a prolonged air leak (persistent after 7 days); prolonged air leaks are more common in patients with upper lobe disease, with marked pleural adhesions, or those on steroids. Air leaks may be minimized by careful intraoperative mobilization and manipulation of the lung, avoidance of excessive lung resection and buttressing of staple lines; large leaks identified at the end of surgery should be addressed before closure by additional stapling, suture plication or surgical glues. Postoperatively, air leaks are managed conservatively by underwater-seal chest drainage, with the avoidance of suction unless there is a large (>40%–50%) or symptomatic pleural space, in which case gentle suction of -10 cmH_2O may be used. Small or moderate leaks usually seal in 72 to 96 hours; continuous, large air leaks, especially in the presence of a large pleural space, may need reoperation, although this should be carefully considered in these frail patients. Patients with prolonged air leaks who are otherwise fully recovered may be discharged with the chest drains connected to a one-way flutter (Heimlich) valve; the chest drains are removed once the air leak has resolved during out-patient follow-up.

RESPIRATORY TRACT INFECTION

Postoperative respiratory tract infections have been reported in up to 50% of patients, although confirmed pneumonia, defined by purulent sputum, fever, elevated white cell count, new infiltrate on the chest radiograph and positive sputum culture, develops in 4% to 18%, but carries a 40% mortality. Respiratory tract infections are managed by ensuring adequate analgesia, early mobilization, aggressive physiotherapy and bronchoscopy or minitracheostomy if indicated. Empirical broad-spectrum antibiotic therapy should be started early, adjusted according to microbiology results, and continued for a 10- to 14-day course; preoperative culture results may be helpful in guiding antibiotic therapy. Empyema in the presence of a persistent pleural space is rare; some authors have even suggested that low-grade contamination of the pleural space is beneficial by encouraging pleural symphysis.

RESPIRATORY FAILURE

Respiratory failure requiring reintubation complicates 12% of cases and has a 40% mortality rate. Early reintubation is usually due to poor pain control, oversedation or inadequate gas exchange with CO_2 retention; late reintubation is indicated for severe pneumonia. Early CO_2 retention may result from surgical compromise of respiratory mechanics outweighing the benefits of LVRS; short-term ventilatory support may allow recovery from the surgical insult, although these patients remain at high risk of postoperative death.

Acute respiratory decompensation may develop secondary to mucous plugging. Excessive mucous production leads to tenacious plugs that require bronchoscopy for proper clearance.

CARDIOVASCULAR COMPLICATIONS

Acute myocardial infarction is rare, with an incidence of 0% to 2% in reported series, most likely because of the extensive cardiac screening in this group of patients. Atrial fibrillation or supraventricular tachycardia develops in 6% of cases and is managed according to standard guidelines.

GASTROINTESTINAL COMPLICATIONS

The incidence of gastrointestinal complications seems to be higher after LVRS than other thoracic surgery, with complications such as gastrointestinal bleeding, ileus or bowel perforation in 7% of patients. Routine acid suppression therapy is recommended to reduce the risks of stress ulcers. Careful assessment is needed in cases of suspected intra-abdominal pathology because steroids may mask the usual signs.

OTHER COMPLICATIONS

Deep sternal wound infection is rare, but if wound infection develops, early, aggressive surgical debridement, flap closure and sternal stabilization is indicated. The incidence of deep venous thrombosis and pulmonary embolism is unknown, but these complications are avoided by early mobilization and routine antithrombotic prophylaxis.

Results

SURGICAL MORTALITY

Surgical mortality remains 4% to 6% in major centres. Early deaths are due to respiratory failure from profound CO_2 retention or massive air leak, haemorrhage or myocardial infarction; later deaths are mainly due to pneumonia.

PROGNOSTIC AND SYMPTOMATIC BENEFITS

If compared with medical therapy, those patients with upper-lobe predominant disease and low postrehabilitation exercise capacity live longer and have an improved health-related quality of life. The advantages in function and quality of life are maintained above the medical group, even though functional improvements return to baseline by 3 years.

Key points

- In selected patients with end-stage emphysema, LVRS prolongs survival and improves breathlessness and quality of life.
- Overall surgical mortality remains at 4% to 6%.
- Pain control, early mobilization and chest physiotherapy are the main facets of postoperative care.
- Complications are common and poorly tolerated; careful attention is vital for the prevention, early identification and aggressive management of complications, with early readmission to critical care if required.

FURTHER READING

DeCamp MM, Blackstone EH, Naunheim KS, *et al.* Patient and surgical factors influencing air leak after lung volume reduction surgery: lessons learned from the National Emphysema Treatment Trial. *Ann Thorac Surg* 2006;82: 197–206.

Geddes D, Davies M, Koyama H, *et al.* Effect of lung volume reduction surgery in patients with severe emphysema. *N Engl J Med* 2000;343:239–245.

Naunheim KS, Wood DE, Krasna MJ, *et al.* Predictors of operative mortality and cardiopulmonary morbidity in the National Emphysema Treatment Trial. *J Thorac Cardiovasc Surg* 2006;131:43–53.

Naunheim KS, Wood DE, Mohsenifar Z, *et al.* Long-term follow-up of patients receiving lung volume reduction surgery versus medical therapy for severe emphysema by the National Emphysema Treatment Trial Research Group. *Ann Thorac Surg* 2006;82:431–443.

Chapter **53**

Chronic thromboembolic pulmonary hypertension and pulmonary endarterectomy

B. THOMSON AND D.P. JENKINS

Introduction

Chronic thromboembolic pulmonary hypertension (CTEPH) is a disease process that develops in 3% to 4% of patients who sustain an acute pulmonary embolism. The process is principally one of organization of thromboembolic material producing an obstructive vasculopathy in the pulmonary vascular bed. The principles of critical care management are similar to any patient with impaired right ventricular (RV) function and pulmonary hypertension. Pulmonary endarterectomy (PEA) is now established as the definitive treatment.

Pathophysiology and natural history

The mechanisms that underlie this process are incompletely understood but may involve:

- in situ propagation of thrombus;
- recurrent embolism;
- organization of thrombus; or
- a secondary obstructive vasculopathy of the pulmonary vascular bed unaffected by embolism itself.

Risk factors for progression to CTEPH include anticardiolipin antibody syndrome, elevated factor VIII levels and splenectomy. Interestingly, other procoagulant states have not been shown to be associated with CTEPH.

The fundamental physiological abnormalities are RV 'pressure overload' and disruption of normal ventilation–perfusion matching. The disease may then progress to RV failure and impairment of gas exchange. This is gradual and initially manifests during exercise, but tends to progress to severely limit the patient, even at rest. As with other forms of pulmonary hypertension, CTEPH confers a poor prognosis when severe.

Clinical features

The clinical diagnosis or suspicion of CTEPH is commonly delayed owing to a lack of awareness of the disease process among clinicians, the insidious onset of symptoms and the subtle nature of early physical signs.

The progression seen in the clinical features reflects a period of compensated pulmonary hypertension that gradually evolves into decompensated cor pulmonale. The terminal phase involves New York Heart Association class IV heart failure and there is a significant incidence of sudden death.

Investigations

The investigations utilized in these patients provide three types of information:

- Initial diagnosis of pulmonary hypertension and cause: transthoracic echocardiography and ventilation–perfusion scanning.
- Detailed anatomic and functional assessment of the nature and severity of the CTEPH: pulmonary angiography, computed tomography, magnetic resonance imaging and right heart catheterization.

Table 53.1 Prognosis in CTEPH in relation to mean pulmonary arterial pressure (MPAP) at the time of diagnosis, without surgery

MPAP (mmHg)	10-year survival (%)
31–40	50
41–50	20
>50	5 (20% 2-year survival in this group)

- Appropriate investigation of known or likely comorbidities, including coronary angiography (>40 years old) in those in whom surgery is contemplated.

Thereafter, a decision regarding operability can be made, usually in a multidisciplinary meeting.

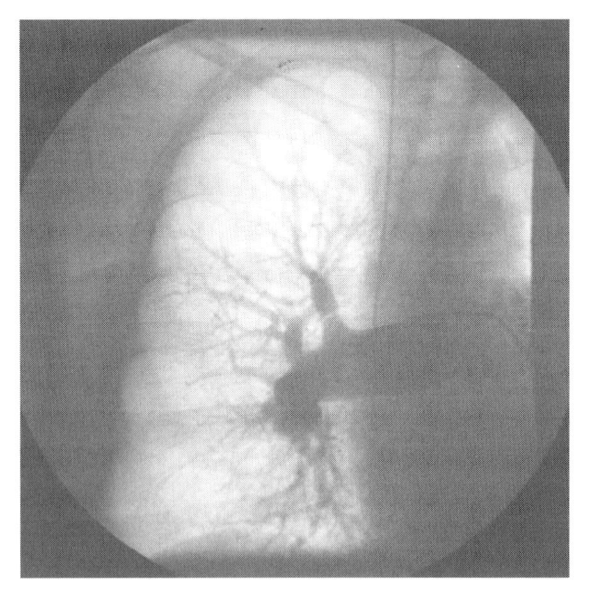

Figure 53.1 Right pulmonary angiogram of a patient with CTEPH demonstrating a classic web in the right upper lobe artery and attenuation and obliteration of the middle and lower lobe vascularity.

Patient selection for operation

Individualized assessment of the risks versus benefits of surgery, taking into account:

- the degree of symptoms experienced (most patients proceeding to surgery are in New York Heart Association class III or IV);
- the expected natural history of the disease process (dependent on the magnitude of elevation of pulmonary vascular resistance – virtually all surgical candidates have a resistance >300 dyne s cm^{-5});
- surgical accessibility of the disease; and
- presence of significant comorbidities.

Table 53.2 Clinical features of chronic thromboembolic pulmonary hypertension

Early phase	Late phase
History	**History**
Documented previous DVT or PE (elicited in ≤50%)	Severe exertional dyspnoea with or without dyspnoea at rest
Minimal to no dyspnoea on exertion	Exertional chest pain
Subtle reduction in exercise tolerance	Syncope/sudden death
Atypical chest pains and palpitations	Haemoptysis (not common)
Physical Signs	**Physical Signs**
Loud P2	Elevated jugular venous pressure
Right ventricular heave and S4	Cyanosis
Pulmonary flow murmur	Congestive hepatomegaly and ascites
Signs of chronic deep venous insufficiency	Ankle oedema with or without anasarca

Abbreviations: DVT, deep venous thrombosis; PE, pulmonary embolism.

Table 53.3 Classification of surgical pathology specimens

Type	Description	Comments
1	Laminated thrombus in main pulmonary artery, needing removal before proceeding with endarterectomy	25%–35% of cases
2	Thickened intima seen in main, lobar and segmental vessels; with or without webs	55%–65% of cases
3	Distal disease confined to segmental and subsegmental vessels	5%–15% of cases; confers higher operative risk & reduced expectation of improved haemodynamics
4	Small vessel disease only	Inoperable disease; if operated on, very high risk of perioperative mortality and morbidity

From Thistlethwaite et al, 2002.

All patients accepted for PEA should have an inferior vena cava filter inserted preoperatively to reduce the chance of further thromboembolic events.

Anaesthesia and surgery

The fundamental aim of the surgery is to perform a true endarterectomy (not thrombectomy) of both pulmonary vascular trees. The success or failure of the operation hinges upon this. Obviously, cardiopulmonary bypass allows perfusion to continue while the pulmonary arteries are dissected, and periods of deep hypothermic circulatory arrest or selective cerebral perfusion reduce bronchial artery perfusion and thus, collateral return to the pulmonary arteries, allowing a clear operative field.

Intensive care management

Most of the general principles of postoperative cardiac surgical care apply to the PEA patient. However, two specific issues impact on the management strategy applied to these patients:

- Keeping the lungs as dry as possible, and
- Minimizing pulmonary vascular resistance.

These two aims are inextricably linked, as maintenance of optimal ventilation–perfusion matching, adequate Pao_2, minimal pulmonary vascular resistance and adequate RV function are all closely interrelated.

Routine care

RESPIRATORY

A ventilation and weaning strategy is employed to avoid episodes of hypoxia and resultant pulmonary vasoconstriction. Additionally, minimizing the mechanical impact of ventilation on pulmonary vascular resistance and on alveolar shear forces is important. In general, pulmonary vascular resistance reaches a nadir at functional residual capacity (FRC). Although raising lung volume above FRC reduces resistance in the pulmonary vessels unrelated to the alveoli (owing to traction–distension effects), the vessels adjacent to the alveoli are compressed. When lung volume is above the FRC, this latter part of the vascular bed predominates on the impact on pulmonary vascular resistance, thus elevating the overall resistance. Thus excessively high ventilation pressures contribute to an elevated pulmonary vascular resistance.

The general aims of ventilation are to maintain (1) a Pao_2 value >12 kPa, (2) normocapnoea, (3) normal acid–base balance and (4) peak airway pressures $\leq$30 cmH_2O. Extubation on the first postoperative day is most common.

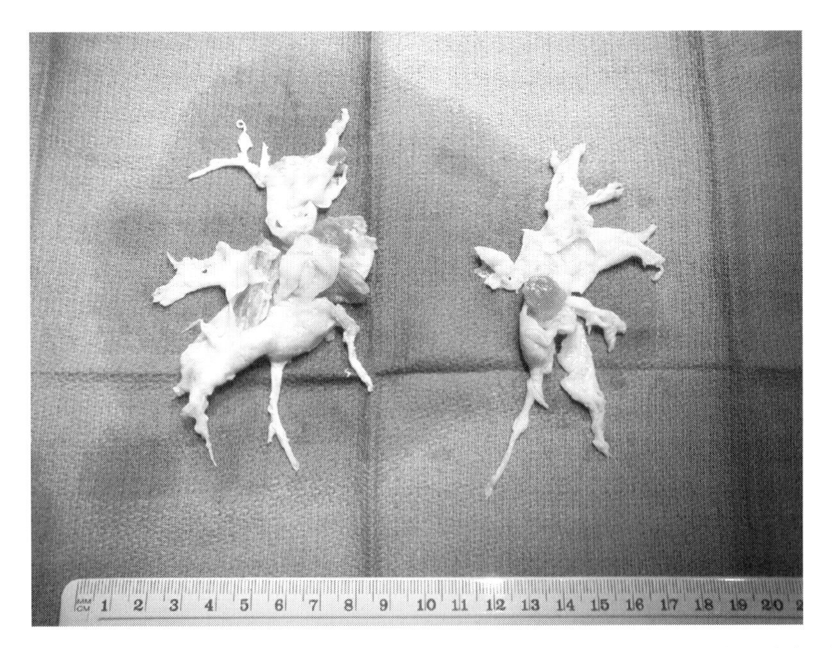

Figure 53.2 Satisfactory PEA specimen. Note the long tapering segmental 'tails' suggestive of good distal disease clearance.

Following admission to critical care, the Fio_2 can usually be reduced in 5% to 10% decrements to 40% over the first 6 to 12 hours. Subsequent to Fio_2 reduction, the positive end-expiratory pressure can be weaned down to +2 cmH_2O.

Routinely obtaining an early chest radiograph is important. Apart from the usual post cardiac surgical features to check for, it is specifically important to assess for early pulmonary oedema and pneumothorax (which is common). One finding that is almost universal in PEA patients is the presence of some diffuse shadowing around the main pulmonary arteries. This is secondary to the surgical dissection itself. Due to the previously mentioned deleterious effects on pulmonary vascular resistance, every effort should be made to avoid peri-extubation hypoxia and respiratory distress at the time of extubation. If gas exchange is borderline, extubation may be immediately followed by mask continuous positive airway pressure to ensure good oxygenation is not interrupted.

CARDIAC

Pulmonary artery catheterization is routine in theatre. It is critical to emphasize that the balloon of the Swan–Ganz catheter must not be inflated and wedged in patients after PEA operation, because they are more prone to pulmonary artery rupture owing to the surgical dissection that has occurred. Haemodynamic calculations are performed regularly, and pulmonary artery wedge pressure may be estimated at 10 each time, to allow comparison of results and calculate pulmonary vascular resistance pre- and postoperatively. This generally allows a reasonably accurate approximation; most PEA patients have well-preserved left ventricular function. Haemodynamic calculations allow comparison with preoperative values as well as providing a means of assessment of the state of pulmonary vascular tone if a clinical change or deterioration occurs in the intensive care unit.

Even with optimal intraoperative RV protection and reduction of pulmonary vascular resistance, the impact of a long bypass time, potential periods of ischaemic arrest of the heart and the preexisting RV hypertrophy with or without dilatation may all limit the inotropic reserve that exists in the early postoperative period. Therefore, despite the surgical reduction of impedance to RV ejection, it is common practice to maintain the patient on 3 to 5 μg/kg/min of dopamine for the first 24 to 48 hours.

RENAL/FLUID BALANCE

Secondary to the general aim of maintaining lung water at a minimum, an aggressive diuresis is maintained, particularly in the first 24 to 48 hours postoperatively. The combination of 40 mg IV furosemide and 12.5 g IV mannitol every 6 hours for the first 36 hours, followed by a reducing dose of IV or oral furosemide commonly achieves this aim. Should significant oliguria persist, apart from the usual measures to optimize pre-renal determinants of urine output, consideration should be given to haemofiltration before volume overload (and hence pulmonary oedema and its consequences) supervenes. If filling is required, then albumin or blood are used. Crystalloid solutions are to be avoided. In practical terms, the average patient is generally rendered 2.5 to 3.5 L negative on fluid balance in the first 48 hours.

ANTICOAGULATION

In the absence of unusual postoperative bleeding, anticoagulation is usually commenced with low-molecular-weight heparin on the second postoperative evening. Warfarin is started at the same time, and heparin may be stopped when the International Normalized Ratio (INR) reaches 2.5, with the therapeutic target range being 2.5 to 3.5. Selected patients with a specific procoagulant diathesis may benefit from a higher target INR range.

Specific problems

REPERFUSION PULMONARY OEDEMA

This complication represents a high permeability form of pulmonary oedema. The onset is usually within the first 24 hours but may occur as late as 72 hours after operation. It manifests as focal or diffuse pulmonary oedema.

Table 53.4 Mechanisms contributing to reperfusion oedema

Sudden reestablishment of pulmonary blood flow in vascular beds that have been subjected to prolonged periods of low or no flow.
Removal of pulmonary vascular endothelium increasing vascular permeability.
Regional heterogeneity of pulmonary vascular resistance (owing to reduction of resistance in areas of successful endarterectomy with other areas having distal inoperable disease) exacerbating hyperaemia in successfully endarterectomized areas – 'steal' phenomenon.
Failure to maintain dry lungs – excessive fluid administration; absence of diuretic response.
Inflammatory reaction to the endarterectomy (primarily neutrophil mediated).

The clinical features observed include a progressively worsening Pao_2:Fio_2 ratio associated with evolution of radiological changes of pulmonary oedema, commonly segmental (and occasionally unilateral) in distribution. This appearance is thought to reflect the maximal effect being manifest in those areas of greatest relative increase in pulmonary vascular perfusion.

Therapy is essentially supportive, with some attempts to ameliorate the associated inflammatory response. Within the limits of maintaining adequate end-organ perfusion, filling pressures should be minimized. Ventilatory strategies include prone positioning, inverse-ratio ventilation, low-volume ventilation, recruitment manoeuvres and higher levels of positive end-expiratory pressure. Although not of proven benefit, corticosteroids are often used empirically. If a patient with reperfusion pulmonary oedema is refractory to all of these

Table 53.5 Mechanisms contributing to persistent pulmonary hypertension and/or right ventricular failure

CTEPH disease process itself
Failure to clear 'surgical' disease
Presence of type 4 disease (inoperable)
Dynamic pulmonary vascular resistance
Pulmonary vascular spasmogens (hypoxia; inappropriate use of vasopressors; effect of mediators released from platelet or fresh frozen plasma transfusions)
High-volume and/or high-pressure ventilation strategy
Incoordinated spontaneous ventilatory efforts (inadequate sedation → 'fighting the ventilator'; turbulent peri-extubation period)
RV function
Poor preoperative RV function
Faulty intraoperative myocardial protection
Inadequate coronary perfusion pressure gradient

Abbreviations: CTEPH, chronic thromboembolic pulmonary hypertension; RV, right ventricular.

interventions, extracorporeal membrane oxygenation (Chapter 21) may be the only option.

PERSISTENT PULMONARY HYPERTENSION AND RIGHT VENTRICULAR FAILURE

Failure to clear enough disease surgically results in persistent pulmonary hypertension. This may lead to rapidly evolving fulminant cardiogenic shock and death in theatre at its most severe. Patients who survive the operation despite a suboptimal reduction in pulmonary vascular resistance (residual >500) suffer a complicated postoperative course.

The presentation is one of systemic hypotension and low cardiac output associated with elevated central venous and mean pulmonary artery pressure. Direct observation (with or without transoesophageal echocardiographic evidence) of impaired RV free wall motion will also be observed.

Early recognition and initiation of management is important; decompensation of RV pump function can be rapid and often irreversible if allowed to develop. The fundamental aims are to:

- initially rest the patient on full bypass if still in theatre;
- optimize loading conditions, guided by observation of haemodynamic trends with or without transoesophageal echocardiography;
- avoid potent doses of vasoconstrictive inotropes (if possible);
- use 'inodilating' agents (e.g. enoximone);
- avoid low coronary perfusion pressures (an intra-aortic balloon pump is often useful in this situation);
- avoid hypoxaemia (a potentially reversible pulmonary vascular spasmogen); and
- consider pulmonary vasodilator therapy.

Intravascular filling to a central venous pressure of 10 to 14 mmHg, targeting a mean arterial pressure of at least 60 mmHg and avoidance of hypoxaemia may allow survival. It must be emphasized that overfilling (generally to a central venous pressure of > 14 to 15 mmHg) commonly results in incremental tricuspid regurgitation, falling forward flow, reduced perfusion pressure gradient across the systemic vascular beds and a spiralling decline. This is to be avoided at all costs as the potential of salvage from this situation is low. In patients who do survive the initial phase, reinstitution of long-term pulmonary vasodilator therapy (e.g. bosentan or sildenafil) is prudent.

PULMONARY HAEMORRHAGE

This feared complication is fortunately rare. It results from inadvertent perforation of the pulmonary arterial wall during endarterectomy. Even a normal pulmonary artery is more friable than a comparable systemic artery. Contributory factors to perforation include calcified and/or very adherent disease, dissecting in too deep a plane, use of excess force and failing to visualize the dissection area clearly.

Careful attention to these factors by the surgeon minimizes the risk as much as possible.

If perforation is recognized at the time of dissection and is sufficiently proximal, it may be repairable with fine sutures. However, unrecognized perforation is more common and this manifests at the time of weaning from cardiopulmonary bypass with massive haemoptysis. This is extremely difficult to manage. Immediate placement of a double-lumen endotracheal tube to isolate the lungs from one another is mandatory to prevent asphyxiation (avoidance of a fall in Pao_2 is particularly important in these patients because hypoxic vasoconstriction could lead to a precipitous rise in pulmonary arterial pressure). There is little to be gained from fibreoptic bronchoscopy at this stage; this is ineffective in airway toilet, may not allow localization of the source of bleeding and delays definitive protection of the contralateral lung. Subsequent single-lung ventilation and awaiting the reversal of systemic anticoagulation may result in arrest of haemorrhage. Even with prompt recognition and management, mortality is high.

Outcomes

The overall in-hospital mortality is generally 5% to 10%. If good disease clearance, haemodynamic improvement and absence of reperfusion pulmonary oedema are achieved, these patients may be discharged from hospital within 7 to 10 days. Long-term functional and survival data suggest a sustained and marked improvement in symptom status in association with approximately 75% 5-year survival. This favourably contrasts with the natural history of the nonoperated condition and with the other competing surgical therapy of lung (with or without heart) transplantation.

Key points

- Careful preoperative selection of surgical candidates is important with respect to surgical accessibility of the disease.
- Complete bilateral endarterectomy while protecting all organs is the surgical aim.
- The most critical facets of intensive care treatment relate to optimally managing:
  - lung water balance;
  - local and systemic inflammatory response to the operation;
  - pulmonary vascular tone;
  - RV function; and
  - determinants of oxygen delivery.

FURTHER READING

Valchanov K, Vuylsteke A. Pulmonary endarterectomy. *Eur J Anaesthesiol* 2006;23: 815–823.

Hoeper MM, Mayer E, Simonneau G, *et al.* Chronic thromboembolic pulmonary hypertension. *Circulation* 2006;113:2011–2020.

Jamieson SW, Kapelanski DP, Sakakibara N, *et al.* Pulmonary endarterectomy: experience and lessons learned in 1500 cases. *Ann Thorac Surg* 2003;76:1457–1464.

Chapter 54

Oesophagectomy

B. DELVAUX, M. DE KOCK AND P.F. LATERRE

Introduction

Surgical pathology of the oesophagus is dominated by cancer; squamous carcinoma and adenocarcinoma are the most common types. The incidence of squamous carcinoma is affected by environmental factors, such as smoking and alcohol consumption. On the other hand, adenocarcinoma is mostly associated with gastro-oesophageal reflux (Barrett's disease) and comprises 50% to 70% of cases in the developed world.

Other oesophageal disease requiring surgical correction and perhaps postoperative critical care includes surgery for motility disorders (achalasia), gastro-oesophageal sphincter pathology, ingestion of caustic or foreign bodies and various other disorders (e.g., Plummer–Vinson, Mallory–Weiss).

Oesophageal surgery leads to significant morbidity and mortality, contributed to by the prolonged and complex surgery itself and the often poor preoperative condition of the patients. Respiratory complications are the most common, and provision of good analgesia is always essential.

Conduct of surgery

The surgical technique chosen determines whether critical care admission is required (which is common) and significantly influences outcome and length of stay. The resection can be limited to the tumour itself (standard oesophagectomy) or may be extended to include lymphadenectomy (radical oesophagectomy). Although it is considered that survival depends on the completeness of the resection, what constitutes an adequate resection margin is still debated. The operative approach may include thoracotomy, laparotomy and/or a cervicotomy (neck incision), according to the location of the tumour and the technique chosen by the surgeon. A transhiatal approach may avoid thoracotomy, but may not allow direct visualization and lymphadenectomy. Another important consideration is the preparation of the replacement oesophageal conduit (stomach, jejunum or colon) and completion of the oesophageal anastomosis.

Analgesia

Adequate treatment of pain is important, not only to alleviate the patient's suffering but also because of its interaction with the inflammatory and immune response. Furthermore, effective analgesia helps to prevent respiratory complications by allowing early mobilization, coughing and physiotherapy. Epidural analgesia is the technique of choice because it provides excellent analgesia even during mobilization or coughing, which allows faster rehabilitation. The epidural catheter is placed at the high thoracic level before surgery and can be kept in place for 24 to 72 hours.

Extubation

The majority of patients are admitted to critical care after surgery with the endotracheal tube in situ, for elective postoperative ventilation. It is routine to exchange the double-lumen endotracheal tube that may have been used in the operating theatre for a single-lumen tube after surgery. Timing of extubation after admission to critical care is controversial, with delayed extubation (for 1 or 2 days) advocated by many teams. This may be beneficial because of the increased risk of reflux and aspiration of acidic contents. However, early extubation may be equally safe and reduce pulmonary complications associated with prolonged tracheal intubation, provided analgesia is good and the patient is cooperative when sedation is discontinued.

Nutrition

Adequate nutrition is a particular problem because of prolonged inadequate diet preoperatively. The disease may not have allowed consumption of sufficient food owing to pain or blockage before surgery, and because of this many patients are admitted some time preoperatively to allow feeding, by enteral tube or parenterally if this is not possible.

Because of this relative lack of nutrients and inability to swallow for some time after the procedure, to allow healing and confirmation of adequacy of anastomosis, nutrition in critical care is of paramount importance.

After oesophageal surgery, enteral nutrition is best given via the jejunal route (a nasojejunal tube should be placed or jejunostomy formed during surgery), and may be started soon after admission to critical care. Tolerance to enteral feeding may need to be built up by increasing the rate of delivery slowly; postoperative ileus is relatively common.

However, complications with the anastomosis may occasionally necessitate a prolonged period of fasting, in which case parenteral nutrition should be commenced, usually the first day after surgery.

Complications

Respiratory

Respiratory complications, and especially postoperative pneumonia, have a high incidence (10%–30%), and are the most important contributor to morbidity and mortality. They are more common in advanced age, poor nutritional status (associated with muscular atrophy) and immunodeficiency (associated with poor nutrition); all factors common in this group of patients. Decreased respiratory function preoperatively, most often assessed by the FEV_1, is also associated with postoperative complications.

Pathophysiology of respiratory dysfunction likely involves several mechanisms.

1. Diaphragmatic dysfunction is common because of the additive effects of general anaesthesia, surgical incision, direct handling and indirect (neurogenic reflex) mechanisms. The poor contraction of the diaphragm and the associated ileus makes atelectasis very common, which may lead to chest infection.
2. Tracheal intubation and mechanical ventilation per se may cause lung damage and provide a route for infection. The involved mechanisms are ventilation/perfusion mismatch, transudation of liquid at the alveolar level, alveolar inflammation (continuous opening and closing), ischaemia and reperfusion of the collapsed lung and local release of mediators of inflammation.
3. Surgical handling of the lung causes oedema and damage, and this may induce a local inflammatory reaction. Nerve lesions (vagus and recurrent laryngeal nerve) are relatively common.
4. Other intraoperative factors include duration of surgery, blood product transfusion, quality of analgesia and pharyngolaryngeal dysfunction.

Acute lung injury is relatively common after oesophageal surgery, although the exact mechanism is not known, and if this dreaded complication develops, it has a very significant effect on mortality.

RESPIRATORY INFECTION

Pneumonia is a leading cause of respiratory complications after oesophageal surgery, occurring in 5% to 25% of patients. Timing of initiation of treatment and appropriate empirical antibiotic therapy are critical.

Atelectasis is almost universal and can develop into overt infection, but may be reduced by 45-degree sitting position, early physiotherapy, non-invasive ventilation if gas exchange is inadequate after tracheal extubation and adequate pain control. Fibreoptic bronchoscopy may be required to clear secretions, and regular treatment may be beneficial.

PULMONARY OEDEMA

Pulmonary oedema is common, and occurs in 10% to 30% of patients. This may be partly due to the increase in pulmonary capillary permeability associated with direct surgical trauma and local release of inflammatory mediators. Lymphatic resorption is also significantly reduced. Hence, fluid management during the intraoperative and immediate postoperative periods is especially critical; overly positive fluid balance is an important risk factor, along with atrial fibrillation.

PLEURAL EFFUSION

Pleural effusion is almost always present on the operated side and is frequently present on the contralateral side also. Such effusions may require drainage if they are thought to be interfering with parlous ventilatory dynamics.

PREVENTION

Although required, mechanical ventilation should be administered in a 'protective' strategy (low tidal volume, reduction of FiO_2 if possible), and weaning/extubation should not be delayed. Epidural analgesia, early intensive physiotherapy and early mobilization may all reduce atelectasis and pneumonia. Patients should rest in bed sitting up to reduce aspiration of gastric contents.

Fluid balance, limiting input to prevent excessive positive balance, is very important.

Surgical technical issues

OESOPHAGEAL CONDUIT NECROSIS, ANASTOMOTIC LEAK AND TRACHEOBRONCHIAL FISTULAE

These are relatively common, occurring in 5% to 10% of patients, and are the most devastating complications. Length of the conduit, compression and, more important, distention seem to be the most important predisposing factors. Leak is most frequent after gastric conduit oesophageal resection, whereas ischaemia and necrosis is most frequent after use of a colon conduit. Necrosis (dead tissue) should be suspected if general inflammatory signs are accompanied by persistent metabolic acidosis or if, after the formation of a gastric conduit, 'coffee-ground' nasogastric drainage persists. The presence of a leak may be indicated if there is a change in the drainage from chest tubes, accompanied by raised inflammatory markers (white cell count, C-reactive protein, erythrocyte sedimentation rate and metabolic acidosis). Barium swallow may not demonstrate a leak soon after surgery and should be delayed for at least 5 to 7 days. Endoscopy may visualize overt ischaemia of the conduit mucosa, however computed tomography of the chest is the investigation of choice and should be performed as soon as these complications are suspected.

In general, anastomotic leak occurs around postoperative day 6 (range, 4–10 days). This may lead to pulmonary abscess, mediastinitis or septic shock. Prompt reoperation is usually required to facilitate closure of the leak and removal of necrosed tissues, together with broad-spectrum antibiotic treatment, which may need to continue for some time.

HAEMOTHORAX, PNEUMOTHORAX AND CHYLOTHORAX

Haemothorax and pneumothorax are relatively common; they may require chest tube insertion or, rarely, reoperation if bleeding is persistent. Chylothorax is rare but devastating; its treatment must be prompt and aggressive, with reexploration required and refashioning of the thoracic duct.

NEUROLOGICAL LESIONS

Damage to nerves within the thoracic cavity may of course occur, and this may lead to prolonged mechanical ventilation and critical care stay. Vagus nerve damage causes ascension of the ipsilateral hemidiaphragm, leading to poor spontaneous breathing mechanics. The recurrent laryngeal nerve may occasionally be damaged, leading to paralysis in abduction of one vocal cord; this causes hoarseness and, most important, impaired swallowing. Laryngeal nerve lesion may require specialist referral and injection of the vocal cord with temporary material to improve glottic closure, or even medialization thyroplasty, a more definitive treatment.

Other complications

Vagotomy at a high level nearly always accompanies oesophagectomy as part of the necessary dissection. It has been shown that cholinergic tonus may influence inflammation and immunity. This may make patients more susceptible to some types of complications, but this hypothesis is under intense investigation and remains to be proven.

Alcohol misuse is common in some patients requiring oesophageal surgery, especially when squamous carcinoma is present, and withdrawal syndrome should be anticipated and managed appropriately.

Key points

- Respiratory complications are the most frequent and serious complications after oesophageal surgery.
- Fluid balance should be strictly controlled.
- Pharyngolaryngeal dysfunction should be suspected and treated.
- Analgesia is best achieved by epidural route.
- Early extubation is safe.
- Early enteral feeding is recommended.

FURTHER READING

Aceto P, Congedo E, Cardone A, *et al.* Postoperative management of elective oesophagectomy for cancer. *Rays* 2005;30:289–294.

Jørgensen H, Wetterslev J, Møiniche S, *et al.* Epidural local anaesthetics versus opioid-based analgesic regimens for postoperative gastrointestinal paralysis, PONV and pain after abdominal surgery. *Cochrane Database of Syst Rev* 2000;4:CD001893.

Chapter 55

Management after heart transplant

J. GOOI AND K. DHITAL

Introduction

The immediate postoperative course after a heart transplant has a profound effect on long-term outcome. This chapter deals with the management of heart transplant recipients in the first 48 to 72 hours in the critical care unit.

The heart transplant recipient has had, above all, a major cardiac procedure on cardiopulmonary bypass (CPB). The main principles in dealing with the postoperative course of any open heart operation, as detailed elsewhere in this book, also apply to heart transplantation. Nevertheless, there are areas where transplantation differs from standard open heart surgery, and these are specifically addressed in this chapter.

Baseline factors

Recipient factors

Before the transplant, the recipient will have undergone thorough assessment and rigorous waiting list surveillance to identify clinical features that may have an impact on both the operation itself and the postoperative course. Two important such features can substantially affect the postoperative course: pulmonary vascular resistance and renal function.

An absolute contraindication to heart transplantation is fixed severely elevated pulmonary vascular resistance. The new heart has a right ventricle (RV) that has never seen pulmonary artery pressure greater than 20 mmHg; it cannot be expected to pump against very high pulmonary artery pressure owing to elevated pulmonary vascular resistance. Many heart transplant recipients have a small degree of elevated pulmonary vascular resistance and, if more than 5 Woods units, this can compromise donor RV function. Such recipients often need perioperative pulmonary vasodilators.

With longstanding chronic low cardiac output (CO) and the use of powerful diuretics, many recipients arrive in the operating room with some degree of renal dysfunction. When the operation itself adds insult to injury, renal function can become worse, and be further impaired by some immunosuppressive drugs. Thus preexisting renal impairment may help to predict the likelihood of postoperative renal complications and may influence the immunosuppressive strategy.

Donor factors

Immediately before the transplant, donor and recipient are matched for blood type and as closely matched as possible for height and weight. Sometimes the matching is less than ideal, and a small donor heart may be expected to sustain a large recipient circulation. On other occasions, the new heart may not be as 'perfect' as one would like; the shortage of donor organs means that borderline hearts are now often used. These may be older or with less good function on haemodynamic monitoring. There is good evidence that satisfactory outcomes can be achieved with such organs, but this means

Table 55.1 Management goals in critical care after cardiac transplantation

Achieving optimal cardiac function and end-organ perfusion
Optimizing respiratory function
Allograft protection
Management of bleeding and coagulopathy
Initiation and maintenance of immunosuppression therapy
Prophylactic antibiotic therapy
Monitoring drug-related side effects
Preparation for rehabilitation and recovery

Table 55.2 Ideal haemodynamic parameters after heart transplantation

Heart rate	80–120 bpm
Mean arterial pressure	60–90 mmHg
Central venous pressure	$\leq$12 mmHg
Pulmonary artery capillary wedge pressure	$\leq$15 mmHg
Cardiac index	>2.2 L min^{-1} m^{-2}
Systemic vascular resistance	800–1,200 dyne s cm^{-5}
Pulmonary vascular resistance	150–250 dyne s cm^{-5}
Urine output	> 0.5 mL/kg per hour

that the heart may need care and coaxing to achieve good haemodynamic function in the early postimplantation period.

The new heart will be recovering from the well-documented deleterious effects of brain stem death on function. These are further exacerbated by a prolonged period of cold ischaemia (during transport in the cool box) and warm ischaemia (during implantation). In principle, the aim is to restore coronary perfusion as quickly as is feasible, up to an arbitrary limit of 4 hours of total ischaemic time. In practice, ischaemic time may exceed this limit owing to a combination of logistic transport difficulties, poor synchronization of donor and recipient procedures, unexpected operative events and slow surgeons. The length of the ischaemic period is a major determinant of short- and long-term outcomes after heart transplantation.

Basic goals

Treatment should also aim at achieving normothermia, normoglycaemia, reducing FiO_2 while maintaining PaO_2 above 10 kPa and $PaCO_2$ at 6 kPa or lower, haemoglobin at 8 g/dL and serum potassium of 4.5 to 5.5 mmol/L.

Bleeding

Heart transplant patients have several risk factors for excessive postoperative bleeding: they may have had previous cardiac operations, sometimes including ventricular assist device (VAD) implantation, and many are taking anticoagulants. Their CPB times are long. There may be liver dysfunction owing to longstanding poor CO. All these conspire to produce post-transplant coagulopathy. Coagulation testing and thromboelastography should be used to guide blood product replacement. Blood products, if necessary, should be leukocyte depleted. Bleeding should be closely monitored with a high index of suspicion of mediastinal and pleural blood collection and cardiac tamponade.

Cardiac function

There is often myocardial dysfunction of the donor heart as a result of ischaemic time and reperfusion injury. This can occur in up to 30% to 50% of patients, although the mortality from early graft failure is less than 2%. Most heart transplant patients return to the critical care unit with infusions of inotropes and vasoactive drugs in progress. The

Table 55.3 Aetiology of low cardiac output syndrome after cardiac transplantation

Aetiology	Common causes
Decreased ventricular preload	Hypovolaemia (bleeding, vasodilatation, vasodilators, sedatives) Cardiac tamponade Positive end-expiratory pressure Right ventricular dysfunction Tension pneumothorax
Decreased myocardial contractility	Ischaemia–reperfusion injury
Hypoxia, hypercarbia, acidosis	
Tachycardia Bradycardia	
Increased afterload	Vasoconstriction Fluid overload
Diastolic dysfunction	
Other problems	Sepsis Anaphylactic reactions Protamine reaction

drugs and their doses depend on the standard institution protocols.

The commonest manifestation is RV dysfunction with tricuspid regurgitation. The RV is thin walled, susceptible to ischaemia–reperfusion injury, often less well protected than the left ventricle (LV) during the operation and less able to cope with increases in afterload. The likelihood of RV dysfunction is also closely related to the degree of pulmonary vascular resistance.

Management of low cardiac output

Myocardial function is often depressed 6 to 8 hours after transplantation owing to oedema and ischaemia–reperfusion injury. This may, in combination with patient factors such as pulmonary hypertension, seriously impair CO. When marginal ventricular function is present, compensatory mechanisms develop from sympathetic autonomic stimulation and endogenous catecholamine production. This increases heart rate as well as arterial and venous tone. All these factors may improve CO or systemic blood pressure but do so at the expense of increased myocardial oxygen demand. This can result in myocardial ischaemia and progressive cardiac dysfunction. In addition to hypotension with high right-sided filling pressures, cardiac dysfunction can manifest as poor peripheral perfusion with pale, cool peripheries and diaphoresis, pulmonary congestion and poor oxygenation, impaired renal perfusion, oliguria and a metabolic acidosis. Diagnosis of low CO state is suspected if:

- cardiac index is 2.0 L min^{-1} m^{-2} or lower;
- pulmonary artery wedge pressure is higher than 20 mmHg;
- systemic vascular resistance is above 1500 dynes s cm^{-5}; and
- oliguria.

As mentioned, RV dysfunction is the commonest cause of low CO after transplantation. It may be exacerbated by inadequate cardiac preservation or by donor–recipient mismatch with the transplantation of a smaller donor heart into a larger recipient.

Table 55.4 Features of right ventricular failure
Elevated central venous pressure
Elevated pulmonary artery pressure
Tricuspid regurgitation
Arrhythmias
Peripheral oedema and ascites
Hepatomegaly with abnormal liver enzyme levels

The LV diastolic dysfunction is usually characterized by elevated left atrial or pulmonary capillary wedge pressures and reflects the increased pressure required to fill the noncompliant LV to maintain CO. Both LV diastolic dysfunction and RV dysfunction usually respond to vasodilating agents such as glyceryltrinitrate and isoprenaline. In addition, decreasing systemic and pulmonary afterload by the use of phosphodiesterase III inhibitors (milrinone or enoximone) can also be extremely useful. When associated with preoperative pulmonary hypertension or high pulmonary vascular resistance, steps should be taken to dilate the pulmonary vasculature and decrease resistance. Intravenous or nebulized prostaglandin-E1 (prostacyclin) or inhaled nitric oxide can be used.

TREATMENT OF LOW CARDIAC OUTPUT SYNDROME

- Look for noncardiac correctable causes (respiratory, acid–base, electrolytes, coagulopathy, bleeding).
- Optimize heart rate at 90 to 100 bpm and ensure sinus rhythm.
- Control arrhythmias by pacing or anti-arrhythmics.
- Optimize preload (pulmonary capillary wedge pressure or left atrial pressure 15–18 mmHg).
- If systemic vascular resistance is above 1500 dynes s cm^{-5}, start a vasodilator.
- If systemic vascular resistance is low, start a vasopressor.
- Assess CO and start inotrope if the cardiac index is 2.0 L min^{-1} m^{-2} or lower in conjunction with systemic vascular resistance.
- If haemoglobin is 8 g/dL or lower, transfuse.
- If pulmonary artery pressure is elevated, use pulmonary vasodilators.

If CO is still not satisfactory, an intra-aortic balloon pump (IABP) should be considered. The use of an IABP can rapidly stabilize the patient as CO may increase by 10% to 20%, mean arterial pressure by 10% to 20% and heart rate and pulmonary capillary wedge pressure decrease by 20% to 30%. By enabling infusions of inotropes to be decreased, an IABP can also improve acid–base states of patients.

If, despite, the maximal use of inotropes and IABP, the patient still remains in a low CO state with persistent acidosis and oliguria, consideration should be given to the implantation of a VAD (Chapter 21).

Management of dysrhythmias

Dysrhythmias, particularly supraventricular, are common after transplantation. Usually they reflect electrolyte imbalance and resolve easily with appropriate correction. However, in the context of myocardial insult with low CO or with RV failure, they are more insidious and may require cardioversion, particularly in the setting of haemodynamic instability. Amiodarone therapy is often required.

Postoperative bradyarrhythmias including forms of heart block can result from a number of causes including surgical trauma, cardiac denervation, myocardial oedema and ischaemia–reperfusion injury. Appropriate heart rate is maintained by atrial or sequential epicardial pacing and by the continuation of isoprenaline infusion if necessary. It is imperative to check the pacing thresholds daily to assess the need for additional transvenous pacing wires or earlier referral for implantation of a permanent system. Persistent arrhythmias should also prompt the exclusion of cardiac rejection.

Table 55.5 Assessment of the patient with low cardiac output

Bedside clinical examination: Temperature, tissue turgor, jugular venous pressure, capillary refill, breath sounds, cardiac murmurs, extremities.
Obtain haemodynamic measurements (assess filling pressures and determine cardiac output and systemic vascular resistance).
Measure mixed venous oxygen saturation.
Analyse arterial blood gases looking for acidosis, hypoxia, hypercarbia and electrolyte levels.
Electrocardiograph – arrhythmias and/or ischaemia.
Chest radiograph: pneumothorax, endotracheal position, mediastinum.
Urine output.
Total chest drainage – suggesting excessive bleeding or tamponade.
A transthoracic or transoesophageal echocardiogram is extremely useful in establishing the nature of the problem, particularly with ruling out tamponade and in guiding appropriate filling pressures.

Renal management

The heart transplant patient often has marginal renal function prior to surgery. The use of CPB with increased fluid retention in the 'third space' and hypoperfusion owing to low CO postoperatively invariably causes a transient decrease in renal function. The additional renal side effects of some immunosuppressive drugs (particularly cyclosporine) make it imperative to maintain careful vigilance over renal function. Diuretic therapy either in the form of regular boluses or as an infusion is used routinely to prevent fluid overload. Because the heart is particularly sensitive to fluctuations in volume status and acid–base balance post-transplantation, early renal replacement therapy should always be considered (Chapter 29).

Pulmonary management and extubation

The management of ventilation and timing of extubation is essentially similar to other cardiac surgery cases. Early extubation, 4 to 6 hours after surgery, is preferred.

Immunosuppression

Protocols for the induction and maintenance of immunosuppression vary. Triple therapy, consisting of cyclosporine, mycophenolate mofetil and prednisolone, is most commonly employed. Prednisolone is usually administered at 1 mg/kg per day in 2 divided doses and may be reduced by 5 mg/d to a maintenance dose of 0.2 mg/kg per day. The mycophenolate mofetil dose is commonly 0.5 to 1.5 g twice daily; this may be reduced if there is gastrointestinal disturbance.

Surveillance of the cardiac allograft commences 7 days post-transplant, when a pulmonary artery flotation catheter and myocardial biopsy are performed. If rejection is noted, pulsed methylprednisolone and an alteration in immunosuppressive regime may be warranted.

Antithymocyte globulin

Immunosuppression induction may be with rabbit antithymocyte globulin (R-ATG); ATG is a purified, polyclonal γ-immunoglobulin with immunosuppressive properties. It is obtained from rabbits (or horses) that have been immunized with human thymocytes. It specifically recognizes and destroys T lymphocytes. Although the exact mechanism of action is not completely understood, it appears to involve T-lymphocyte clearance from the circulation and modulation of T-lymphocyte activity. During treatment (which usually commences at the time of surgery and continues for 3 days) $CD3^+$ counts should be maintained between 50 and 100×10^6.

Cyclosporine

Cyclosporine is not started during R-ATG treatment. Intravenous administration may be required if oral

Table 55.6 T-cell count and rabbit antithymocyte globulin dosing protocol

Absolute CD3 count ($\times 10^6$/L)	Rabbit antithymocyte globulin dose (mg/kg body weight)
>100	1.0
75–100	0.75
50–75	0.50
25–50	0.25
≤25	0

feeding is not established, and dosage should be reduced if renal function is compromised. Plasma cyclosporine level should be checked, and after 1 week of treatment, the level should be 250 to 350 μg/L. In patients with ongoing chronic renal impairment or those whose renal function is worsened by cyclosporine, sirolimus may be administered as an alternative.

Cytomegalovirus

The cytomegalovirus and toxoplasmosis status of both the donor and recipient are important as these infections can be transmitted to the recipient with the donor organ. If the donor is cytomegalovirus positive and the recipient negative (a mismatch), ganciclovir should be administered immediately after surgery (5 mg/kg twice daily IV adjusted for renal function) and converted to 1 g three times a day when the patient is taking oral medications. Sulfadiazine and pyrimethamine treatment may be required if toxoplasmosis is detected by polymerase chain reaction.

Other organ systems

Neurological problems

Neurological dysfunction is unfortunately common after cardiac transplantation. Preexisting peripheral vascular disease, left atrial or ventricular thrombi or VAD cannulae predispose to thromboembolic strokes or watershed infarcts. Prolonged coagulopathy or requirement for anticoagulation make intracerebral haemorrhage more likely.

Gastrointestinal dysfunction

A proton pump inhibitor is normally used for peptic ulcer prophylaxis, but ulceration and gastritis can still occur and cause gastrointestinal bleeding. Low CO syndrome and subsystem organ failure can also predispose patients to pancreatitis, cholecystitis or hepatic dysfunction. In addition, high-dose inotropes and low CO can predispose to paralytic ileus and intestinal ischaemia that can cause major morbidity.

Other considerations

Discharge from critical care generally occurs once the patient is haemodynamically stable, on low-dose inotropes only and on minimal oxygen. Once discharged from critical care, the patients continue a rigorous program of physiotherapy, nutritional support and continued transplant education, particularly with respect to medication, to facilitate independence and discharge from hospital.

Key points

- Preexisting pulmonary hypertension is a strong risk factor for RV dysfunction and failure after transplantation.
- Low CO syndrome is relatively common; haemodynamic monitoring should guide inotropic therapy and mechanical support may be required.
- Prolonged bradycardia or heart block after transplantation may require permanent pacemaker implantation.
- Immunosuppression induction and maintenance are very important and must not be omitted; choice of agent and dose should be regularly assessed.

Chapter 56

Management after lung transplant

L. SPENCER, C. LEONARD AND N. YONAN

Introduction

Lung transplantation has now become an accepted treatment option for patients with end-stage lung disease.

The lung transplant 5-year survival is lower than other solid organ transplants and is currently at 50% or lower.

Improvements in survival have occurred recently, and these have been mainly in the early post-transplant period, probably reflecting better patient selection, surgical skill and critical care.

Recipient selection

Meticulous preoperative assessment and selection is vital. The number of lung transplants performed is limited primarily by donor organ supply. Generally, recipients should have single organ failure only. Furthermore, there should be no evidence of uncontrolled systemic active infection at the time of transplantation.

Postoperative management

Respiratory

After transplantation, extubation should generally take place after 12 to 24 hours, provided patients are stable with good gases and minimal pressure support. Earlier extubation may be associated with increased incidence of hypoxaemia, hypercapnia and respiratory distress, and does not permit bronchoscopic clearance of secretions if required. Pulmonary oedema, accumulation of secretions and pneumothorax must be suspected if oxygenation and ventilation prove difficult. Occlusion or narrowing of the pulmonary venous anastomosis can also cause chest radiograph shadowing, poor oxygenation and pulmonary oedema; transoesophageal echocardiography may be diagnostic. Reperfusion injury should be suspected if other diagnoses have been ruled out, and may present 6 to 12 hours after surgery.

Pain relief is an important feature postoperatively, and epidural infusion may be most effective and allow earlier extubation if clam shell or thoracotomy incisions have been performed. If the epidural has not been sited intraoperatively, it can be inserted in critical care before stopping sedation, providing clotting and full blood count have been checked.

Chest drains are removed when there is no documented air leak and fluid drainage is 100 mL or less over 24 hours.

Noninvasive ventilation or continuous positive airway pressure (Chapter 24) may be used after extubation if oxygenation becomes suboptimal.

Surveillance bronchoscopy is often employed to ensure good clearance of secretions and to allow inspection of bronchial anastomoses. Ischaemic airway injury may be seen, but is managed expectantly. Lung biopsy is performed on occasion to allow histological investigation for rejection and signs of infection; bronchoscopic lavage also allows more accurate microbiological diagnosis.

Table 56.1 Common indications for lung transplantation

Obstructive lung disease (COPD, obliterative bronchiolitis)
Interstitial/fibrotic lung disease (idiopathic pulmonary fibrosis, sarcoid, extrinsic allergic alveolitis, lymphangioleiomyomatosis, histiocytosis X, connective tissue disease-related interstitial lung disease)
Suppurative lung disease (CF, non-CF bronchiectasis)
Pulmonary vascular disease (primary pulmonary hypertension)
Others (cancer, chronic lung rejection, LAM, congenital heart disease)

Abbreviations: CF, cystic fibrosis; COPD, chronic obstructive pulmonary disease.

Cardiovascular

A pulmonary artery catheter (Chapter 12) is recommended to allow regular monitoring of pulmonary pressure and mixed venous saturation. Pulmonary hypertension should be controlled; nebulized prostacyclin may be effective and is relatively easy to administer. Decreasing mixed venous saturation may be an early indicator of poor perfusion or graft function, and should prompt further investigation such as CO studies to guide optimization of therapy. Inotropic support is commonly required after lung transplantation, despite apparently normal cardiac function preoperatively, although low-dose dopamine alone may be sufficient. Isoprenaline infusion is routinely administered to ensure adequate heart rate and reduce pulmonary arterial pressure.

Immunosuppression

INDUCTION IMMUNOSUPPRESSION

Induction treatment is often employed to buy time until maintenance immunosuppression takes effect. Rabbit antithymocyte globulin is most commonly used, but more recently interleukin-2 receptor blocking antibodies such as daclizumab or

Table 56.2 Indications for heart–lung transplantation

Complex congenital heart disease
Primary pulmonary hypertension
Conditions in Table 56.1 with poor cardiac function

basiliximab have been used. However, a higher incidence of infection such as cytomegalovirus (CMV) may offset the lower rates of acute rejection after induction therapy. High-dose intravenous prednisolone is also administered for the first 24 hours.

MAINTENANCE IMMUNOSUPPRESSION

Triple therapy using corticosteroid with azathioprine or mycophenolate and cyclosporine or tacrolimus is usually started 24 hours postoperatively.

Cyclosporine levels may be checked 2 hours post dose to ensure adequate dosing and minimize the risk of renal impairment.

Tacrolimus may result in high blood sugars but does not increase cholesterol levels. There is a minor issue with intravenous and nasogastric administration; it cannot be given through the standard giving sets. Mycophenolate mofetil (IV or oral) or azathioprine do not improve outcome when compared with azathioprine.

Everolimus and sirolimus are alternatives, but care is needed owing to the risk of wound dehiscence in the early postoperative period. These agents should not be started in lung transplant recipients before bronchial healing has been documented (which usually occurs by 6 weeks).

Complications

Bleeding

Haemorrhage after lung transplantation is more common if cardiopulmonary bypass (CPB) is used intraoperatively. Other predisposing conditions include cystic fibrosis, bronchiectasis, sarcoidosis

Table 56.3 Percentage alive at 1, 3, 5, 7, and 10 years post lung transplant

Year	Alpha-1	CF	COPD	IPF	PPH	Sarcoidosis
1	75.7	80.6	81.3	69.4	65.4	67.6
3	60.2	65.2	63.4	53.7	55.5	54.1
5	50.5	53.8	48.4	42.1	46.1	47.3
7	42.2	44.7	35.3	32.8	37.1	42.2
10	31.3	32.1	19.0	15.4	25.5	32.8

Based on International Society of Heart Lung Transplantation data, 2006.
This demonstrates disease-specific impacts on survival, for example, survival in patients with idiopathic pulmonary fibrosis (IPF) is worse than in young patients with cystic fibrosis (CF).
Abbreviations: COPD, chronic obstructive pulmonary disease; PPH, primary pulmonary hypertension.

and previous thoracic surgery. Return to theatre and possibly packing the chest cavity may be required. Management of postoperative bleeding is based on full assessment of coagulation status and thromboelastograph may be particularly useful.

Reperfusion injury

Risk factors for reperfusion injury after lung transplantation are:

- long ischaemic time, particularly warm ischaemia;
- high preoperative pulmonary artery pressures;
- borderline donor organ quality; and
- older donors.

Reperfusion injury presents with increased oxygen requirement, elevated pulmonary artery pressures and ventilatory difficulties. The clinical pattern is similar to pulmonary oedema, and the chest radiograph often shows diffuse haziness. Treatment may include keeping the patient relatively intravascularly dry and minimizing the infusion of crystalloid or colloids. Oedema fluid may be present

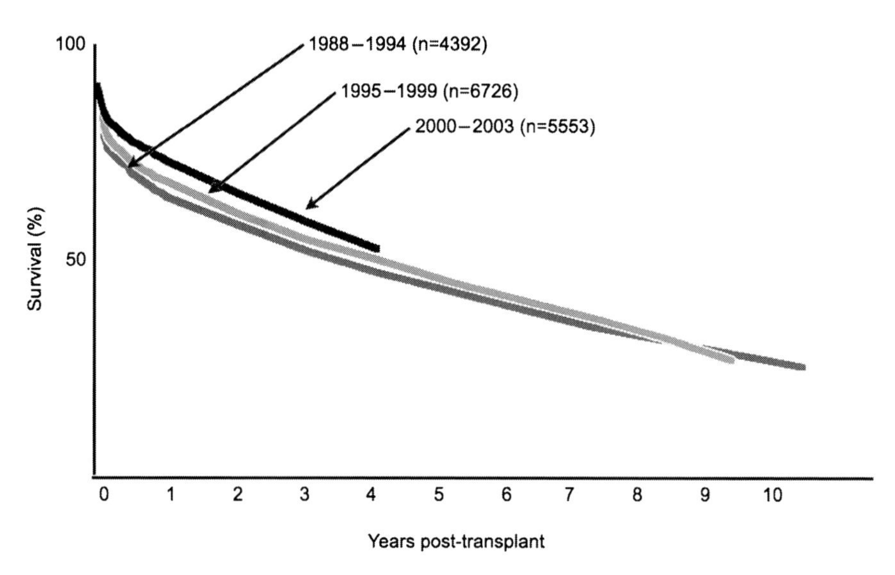

Figure 56.1 Lung transplantation: 5-year survival.

and suction of the endotracheal tube should be discouraged while ensuring maintenance of positive end-expiratory pressure (7.5–10 mmH_2O). Invasive ventilation may necessitate deeper sedation. If severe, extracorporeal circulation (Chapter 28) may be required; nitric oxide treatment has been advocated, but has not been shown to reduce mortality.

Native lung hyperinflation

If single lung transplantation has taken place, particularly as a treatment for emphysema, there is a risk of hyperinflation of the native and excessively compliant emphysematous lung at the expense of the transplanted lung. The native lung can, on occasion, cross the midline and cause cardiac tamponade and haemodynamic instability. Reintubation with double-lumen endotracheal tube and selective ventilation (using two ventilators; Chapter 25) may be required.

Infection

Bacterial and viral infections are common after lung transplantation. Less common and of later onset are protozoal infections (mainly *Pneumocystis carinii* and toxoplasmosis). Fungal infections with *Candida* or *Aspergillus* are also relatively common.

Early postoperative bacterial pneumonia, usually due to Gram-negative organisms, is the most common infectious complication affecting at least 35% of patients. Preoperative recipient sputum cultures can, if available, help to guide antibiotic choice. C-reactive protein and white cell count should be measured daily. Routine fungal prophylaxis with fluconazole and inhaled amphotericin is commonly used. Pneumocystis prophylaxis with cotrimoxazole is required for life.

Cytomegalovirus infection or reactivation is a major problem after transplantation. It is usually delayed until a few weeks after surgery and thus hopefully after the patient has left critical care. However, in the setting of preoperative immunosuppression, it may present much earlier. The severity of the problem depends on donor-recipient CMV matching. If the recipient is CMV negative but the donor was CMV positive, the risk of infection is high. This is called a primary CMV mismatch and ganciclovir should be administered for up to 90 days. Quantitative polymerase chain reaction analysis may allow measurement of CMV load.

Hyperacute rejection

A small percentage of patients who have preformed anti-human leukocyte antibodies are at risk of hyperacute rejection. This can result in rapid primary graft failure. This condition is rare, but may necessitate plasmapheresis, antithymocyte globulin and the monoclonal anti-B-cell drug rituximab. Mortality remains high.

Airway complications

Bronchial anastomotic dehiscence may occur after lung transplantation but bronchial stenoses are far more common. These usually present some months after surgery, and may require bronchoscopic dilatation or stenting.

Renal impairment

The calcineurin inhibitors (cyclosporine and tacrolimus) are nephrotoxic and this action may be aggravated by the stress of prolonged surgery and long periods of CPB. Renal replacement therapy may be required. Renal function often improves, although the serum creatinine level may remain elevated.

Gastrointestinal complications

Enteral nutrition should be given early to maintain muscle mass, general strength, immune status and preserve bowel integrity. However, there is an increased recognition of the frequency of gastric aspiration after transplantation surgery and this may have a potential role in chronic rejection. Antireflux surgery such as pretransplantation fundoplication is performed in some centres, but gastric and oesophageal dysmotility after transplant is ill-defined and may be multifactorial. Upright feeding and prophylactic proton pump inhibitors should certainly be employed.

Key points

- Extubation after lung transplantation may be delayed for 12 to 24 hours because of the relatively high incidence of early reperfusion injury.
- Epidural analgesia is preferred after clamshell or thoracotomy incision.
- Immunosuppressive therapy is very important and should not be omitted. Intraoperative induction is followed by long-term maintenance therapy, and should be supervised by specialist teams.
- Infection is common postoperatively, and accurate diagnosis and prompt treatment are essential in the face of immunosuppression.

Chapter 57

Prolonged critical care after cardiac surgery

J. MOORE AND J. EDDLESTON

Introduction

With advances in surgical and anaesthetic practice, the majority of patients undergoing cardiac surgery spend less than 24 hours in critical care. However, a proportion (between 4.8% and 16%) are admitted for longer than 5 days. This is more likely in the increasingly prevalent older patient population, who often have comorbidities. In addition, the development of less invasive surgery has permitted higher risk patients to be accepted for surgery.

For patients with a complicated critical care stay, surgical mortality in terms of 30-day or in-hospital mortality only partially reflects the overall outcome. Longer term mortality and morbidity provide a better analysis of the benefit of surgery.

Mortality

In the mid 1990s, authors began to examine the long-term mortality of cardiac surgical patients requiring prolonged critical care treatment. A number of studies have been published. In these studies, long-stay patients represented around 5% of those who underwent cardiac surgery, but accounted for 50% of the hospital critical care days and consumed 48% of the total critical care resources and 23% of the hospital direct costs. Early mortality (within 10 days) appears related to the patient risk profile and to the type of operation performed. A late increase in mortality is noted for those patients remaining in critical care, which is due to complications such as ventilator-associated pneumonia and sepsis.

The survival curves for those patients with a prolonged critical care stay show a marked decline in the first 6 months of follow-up. This reflects the high critical care and hospital mortality of these patients secondary to organ failure. After 6 months, however, long- and short-stay patients become comparable.

It is noteworthy that high-risk surgical patients who survive the first few perioperative months have a better long-term outcome than medically treated patients, because of the corrective nature of the surgery. Patients and their surgeons need to be aware of this, to aid their understanding and decision making.

Risk factors

Various risk factors for increased mortality and prolonged critical care have been identified. Overall, respiratory failure and acute renal failure appear to be the most important factors in predicting prolonged critical care stay. Attempts have been made to identify patients who will not benefit from prolonged critical care. Predictive indices based on patient baseline characteristics and organ failure scoring have been devised. Although they identify high-risk patient groups, they do not reliably predict individual patient outcomes. Interestingly, retrospective studies have demonstrated that identification of patients whose care is deemed futile, leading to withdrawal of critical care, does not result in a significant improvement in resource utilization.

Table 57.1 Cumulative mortality for cardiac patients requiring prolonged critical care

Study	Hospital (%)	6 months (%)	Long-term (%)
Nielsen *et al* (1997): 96 patients staying >5 days in critical care	35%	44%	45% (12 mos)
Bashour *et al* (2000): 142 patients staying >10 days in critical care	33%	51%	64% (30.6 mos)
Hein *et al* (2006): 685 patients staying >3 days in critical care	19%		34% (36 mos)

Morbidity

It is well recognized that patients with prolonged critical care stay have an increased mortality and are more likely to have poor functional status after recovery. However, the literature is scarce regarding long-term morbidity resulting from critical care in cardiac patients. The specific morbidity associated with cardiac surgery must be considered together with the problems commonly encountered by patients after critical care in general.

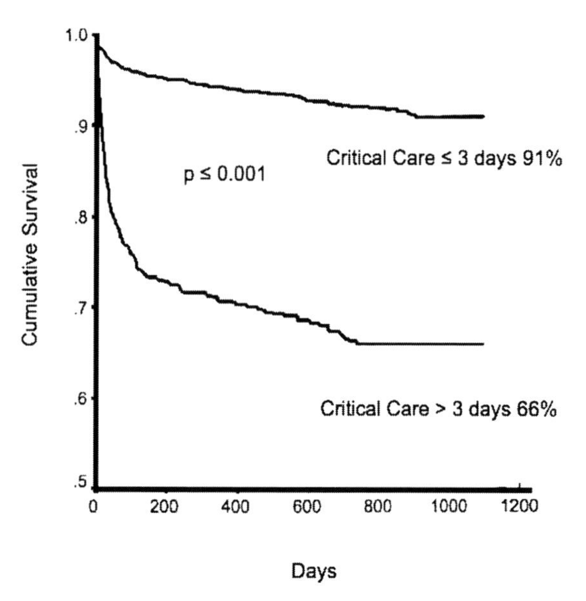

Figure 57.1 Kaplan–Meier survival curve for 3 years of follow-up for patients ($n = 651$) with a critical care stay of longer than 3 days and patients ($n = 1{,}912$) with a critical care stay 3 days or less. There is a large mortality disadvantage in the first 6 months for those requiring longer than 3 days in critical care. Reprinted by permission from Elsevier.

Neurological and cognitive complications

Neurological injury after cardiac surgery can be devastating, and is a common cause of prolonged stay in critical care. Adverse neurological outcome can be divided into two categories:

- type I includes stroke, transient ischaemic attacks and coma; and

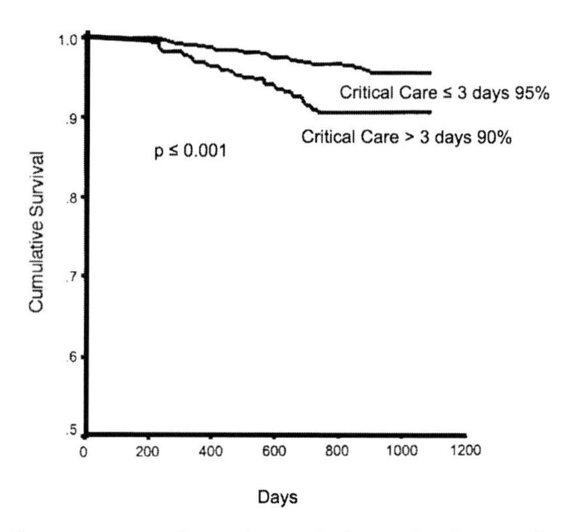

Figure 57.2 Kaplan–Meier survival curve for the period 6 months after surgery until 3 years follow-up, with a critical care stay 3 days or less and greater than 3 days. Note the improvement in survival as the two groups become more comparable. Reprinted by permission from Elsevier.

- type II consists of intellectual deterioration, cognitive dysfunction and memory deficits. This is more common.

Up to 69% of patients suffering type I injury require admission to a long-term care facility. Stroke affects 2% to 5% of patients; only 39% of these are living with minimal disability at 5 years (61% have major disability). Intellectual deterioration by itself is common, with 22% of patients having evidence of neurological impairment after 2 years. Psychological and cognitive difficulties occur in up to 30% of patients attending critical care follow-up clinics. Patients may complain of difficulties with concentration and short-term memory, and inability to perform simple mental tasks. The psychological consequences of critical illness (anxiety, depression, post-traumatic stress disorder) can be equally important. The effect on the family must not be overlooked. Adverse psychological sequelae are commonly reported in families of critical care patients. Rehabilitation programmes must therefore also include close family members.

Physical impact of critical illness

Physical recovery from critical illness can take over a year, particularly in those over 50 years of age.

Table 57.2 Common physical problems after a period in the critical care unit

Weakness	Insomnia
Weight loss	Impotence
Fatigue	Skin and nail changes
Poor appetite	Hair loss
Painful joints	Pruritus
Voice and taste changes	Amenorrhoea
Peripheral neuropathy	

From Intensive Care After Care by R Griffiths and C Jones. Reprinted by permission from Elsevier Science.

Patients invariably lose up to 2% of lean body muscle mass per day in critical care, become cachectic and deconditioned. Appetite is depressed for some time, and the recovery of body mass is slow. Weakness and lack of coordination can be debilitating, requiring considerable effort by the patient to retrain the muscles.

Critical illness neuropathy and myopathy are almost universal in patients who are critically ill for longer than 7 days. The clinical manifestations are severe weakness and loss of axonal conduction on electromyography, which may translate into difficulty weaning from mechanical ventilation. The aetiology remains uncertain, although neuromuscular blockers, steroids and the peripheral neurological manifestation of multiple organ dysfunctions have been suggested as potential causes. Recovery may take many months, and persistent neurophysiological abnormalities have been detected in over 90% of survivors of prolonged critical illness at 5 years.

Breathlessness is a common symptom reported by critical care survivors. Possible causes include progression of preexisting lung disease, cyst formation, bronchiectasis, pulmonary fibrosis, phrenic nerve palsy or simply muscle weakness. Acute lung injury complicating critical care may continue to cause a reduction in respiratory function for up to 2 years after critical care discharge. Most acute lung injury survivors have abnormal pulmonary function tests if tested in the first few months of recovery, which usually reach a plateau after 6 to 9 months. They generally demonstrate a restrictive ventilatory defect, with some impairment of diffusion capacity. Associated with these abnormalities is a persistence of fibrotic changes on computed tomography.

Dysphagia has been reported in over 50% of patients ventilated for longer than 24 hours. After discharge, patients remain at risk of a reduced nutritional intake and may continue to require nasogastric supplementation.

Because of prolonged immobility, patients are at risk of contractures, particularly of the shoulders, hands, hips and ankles. They find mobilizing difficult and may need mobility aids for some time.

Sexual dysfunction

Follow-up studies have found that 26% of patients report sexual dysfunction at 2 months and 16% at 1 year after critical care stay. This lack of a sexual relationship can have a major impact on quality of life (QOL), with an adverse effect on close relationships. This can increase the feeling of isolation and reduce the patient's sense of well-being. It may also often go unrecognized, because patients may feel too embarrassed to talk about such problems. Sexual dysfunction is often put down to psychological issues, such as a concern that sexual activity may precipitate a relapse of the illness. However, it is important to look for potentially treatable medical conditions (diabetes) and the side effects of commonly used drugs (β-blockers, antidepressants). Men may describe impotence – a lack of desire or difficulty maintaining an erection. Management along erectile dysfunction guidelines should be helpful and may include pharmacological agents. Women may describe a lack of libido and treatment may require more specialist advice.

Quality of life

The success of cardiac surgery has traditionally been measured by survival rate, looking at hospital or 30-day mortality. However, after cardiac surgery, mortality is low and statistical comparison is difficult. Also, patients with the most preoperative morbidity are often the ones who stand to benefit most from their surgery. More recently, the focus has begun to change, and QOL is being increasingly recognized as central to the definition of success. There is no agreed definition about what QOL actually represents, but it can be summarized as a person's sense of well-being that stems from satisfaction or dissatisfaction with the areas of life that are important to him or her. Presented generally in the form of a questionnaire, a QOL tool may be a generic health outcome tool or designed specifically for a particular condition or patient group. There is currently no specific QOL measure designed for cardiac surgical patients. However, the Short Form Health Survey (SF-36) and the Nottingham Health Profile (NHP) have been used in a number of published cardiac surgery studies, and have been validated in a variety of patient populations. The SF-36 and NHP questionnaires are reasonably concise (should take about 45 minutes) and enjoy favourable patient response. They may be self-administered, conducted by telephone or by face-to-face interview.

Most studies of QOL in cardiac surgery have shown improvements after coronary and valve surgery. Compared with the general population, critical care survivors have lower QOL for all domains except pain. Although these improve over time, they remain lower than the general population levels throughout long-term follow-up (up to 14 years). It would be interesting to see if this is also true in long-term follow-up of cardiac critical care patients.

Relatives' perspective

Caregivers have frequently reported that they perceive cardiac surgery as a major life event for the patient and themselves. Partners may have to adopt a new role within the family after the surgery. They look out for any symptoms of deterioration and may supervise or administer medication. They also support the patient and may assume responsibility for tasks of everyday life within the family. Often they feel alone in this situation and describe not receiving adequate support from health care services. Not surprisingly, financial worries are common. Relatives of critical care patients may even report higher anxiety and depression scores than the patients themselves. This can partly be explained by the fact that patients often suffer from some amnesia around the

Table 57.3 Short Form Health Survey health concepts: Number of items and summary of content

Concepts	No. of items	Summary of Content
Physical functioning	10	Extent to which health limits physical activities such as self-care, walking, climbing stairs.
Social functioning	2	Extent to which physical health or emotional problems interfere with normal social activities.
Role limitation		
Physical	4	Extent to which physical health interferes with work or other daily activities, including accomplishing less than wanted, or difficulties in performing activities.
Emotional	3	Extent to which emotional problems interfere with work of other daily activities.
Mental health	5	General mental health, including depression, anxiety.
Energy/vitality	4	Feeling energetic versus feeling tired and worn out.
Pain	2	Intensity of pain and effect of pain on normal work, both inside and outside the home.
General health	5	Personal evaluation of health, including current health, health outlook and resistance to ill health.
Change in health		Further unscaled single item asking respondents about health change over the past year.

Note. The SF-36 measures 8 health outcomes through a 36-item questionnaire. This generates a score for each heath concept from 0 to 100 (best possible). There is a summary score for the physical and mental components of the questionnaire. (Change in health is not included in the final score.)

time of their critical care admission, and, once recovered, may not realize how ill they were.

After discharge from intensive care, patients often have unrealistic expectations of their capabilities, which may lead to frustration and conflict.

Relatives may not spontaneously request support. It is therefore important to pay attention to the needs of the family. These should be addressed during the rehabilitation phase of intensive and cardiac care follow-up.

Interventions

Patients having cardiac surgery are usually entered into cardiac rehabilitation programs. However, those with prolonged critical care stays have needs that are quite different from those with uncomplicated surgery, and a more tailored program is required. They may benefit from a hybrid of cardiac and intensive care rehabilitation. The emphasis shifts further towards the critical care-based regime as the original cardiac surgery becomes a secondary factor.

Cardiac-based rehabilitation

Programs for rehabilitation of the cardiac patient are well established and should be offered to every patient after cardiac surgery. Randomized controlled trials have demonstrated their efficacy.

Table 57.4 Cardiac rehabilitation program

Prehabilitation	Information for the patient is provided by the primary care team or during pre-hospital visit, before treatment (may or may not be offered in all areas).
Inpatient	Initial advice on lifestyle, e.g. smoking cessation, diet, alcohol, exercise. If service in place, referral sent to community nurses.
Primary care based	Early postdischarge. May include assessment by community nurses including physical, psychological and social needs. General practitioner services.
Formal exercise and education program	At 2–8 weeks postdischarge, depending on procedure. As Phase 2 plus structured exercise sessions and access to relevant support and advice. May take place within hospital or community setting.
Long-term maintenance and risk factor modification	Long-term follow-up in primary care. Annual patient reviews, patient satisfaction survey, support groups. Continuation of lifestyle changes and referral to specialist advice as required, e.g. smoking cessation, diet.

The proportion of patients participating in cardiac rehabilitation, however, has remained low. This may partially be explained by a lack of resources, but also by patient motivation and paradoxically improved health. To reduce scepticism about such programmes, patient and relative education should be improved along with an emphasis on psychological support.

- *Prehabilitation* is provided by the primary care team or hospital rehabilitation teams on pre-procedure visits. It consists of an explanation of the medical procedure and postoperative care, together with orientation by visits to the cardiac surgical ward and critical care.
- *Rehabilitation* starts during the hospital admission, and information needs to be given to patients as soon as possible, with a multidisciplinary approach involving nurses, physiotherapists, dieticians, occupational therapists and medical staff.
- *Rehabilitation after discharge* until the start of the exercise/education program at 4 to 6 weeks is also important. This convalescence period can be a difficult time for both patients and families. Partners who monitor patient's daily activities may show a tendency towards overprotection.

Primary care services are an important part of the process, and may involve regular structured community health nurse home visits as well as close liaison with general practitioners. They should support both patients and relatives before and during the rehabilitation, education and exercise programme. Patients are usually seen in the surgical outpatient department 6 weeks after surgery. This allows a detailed assessment of patients' early postoperative recovery, including wound healing and adjustment of medication. After 4 to 6 weeks, patients should enter the formal cardiac rehabilitation program. This aims to help participants achieve lifestyle changes that modify risk factors, using a combination of exercise, education, counselling and support.

There is some evidence that the inclusion of partners and close family members in the rehabilitation process can influence outcome. This needs to be tailored to both the perceived needs of the patient and the patient's partner and family.

Critical care intervention

Ideally, the rehabilitation process should begin while the patient is in the critical care unit. Traditionally, physiotherapy on critical care has focused

Table 57.5 Aims of cardiac rehabilitation program

Improvement in exercise tolerance and physical work capacity
Improvement in blood lipid levels and global risk profile
Reduction in cigarette smoking
Improvement in psychosocial well-being
Attenuation of the atherosclerotic process
Reduced hospitalization
Decreased morbidity and total mortality

on clearing secretions and improving respiratory function. Evidence from ventilation rehabilitation units suggests that limb and trunk physiotherapy improves strength and reduces fatigability. This may help to wean patients from ventilatory support, improve muscle strength and can reduce the incidence of contractures. Adequate nutrition is essential, and risk factors for critical illness polyneuropathy should be minimized (muscle relaxants and high-dose steroids). Optimal glycaemic control may also reduce the effects of critical illness polymyopathy.

From critical care unit to the ward

The period after discharge from critical care can be challenging for patients and caregivers, with the move to the ward leading to less monitoring and lower staffing levels. Interviews of critical care survivors have identified this period as a major source of stress and it has been termed 'transfer anxiety.' There is potential for a gap in a patient's rehabilitation as a period of transition takes place. Critical care follow-up services can help this readjustment, while also trying to prevent readmission to critical care, reduce the hospital ward stay and promote physical and psychological recovery. Multidisciplinary follow-up teams may be beneficial, with input from doctors, nurses, physiotherapists, speech therapists, psychologists and occupational therapists contributing to a smooth recovery. Close collaboration allows a coordinated approach to ongoing rehabilitation whilst maintaining links with critical care.

Rehabilitation for critical care patients

It is known from work in chronic obstructive airways disease and after myocardial infarction that rehabilitation consisting of exercise and psychological support improves recovery and encourages coping behaviour. In 1990, the Intensive Care Research Group looked at the follow-up of patients recovering from a critical illness. This developed into a structured follow-up process, with ward visits before discharge, a rehabilitation program and a dedicated outpatient clinic.

Key points

- Cardiac surgical patients with prolonged critical care stay have a higher mortality in the first 6 months. Thereafter, survival is comparable with short-stay patients.
- To address the morbidity of patients and relatives, a multidisciplinary approach is required.
- Hospital recovery both in critical care and on the ward requires active physical rehabilitation, with mechanisms to identify and treat cognitive and psychological morbidity.
- After discharge, outpatient support is required, and should be shared between hospital and primary care, with the continued inclusion of relatives.

FURTHER READING

Bashour CA, Yared J-P, Ryan TA, *et al.* Long-term survival and functional capacity in cardiac surgery patients after prolonged intensive care. *Crit Care Med* 2000;28:3847–3853.

Caine N, Harrison SC, Sharples LD, *et al.* Prospective study of quality of life before and after coronary artery bypass grafting. *BMJ* 1991;302:511–516.

Holmes L, Loughhead K, Treasure T, *et al.* Which patients will not benefit from further intensive care after cardiac surgery? *Lancet* 1994;344: 1200–1202.

Jones C, Skirrow P, Griffiths RD, *et al.* Rehabilitation after critical illness: a randomized, controlled trial. *Crit Care Med* 2003;31:2456–2461.

Chapter 58

Palliative care

S.J. HARPER AND L. CHAPMAN

Introduction

Patients admitted to critical care units share a common characteristic: without invasive organ support and monitoring they will die. The majority recover; some die quickly even with treatment; a third group are supported while their prognosis remains unclear. They continue to receive treatment until either they improve or until it becomes apparent that they are not going to survive. At some point, we all confront the question, 'Is it appropriate to continue aggressive support in the face of increasing futility of treatment?'

The aim of this chapter is to describe the process of dying in this environment and how to deal with the challenges presented. It does not explore the decision-making processes and ethical conundrums of identifying and dealing with patients who are dying in the intensive care unit.

Epidemiology

A greater number of people die in hospital than at home. Of all patients dying in hospital, 10% die in critical care units. Mortality rates are about 20% to 30% in critical care units admitting general adult patients. Up to 70% of those patients who die have treatment withheld or withdrawn. However, there is large variation in the proportion of patients for whom treatment is withheld or withdrawn and in the way patients are managed during the dying process. Up to 70% of families describe patients suffering pain and discomfort in the days before death.

It is imperative that critical care clinicians have training and gain expertise in dealing with the palliative care of these patients. Palliative care, as described by the World Health Organization in 2002, is 'the active, holistic care of patients with advanced progressive illness. Management of pain and other symptoms and provision of psychological, social and spiritual support is paramount. The goal of good palliative care is to achieve the best quality of life possible for patients and their families.'

Barriers to improved end-of-life care in critical care

Diagnosing dying on critical care

Patients are admitted to critical care in the hope that they will recover. One of the first challenges, then, is to identify those patients who will not. There is no controlled evidence to show that prognostic models improve end-of-life decision making for individual patients. Clinicians may find it beneficial to have an objective estimate of survival, but they are better used alongside clinical experience in the decision-making process.

It is hard to define the moment at which death becomes inevitable and further treatment futile, and it is frequently difficult for families and clinicians to accept that inevitability. Without making this difficult decision, end-of-life care cannot be explored.

Surrogate decision making

Patients are frequently required to make decisions about their treatment, some of which involve end-of-life care and choosing to forego treatment. The situation in critical care is often more complex; the majority of patients are comatose and therefore lack capacity. Patients in critical care units may be unconscious because of their primary pathology or sedated to enable treatment. Only about 5% of patients are able to participate in end-of-life discussions. The wishes of the other 95% are less clear, as advance directives are seldom available, and may not be specific to the clinical situation. Therefore, family members may be required to act as surrogate decision makers.

Some families are uncomfortable with the burden of decision making for their relative in the midst of grief, and may have unrealistic expectations of their relative's ongoing treatment. In our multicultural environment, we recognize that for some cultures it may not be acceptable to withdraw or withhold treatment. Occasionally, surrogate decision makers may not be available, leaving medical staff to try to decide the patient's wishes with no personal knowledge of the patient; in these cases, the hospital legal department should be contacted for advice about involving an independent mental capacity advocate. Ideally, the decisions reached should be a balance between the patient's previously stated wishes, inferences based on their beliefs and values (guided by a surrogate) and the best interests of the patient, as judged by clinicians.

Mode of death

For expected deaths in progressive illness, it is usual for people to die after a period of decline due to a progressive illness, and to some extent the disease trajectory can be predicted. This enables clinicians to foresee the likely course of an illness and inform the patient and their family accordingly. This empowers patients to make decisions about their ongoing treatment and future place of care.

A critical care death is different from deaths occurring elsewhere, even within a hospital setting. The majority of people who die in critical care units (studies suggest approximately 70%) do so after life-sustaining treatment has been withdrawn or withheld. Withdrawing treatment on a ward-based patient may mean stopping antibiotics or intravenous fluids, and they will continue to die slowly over a number of days. Withdrawing treatment in critical care units can have a much more immediate effect, especially if the patient's cardiovascular system is being supported by large amounts of inotropes and their respiratory function is controlled by a ventilator. The result of this situation is that, regardless of the event precipitating critical care admission, the time from diagnosis of dying to actual death in the majority of patients is likely to be short. As a consequence, the time frame for provision of effective end-of-life care, within which patients and their families must approach impending death, is brief and on average little more than 4 hours.

Conflict between medical teams

Most critical care units are run by specialists who meet their patients for the first time in a state of extreme illness. Doctors who refer patients for critical care may have a longstanding relationship with their patients, and that sometimes makes it hard for them to accept that the patient is dying. Conflict between medical teams about whether ongoing treatment is appropriate is another of the barriers to giving these patients good end-of-life care.

Death-denying culture

All patients are admitted to critical care with the hope of reversing the disease process and clinicians can sometimes lose sight of the fact that certain deaths are inevitable. Perhaps more than

Table 58.1 Barriers to providing optimal end-of-life care in the intensive care unit
1. Difficulty in diagnosing dying
2. Mental capacity of patients: designating surrogates
3. Discomfort with mode of death
4. Conflict amongst staff, family
5. 21st-century 'death-denying' culture
6. Lack of protocol/guidelines for staff

in other branches of medicine, the ethos on critical care is to view death as a failure. A change in culture is required for critical care staff to see the care given to a dying patient, which enables them to have a comfortable and dignified death, as a vital element of their job that deserves to be recognized.

Lack of protocol for the critical care team

The different members of the critical care team approach end-of-life care from different perspectives.

- Nursing staff are dedicated to caring for patients and may have a holistic view of the needs of the patient and the family unit.
- Doctors are more frequently engaged in problem solving, centred around the primary physiological problems of the disease.

Conflict may arise from different perceptions about reversibility of disease and the burden of treatment. Nurses may be uncomfortable about the temporal relationship between discontinuing inotropes and ventilation, and the time of death. Additionally, the medicolegal environment may make doctors and nurses feel vulnerable about withdrawing and withholding treatment. Some clinicians worry about the 'double effect' of giving sedative and analgesic medications that they (often) believe may hasten the moment of death. Good and open communication within the team, ensuring that all views are heard, and clear standardized guidance on treatment can prevent some of these problems arising.

Even when clinical staff agree about the prognosis and the need to change emphasis from aggressive treatment to calm palliation, there is a vast difference documented in the way that doctors approach withdrawal of treatment in these critically ill patients. A lack of protocol and guidance at this difficult time can lead to reduced confidence in the proactive management of dying patients. This in turn can impact on the information and support given to families and the symptom control offered to patients.

Goals in dealing with dying patients

Patients, families and medical staff may have different focuses at the end of life, but with the common overall aim of providing compassionate care. Patients may have concerns about being a burden to their families and do not want to be alone. Families want their relatives not to suffer. Sometimes they want to be intimately involved in end-of-life discussions and care giving, and sometimes they do not. The goals of care for patients dying on critical care wards are no different than for patients dying elsewhere. The important issues to address are symptom control, insight into condition, psychological and spiritual support, and communication.

The Liverpool Care Pathway for Dying patients (LCP), which was developed at the Royal Liverpool University Hospital and the Marie Curie Hospice in Liverpool (UK), has been adapted to address these issues in the critical care environment. It incorporates multiprofessional evidence-based practice and appropriate guidelines related to end-of-life care. The LCP provides a template for the process of care and has been designed to replace other documentation in this phase of the illness. It also gives specific instructions for rationalizing interventions and for prescribing analgesia, sedation and other

Table 58.2 Initial assessment and care goals

Comfort measures	
Goal 1	Current medication assessed and nonessentials discontinued
Goal 2	IV medication written up according to agreed guidelines
Goal 3	Discontinue inappropriate interventions
Psychological insight	
Goal 4	Patient/family's ability to communicate in English assessed
Goal 5	Patient/family's insight into condition assessed
Religious/spiritual support	
Goal 6	Religious/spiritual needs assessed with patient/family
Communication	
Goal 7	Identify how family is to be informed of impending death
Goal 8	Family given hospital facilities leaflet
Goal 9	GP practice is aware of patient's condition
Summary	
Goal 10	Plan of care explained and discussed with patient/family
Goal 11	Family expresses understanding of plan of care

medications for symptom control, which has proved helpful for patients, families and staff.

Initial assessment and care of the dying critical care patient

Dying in this environment is a process. As the focus of care changes from providing cure to providing comfort, good communication is key. Thus, the first item documented in the LCP is that the multidisciplinary team agree that the patient is dying. This may take several days, taking into account physiological, biochemical and any other prognostic indicators. It is essential to involve the family and, if possible, the patient in these discussions.

Once the decision has been reached that a patient is dying, the active care of the patient should include prespecified goals.

Dying in critical care

When it is agreed that the patient is dying, treatment refocuses from aggressive intervention to preserve life to that of improving comfort for both patient and family. Explanation and communication with the family and, where possible, the patient, is vital. The fact that the patient is now dying, the likely course of the illness, the do not attempt resuscitation order and the plan of care are explained in as sensitive and understandable a way as possible. Spiritual needs of the patient and family are addressed. They should be able to discuss any outstanding issues about care, and about their feelings about their role in treatment limitation. The family should be prepared for uncertainty about the precise time of death after treatment withdrawal. Nursing support is vital during the interview with medical staff and during the process of dying. When possible, the general practitioner practice should be informed that the patient is dying, because it may need to support other members of the family.

The underlying diagnosis is documented, as is the baseline physical condition of the patient. Then, investigations and interventions are discontinued, as are nonessential medications, including fluids and nutrition. In some cases, staff or families may be

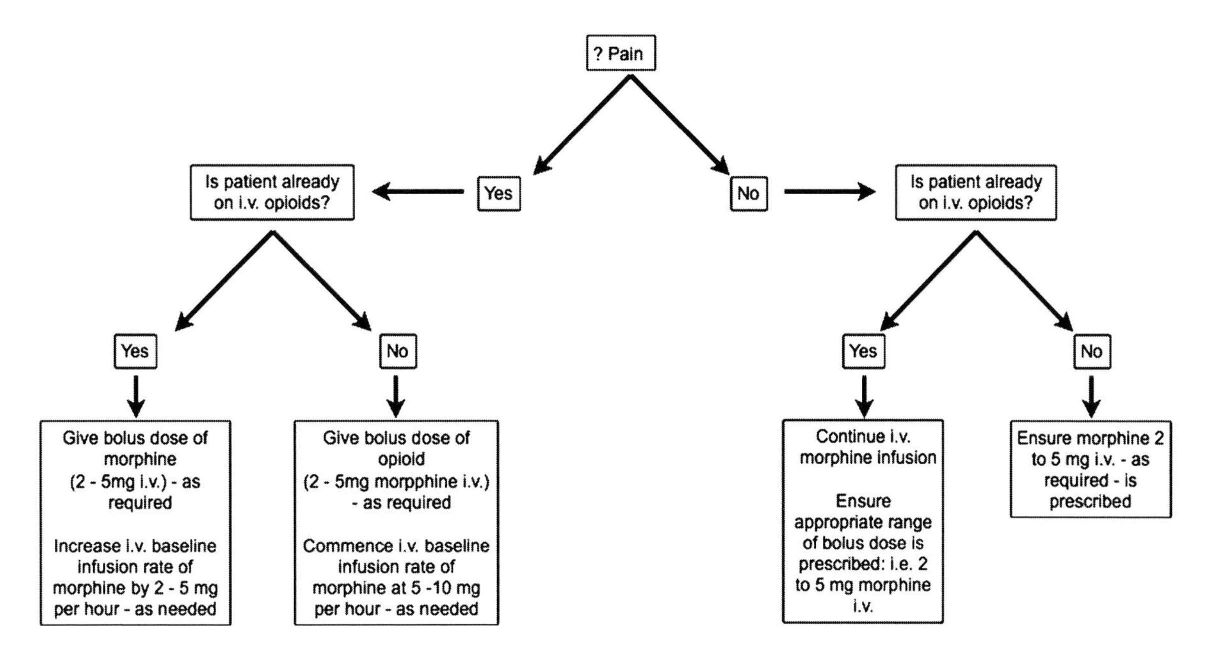

Figure 58.1 Example of guideline for pain control.

uncomfortable about stopping certain treatments, for example, IV fluids. Although there is no obligation to provide futile care to patients, it is best to discuss with families and reach agreement about what will provide the greatest patient comfort. The actual process of treatment withdrawal is a very contentious subject, with individual units, and perhaps clinicians, having their own approach. Guiding principles can be described, but not specific steps.

Sedative medications are continued or infusions started. They are titrated to effect, with the goal that the patient is comfortable and not agitated. Analgesics are similarly titrated if required, to ensure the patient does not appear to be in pain. Neuromuscular blocking agents have no place in this situation.

Nasogastric tubes are removed, unless the clinician anticipates that this will lead to vomiting. Because of the possibility of air hunger in dying patients, mechanical ventilation should be maintained, but without positive end-expiratory pressure and without added oxygen. Implantable cardiac defibrillators are deactivated.

Monitoring may be discontinued, to allow family the opportunity to sit with their relative, to touch and communicate as naturally as possible. Where possible, the patient is nursed in a side room or a separate part of the unit so that families can have unrestricted access and other patients may not be distressed; at the very least, curtains are drawn around the bed space for privacy. Observations should be less frequent and focus on symptom control rather than physiological parameters. In some cases, patients are extubated if they are not ventilator dependent. This must be discussed with and described to the family so that they are prepared for signs of respiratory obstruction and respiratory secretions.

Care after death

After death, the doctor documents the fact and time of death, and critical care staff speak to the family; the patient is laid out according to hospital policy

Table 58.3 Referring deaths to the coroner

Refer to the coroner if the death:
1. is of uncertain cause
2. was violent or unnatural cause or suspicious
3. is due to accident
4. occurred during surgery
5. is due to industrial disease or employment
6. is due to abortion
7. is due to suicide
8. occurred in police custody
Note that any death in hospital may be referred in the future.
If in doubt, discuss it with the coroner's office.

and cultural requirements, and the general practitioner informed. When appropriate, the coroner or other designated authority is also informed.

Once the patient has died, different units have different approaches in their support for bereaved families. Some refer them to counselling or bereavement services, some back to their own doctors, some send sympathy cards and others encourage self-help groups of those who have had relatives die on critical care.

Other considerations

There are other areas where specialist palliative care teams can work together with critical care to improve care of patients. In rare instances, families may wish to take family members home from the critical care unit to die. When patients and families are motivated it is possible, in liaison with community services, to fulfill these wishes; each case requires tailoring according to individual circumstances.

Finally, with the genesis of critical care outreach teams on wards, another area where palliative care and critical care can work together is apparent. Frequently, outreach teams assess patients who are not suitable or who do not wish to have aggressive treatment, including mechanical ventilation and critical care. In these instances, input from palliative care to ensure symptom control and compassionate care is invaluable.

Key points

- Communication at all levels is of key importance.
- Patient assessment, symptom control and documentation of decision making and care are critical; a holistic approach should be taken.
- Palliative care involves caring for patients, families and staff and facilitating a 'good death' for dying patients.

FURTHER READING

Curtis JR, Rubenfeld JD. *Managing death in the ICU: The transition from cure to comfort.* Oxford: Oxford University Press; 2000.

Ellershaw JE, Wilkinson S. *Care of the dying: A pathway to excellence.* Oxford: Oxford University Press; 2003.

Marie Curie Institute [homepage on the Internet]. Liverpool care pathway. Available at: www.mcpcil.org.uk.

Truog RD, Cist AF, Brackett SE, *et al.* Recommendations for end-of-life care in the intensive care unit: The Ethics Committee of the Society of Critical Care Medicine. *Crit Care Med* 2001;29:2332–2348.

SECTION 5 Discharge and Follow-up from Cardiothoracic Critical Care

Chapter 59

Discharge

D.E.P. BRAMLEY AND A.A. KLEIN

Introduction

Discharge is not a single event, but a process that involves careful planning and the involvement of medical, nursing and ancillary staff in a multidisciplinary team. Critical care represents only one part of the patient pathway from surgery to recovery and successful discharge is achieved when this continuum of care is acknowledged and appropriate planning for the next step is undertaken. Safe and timely discharge from the critical care unit after surgery can have a major impact on patient outcomes with failure to plan adequately leading to increased mortality and high rates of readmission.

It is important to recognize that discharge criteria are not simply the inverse of admission criteria and they must reflect the resources of the next level of care, staff skill levels and institutional guidelines. Critical care pathways and protocols can clarify expected progression for individual cases and aid discharge planning, which should commence at or before the time of admission.

Discharge planning

The move from the critical care unit to the next point of care is a key transition for patients after cardiothoracic surgery. The process of discharge planning is dynamic, multidisciplinary, goal directed and promotes continuity of care. The discharge plan is the mechanism that facilitates a patient's progression through the intensive care unit to the next level of care and beyond.

In addition to the medical needs of the patient, there are several factors to consider.

Where patients are discharged to

Cardiothoracic patients have unique requirements and should be discharged to specialist clinical areas acquainted with the provision of postoperative care. Familiarity with intrathoracic drains, epicardial pacing wires and urinary and central venous access catheters is essential. Ward staff should also be trained to prevent and recognize common complications. These include, but are not limited to, arrhythmias, respiratory complications, pneumothorax, postoperative myocardial infarction, cardiac tamponade and deep venous thrombosis. Many hospitals have a dedicated cardiothoracic ward where the necessary skills and equipment are concentrated.

Another option is the 'step-down' or intermediate care unit where specialist care can be provided without consuming the resources of the critical care unit. Studies have shown such units reduce critical care length of stay without increasing hospital length of stay, do not impact negatively on patient outcomes and improve patient satisfaction by providing a quieter physical environment. The intermediate care unit may reduce hospital costs by decreasing staffing to levels appropriate for the continuing care of the patient and potentially frees the operating schedule from being critical care dependent. Less commonly, patients with special circumstances

Table 59.1 A definition of discharge planning
A process that coordinates all members of the health care team, utilizing their specific skills to achieve continuity of care through key transitions and optimal outcomes for the patient and health care service.

may be discharged to other facilities such as palliative, respiratory or long-term residential care units.

When patients experience noncardiothoracic complications, transfer to a general critical care unit or another hospital may be appropriate. In each case, early planning with clear and frequent communication between the respective care teams is essential to ensure continuity of care.

When patients are discharged

Timing of discharge from the critical care unit has been shown to significantly affect patient outcomes. Mortality may be increased when patients are discharged inappropriately early and rates of readmission are increased.

The practice of 'fast-track' management of cardiac patients and the pressure to further reduce critical care length of stay increases the potential for readmission if cases are not selected carefully. Emergency cases and limited resources may also necessitate triage and early discharge of patients.

The converse situation of an unnecessarily extended stay in the critical care unit is also undesirable. As well as being an inappropriate use of a limited and costly resource, patient well-being may be compromised owing to impaired sleep, emotional strain and restricted visitation policies.

Table 59.2 Goals of discharge planning
Achieve optimal outcome for patients.
Facilitate continuity of care.
Prevent complications and readmission.
Avoid inappropriate delay and 'bed-blocking.'
Maximize efficiency of resource utilization.

The time of day is also important with those being discharged at night having a higher mortality rate. This may reflect the lack of discharge planning, emergency pressure for critical care beds or the lack of appropriate resources on the ward at night. Where possible, discharge from the critical care unit should occur during the day when staffing levels are adequate and all necessary services available.

Who is involved in discharge planning

Medical staff including the surgeon and critical care specialist are necessarily involved in the decision-making process for planning an appropriate discharge, but it is frequently the nursing staff who assume the lead role in coordinating the team members. Some units will employ a dedicated discharge coordinator to facilitate communication between the health care providers.

Ancillary staff including physiotherapists, social workers, pharmacists and dieticians all have a crucial and ongoing role in patient care beyond the critical care unit and should be involved in any discharge planning.

The patient and their family must also be engaged in the discharge planning process. The experience of critical care is associated with physical and psychosocial effects, which may persist beyond discharge. The anxiety that patients experience may, in part, be related to unrealistic expectations for their care beyond the critical care unit. Frequent education and ongoing communication about progress can serve to prepare patients and their families for subsequent care and recovery, and has been shown to improve patient satisfaction levels.

How patients are discharged

A smooth transition from critical care unit to the next level of care clearly involves coordinating a large number of people. The high volume and repetitive nature of cardiac surgical cases mean clinical care pathways are particularly well suited, with predefined criteria marking patient progress. Such pathways also ensure staff in different clinical areas have similar goals for current and ongoing care. As a discharge tool, they serve to manage expectations and aid in preparing staff and patients for the transition to post critical care.

Practical issues must also be addressed and the receiving facility needs adequate notice so that preparations may be made. These include ensuring a bed space is free and that the necessary staff and equipment are available to continue to meet the patient's care needs. Additional requirements for the actual transfer may include porters or clinical assistants, essential equipment (e.g. monitoring, oxygen cylinders, emergency drugs) and a medical or nursing escort as appropriate.

There should be an adequate and succinct handover each time there is a transfer of responsibility for patient care. Medical and nursing staff should communicate directly with their colleagues about the patient history and subsequent progress from surgery to critical care unit, highlighting any problems encountered during the stay and any issues for ongoing care. Documentation should be provided to summarize this information.

The discharge summary

A clearly written discharge summary is an essential document that serves as both a record of treatment received while in the critical care and a plan for ongoing intervention. It improves communication and provides a reference point for clinicians and other staff.

A pro-forma may be used and the summary should include:

- patient demographics;
- details of surgical procedure including any prosthetic devices employed;
- past medical and surgical history;
- medications and allergies; and
- critical care summary, including duration of ventilation, details of mechanical or inotropic support and any complications.

The discharge summary should preferably be typed or dictated to avoid errors associated with illegible handwriting. The increasing implementation of computerized clinical information systems in critical care environments may mean that much of the necessary data can be generated automatically. This has the potential to reduce the time it takes to produce a summary and to increase the accuracy and detail of the information contained.

Discharge criteria

No single list of discharge criteria is applicable to all patients or institutions and each critical care unit needs to develop a discharge policy that reflects the available resources and staff skill levels of the receiving ward.

In general terms, the discharge criteria of the intensive care unit are similar to the admission criteria of the next level of care. Locally developed objective criteria, when used in conjunction with a critical care pathway, aid the process of identifying patients who are suitable for discharge from the critical care unit. Well-defined discharge criteria may result in decreased length of stay without compromising quality of care. Additional advantages include ensuring consistency of practice between different staff, improving communication with patients and managing their expectations, facilitating discharge planning and identifying areas that may require particular attention during subsequent care.

The multiple factors that must be considered and the complexity of postsurgical care demand the use of a systematic approach when devising a list of relevant discharge criteria.

These arbitrary divisions ensure key areas are addressed; however, when devising and applying individual criteria, the broader context of the patient's recovery must be borne in mind. Clinicians must ask themselves:

Table 59.3 Areas for assessment before discharge

Medical
Cardiovascular
Haemodynamically stable
Minimal or no inotropes
No mechanical circulatory support
Stable rhythm
Respiratory
Patient able to maintain and protect airway
Oxygen saturation >95% on Fio_2 ≤0.6
No requirement for mechanical ventilatory support
Metabolic and endocrine
Normalized acid–base status
Serum electrolytes in normal range
Blood glucose controlled
Genitourinary
Adequate urine output
Stable or improving renal function
Gastrointestinal
Evidence of return of bowel function
Adequate nutrition possible
Neurological
Stable or improving neurological status
Adequate pain control
Surgical
Pacing wires
No ongoing bleeding or air leak from drains
Surgical wound site clean
Adequate function of bypass grafts or prosthetic valves
Practical
Patient mobility and self-care adequate for destination
Medication appropriate for administration outside monitored environment
Discharge documentation and handover complete
Bed and transport available
Patient and family aware of discharge plan and new location within the hospital

- Is the patient recovering as expected?
- Is the discharge destination appropriate?
- Is discharge from the critical care safe for this patient?

Readmission to critical care after cardiac surgery

Patients who are readmitted have a median length of stay in the critical care unit of up to 7 days and a hospital stay that may be three times that of patients with an uncomplicated course. Mortality increases dramatically from 1% to 2% up to more than 30% in some series. Clearly, readmission has significant implications for utilization of critical care beds and for patient outcomes. The major cause of readmission is pulmonary complications, which account for up to 50% of cases. They include refractory hypoxia, hypercarbia and subjective respiratory distress. Most commonly the deterioration is non-specific, but important causes are pneumothorax, pleural effusions, atelectasis, aspiration and exacerbation of chronic obstructive pulmonary disease. Cardiovascular instability (including that due to dysrhythmias) and heart failure accounts for approximately 20% to 25% with a proportion being due to perioperative myocardial infarction and angina, tamponade and cardiac arrest. Those patients who return to the operating theatre for whatever reason may also be readmitted to the critical care unit. Additional reasons for readmission are renal dysfunction, sepsis and wound dehiscence, neurological events and gastrointestinal bleeding. Awareness of these causes enables complications to be identified early or potentially avoided.

Predicting those at risk of readmission

Attempts have been made to identify those factors that may predict patients at risk of readmission. The use of multivariate logistic regression models to look at preoperative, intraoperative and postoperative variables associated with subsequent readmission has demonstrated some important independent predictors, albeit inconsistently. It is prudent to remember that the presence of such factors does not universally imply causality, but they do serve to alert the clinician to those patients who are likely to have complex discharge needs.

Table 59.4 Causes of readmission to critical care

Pulmonary complications
Cardiovascular instability, including dysrhythmias
Return to the operating room
Renal dysfunction
Sepsis
Neurological events
Gastrointestinal bleeding/ulceration

Patients with complex discharge needs

Respiratory support beyond the critical care unit

The vast majority of patients require mechanical ventilatory support only as an interim measure until the cause of respiratory failure resolves. In the surgical setting, this is usually the residual effects of anaesthesia maintained until bleeding has settled and the patient is rewarmed. Uncommonly, patients have an ongoing requirement for mechanical support, whether invasive or noninvasive. Examples include loss of central respiratory drive owing to cerebrovascular accident, failure to wean after acute respiratory failure in severely unwell individuals and patients with chronic comorbid disorders such as chronic obstructive pulmonary disease or progressive neuromuscular diseases. Facilities for ongoing care range from specialized respiratory care units through to home-based care with available medical resources and costs generally being inversely related to patient independence and quality of life. To be suitable for discharge to an intermediate care facility for weaning, nonrespiratory organ dysfunction must be satisfactory and ventilator settings should be stable and oxygenation adequate. Of paramount importance is that the airway must be secure (either tracheostomy with sufficiently mature stoma to enable airway exchange or established noninvasive ventilation regimen with minimum risk of aspiration).

For discharge to a long-term care facility where quality of life and not weaning is the primary goal, there must be demonstrated medical and respiratory stability and additional psychological preparedness. Either circumstance requires specialist involvement.

Mechanical circulatory support beyond critical care

The prevalence of intractable heart failure and the delay to transplantation as an ultimate therapy have seen the increasing use of mechanical circulatory support devices. They may be used as a bridge to recovery, a bridge to transplantation or as a destination therapy.

The prospect that a patient with a total artificial heart or left ventricular assist device could leave the critical care setting would have been unthinkable only a few years ago, but ongoing technological advancement has led to smaller, more reliable systems such that discharge from the critical care unit may not only be acceptable but expected. This is particularly the case as devices may be intended for use over periods ranging from months to years.

After implantation, a significant period of postoperative stabilization in the critical care unit is expected. Initial discharge should be to an intermediate care unit or specialist care ward with expertise in device management and ready access to critical care facilities and the operating suite. To be suitable for discharge, there must be no evidence of bleeding, infection or thromboembolism. There must also be demonstrated cardiovascular and device stability with adequate noncardiac organ perfusion and function. For subsequent discharge to the home environment, there must be a period of patient and family training with a stepwise progression to relative independence.

Emergency discharge and triage

The relative shortage of critical care beds means that demand on occasion outstrips supply, and staff are forced to make difficult decisions about allocation of intensive care resources. This may be the case where emergency cases accumulate or in combined medical and cardiothoracic units when medical cases encroach on allocated surgical beds. Units may deal with fluctuations in demand by cancelling elective operations or by providing additional beds staffed by on-call teams. On occasion, patients may need to be discharged earlier than expected. Any decision about triaging patients for discharge must incorporate consideration of the health of those requiring admission. Senior staff should be involved in the decision making, which should be guided by an ethical and transparent framework. In practice, three groups of patients can usually be identified:

- discharge ready,
- potentially discharge ready, and
- not appropriate for discharge.

The difficulty arises in examining the group of patients that are potentially suitable. The clinician should bear in mind the common causes for readmission (i.e., pulmonary) and be aware of the resources of the next level of care. It may be possible to provide additional staff to the ward environment to facilitate care of a patient that would otherwise occupy a critical care bed.

Critical care outreach services

Improved continuity of care may be achieved with specially trained liaison staff conducting regular follow-up of all recently discharged patients. This may provide the greatest benefit to those patients with the complex needs as discussed (Chapter 60).

Key points

- Discharge planning improves patient outcomes and reduces readmission rates.
- A multidisciplinary approach is required to achieve continuity of care.
- Discharge criteria must reflect hospital resources and staff expertise.
- A written discharge summary is an essential document.

FURTHER READING

American College of Chest Physicians [homepage on the Internet]. Consensus statement on mechanical ventilation beyond the ICU. Available at: www.chestnet.org.

Goldhill DR. Preventing surgical deaths: critical care and intensive care outreach services in the postoperative period. *Br J Anaesth* 2005;95: 88–94.

Guidelines for intensive care unit admission, discharge, and triage. Task Force of the American College of Critical Care Medicine, Society of Critical Care Medicine. *Crit Care Med* 1999;27: 633–638.

Chapter 60

Outreach: Critical care without walls

P. HOLDER AND B.H. CUTHBERTSON

Introduction

The way in which we provide critical care is changing. However, resources are limited, and are likely to remain so. Outcomes are improving, and many clinicians feel that the care of sick patients outside of the critical care itself is an area that could be significantly improved. Therefore, critical care outreach has been developed, and is mainly managed by the medical and nursing staff on the critical care units.

Theory

Outreach involves exporting skills and knowledge from the critical care area into the general ward environment. The purpose is early recognition of signs and symptoms that may predict deterioration in the patient's condition and, by timely intervention, reversing the deterioration and therefore avoiding critical care admission, major morbidity or death. However, if admission to the critical care is required, early recognition allows timely transfer, which minimizes patient risk and optimizes outcome. This approach should theoretically also improve overall care on the general ward, allowing earlier safe discharge of critical care patients.

The team

The idea of critical care outreach has been suggested in many forms. The 'medical emergency team' (MET) concept was developed in Liverpool, New South Wales (Australia) in 1989. This concept involves ward staff contacting a team of senior medical and nursing staff from critical care areas when a set of physiological parameters are breached or whenever concern is expressed, so-called track-and-trigger systems. The composition of the outreach team should be multidisciplinary and it should be led by a qualified critical care practitioner who may or not be a doctor. Many models of outreach have been developed across hospitals and countries, and a unified definition does not exist.

The evidence

Of the many published studies on outreach, the MERIT study represents the best available evidence in the sphere of outreach, involving more patients than all other studies combined. In 23 participating centres, patients were randomised to receive treatment by MET or management entirely as previously. Education of staff was implemented before the start of the trial and reinforced during it. The MET consisted of at least one doctor and a nurse. The trial failed to demonstrate any significant reduction in the incidence of the study outcomes (cardiac arrest, unexpected death or unplanned critical care admission). The study, however, may not have been sufficiently powered to detect a difference and there was variability among the centres in the adequacy of response to changes in vital signs and in the completeness of documentation. The major impact of the trial was to emphasize the importance of staff education.

Table 60.1 Medical emergency team (MET) calling criteria

Airway
If threatened
Breathing
All respiratory arrests
Respiratory rate ≤5 breaths per minute
Respiratory rate >36 breaths per minute
Circulation
All cardiac arrests
Pulse rate ≤40 beats per minute
Pulse rate >140 beats per minute
Systolic blood pressure ≤90 mmHg
Neurology
Sudden fall in level of consciousness (fall in Glasgow Coma Scale of >2 points)
Repeated or extended seizures
Other
Any patient you are worried about that does not fit the above criteria

Although outreach is not yet proven to be beneficial, there is no doubt that the current care of sick patients on the wards is deficient in many areas. Adverse events are often preceded by a period of physiological instability. It has been shown that the recognition and documentation of these precedents is inadequate. There is also evidence that the response by caregivers to physiological deterioration may be deficient. There are various documented explanations for these failings:

- recording of physiological parameters may be insufficient in completeness and frequency;
- disempowered nursing staff may record continuing deterioration without directly intervening;
- junior medical staff may have had little formal training in the increasingly complex areas of resuscitation of the critically ill; and
- senior medical staff may not be always available in the hospital when patients deteriorate.

There is therefore a sound common sense argument for supplementing the provision of care on the ward for the sickest patients with input from experienced critical care teams.

What can outreach offer?

It is important that the deteriorating patient is recognized as early as possible. This requires the use of track-and-trigger systems of monitoring that help to identify the deteriorating patient. In general, the systems rely on the recording of physiological parameters at set intervals and provide criteria for recognition of deterioration and triggering a call to the outreach team. Such systems should be used in all clinical in-patient areas. Several systems are available and the choice of system may depend on local preference, but, regardless of the system chosen, there must be formal training of ward staff in monitoring and in the trigger criteria. Outreach teams themselves should participate in the implementation of the system and in the education of staff throughout the process.

The outreach team should ideally be available 24 hours a day and, once called, should aim to see all referrals within 30 minutes. The team should be adequately senior and experienced to fulfill the following duties.

The basic skills required by the outreach team are

- airway protection;
- appropriate use of oxygen therapy;
- fluid resuscitation; and
- recognition of the requirement for higher levels of care when necessary.

These skills are widely available in critical care areas. Therefore, it seems appropriate that critical care nurses form the core of the team, but a truly multidisciplinary approach should include input from senior physicians and physiotherapists. This obviously has important resource implications, especially in view of the failure to prove the benefits of outreach teams scientifically.

Table 60.2 Outreach team duties

Review all referrals promptly.
Advise on patient care.
Enable extra staff to be provided on ward if required.
Advise on admission to another unit.
Expedite admission to high-dependency unit/critical care unit if required.
Advise on referral to other specialist teams.
Education of ward staff, both nursing and medical.
Audit of referrals, admissions to critical care unit and incidence of cardiac arrest.

Liaison with ward staff

There is a risk that the provision of an outreach service may alienate ward staff. Nurses may feel threatened when instructed in how to provide care and medical teams may feel that they do not need advice in how to do their jobs. Therefore, one of the most important requirements of the outreach team is to involve other disciplines in the decision-making process and allow the team already looking after the patient to continue to do so, but with advice, assistance and reassurance. The ward nurses should be encouraged to call the team by offering support and training, giving their role more scope for development and providing additional resources when required.

Rotation of junior medical staff through the outreach team helps with integration and prevents resentment. Again, education and communication are paramount, with particular care needed to avoid alienating consultant staff in other disciplines. Where consultants have regular input into the critical care areas, such multidisciplinary team working will be easier to implement.

Key points

- Outreach is not yet proven but makes sense
- An outreach program has four aims:
  - to avert critical care unit admissions where possible by recognizing and reversing deterioration;
  - to ensure timely recognition and critical care unit admission for patients who truly need it;
  - to enable critical care unit discharges; and
  - to improve the standard of care on the wards by wider dissemination of some critical care skills.
- Critical care nurses are ideally suited for work within the multidisciplinary outreach team.
- Education of and liaison with ward staff is paramount in achieving the success of an outreach team.

FURTHER READING

Hillman K, Chen J, Cretikos, *et al*. Introduction of the medical emergency team (MET) system: a cluster randomised trial. *Lancet* 2005;365: 2091–2097.

Lee A, Bishop G, Hillman K, *et al*. The medical emergency team. *Anaesth Intensive Care* 1995;23: 183–186.

Chapter 61

Follow-up

J.A. GRIFFITHS AND S.J. BRETT

Introduction

Although mortality and survival are easy to understand and measure, survival alone is an incomplete endpoint for the recovery from critical illness or major surgery. Therefore, patient outcome from critical care treatment is not only described in terms of longer term survival ('mortality' outcomes), but also incorporates quality of life and neuropsychological and functional status ('nonmortality' outcomes). Assessment of these broader long-term outcome measures requires organized long-term follow-up that often extends to 12 months after hospital discharge. Critical care follow-up clinics have highlighted the variety of physical, psychological and psychosocial complaints experienced by patients as they recover from their critical care experience and treatment.

Patients requiring more than a 2- to 3-day critical care stay after cardiothoracic surgery tend to experience similar long-term outcomes to noncardiac patients. This chapter focuses on some of these long-term, patient-centred outcomes.

Mortality

In the United Kingdom, the mortality at critical care discharge exceeds 20%, and at hospital discharge, it exceeds 30%. Longer term survival rates are commonly represented by a Kaplan–Meier survival curve.

A very simplistic survival curve for a critical care population shows a very high initial mortality that gradually diminishes with time. The effects of critical illness and the underlying pathophysiological process on mortality are no longer present when the survival curve parallels that of a comparable patient cohort. The survival time corresponding to any proportion of the patient cohort is easily calculated, and survival curves of different cohorts can be compared.

Long-term survival analysis has demonstrated a significantly lower survival in patients with longer critical care stay (>3 days).

Nonmortality outcomes

A variety of instruments that assess functional status, neuropsychological impact and quality of life have been used to determine an individual patient's recovery from illness. Nearly all of the outcome measures that have been used in the setting of intensive care follow-up have been developed for use in other patient populations; few are critical care specific. Results must therefore be interpreted with caution.

Critical care outcome studies are often difficult to compare because they frequently include a different case mix of patients and employ a variety of outcome measures that are administered at different follow-up time points. However, extended follow-up of critical care survivors has provided a wealth of information on the common physical and psychological problems encountered during the recovery period. These are described herein.

Table 61.1 Physical and psychosocial limitations experienced after discharge from a critical care unit

Physical	Psychosocial
Neuropathies	Amnesia and memory difficulties
Neuromuscular weakness	Paranoia and delusions
Muscle wasting	Anxiety
Erectile dysfunction	Panic attacks
Difficulty swallowing	Depression
Joint stiffness	Guilt and anger
Sleep disturbances	Post-traumatic stress disorder
Breathlessness	Recurrent nightmares
Weight loss	Concentration difficulties
Pain	Reduced confidence
Fatigue	Family conflict
Appetite loss	Reduced libido
Changes in the ability to taste	Irritability
Hair loss	Financial difficulties

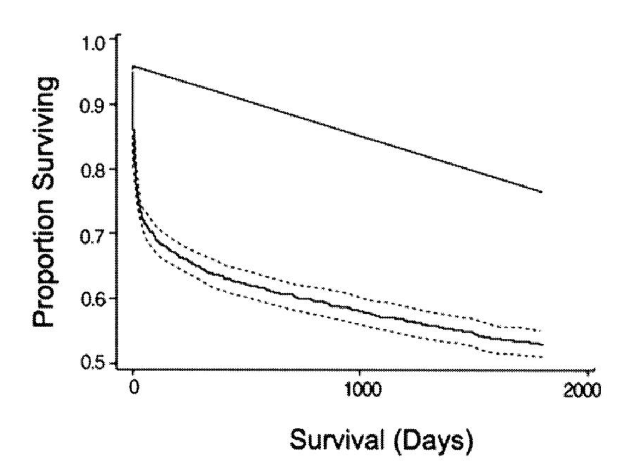

Figure 61.1 Kaplan–Meier survival curve model for critical care patients. The dashed lines represent the 95% confidence interval for the survival line. The straight line represents the survival of the same cohort of patients if they were subjected to the same age- and gender-adjusted mortality rates of the normal population. (From Wright *et al.*, *Anaesthesia* 2002;58:637–642.)

Physical impairment and disability

NUTRITION

The nutritional challenge of intensive care has been recognized for a long time. Prolonged critical care treatment is associated with a dramatic loss of muscle mass. Losses of 2% lean body mass per day have been reported, which can leave the patient with a formidable energy and protein deficit. Weakness, depression, breathlessness, altered taste perception and dysfunction of gut-derived appetite regulatory hormones further reduce a patient's appetite during recovery. In certain circumstances, recovery of weight lost during critical illness may not be complete at 12 months.

STRENGTH AND THE MUSCULOSKELETAL SYSTEM

Muscle wasting, joint stiffness (commonly due to heterotropic ossification), joint pain, weakness and reduced cough power are listed among the physical complaints reported after critical care treatment. Critical illness neuropathy is a well-recognized axonal neuropathy occurring in critical care patients. Numerous factors have been implicated including muscle relaxant drugs, steroids,

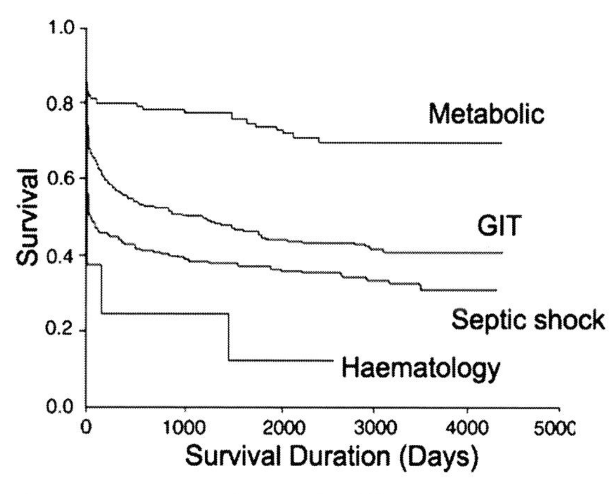

Figure 61.2 Survival curves for different patient groups. (From Wright *et al.*, *Anaesthesia* 2002;58:637–642.)

Table 61.2 Patient-centred outcomes after critical care

Mortality outcomes
Critical care discharge
Hospital discharge
Survival up to different time points (28 days, 3 or 6 months, 1 or 5 years)
Nonmortality outcomes
Physical impairment and disability
Physical functional status
Mental function
Neuropsychological function
Recovery
Health-related quality of life

sepsis, metabolic, glycaemic and nutritional disturbances. As yet, insufficient evidence is available to attribute cause, and little information is available regarding its prevention or treatment. Although recovery can be anticipated within a few months in milder cases, more severe forms can have devastating consequences. Poor recovery is correlated with longer length of stay in the critical care unit, longer duration of sepsis and greater weight loss.

BREATHLESSNESS

Breathlessness on exertion is a common symptom reported by critical care survivors. The possible causes include muscle weakness, neuropathy, pulmonary fibrosis, progression of premorbid respiratory and cardiac disease as well as psychological factors.

SEQUELAE OF TRACHEOSTOMY

Percutaneous techniques, coupled with changes in sedation practice and advances in ventilatory support, have resulted in an increasing number of patients receiving a tracheostomy earlier in their critical care stay. Lung function tests, nasoendoscopy and magnetic resonance imaging have been used to assess the long-term sequelae of tracheostomies; long-term follow-up studies suggest a favourable outcome. The most common complaints are minor cosmetic problems, such as scar tethering, which is easily dealt with in outpatients under local anaesthetic. The incidence of significant complications such as tracheal stenosis remains extremely low.

SEXUAL DYSFUNCTION

Sexual dysfunction is caused by a variety of conditions, with even more differences between men and women. In males, sexual dysfunction normally refers to erectile dysfunction and a large proportion of patients with cardiovascular disorders suffer from erectile dysfunction. Premature ejaculation, anorgasmy and reduced desire are also common. In women, sexual dysfunction often represents lack of vaginal lubrication, anorgasmy and painful intercourse or reduced arousal caused by lack of libido. Cardiac patients are both at particular risk for sexual dysfunction, and are potentially a difficult group to treat for the following reasons:

- Fear, especially after a cardiac event such as a myocardial infarction, or symptoms of chest pain or after a procedure such as a cardiac catheterization or bypass surgery.
- Concomitant medication such as β-blockers.
- Risk factors associated with the development of erectile dysfunction are those associated with atherosclerosis (e.g. diabetes, smoking, hypertension, hypercholesterolaemia).
- Performance capability: most patients with preserved left ventricular function after myocardial infarction can resume sexual activity. However, even after successful balloon angioplasty or bypass surgery, one third of men believe that they should not be sexually active to prevent further damage to their heart.
- Medication interaction: the absolute contraindication for all phosphodiesterase

Table 61.3 Psychological disturbances that may occur in critical care unit patients after hospital discharge

Grief reactions
Social isolation
Anxiety
Depression
Irritability
Memory disturbances
Agoraphobia
Panic and confusion
Anger and conflict
Fear of dying
Guilt
Post-traumatic stress disorder
Sexual dysfunction and dissatisfaction

type-5 inhibitors used to treat erectile dysfunction (e.g. Viagra, Levitra, Cialis) is the concurrent use of nitric oxide-donating agents such as nitrates.

Although most cases of sexual dysfunction can be treated with pharmacological or psychological interventions, medical practitioners rarely seek the presence of sexual dysfunction or offer referral or treatment. If sexual dysfunction goes unrecognized, it can have a considerable effect on a patient's quality of life and can lead to relationship difficulties and even marital breakdown.

Mental function

Many critical care patients experience psychological problems for months and even years after their critical care treatment.

Many factors potentially influence the future mental health outcomes of critical care survivors, including the presence of preexisting psychological, psychiatric or personality disorders, critical care sedation policy, sleep disturbance, delirium and memory.

DELIRIUM AND ITS CONSEQUENCES

The true incidence of delirium in the critical care unit is unknown. Various terms have been used in the literature to describe this condition, including 'intensive care syndrome' and 'ICU psychosis.' Estimates reported in the literature suggest that the incidence of delirium within surgical critical care patients is 40%; the incidence may be as high as 60% in older patients. Delirium may be obvious in some patients and easy to diagnose, but withdrawn or hypoactive delirium is likely to evade diagnosis while having the same impact. Importantly, the recent validation of the Confusion Assessment Method for the Intensive Care Unit tool has aided the bedside assessment of delirium in critical care patients and should prove a valuable research tool in future long-term studies.

Delirium is often accompanied by profound amnesia of events occurring during and preceding the confusional state. The amnesia results in fragmented and frequently distorted memories – commonly termed 'delusional memory.' The state between sleep and wakefulness predisposes to hallucinations and creates a mental environment favouring the development of paranoid delusions. Nightmares, dreams and hallucinations have all been described during recovery, and can be the source of considerable long-term psychological distress.

ANXIETY AND DEPRESSION

Studies of survivors of general critical care treatment have estimated the prevalence of clinically significant anxiety and depression to range from 30% to

50% in the short term to 20% to 30% in the long term. Patients are more likely to suffer from anxiety and depression if they cannot recall any factual memory for their critical care experience, but retain a delusional, fragmented memory. The rate of clinical depression in long-term survivors of acute lung injury has been estimated at 67%, and seems to correlate with the number of days pharmacologically sedated.

Neuropsychological function

COGNITIVE DYSFUNCTION

Impairment of cognitive dysfunction is an important outcome from critical care treatment and is common in survivors of cardiac surgery. This cognitive dysfunction is of a similar level to that associated with mild dementia.

In many studies, the greatest indices of cognitive deficit are observed for immediate memory and attention. Another important aspect of cognitive performance is executive function, which is an umbrella term for a range of abilities that enables us to assimilate information, analyse that information, follow rules and make decisions. In neurological patients, it is well established that executive dysfunction presents a major obstacle to the return to premorbid levels of socioeconomic functioning. Indeed, adverse neurological outcome has important financial, social and care implications for patients, their families and society.

Functional status

Functional status is a measure of a person's physical and mental capability, and describes the ability to perform tasks in daily life. It is objectively assessed and two of the most commonly used and relevant generic measures for physical function are the Karnosky Index and Katz's Activities of Daily Living. Unsurprisingly, elderly patients discharged from general critical care exhibit decreased activities of daily living, which may reach premorbid levels approximately 6 to 12 months after discharge. Higher survival rates have been reported in those patients with higher pre-critical care admission Karnofsky Index scores.

Quality of life and heath-related quality of life

The term 'quality of life' is not a precise concept. Quality of life is a subjective, multidimensional concept comprising five major domains:

- physical status and functional abilities;
- psychological status and well-being;
- social interactions;
- economic and/or vocational status and factors; and
- religious and/or spiritual status.

Because this conceptualization of quality of life is broad, health care researchers commonly restrict their focus to the dimensions associated with illness and treatment, using the term 'health-related quality of life' (HRQOL).

The identified attributes of HRQOL are clustered in domains of physical, psychological and social function. The physical domain contains physical complaints, and the capability to perform activities. Complaints can be symptoms (pain, nausea), whereas activities concern a wide range of aspects like mobility and eating. Cognitive functioning (memory, orientation) and emotion (anxiety, depression) are elements of the psychological domain. The extent and quality of social contacts and activities (work, hobbies) are aspects of social function.

HEALTH-RELATED QUALITY-OF-LIFE SCORES BEFORE CRITICAL CARE

Several studies have retrospectively estimated HRQOL scores before admission to critical care by interviewing patients or relatives either during critical care stay or at some stage after discharge. Surgical critical care patients have been demonstrated

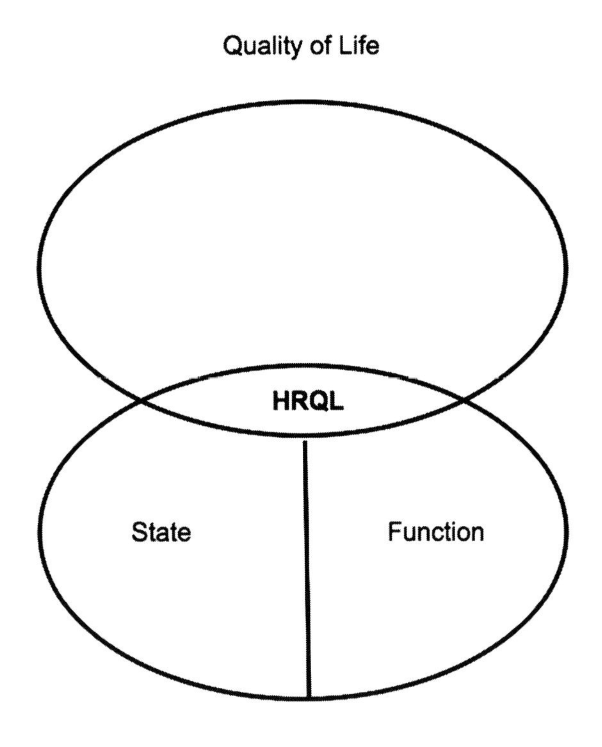

Figure 61.3 Health-related quality-of-life. The *upper ellipse* represents all aspects that are of value to patients and their quality of life. The *lower ellipse* represents health status measurements, and is divided in to *state* (e.g. cardiac ejection fraction) and *function* (e.g. treadmill exercise tolerance test). The intersection *HRQL* represents the aspects of health status that patients value and are also part of their quality of life. Hence, HRQOL is partly subjective, and not necessarily generalizable (Adapted from Heyland *et al.*)

to display a reduced pre-critical care HRQOL when compared with population averages, and there is a significant correlation between burden of premorbid disease and HRQOL.

HEALTH-RELATED QUALITY-OF-LIFE SCORES AFTER CRITICAL CARE STAY

The 6-month HRQOL of survivors of general critical care treatment has been shown to be predominantly a function of admission diagnosis. Overall HRQOL are moderate, albeit lower than population averages. Studies have shown that up to two thirds of critical care survivors have more health problems, are more anxiously depressed, are more dependent on others and engage in less sexual activity than a random community sample. In an ever-aging population, it is interesting to note that the long-term HRQOL of elderly survivors of critical care treatment is little influenced by age. A comparison of patients aged 65 to 74 years and those 75 years or older demonstrated no significant differences in HRQOL scores.

CHANGES IN HEALTH-RELATED QUALITY-OF-LIFE SCORES

Several studies have estimated pre-critical care HRQOL scores and compared these with scores measured after critical care discharge. On the whole, HRQOL decreases for patients who experience emergency admissions to critical care or suffer acute pathologies. Patients who enjoy a normal quality of life before critical care admission suffer significant decreases after their illness. Those with preexisting morbidity show some improvement in their quality of life 6 months after critical care admission, principally by improvements in mental health, vitality and social functioning.

Social and family consequences

Family members often exhibit significant degrees of anxiety and depression while their relative is being treated on the critical care ward. Survivors may experience guilt as they become aware of the strain placed on their family, which adds to the overall psychological burden. A 'ripple' effect is often seen, where the processes affecting an individual patient spread to involve the people in immediate contact with that patient, commonly their family and close friends. It is therefore imperative that multidisciplinary critical care follow-up also addresses

Table 61.4 Commonly applied generic measures of physical and psychological outcomes

Hospital Anxiety and Depression Scale (HADS)

The HADS is a questionnaire composed of statements relevant to either generalized anxiety or depression. The HADS has been validated in a variety of settings and centres to provide a reliable and simple tool for the measurement of mental function.

Short-Form Health Survey – 36 items (SF-36)

The SF-36 is a generic, self-administered general health status survey with 36 questions aggregated into 8 domains/dimensions: General Health, Physical Functioning, Role Physical, Role Emotional, Social Functioning, Bodily Pain, Vitality and Mental Health. Each is scored from 0 (worst score) to 100 (best score). The SF-36 has been found to be reliable, stable over time and valid in the critical care setting.

EuroQol five-dimension (EQ-5D)

The EQ-5D questionnaire is a simple, standardized generic instrument designed to measure health outcome. The EQ-5D comprises two parts: the EQ-5D self-classifier, a self-reported description of health problems according to a 5-dimensional classification – mobility, self-care, usual activities, pain/discomfort and anxiety/depression; and the EQ VAS, a self-rated health status using a visual analogue scale (VAS) to record perceptions of the patient's own current overall health. The EQ-5D has been specifically designed to complement other quality-of-life measures such as the SF-36.

Karnofsky Performance Status (KPS) and Karnofsky Index

KPS is a simple, objective measure of physical functional status. The Karnofsky index ranges in units of 10 from 0 (death) to 100, where 100 = no limitations, >80 indicates the ability to carry on normal activities independently, and ≤80 suggests disability in physical performance. KPS has been validated and recommended as a reliable measure of physical performance in HRQOL.

the needs of the family members during the recovery period.

Extended critical care follow-up

The burden that prolonged critical care treatment imposes on a patient's physical and psychological well-being as they try to recover from their critical care experience has been termed 'dishabilitation.' Extended critical care follow-up aims to ameliorate this burden by improving and speeding up the quality of recovery.

Although conclusive interventional studies demonstrating the benefits of extended critical care follow-up are currently lacking, patients and their relatives consistently report high levels of satisfaction with the service. A pioneering group have demonstrated an improved psychological outcome in survivors of critical care treatment through the use of a self-directed, critical care rehabilitation manual. It is an exciting prospect that the critical care follow-up research agenda remains in its infancy.

Table 61.5 Objectives of extended critical care follow-up

Explanation of critical illness

Opportunity for discussion and questions
Opportunity for audit and information gathering to aid service improvement
Identification of critical illness specific morbidity
Surveillance of physical and psychological morbidities identified
Research

Key points

- Extended follow-up of survivors of critical illness is increasingly recognized as an important goal for critical care practitioners.
- Extended follow-up of survivors of critical illness has demonstrated that many patients suffer from physical and psychological morbidities that ultimately affect their HRQOL.
- The burden of critical illness often extends to involve the relatives.
- Identifying the common and important problems experienced by survivors of critical illness enables patient directed tailored rehabilitative programs to be formulated to speed up and improve the quality of recovery.

FURTHER READING

Broomhead LR, Brett SJ. Intensive care follow-up – what has it told us? *Crit Care* 2002;6:411–417.

Cheung AM, Tansey CM, Tomlinson G, *et al.* Two-year outcomes, health care use, and costs of survivors of acute respiratory distress syndrome. *Am J Respir Crit Care Med* 2006;174:538–544

Cuthbertson BH, Hull A, Strachan M, *et al.* Post-traumatic stress disorder after critical illness requiring general intensive care. *Intensive Care Med* 2004;30:450–455.

Herridge MS, Cheung AM, Tansey CM, *et al.* One-year outcomes in survivors of the acute respiratory distress syndrome. *N Engl J Med* 2003;348:683–693.

SECTION 6 Structure and Organization in Cardiothoracic Critical Care

Chapter 62

Cardiothoracic critical care nursing

A.M. INGLE, M. SCREATON
AND J. OSGATHORP

Introduction

Nursing the critically ill cardiothoracic patient requires advanced skills in assessment as well as in-depth knowledge of nursing practice, cardiovascular physiology, technology and pharmacology used in critical care. The nurse's role is essential to helping patients and their families cope with life-threatening illness and its treatment.

The cardiothoracic critical care unit has evolved alongside rapid advances in diagnostic modalities and therapeutic intervention in the fields of clinical cardiology and cardiac surgery. These changes have led to a progressive and aggressive specialist field in which very sick patients receive often complex care that is usually delivered and managed by the nurse at the bedside.

The workforce

The most notable difference between critical care and a general ward is that the former has a much higher nurse-to-patient ratio, which reflects the dependency of patients in this setting. Historically, this ratio has been one to one, but tight adherence to this principle is being challenged. The pivotal role in delivering critical care is that of the bedside registered nurse. In this, the bedside nurse is supported by health care support workers, supervised by a senior nurse and guided by an education team.

The bedside critical care nurse

In addition to basic education, such nurses have been specifically trained in critical care and most have completed a specialized critical care course. The primary role of the nurse is to provide continuous nursing vigilance of vital signs, assess change, adjust medication as appropriate and communicate with the nurse in charge and the rest of the multidisciplinary team when necessary. Part of the responsibility for the safety of the patient includes ensuring emergency equipment is present and working, alarm limits are set on monitors and transducers are calibrated. Of course, all this is in addition to delivering basic nursing care, including communication with the patient and the family. This can be challenging in the frenetic environment of high-tech equipment, powerful drugs and multiple timed tasks.

The degree of autonomy varies. In some units, experienced bedside nurses work to guidelines and protocols when caring for patients after surgery. They manage weaning from ventilation, tracheal extubation, fluid balance and haemodynamic interventions. In other units, this role is restricted to more advanced critical care practitioners. Although the primary focus is the allocated patient, the critical care bedside nurse must be able to respond quickly to the changing needs of the unit, such as assisting with unexpected events, facilitating quick turnover of patients and change in allocation when necessary.

The health care support worker

Health care support workers are a valuable and essential part of the workforce in critical care. Although they are not registered nurses, they support the registered nurse in delivering patient care. This is usually by performing specific delegated tasks for which they have received appropriate, competency-based training.

The range of such tasks depends on training and the requirements of the service in a particular unit. It ranges from housekeeping tasks (ordering supplies, and cleaning and tidying the clinical area) to assisting in direct patient care, such as positioning, personal hygiene and nutritional needs.

The senior nurse

Depending on the size of the unit, there may be one or more senior critical care nurses leading the nursing team. An essential part of their role is to have an overview of the patients being cared for by their team. They participate in multidisciplinary ward rounds and deploy the team so as to ensure the most appropriate, safe and effective use of the available skills. During handover, the senior nurse allocates nurses to patients for the forthcoming shift and ensures the comprehensive transfer of clinical information. After handover, the senior nurse remains visible and available to patients, relatives and staff and continues to provide support and guidance to the team, especially during moments of crisis. In addition to all this, the senior nurse is pivotal in the coordination of admission, transfer and discharge of patients. This requires regular review of the bed state and liaison with other departments and hospitals.

The nurse manager

Critical care units vary in staffing structure, but are traditionally headed by a clinical manager who carries responsibility for service delivery, budgetary management, recruitment, retention, appraisal and individual performance review as well as handling complaints. Alongside this is the responsibility for leadership and development of the nursing service to ensure the highest standards of clinical care. This is achieved through supporting, developing and implementing policies, strong commitment to education and training, and supporting research and audit projects. Prevention of hospital-acquired infection is a priority for the nurse manager who is able to raise issues of concern at unit and hospital levels.

The educator

Critical care is a rapidly evolving specialty. New technology is frequently introduced and maintaining and updating skills is always a challenge. For this reason, many units have dedicated in-house education teams who provide comprehensive training programs for existing staff as well as new recruits. Educational development has a high profile in cardiothoracic critical care from induction to the most senior level, and educators play a crucial role in the development, implementation and review of the guidelines and protocols for the unit.

Advanced nursing roles

The two main drivers for developing these roles are to deliver patient care more responsively and to improve recruitment and retention of trained staff by enhancing the practice of nursing itself. Role development at the medical–nursing interface has resulted in the advancement of nursing roles throughout health care. The roles encompass many job titles, such as clinical nurse specialists, nurse practitioners, advanced nurse practitioners, critical care practitioners and nurse consultants. Whatever the title, the net result is that the responsibilities and duties of the more senior nurses have increased dramatically. In cardiothoracic critical care, such advanced nurses practice within specific guidelines and make decisions autonomously. For example, in the care of the postoperative cardiac surgical patient, the advanced nurse manages ventilation, cardiovascular problems, haemostasis, fluid and electrolyte balance, chest drains and drug prescription within defined guidelines.

Key points

- The cardiothoracic critical care nurse is an integral part of the multidisciplinary team.
- Nursing is provided by a range of staff all of whom require specialist education and skills.
- Strong leadership of a motivated and well-organized team is essential.
- Advanced roles allow nurses to practice more independently and to deliver patient care more responsively.

FURTHER READING

Adam SK, Osborne S. *Critical care nursing: Science and practice*. Oxford: Oxford University Press; 2005.

Cutler L, Robson W. *Critical Care Outreach*. London: John Wiley & Sons Ltd; 2006.

Department of Health [homepage on the Internet]. Comprehensive critical care: A review of adult critical care services. London: Department of Health. Available at: www.dh.gov.uk.

Chapter 63

Physiotherapy

A. BRICE, D. DYKES AND A. HARVEY

Introduction

The aims of respiratory physiotherapy include mobilization and aid in expectoration of bronchopulmonary secretions, improving the efficiency of ventilation and maintaining or improving exercise tolerance. Physiotherapy has a key role to play in the prevention and treatment of respiratory complications after cardiac surgery.

This chapter starts by detailing the possible effects of cardiac surgery and general anaesthesia on the respiratory system. It then discusses the physiological basis and current evidence for the most commonly used physiotherapy techniques in the cardiac critical care unit. The management of both the spontaneously ventilating and intubated patient is considered.

Respiratory complications after cardiac surgery

It is well recognized that left lower lobe collapse occurs in the majority of patients after cardiac surgery. Reasons for this include:

- perioperative compression of the lobe;
- occasional injury to the phrenic nerve; and
- postoperative pain.

Other contributory factors leading to postoperative atelectasis include:

- the effects of the median sternotomy/thoracotomy incision;
- internal mammary artery dissection;
- the use of cardiopulmonary bypass; and
- prolonged recumbency.

A certain amount of micro-atelectasis after surgery is inevitable, partly due to a reduction in functional residual capacity (FRC) secondary to general anaesthesia. If FRC falls below closing volume, then atelectasis occurs in the dependent lung. The efficiency of the mucociliary escalator (composed of mucus-secreting goblet cells, cilia and a viscous mucus gel layer) is also reduced. Cilia move the mucus layer towards the larynx where it is either swallowed or expectorated. This process is affected by a variety of factors, including breathing dry gases. Respiratory muscle strength and vital capacity can be reduced after cardiac surgery and this adversely affects cough efficiency, leading to sputum retention and further atelectasis.

Physiotherapy techniques in the spontaneously breathing patient

Therapeutic body positioning

Body positioning is used to:

- improve ventilation/perfusion (V/Q) matching;
- increase lung volumes;
- aid airway clearance (postural drainage); and
- decrease the work of breathing.

V/Q MATCHING

The position most appropriate for V/Q matching should be selected to optimize oxygenation. For example, a patient with unilateral lung disease

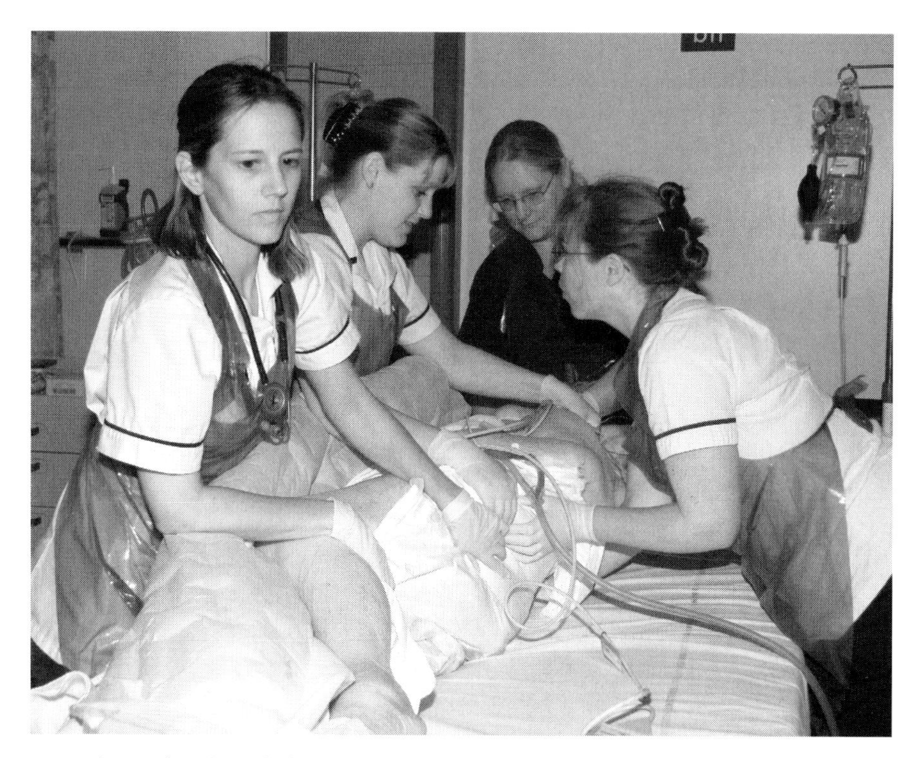

Figure 63.1 Patient being placed in side lying position.

should be positioned in side lying with the affected lung uppermost as V/Q is optimal in the dependent (unaffected) lung. However, regular repositioning should be encouraged because intercellular fluids, lymphatic fluids and secretions migrate, and may adversely affect the dependent lung.

OPTIMIZING LUNG VOLUMES

One method of optimizing lung volumes is to transfer the patient out of bed at the earliest opportunity: FRC is greater when sitting in a chair or side lying compared with slumped sitting in bed. Some patients, such as those with an intra-aortic balloon pump, cannot sit but can be positioned in side lying to optimize gas exchange.

Side lying and deep breathing exercises may help to recruit areas of collapse in the uppermost lung. This is because the weight of the mediastinum and lung results in an expanding force that pulls on the elastic tissue, encouraging collapsed alveoli to inflate.

POSTURAL DRAINAGE

Postural drainage is the use of gravity to aid the drainage of secretions from peripheral lung units to more proximal airways. A number of positions, which may include a head-down tilt, can be used to drain specific bronchopulmonary segments. For patients with vascular instability, these positions may need to be modified.

WORK OF BREATHING

Positioning can be used to reduce the work of breathing in the breathless patient:

- Forward lean sitting: leaning forward increases the curvature of the anterior portion of the diaphragm owing to increased pressure from the abdominal contents. This improves the length–tension status of the diaphragm to facilitate its contraction.
- High side lying: side lying with the head elevated may also increase the curvature of the dependent hemidiaphragm.

Techniques such as breathing control and intermittent positive pressure breathing can be used in these positions.

Airway clearance

A number of airway clearance techniques exist, some of which may involve the use of devices such as the Flutter, the Acapella and positive expiratory pressure. Much of the research in airway clearance techniques has been done in respiratory patients with chronic sputum production. There is only limited evidence in the cardiac surgery population. However, these techniques may be indicated for patients with preexisting hypersecretory lung diseases and for patients who develop a productive chest infection. Adequate analgesia before intervention is critical. Airway clearance techniques cannot be effective if pain prevents the patient from taking the deep breath necessary to generate an effective cough. In addition, the patient should be taught to support their wound while coughing because this may help to reduce pain, and also increases confidence. A comprehensive assessment to identify the exact cause of the patient's inability to clear excess secretions is required. The most appropriate airway clearance techniques should be selected, taking into account patient compliance and available resources.

ACTIVE CYCLE OF BREATHING TECHNIQUES

This consists of a cycle of different breathing techniques that include thoracic expansion exercises, breathing control and the forced expiration technique.

Thoracic expansion exercises aim to increase lung volume by increasing airflow through collateral channels of ventilation. This enables air to move behind secretions to mobilize them to the more proximal airways. An end-inspiratory hold may be performed to further encourage collateral flow. If appropriate, manual techniques can be carried out simultaneously.

Breathing control involves tidal volume breathing, encouraging relaxation of the upper chest and shoulders. This is done to prevent hyperventilation, bronchospasm and fatigue.

The forced expiration technique involves a combination of up to two forced expirations (called huffs) followed by periods of breathing control. The patient is encouraged to adapt the huffs according to the location of secretions. Huffing to low lung volumes encourages movement of distal secretions, whereas huffing from higher lung volumes encourages movement of more proximal secretions.

INTERMITTENT POSITIVE PRESSURE BREATHING

Using a pressure-cycled device, the patient triggers a breath in (via a mouthpiece or facemask), and is given positive airway pressure throughout inspiration, returning to atmospheric pressure on expiration. Physiological effects of intermittent positive pressure breathing include:

- increased tidal volume;
- increased minute ventilation;
- improved gaseous exchange; and
- reduced work of breathing.

By increasing lung volumes, intermittent positive pressure breathing also enhances cough effectiveness and aids secretion clearance. The mechanical effects are short lived (lasting less than 1 hour) and so continuous positive airway pressure (CPAP) may be used in between sessions to maintain alveolar recruitment. As with noninvasive ventilation, intermittent positive pressure breathing can reduce the work of breathing, but only if the patient is relaxed and the settings are appropriate to optimize synchronization.

NASOPHARYNGEAL SUCTION

If other techniques have failed to clear secretions, nasopharyngeal suctioning may be indicated. This technique is traumatic and should only be used if retained secretions are compromising gaseous exchange or increasing the work of breathing. A nasopharyngeal airway may be

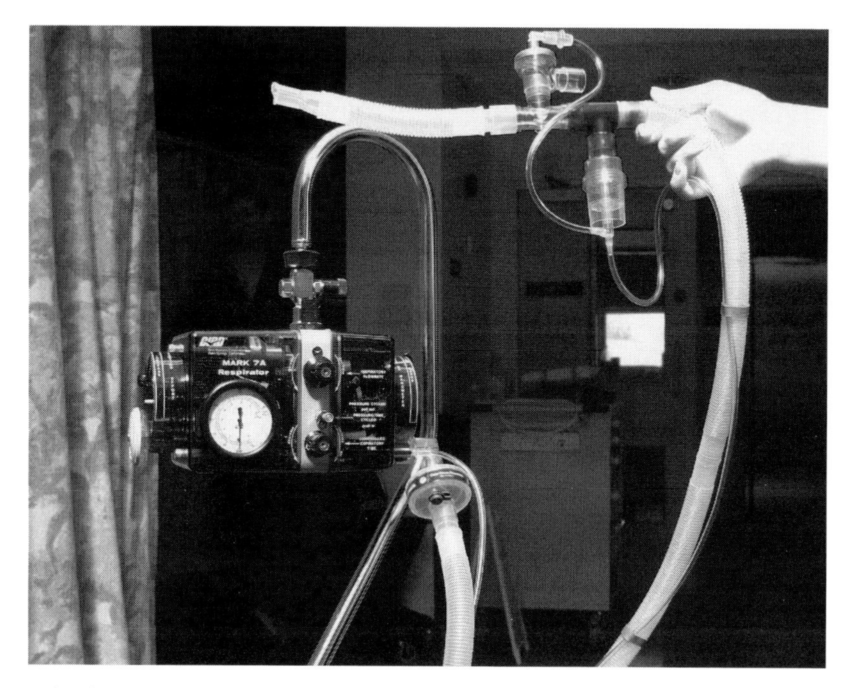

Figure 63.2 Example of intermittent positive pressure breathing machine – Bird ventilator.

inserted and left in situ to aid the passage of a suction catheter. A mini-tracheostomy can be considered if repeated nasopharyngeal suction is required, but this requires careful consideration because it carries some risk.

Techniques to increase lung volume

Historically, deep breathing exercises, supported coughing and early mobilization have been routinely performed after cardiac surgery to prevent postoperative pulmonary complications. However, research has shown that the removal of deep breathing exercises does not affect patient outcome. Early mobilization and teaching a supported huff/cough are now the key components of the physiotherapy management plan in routine cardiac surgery patients.

DEEP BREATHING EXERCISES

Deep breathing exercises should be reserved for patients who are too unwell to sit up in a chair or mobilize, or who have developed a pulmonary complication, and should be carried out in a position that also enhances lung volumes – side lying, sitting or standing.

EARLY MOBILIZATION

All patients should be comprehensively assessed before mobilizing, and closely monitored throughout. Haemodynamic instability is a contraindication to early mobilization. The routine postoperative cardiac patient should be sat out of bed on the first postoperative day. Some patients may also be able to tolerate marching on the spot on this day, and this should particularly be encouraged in those with significant atelectasis and/or retained secretions.

The aim of mobilization is to increase minute ventilation and in particular tidal volume. Therefore, the patient should be instructed to ambulate at a pace that induces a comfortable level of shortness of breath. If this pace cannot be achieved, then deep breathing exercises should be performed while mobilizing.

INCENTIVE SPIROMETRY

An incentive spirometer is a mechanical device that aims to reduce postoperative respiratory complications by increasing lung volumes: the patient takes a slow deep breath in and receives visual feedback. There is, however, no proven benefit when compared with early mobilization or deep breathing exercises in the improvement of lung volumes or in the prevention of postoperative complications.

CONTINUOUS POSITIVE AIRWAY PRESSURE

Continuous positive airway pressure maintains positive pressure within the lungs throughout inspiration and expiration. It increases FRC, leading to a reduction in shunt, improved arterial saturation and lung compliance and a decrease in the work of breathing. It is useful in patients with postoperative atelectasis who require high concentrations of inspired oxygen. The optimal treatment regime for CPAP after cardiac surgery has not been established. Although intermittent CPAP is not ideal, this is sometimes the only solution in a poorly compliant patient. The compliant patient should be encouraged to march on the spot with the CPAP to maximize alveolar recruitment.

Physiotherapy techniques in mechanically ventilated patients

Positioning

The aims of positioning the intubated patient are to:

- optimize oxygen transport by improving V/Q matching;
- increase lung volumes;
- reduce the work of breathing; and
- assist with secretion clearance.

Mechanical ventilation often causes V/Q mismatching with preferential ventilation of the non-dependent lung regions; perfusion is greater in the dependent regions. When weaning from mechanical ventilation, upright sitting is encouraged to improve lung volume and reduce the work of breathing. Despite a sound physiological rationale for the use of positioning in the critically ill patient, there is limited evidence to support its effectiveness.

With unilateral lung disease, the patient should be positioned in side lying with the affected lung uppermost. Secretion clearance may also be assisted due to gravity-assisted drainage. In addition, oxygenation may improve as the unaffected lung will be well perfused. Prone positioning may be used to improve V/Q matching, redistribute oedema and increase FRC in those patients who develop acute respiratory distress syndrome after cardiac surgery. Short-term improvements in oxygenation have been reported. Special care must be taken of the endotracheal tube when proning the patient, and this should only be performed by appropriately trained staff.

Suction

Suctioning is performed to maintain endotracheal tube patency, as well as to clear excess secretions. Secretion accumulation may be indicated by increased peak airway pressures or reduced tidal volumes on the ventilator.

The suction catheter should be no more than half the diameter of the endotracheal tube, and adequate preoxygenation should be ensured to prevent hypoxaemia. Great care should be taken in anticoagulated patients; occult bleeding may be more common.

Manual hyperinflation

Manual hyperinflation is the technique of manually inflating a patient's lungs to a tidal volume 50% greater than that delivered by the ventilator while keeping the airway pressure between 20 and 40 cmH_2O. The technique, commonly known as 'bagging' or 'bag squeezing,' involves using a 2-L rebreathing circuit connected to a flow of 10 to 15 L of oxygen. Manual hyperinflation is performed with a slow deep inspiration to encourage the inflation of slower filling alveoli. The increase in tidal volume increases lung recruitment and enhances

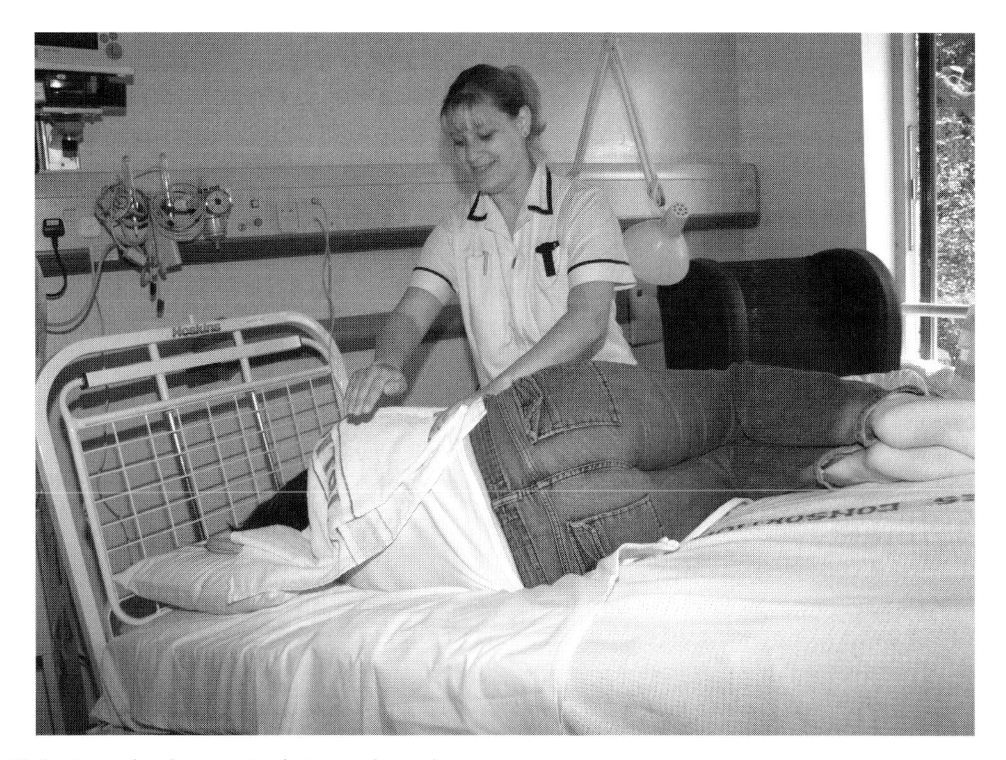

Figure 63.3 Example of percussion being performed.

interdependence (the effect of the expanding forces exerted between adjacent alveoli) because it is greater at high lung volumes. A 3-second end-inspiratory pause should be utilized to further encourage collateral flow, followed by a 'quick expiratory release' to maximize expiratory flow rate and facilitate movement of sputum towards the central airways. Manual hyperinflation has been shown to:

- increase lung compliance;
- improve gas exchange;
- aid the resolution of acute lobar atelectasis; and
- aid airway clearance.

To optimize treatment, manual hyperinflation should be performed in side lying with the affected lung uppermost. In addition, it should always be performed with a manometer and volumeter in the circuit to avoid barotrauma and/or volutrauma. Alternatively, ventilator hyperinflation may be employed by increasing the tidal volume on the ventilator and using the inspiratory hold button.

Manual techniques

There is little evidence to support the use of manual techniques such as percussion (chest clapping) or vibrations (shaking of the chest on expiration), but they might at times be clinically useful when all other techniques have proved ineffective.

Rehabilitation

Many long-term critical care patients go on to develop muscle weakness as a result of disuse atrophy, exacerbated by poor nutritional status before admission, increased catabolic states (infection) and use of steroids or muscle relaxants. Orthostatic intolerance also develops and appears to be the result of the loss of gravitational stimulation rather than the lack of exercise. The aims of rehabilitation are therefore to:

- increase functional independence;
- minimize adverse effects such as muscle atrophy and joint stiffness;

- improve psychological well-being;
- aid weaning from mechanical ventilation; and
- decrease the length of stay on critical care.

For patients who are fully sedated, rehabilitation is limited to the assessment of the passive range of movement of peripheral joints. If muscle shortening is evident, then the appropriate muscle will either be positioned so it is on a prolonged stretch, or splinting may be used. Once patients are awake, the physiotherapist teaches active upper and lower limb exercises to increase muscle strength. In addition, the physiotherapist starts to sit the patient over the edge of the bed. If tolerated, the patient may then be considered to be suitable to sit out in a chair. If the patient has profound muscle weakness, this is achieved with the aid of a hoist.

There are a number of adjuncts to assist with the rehabilitation process:

- A tilt table allows the patient to be subjected to a gravitational stress, but it is largely a passive process because the patient is strapped onto the table.
- A standing hoist or standing frame allows the patient to be erect but requires some lower limb strength.

Any rehabilitation program should be planned in conjunction with the whole multidisciplinary team to optimize outcomes.

Key points

- Physiotherapists need to formulate an appropriate treatment plan, in collaboration with the multidisciplinary team.
- Positioning can be used to increase lung volumes, improve V/Q matching, optimize airway clearance and decrease work of breathing.
- Early mobilization is essential.

FURTHER READING

Pryor JA, Prasad NH. *Physiotherapy for respiratory and cardiac problems: Adults and paediatrics.* London: Churchill Livingstone; 2002.

Sorenson HM, Shelledy DC; AARC. AARC clinical practice guideline. Intermittent positive pressure breathing. *Respir Care* 2003, 38:1189–1195.

Stiller K. Physiotherapy in intensive care: towards an evidence-based practice. *Chest* 2000;118: 1801–1813.

Chapter 64

Clinical pharmacy

L. BARROW

Introduction

The critical care pharmacist, as part of the multidisciplinary team, may initiate, monitor, evaluate and individualize pharmacotherapy for each patient. The traditional role of supplying medications, although still fundamentally important, is now only a small part of the pharmacist's contribution to the patient's care. The pharmacist is responsible for confirming whether the patient is getting the right drug, at the correct dose, by the appropriate route and at the right time. Drug interactions should be identified and drug doses adjusted according to kidney or liver function. A thorough knowledge of changes that can occur in drug handling and the use of therapeutic drug monitoring is also essential.

In a climate of rising health costs, the evaluation of cost effectiveness of treatments must be assessed, as should medication usage through drug utilization evaluation. Pharmacists provide up-to-date medicines information and education to all health professionals. Their role in developing procedures and policies encourages the safe use of medicines, helping to prevent medication errors.

Routine care

After elective cardiac or thoracic surgery, patients are expected to have a routine recovery. The pharmacist's role is to check that standard postoperative medications are prescribed and the patient's regular medications are correctly charted. The expected transitory postoperative renal impairment requires the temporary withholding of medications that impact on renal function.

In contrast, essential drugs such as anti-parkinsonian drugs, anti-epileptics and glaucoma eye drops should not be stopped. The pharmacist should ensure that their administration is continued and an alternative route should be proposed if oral administration is not possible. Patients undergoing surgery with cardiopulmonary bypass are often fluid overloaded and may routinely receive an IV diuretic (e.g. furosemide). Significant amounts of potassium are also excreted and the potassium level must be strictly monitored and maintained within predefined limits.

Constipation may be overlooked and the addition of a laxative should be instituted; postoperative intravenous opioids are administered, often concurrently with inotropes, causing a decrease in gut motility. The laxative should be continued as long as opioid analgesia is required.

There is no firm evidence for the routine administration of acid-suppressing medications for gastrointestinal protection, for all postoperative cardiothoracic surgical patients. Certain risk factors increase the likelihood of stress-related mucosal disease and it is in these patients that a H_2 antagonist or a proton pump inhibitor should be administered (the most commonly used drug is omeprazole). Initially, this needs to be given intravenously, but when

Table 64.1 Example of commonly used drugs with possible renal toxicity
Nonsteroidal anti-inflammatory drugs
Angiotensin-converting enzyme inhibitors
Angiotensin 2 antagonists

nutrition is being absorbed it may be given via the oral/nasogastric route.

Many clinical situations dictate the use of anticoagulation and the pharmacist can advise on appropriate dosing and monitoring. Drugs can be expensive and cost–benefit analysis should influence drug choice.

Medications such as amiodarone have significant drug interactions and dose adjustment may be required. Warfarin, erythromycin, calcium channel blockers and some β-blockers interact with amiodarone.

Table 64.2 Risk factors for stress-related gastrointestinal haemorrhage
Respiratory support >24 hours
Hypotension, use of >2 inotropes
Sepsis (evidence of clinical infection)
Renal failure (acute or chronic)
Hepatic failure
Coagulopathy/low platelets
Anticoagulant therapy
Corticosteroid administration

Specialist care

Inotropes, chronotropes and vasoactive drugs are commonly used on a cardiothoracic critical care unit and a good understanding of the pharmacology of these drugs is fundamental. Standard

Table 64.3 Various drugs interactions with amiodarone

Tricyclic antidepressants	Increased risk of ventricular arrhythmias
β-Blockers	Increased risk of bradycardia and atrioventricular block
Warfarin	Enhanced anticoagulant effect
Digoxin	Increased plasma levels digoxin
Diuretics	Care to avoid hypokalaemia
Erythromycin	Increased risk of ventricular arrhythmias
Haloperidol	Increased risk of ventricular arrhythmias
Lithium	Increased risk of ventricular arrhythmias
Phenytoin	Increased plasma levels phenytoin
Simvastatin	Increased risk of myopathy
Sotalol	Increased risk of ventricular arrhythmias
Levothyroxine	Monitor thyroid function closely
Trimethoprim	Increased risk of ventricular arrhythmias

Table 64.4 Relevant drug level

Aminophylline	10–20 μg/mL
Digoxin	0.8–2.0 ng/mL
Gentamicin	Peak, 4–10 μg/mL; trough, 0.5–2 μg/mL
Phenytoin	10–20 μg/mL
Vancomycin	Peak, 20–40 μg/mL; trough, 5–15 μg/mL

preparations are useful to avoid errors of dilutions. Incompatibility in infusion lines is important as precipitation before administration can have dramatic consequences.

In some cases, the pharmacist must be able to work out different preparations to respond to clinicians' requests (such as decreasing the volume of fluid administered to the patient).

New therapies are constantly being evaluated and the pharmacist must be able to support the clinical team in the search of the best available treatment, while ensuring that costs remain contained.

Monitoring of drug levels

This is an important area of pharmacist responsibility on critical care with the other team members. Trough levels should be measured immediately before the next dose.

VANCOMYCIN

In patients with normal renal function, trough levels should be measured before the third to fifth doses and immediately before the dose. Then, if necessary, adjust dosing interval, not the dose itself. If renal function remains stable, trough levels should be measured twice weekly thereafter. Peak levels are usually not required. It is not necessary to wait for the results of the level before giving a single further dose, unless renal function is abnormal or previous levels have been high. If renal function is fluctuating, measure trough levels daily.

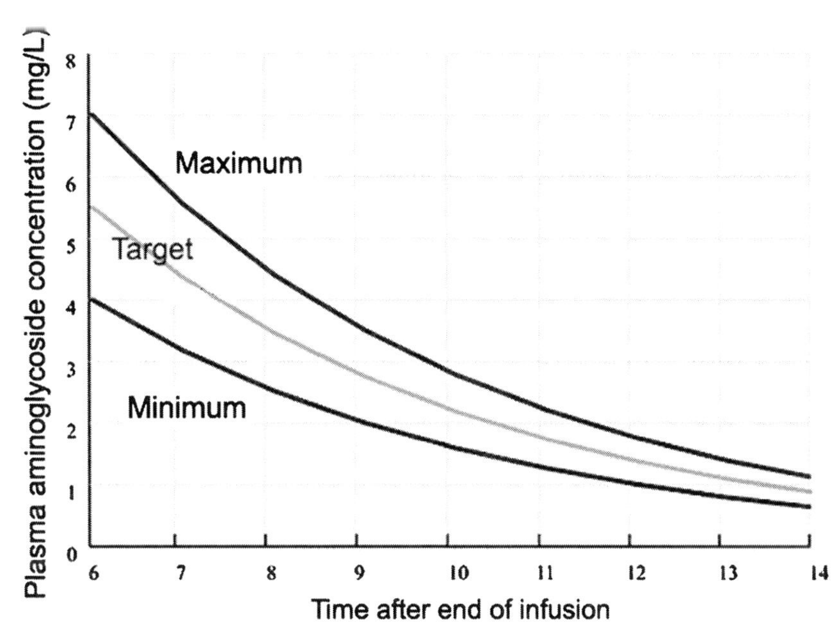

Figure 64.1 Examples of curve allowing drug blood level monitoring: aminoglycoside plasma concentration versus time for once-daily dosing

GENTAMICIN

For patients with normal renal function, give 4 to 6 mg/kg per day once daily. Plasma level should be measured between 6 and 14 hours after the end of the infusion of the first dose. This plasma concentration is then compared to Fig. 64.1.

Dosage adjustment should be applied after the first dose. It should be repeated daily if the clinical state, especially renal function, is unstable and otherwise every 3 to 5 days. If renal function is abnormal, the total dose should be divided into two to three doses daily and peak and trough plasma levels should be monitored. Plasma levels are done immediately before the third dose (trough) and 30 minutes after completion of the third dose (peak). This should be repeated every 3 to 5 days, or more frequently if renal function is unstable.

Drug compatibility

A critically ill patient may have several intravenous drugs being infused concurrently and drug compatibility is an important consideration. Various textbooks are available to aid safe and effective administration of most intravenous drugs.

Where no information is available, it should be assumed that the drug combination is incompatible. The pharmacist needs to be able to advise which drugs can be administered in combination or if necessary, via another route of administration.

Renal replacement therapy

When renal replacement therapy is required, the pharmacist may be able to advise on the procurement of the best available replacement fluid. Drug dosage adjustment is often necessary and this depends on the continuous venovenous haemofiltration circuit used, including the type of membrane in the circuit.

The pharmacist is an invaluable source of information in this area and may help in preventing accumulation of active drug, drug metabolites or underdosing.

Table 64.5 Examples of drug compatibility relevant in cardiac critical care

Insulin	Compatible only with amiodarone, calcium, dobutamine, folic acid, gentamicin, heparin, hydrocortisone, imipenem, magnesium, midazolam, morphine, nitroglycerin, nitroprusside, KCl, potassium phosphate, propofol, ranitidine, sodium bicarbonate, thiamine, vancomycin
Noradrenaline	*Not* compatible with insulin, aminophylline, phenytoin, sodium bicarbonate
Dopamine	*Not* compatible with sodium bicarbonate, insulin
Propofol	*Not* compatible with methylprednisolone, verapamil
Enoximone	*Not* compatible with any other IV drugs

Route of administration

The absorption of oral medications may be significantly altered if the patient is receiving intravenous inotropes, because hypoperfusion secondary to vasoconstriction may affect the stomach. Where patients require administration of medication by an enteral tube, the pharmacist should provide advice on timing the administration of certain medications separate from the enteral feed owing to the possibility of drug–food interactions. Other clinical considerations for these patients include the conversion of oral tablets to an equivalent suspension dose and the continuation of drugs of critical therapeutic importance such as anti-epileptics. Osmolar effects as a result of drugs and enteral feeds need to be considered to avoid diarrhoea. When high osmolar solutions are administered via a nasojejunal tube, there is a higher risk of diarrhoea because the buffering effect of stomach contents is lost.

The administration of drugs via a percutaneous endoscopic gastrostomy tube requires, where

Table 64.6 Characteristics of drugs removal by renal replacement therapy

Molecular weight	
	Low molecular weight favours removal (≤500 Da)
	500–2,000 Da – inadequately removed by RRT
	>2,000 Da – not removable by conventional RRT
Protein binding	
	Low protein binding favours removal – more free drug available, therefore more available to cross the dialysis membrane
Volume of distribution	
	Low apparent volume of distribution favours removal; if ≤1 L/kg there may well be significant removal, if >2 L/kg then removal will probably be insignificant
Solubility	
	High water solubility favours removal by the aqueous dialysate
	Lipid soluble drugs tend to have large volume of distribution and therefore be less concentrated in blood which is where RRT takes place
Renal clearance	
	A high degree of renal clearance in patients with normal renal function, favours removal

Abbreviation: RRT, renal replacement therapy.

possible, the substitution of tablets or capsules to liquid or suspension forms of the medication. The pharmacist in conjunction with the dietitian plays an important role in providing appropriate total parenteral nutrition. Ensuring compatibility of electrolyte concentrations prevents fine precipitation or cracking of the emulsion and administration of particles that are visually undetectable.

Guidelines

The pharmacist promotes existing national and local guidelines and monitors efficacy of treatment, providing alternative options if necessary.

Key points

- The pharmacist's role on a cardiothoracic critical care unit is diverse and important as part of the multidisciplinary team.
- A proactive approach is necessary to ensure safe and affective administration of medication.
- Particular care is needed when renal replacement therapy is in progress.
- Poor absorption of oral drugs must always be borne in mind during critical illness.
- Drug compatibility when multiple infusions are in progress is a serious concern.
- Monitoring of biochemistry and drug levels is necessary to ensure safety.

FURTHER READING

Ashley C, Currrie A. *The renal drug handbook.* Abingdon, UK: Radcliffe Publishing; 2003.

Stockley I. *Stockley's drug interactions*. London: Pharmaceutical Press; 2005.

Trissel LA. *Handbook on injectable drugs*. London: Transatlantic Publishing; 2004.

Chapter 65

Evidence-based design of the cardiothoracic critical care unit

D.K. HAMILTON AND R.S. ULRICH

Introduction

Critical care units are the locus of some of the most important and complex clinical episodes in the hospital, and as such deserve careful attention to design. There is a growing body of evidence relating the physical environment to outcomes.

Key issues in the design of future cardiothoracic critical care units

Typical geometries

Selecting a geometric floor plan to increase observation of patients and to reduce the travel distance of staff while performing their duties in a critical care unit is important. Each patient bed should have an exterior window.

Although the intuitive response is often to suggest a variation of circular forms, careful study of unit shape has shown that there is no single ideal geometry. Good floor designs have been demonstrated in semi-circles, hexagons, octagons, squares and diamonds, along with some irregular shapes. A strong recommendation is to limit unit size to the range of 7 to 10 beds, breaking larger units into pods or clusters of smaller numbers. The most successful designs are symmetrical, or nearly so, and efficiently compact.

Patient safety

The Institute of Medicine has indicated that nearly 100,000 preventable deaths occur annually in hospitals in the United States. These can often be attributed to error, hospital-acquired infections, and in some cases, falls.

Latent environmental conditions such as noise increase staff fatigue and job strain, erode performance and heighten the risk for error. Workplace design should reduce latent environmental conditions through measures such as noise control, reduced distractions, adjustable task lighting, convenient location of washbasins and fresh air.

Infection is a danger to staff as well as patients. Contagious spread can be reduced by careful design of the air handling system and filtration. To reduce the threat of airborne pathogens and negative impacts from hazardous chemicals, critical care units should be designed to minimize unfiltered or recirculated air and to receive higher quantities of fresh air to accomplish more frequent air changes and to maintain air quality at higher levels. Design to enhance staff hand hygiene is a key priority; low rates of hand cleaning have a causal link with infection transmission. Evidence suggests that hand washing compliance improves if the design incorporates sinks with deep bowls and hands-free operation, along with alcohol gel or hand rub dispensers, installed in the line of sight of staff members and close to their work paths as they enter patient rooms or approach patients. Every object or device touched by the patient, family member, physician or staff member can become a reservoir for colonization and contact spread of pathogens. Ubiquitous items, such as computer keyboards or monitor controls, may be especially difficult to decontaminate. Design of surfaces in the clinical areas to reduce the chance of harbouring moisture is important. Durable, cleanable materials with antimicrobial characteristics should be specified.

Advantages of single rooms with respect to infection control include:

- separation of patients from other potentially infected patients;
- facilitation of thorough cleaning after discharge, lessening risk from environmental surfaces serving as pathogen reservoirs;
- superiority in reducing airborne spread through measures such as air changes, filtration, creation of negative pressure;
- application of positive pressure to safeguard an immunocompromised individual from aerial pathogens in adjacent spaces;
- elimination of time consuming and potentially risky patient transfers around the critical care unit due to development of new infection.

Falls are a problem for patients who are ambulatory, or for whom an attempt to leave the bed is likely. Although some technological interventions are available, the best insurance against falls is observation by the nursing staff or family. Design responses include decentralized staff positions, family presence in the room, short paths to the toilet with a continuous handrail and extra wide doorways into patient toilets so staff can assist patients all the way to their destination.

Toilets are rarely used by cardiac surgery patients in critical care. By the time patients are able to use a toilet, they are likely to be transferred off the unit. For this reason, the toilet is most often used for bedpan dumping and cleaning. Evidence suggests that this cleaning activity is a source of aerosols that distribute pathogens from the human waste. A more successful solution to the bedpan cleaning problem is the deep flushing rim clinical sink, and the safest alternative is the use of a macerator, which disposes of waste in papiér maché pans and basins in a sealed chamber.

Choice of life support system

Technological support for the patient includes monitors, medical gas supply, suction, electrical sockets and communications. It can also include a variety of infusion pumps, ventilators or other medical equipment devices.

The 'headwall' configuration, in which monitors and equipment outlets are placed on the wall flanking the patient's head, is the most common choice of life support system. Manufactured systems are ubiquitous despite the fact that most custom installations by a contractor are more economical. The manufactured systems offer the appeal of flexibility that is rarely utilized once the initial set-up to match staff preferences is completed. The principal disadvantage of a headwall configuration is the need to pull the bed away from the wall and step over the various umbilicals in a crisis or cardiac arrest to access the patient's airway.

The 'power column' configuration takes the monitor and utilities off the wall, locating them in a columnar unit that stands diagonally off the head of the bed. This configuration allows for immediate, continuous access to the head and airway in a crisis.

In recent years, 'pendant' systems have appeared. They are suspended from the ceiling and can be rotated to multiple positions. The advantage of such systems is the flexibility to move the life support components as needed, as in the case of procedures at the bedside, or to reorient the bed. The decision about life support systems and space for equipment governs the size of the patient room. For the purpose of future flexibility, it could be wise to plan for the largest likely model, even if a conventional headwall is used.

Staff safety

Nursing has been shown to be a more dangerous profession than construction in some studies. The

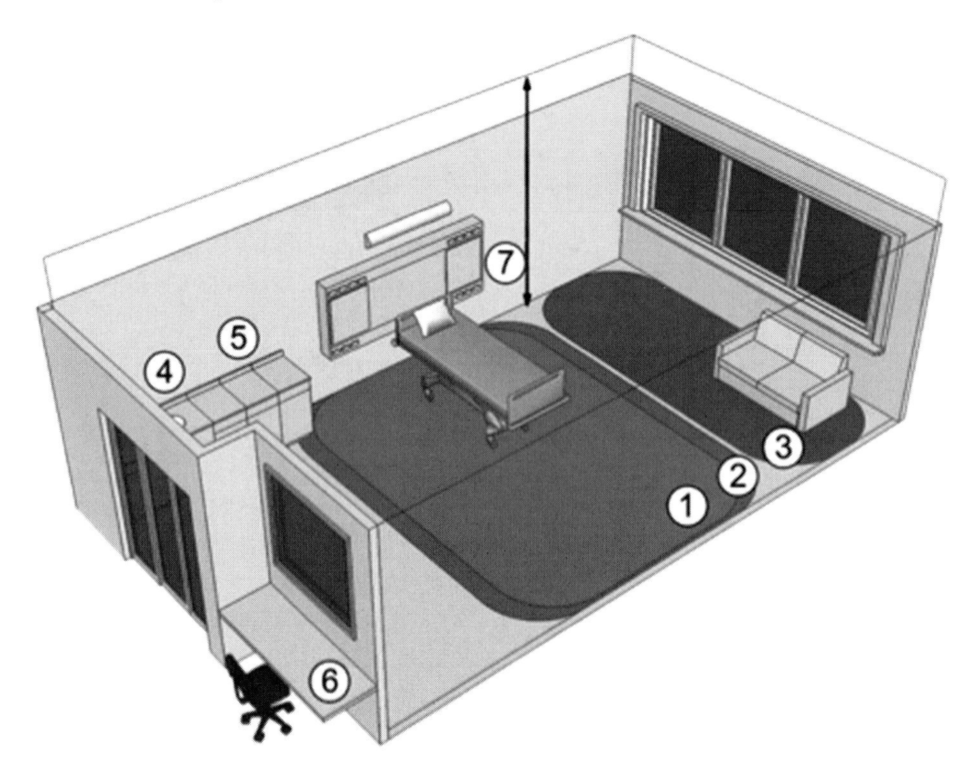

Figure 65.1 Headwall life-support system. (1) Patient zone; (2) bariatric patient zone; (3) family zone; (4) hygiene zone; (5) clinical zone; (6) charting substation; (7) ceiling height: 2.7 to 3.3 metres.

most prevalent staff injuries are lower back injuries associated with the lifting of patients. Based on calculations of cost of injuries, cost of installation and return on investment, many hospitals and critical care units have adopted a policy to include mechanical patient lifts in every patient room, or to provide ready access to mobile lifts.

Design of disposal containers and their mounting locations can contribute to the reduction of needle stick injuries. Location of eyewash deluge showers can address accidental exposure to dangerous chemicals.

Isolation of cardiothoracic patients is normally planned as a component of every unit design. The physical implications of isolation precautions can range from separate filtered air handling systems that can deliver positive or negative pressure protected from the unit with an anteroom, to a simple alcove for isolation supplies outside the door of a negative pressure patient room. Canadian planners responding to the SARS epidemic have suggested that the general mechanical system might need to be shut down in the case of a pandemic situation if the air supply to each patient room is not recirculated. In an era of pandemic threats from mutating viruses and resistant strains of viruses, future critical care units designs may well have significantly greater levels of isolation capability.

Decentralized care giving

A current design trend is the location of satellite stations for nurses and other clinical staff close to the bedside. In the critical care unit, this has taken the form of documentation stations inside the patient room, just outside the room or pairs of rooms and clusters of patient rooms. Robust versions of these stations may have documentation, communications, clean and soiled supplies, medication

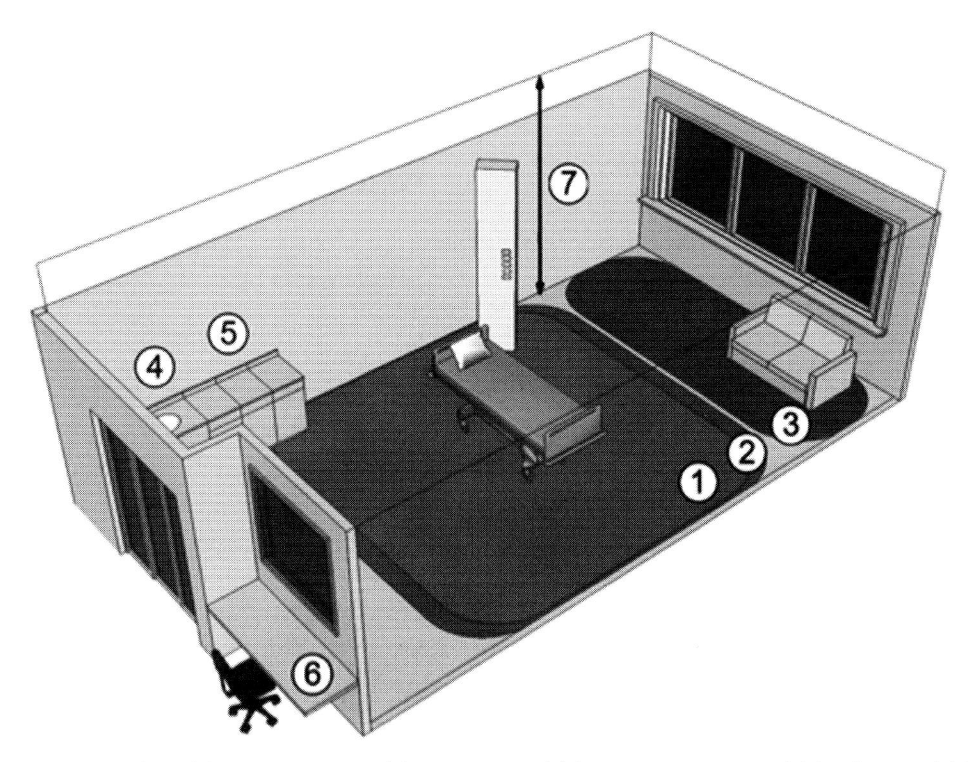

Figure 65.2 Power column life-support system. (1) Patient zone; (2) bariatric patient zone; (3) family zone; (4) hygiene zone; (5) clinical zone; (6) charting substation; (7) ceiling height: 2.7 to 3. 3 metres.

storage and hand hygiene capability. The advantage of these configurations is the increase in ability to observe the patient and the potential for important reductions in the amount of walking required of staff. It is important to localize supply storage; centralized storage can negate the benefit of decentralized care giving by requiring nurses to spend much of their time walking up and down halls engaged in wasteful fetching. There is convincing evidence that the combination of decentralized nurse stations and single rooms does not require higher nurse staffing than conventional units with centralized stations and multi-bed rooms.

Point-of-care technologies

An aspect of decentralized care giving and improved response is the ability to perform tests and obtain the results at the point of care. Advances in integration of technologies and information systems allow simplification of documentation and predictive clinical analysis. As device intercommunication becomes more widely available, space for testing equipment and information systems must be considered.

Response to staff shortages

The nearly universal and increasing shortage of skilled critical care staff suggests the need to do more with fewer human resources. Designs that offer increased efficiency and productivity will be prized; reduction of fatigue and stress for the staff will contribute to improved performance.

Electronic and camera-based models of critical care unit management and clinical observation are

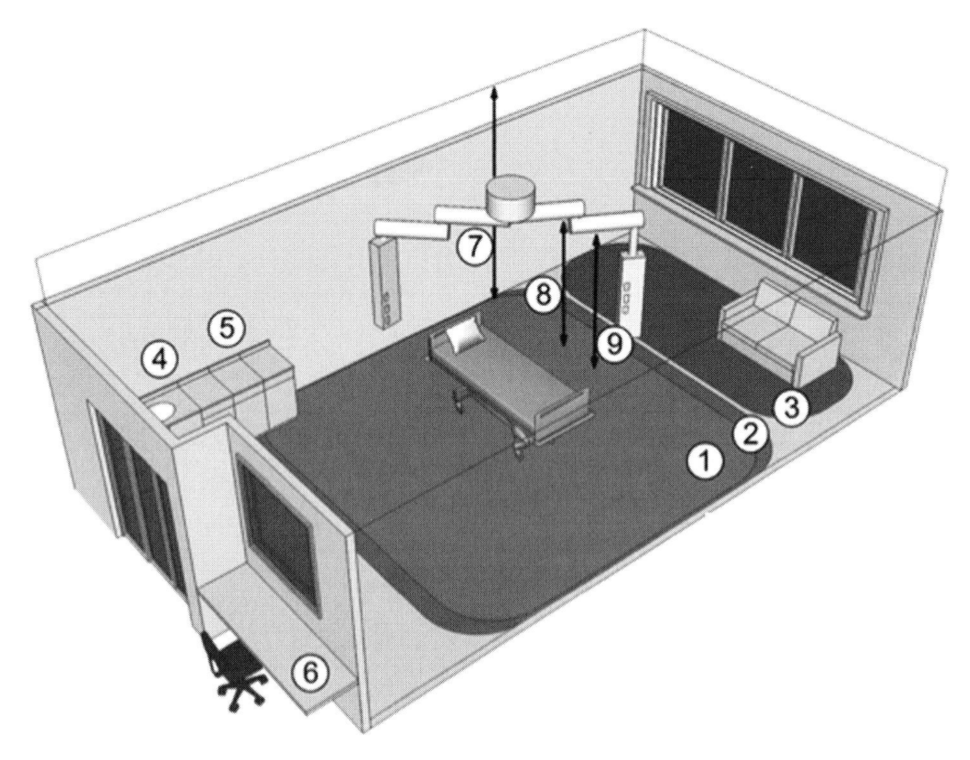

Figure 65.3 Pendant mounted life-support system. (1) Patient zone; (2) bariatric patient zone; (3) family zone; (4) hygiene zone; (5) clinical zone; (6) charting substation; (7) ceiling height: 2.7 to 3.3. metres; (8) clearance: 2.4 to 3.0 metres; (9) clearance: 2.1. to 2.7 metres.

appearing in greater numbers and early evidence suggests that the clinical and financial outcomes are positive. The ability for intensivists and clinical specialists to cover larger numbers of patients with the support of technology is likely to grow in importance.

Performance improvement

It is possible to relate many quality and performance measures to environmental factors. Evidence-based design of the environment has been shown to favourably impact infection rates, error rates, patient pain and intake of analgesics, length of stay, staff fatigue and turnover, financial performance and a variety of patient and staff satisfaction measures. Stress is known to exacerbate many clinical conditions and worsen satisfaction and performance. For this reason, a theory of supportive health care design focuses on stress reduction as one path to improved outcomes.

Noise is a major problem in the critical care environment and recent studies show it may have more serious effects than previously understood. Noise in critical care is associated with sleep loss and fragmentation, elevated blood pressure and heart rate, worse rates of recovery from myocardial infarction and decreased oxygen saturation; it also seems to contribute to critical care delirium or psychosis and staff burnout. Location and control of monitor alarms, along with the use of sound-absorptive materials help to reduce noise. Single patient rooms are important for reducing noise and the indignity and stress related to exposure in the undressed state and also eliminate the privacy violations and other problems associated with mixed-gender accommodation during times of high bed occupancy rates.

Critical care patients experience loss of control in their lives. Elements to enhance personal control such as a nurse call, thermostat, window blinds, telephone and entertainment systems may contribute to reducing patient stress. Research has consistently shown that access to nature, views of nature or positive and realistic representations of nature subjects can reduce stress for patients and staff. Other positive distractions, such as music, appear to have similar stress-reducing effects. Well-controlled prospective studies suggest that both views of nature and exposure to daylight lessen pain in patients.

Effective communication with patients and their families can be a factor in reducing stress and anxiety, but it can also play a role in improved patient safety by alerting the family to be careful observers of the patient's condition and to serve as another important checkpoint for accuracy. There should be designated space to provide privacy for discussions in a quiet area.

Changing technology

The environment of critical care is impacted by changes in technology at a pace that equals or exceeds the rate of change in any other area of the hospital. In some cases, the equipment is becoming miniaturized, but in other cases, new devices are being introduced that take up much more room. New imaging devices are being developed to make fluoroscopy, computed tomography, magnetic resonance imaging and other sophisticated technologies into portable machines that could be used on the unit or in the patient room. One prudent design response to change is to provide a robust and expandable utility infrastructure to support the unknown mechanical, electrical, communications, medical gas and plumbing requirements of the future. Another strategy is to design rooms on the unit to 'loose fit' standards that could accommodate multiple functions and unanticipated equipment rather than base the project brief or programme of space requirements on the minimum sizes to meet the current need.

Flexibility

The ability to respond to changing technology and treatment modalities is highly prized in the health care setting. Adaptable flexibility is the ability for a space to adapt with little or no time, effort or cost to a new activity as in the case of a patient room capable of supporting surgical procedures. Convertible flexibility is the ability for a space to be converted to another purpose after a modest time and effort without enormous cost (e.g. storage room to patient room).

Anticipation of future needs can lead to the use of 'shell space,' which is structured and enclosed but not fitted out for use. 'Soft space' strategies for change anticipate future expansion of the critical care unit by adjacent locations for departments or functions that can be easily relocated. Another strategy for flexibility is the use of a 'loose fit' concept for design, which utilizes generous room sizes and creates the capacity for some future change within the original boundaries of the department or unit.

Access for the cardiac arrest team and work space in a crisis intervention such as chest reopening is a critical design consideration. The ability to perform procedures in the patient room can be an important way to reduce dangerous transfers.

Family presence

There is evidence that the presence of family during critical interventions in the critical care unit improves satisfaction with care. Enhanced communications with family is an important element of quality and satisfaction. Research has begun to indicate the importance of social support for patients in the critical care setting. Evidence suggests, for example, that postsurgical cardiac patients survive longer if they have strong social support. Space to accommodate family members in the patient room and amenities like sleeper chairs and Internet connections should be provided.

Key points

- Care of the critically ill patient can be more effective in a properly designed and supportive environment.
- The critical care unit should be designed to account for the key issues of safety, efficiency, interdisciplinary teamwork, and thoughtful concern for the patient and their family.

FURTHER READING

Blomkvist V, Eriksen CA, Theorell T, *et al.* Acoustics and psychosocial environment in intensive coronary care. *Occup Environ Med* 2005;2: 132–139.

Ulrich RS. Evidence-based healthcare architecture. *Lancet* 2004;368:S38–S39.

Ulrich RS, Zimring C, Joseph A, *et al.* The role of the physical environment in the hospital of the 21st century: A once-in-a-lifetime opportunity. Concord, CA: The Center for Health Design. Available at: www.healthdesign.org and www.rwjf.org.

Wilson APR, Ridgeway GL. Reducing hospital-acquired infections by design: the new University London Hospital. *J Hosp Infect* 2006; 62:264–269.

Chapter 66

Clinical information systems

R.J. BOSMAN

Introduction

Critical care is a highly technical environment that has greatly benefited from advances in computer technology such as accurate monitoring with automated pattern recognition and alarms, or algorithm-driven ventilators. Integrating and organizing the vast amount of information related to a specific patient is a daily challenge for the critical care doctor. Medical records are notorious for their illegible handwriting, errors, omissions and dispersion of information resulting in an incomplete representation for the caregiver. Incomplete information can lead to delayed, duplicate or erroneous medical treatment. Nurses and others caregivers spend a lot of time collecting and organizing all relevant information so that it can be comprehensively appraised and acted on.

It has long been recognized that computers may help to organize and render information in critical care but it is only since the start of the 21st century that units have started to systematically equip themselves. This increase can be attributed to the awareness that Clinical Information Systems (CIS) can improve efficiency while simultaneously improving patient outcome, and may reduce staff workload. As a result, the work area at the bedside is changing: paper charts are being replaced by computers running sophisticated software. Physicians no longer prescribe on paper, but send their prescriptions electronically to the pharmacy; nurses validate the patient's vital signs in the computer and receive notification that new laboratory results have become available. Radiographs are no longer hunted for, but are presented at the bedside monitor.

Definitions

A CIS can be described as a gateway to all of the available data of a patient. The CIS can exist in the form of one application, or a combination of applications presenting themselves with one user interface. The CIS integrates vital signs, order entry, clinical documentation (medical history, examination and progress notes), laboratory and microbiology results, radiology examinations, decision support and billing.

The patient-centred electronic medical record (EMR) is the heart of the CIS. This nucleus mainly receives information from context systems (registration, managed care and medical vocabularies), sharing information with cooperating systems (pharmacy and laboratory) and sending information to subscriber systems (financial and reporting). Bedside devices like monitors and ventilators append their signals directly to the EMR.

The electronic health record includes general health-related information, which encompasses health and health-related administrative data from all CIS. The 'National Spine' in England, currently in development, aims to provide lifelong care records for every patient in England. The task is

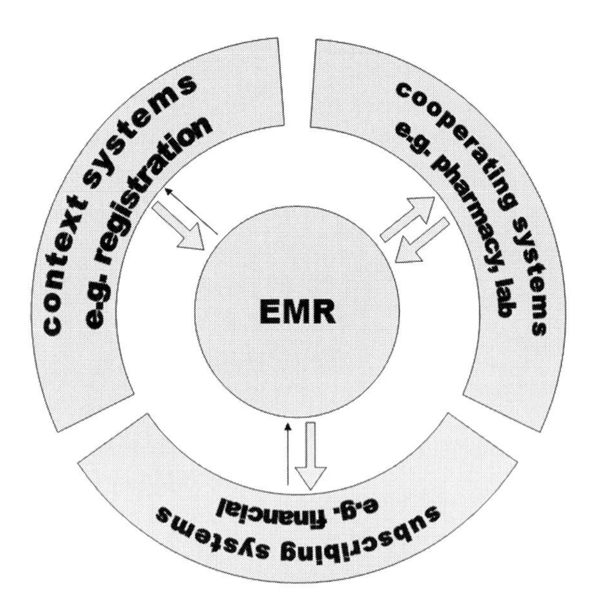

Figure 66.1 Schematic representation of the relation between the EMR and the contributing systems.

ambitious and indeed the world's biggest nonmilitary IT project ever.

Computer-aided physician order entry (CPOE) allows interaction between clinicians and CIS with warnings regarding allergies, drug interactions, deviation from the hospital standard, relevant abnormal laboratory results and so on. The term 'Patient Data Management System' (PDMS) is another term for CIS, usually restricted to critical care.

History

Although the health care industry started using computers in the early 1960s, these installations were mainly intended for administrative and financial purposes. Critical care physicians were the first to understand that the processing abilities of computers would be useful in a data-driven environment, and clinical applications of computers in hospitals started to be seen in the early 1970s. The growth in popularity of the personal computer from the end of the 1980s to the present, coupled with the increase in computing power, facilitated the migration from industrial-based operating systems to a user-friendly interface.

Advantages

Many advantages have been attributed to CIS but few have so far been proven true in clinical trials.

Data quality and quantity

It is estimated that up to 50,000 data-points per 24 hours are obtained from bedside monitors, ventilators, infusion pumps, renal replacement devices and organ assist devices, together with laboratory data and clinical documentation (assuming that continuous items are sampled every minute). Complete manual registration is clearly impossible. Accuracy depends on the person recording the information; a large amount of data are lost and errors are present in approximately 20% of the record. Manual charting shows less variability compared with a continuous record, with 'clipping' of extremes. The connection between the bedside devices and the CIS allows a continuous record of accurate data into the database.

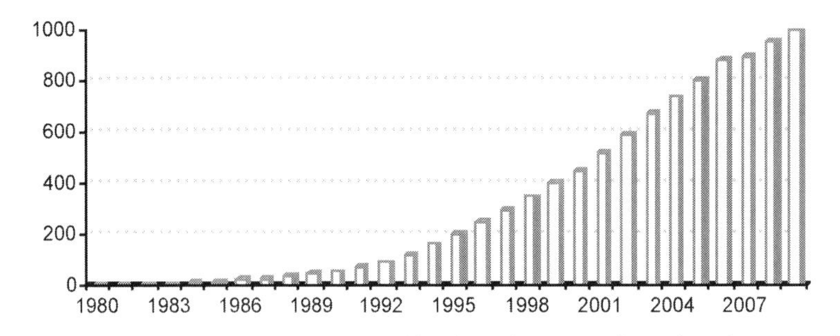

Figure 66.2 Estimated number of personal computers worldwide with projected numbers for years after 2006.

Time savings

With paper charting, nurses spend approximately 15% to 30% of their time on documentation and charting of vital signs. Reduction of charting time is a powerful argument used by the industry to promote the use of CIS. Although this was not initially confirmed, recent trends seem to indicate that use of CIS increases time devoted to direct patient care. The impact of a CIS on physician time is unclear, but it is thought that the possible small increase in data entry is a small burden considering the benefits of integrated prescription support, data analysing, automatic billing and so on.

Error reduction

In 1999, the American Institute of Medicine reported that between 44,000 and 98,000 people die each year in the United States alone as the result of medical errors, approximately half of them attributable to medication errors. A subsequent publication stated that information technology should be part of the approach to deal with the problem. Ordering through a CPOE can reduce the number of medication errors if the system is well integrated in the complex critical care environment. On the other hand, it is possible to increase the number of medication errors by introducing an ill-designed CIS. Other benefits of well-designed CIS include elimination of illegible handwriting, data integrity checks, improved documentation and less chance of data losses. The integration of multiple signals from various sources allows a problem-orientated approach, leading to better understanding of impending deviations or problems.

Expert system

The integration of monitored data from multiple sources, coupled with processor power, allows for the creation of so-called intelligent systems. Whereas the bedside monitor can generate an alarm when detecting a change in ST segment, a CIS has the possibility to integrate this ST-segment change to a change in treatment and highlight this combination to the physician. The CIS can alert the physician that a change in drug dosage is required or has been missed or further intervention is required.

Telemedicine

Telemedicine is a care relation between the care provider (physician or nurse) and the care requester (patient or physician/nurse on behalf of the patient) where the two parties are geographically separate. Although at first sight, telemedicine seems irrelevant in critical care, it is not uncommon in practice for critical care physicians to manage patients from a remote location, talking on the phone to the nurse or resident or evaluating investigations.

Remotely supervised critical care units may be a solution to the shortage of trained intensivists in some countries. The specialist may have access to the monitor, chart, laboratory results and radiographs of the patients and have a direct audio/video connection to the bedside nurse. This has proven to be better (with shorter length of stay and reduced mortality) when compared with a situation where intensivists were only available during 'office hours.'

Disadvantages

Despite all the advantages, three main disadvantages can readily be identified: initial procurement process and acceptance, financial aspects and privacy regulations.

Selection, implementation and acceptance

Selecting a CIS requires extensive knowledge of the structure and workflow of the current organization. This includes identification of areas where patient outcome or care can be improved. A CIS has to be customized according to the workflow of the specific unit and hospital. The way the old 'paper' workflow is translated into the CIS is one of the major determinants of a successful implementation. Great care should be given to adapt the CIS to existing practice; however, it must be recognized

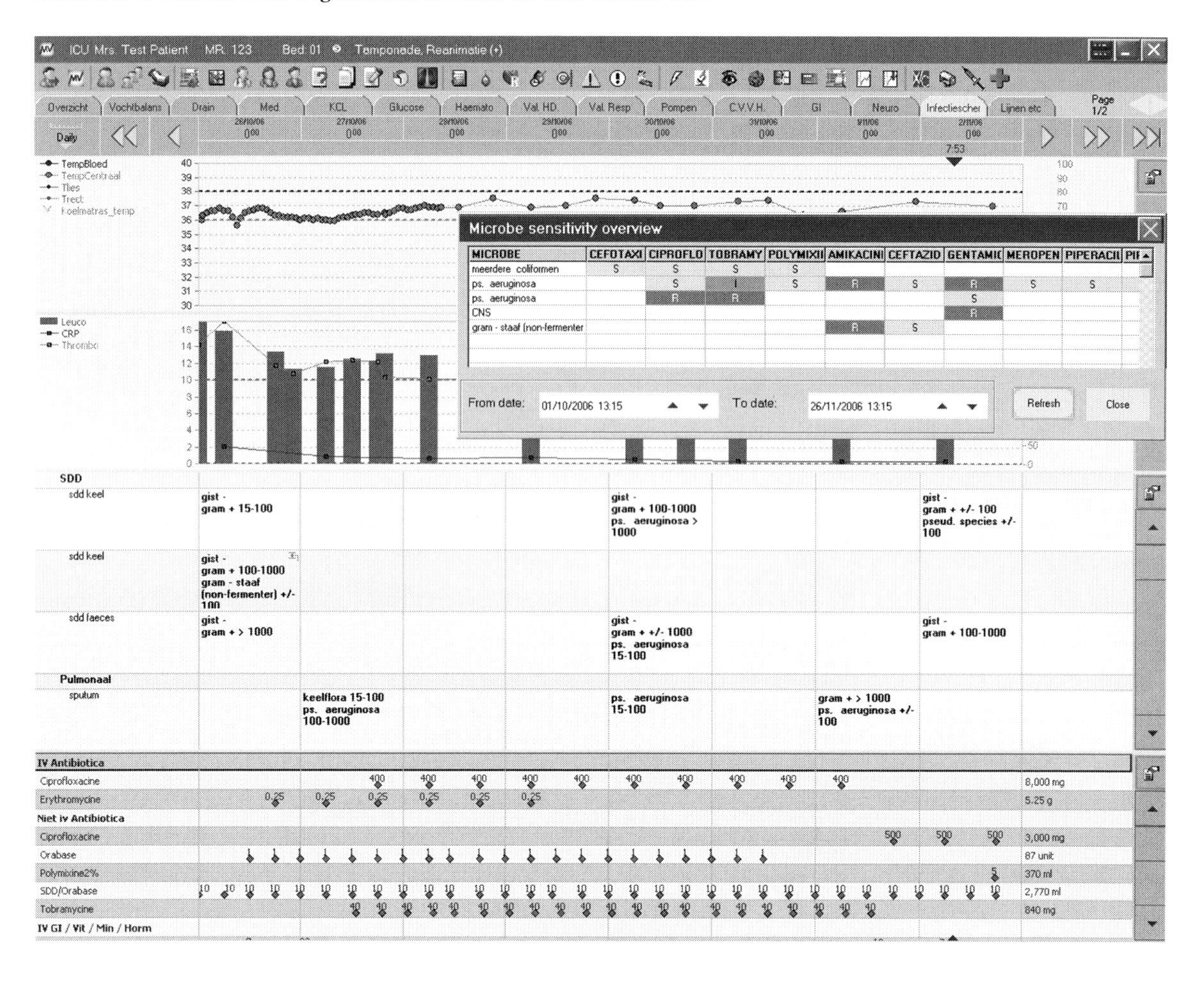

Figure 66.3 Example of a problem-orientated presentation: patient's temperature, laboratory results are combined with microbiology results and antibiotic use, creating an infection-orientated view.

that changes in working pattern will occur after the adoption of a CIS. Factors affecting acceptance are reliability of the system, responsiveness, intuitive user interface, ownership and a sense of added value, such as increased patient safety. Resistance to change is a major hindrance during this process and selecting and implementing a CIS is a labour intensive task!

Costs

The financial cost of implementing a CIS is substantial and must include personnel cost, including time required to develop the database and train other users. Once the CIS is in use, the costs can be ascribed to annual software maintenance fees and hardware depreciation. Keeping the CIS up to date and implementing new developments requires a dedicated team.

Privacy

Patient privacy can be infringed either by illegitimate users ('hacking') or through inappropriate access by legitimate users ('peeping').The first must be addressed by the IT security features of the institution; the second requires appropriate organizational procedures and adaptable software.

Future

The sky is the limit! But delays and setbacks make the path to heaven a long one!

Radiofrequency identification

Enhanced patient safety and ease of use are the advantages of radiofrequency identification technology that allows tagging patients, drugs, equipment and automatic recognition by computers.

Data presentation

Dynamic screens can display only the relevant information based on patient's condition, user and other parameters.

Intelligence

Integration of the information and cross reference to powerful databases might lead to the computer generating its own hypothesis in clinical scenarios.

Key points

- The problems in the procurement process of a CIS should not be underestimated.
- Acceptance of a CIS should be promoted by active involvement of the end-users.
- A CIS can improve patient safety.
- A CIS can result in time saving for all users, but is very dependent on customization.
- Every measure must be taken to guarantee patient privacy.

FURTHER READING

EuroSOCAP [homepage on the Internet]. European Standards on Confidentiality and Privacy in Healthcare Among Vulnerable Patient Population. Available at: www.eurosocap.org.

Kohn KT, Corrigan JM, Donaldson MS. *To err is human: Building a safer health system*. Washington, DC: National Academy Press; 2000.

Wong DH, Gallegos Y, Weinger MB, *et al.* Changes in intensive care unit nurse task activity after installation of a third-generation intensive care unit information system. *Crit Care Med* 2003;31: 2488–2494.

Chapter 67

Resource management

D. CHENG

Introduction

Cardiac surgery and cardiac critical care are expensive endeavours. Intraoperative costs of coronary artery bypass grafting (CABG) and cardiac valve operations are among the highest when compared with other surgical procedures. Once the surgical procedure has finished, the costs continue to rise because of the expensive postoperative care provided in the critical care unit. Although the proportionate use of CABG to treat coronary artery disease is declining owing to increasing numbers of percutaneous coronary interventions, there are still many cardiac surgical operations performed each year worldwide. The profile of patients presenting has changed, and cardiac surgery is increasingly performed on elderly patients with extensive coronary artery disease and numerous medical comorbidities. These patients can be expected to have lengthier recovery periods and an increased chance of postoperative complications, further increasing costs.

Coinciding with the high demand for cardiac surgical procedures and critical care are institutional and societal pressures to contain costs within the health care arena. The motto of health care management since the 1990s has been to 'do more with less.' The aim is therefore to attain the best possible combination of excellent clinical outcomes, patient safety and cost containment.

Factors influencing the cost of cardiac surgery

The strongest predictors of cost for cardiac surgical patients are:

1. hospital length of stay (LOS);
2. critical care LOS;
3. operating room time;
4. patient age; and
5. postoperative complications (such as sternal wound infection, respiratory failure, left ventricular failure, and death).

Patient risk factors

Numerous scoring systems have been devised to calculate a patient's predicted mortality preoperatively. However, these scoring systems do not necessarily reflect risk factors associated with an increased LOS. Because critical care and hospital LOS are such important factors for computing the resources consumed, these scoring systems do not reliably predict resource utilization.

Instead of looking at mortality, an alternative approach is to look at the impact of preoperative patient risk factors on important postoperative adverse events that are associated with a prolonged LOS.

The Toronto Risk Score (TRS) for adverse events following cardiac surgery has a very good predictive

Table 67.1 The adverse events that prolong length of stay

Perioperative myocardial infarction (defined by electrocardiography and enzymatic criteria)
Low cardiac output syndrome (cardiac index <2.1 L min^{-1} m^{-2} and a systolic blood pressure <90 mmHg lasting >15 minutes despite adequate preload)
Perioperative stroke
New postoperative renal failure (requiring dialysis)
Deep sternal wound infection

ability to estimate critical care and hospital LOS, and adverse events.

When stratified into risk groups according to the TRS, important information regarding expected mortality and adverse event incidence can be determined accurately.

For instance, a common issue in critical care is a lack of beds for new patients caused by patients who have suffered adverse events and are therefore not yet ready to go to the hospital ward. This situation prevents any further surgery from being performed until patients are transferred out, resulting in cancelled operations, a backlog of patients and a subsequent increase in costs. Calculating the TRS allows intensivists, surgeons and hospital administrators to predict which patients will need additional recovery time in the critical care unit. This approach is only possible if the teams communicate well and a central booking system operates that takes this into account when scheduling surgical cases.

Table 67.2 Toronto Risk Score for adverse events after cardiac surgery

Variable	Weight
Age	
65–74 years	1
≥75 years	2
Female gender	2
LV grade 3 (LVEF 20%–40%)	2
LV grade 4 (LVEF <20%)	3
Urgent priority	1
Emergent priority	6
MI ≤1 month before operation	1
Redo CABG	4
Triple vessel disease	1
Left main disease	1
Congestive heart failure	2
Renal insufficiency	2
Diabetes	1
Peripheral vascular disease	1
Hypertension	1
Complex valve	2
Other pathology	2

Risk weights are summed to calculate the Toronto Risk Score. A complex valve includes two valves, valve + CABG, or any other procedure on the heart in addition to one valve.
Abbreviations: CABG, coronary artery bypass grafting; LV, left ventricle; LVEF, left ventricular ejection fraction; MI, myocardial infarction.
From Ivanov et al.

Anaesthesia factors

Perioperative anaesthetic management, the individual anaesthetist and postoperative critical care management can all influence the postoperative outcome of patients. One of the biggest changes in the anaesthetic management of patients undergoing cardiac surgery in recent years has been the switch from prolonged postoperative mechanical ventilation to early tracheal extubation, which has been facilitated by the use of a balanced anaesthetic technique consisting of short-acting intravenous anaesthetics such as propofol, low-to moderate-dose opioids, intermediate-duration muscle relaxants and

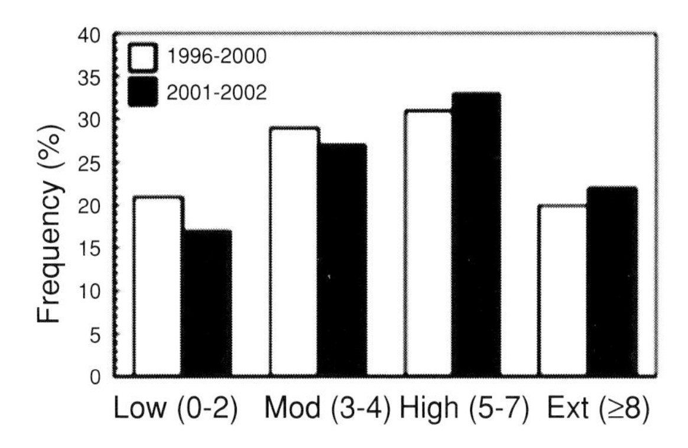

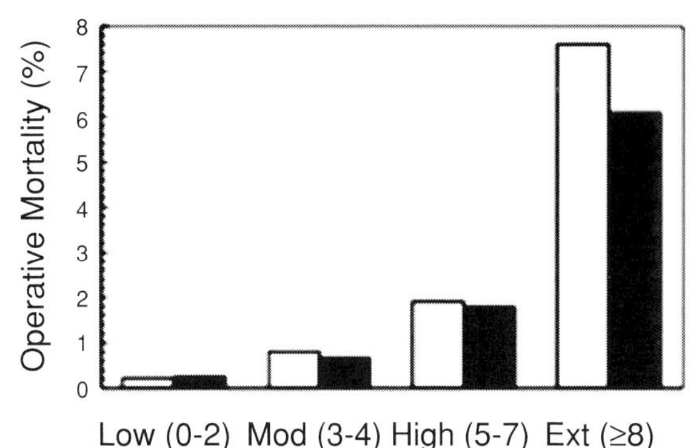

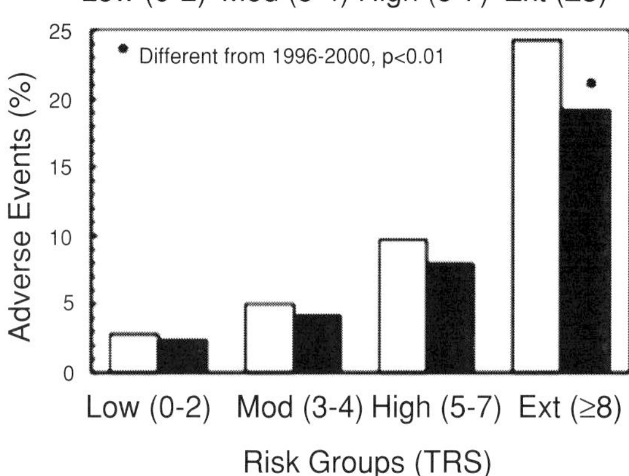

Figure 67.1 (*Top panel*) Proportion of patients in each risk stratum of the Toronto Risk Scoring (1996–2000) and validation data set (2001–2002). (*Middle panel*) Risk-stratified operative mortality. (*Bottom panel*) Incidence of adverse events.

poorly soluble volatile anaesthetics. Less bleeding occurs postoperatively because of an increased use of antifibrinolytic drugs, and early use of antidysrhythmic drugs can reduce the incidence of postoperative rhythm disturbances. All of these factors can promote a faster recovery, reducing LOS and cost. Resource utilization increases in patients monitored with a pulmonary artery catheter (PAC), but the good news is that the routine use of a PAC for uncomplicated cardiac surgery is becoming less and less common in both North America and Europe. This may principally be due to the rise of intraoperative transoesophageal echocardiography as a standard monitor intraoperatively and insertion of a PAC only when indicated.

Surgical Factors

Advances in surgical technique have also contributed to a shorter LOS in the critical care unit and decreased overall costs by avoiding prolonged cardiopulmonary bypass duration, deep systemic hypothermia, postoperative bleeding and neurological morbidity. Other changes, such as improved myocardial protection, allow the myocardium to regain normal systolic and diastolic function sooner.

Postcardiac surgery recovery

Numerous aspects of the postoperative management of a cardiac surgical patient can influence overall cost and quality of care. These include:

- model of care;
- management of pain; and
- diagnosis of postoperative haemodynamic disturbances.

The concept of providing graded levels of care for postoperative cardiac surgical patients can be categorized by patient flow:

- *Conventional model*: Conventional flow of patients from the operating room to a critical care unit, then to a freestanding intermediate care unit, and then to the ward.
- *Parallel model*: Freestanding intermediate care unit, which directly admits postoperative cardiac patients and operates in parallel to an independent medical–surgical critical care unit.
- *Integrated model*: A fully integrated intermediate care unit/critical care unit. Patients are admitted

directly from the operating room and recover with a flexible nursing ratio depending on the patient's acuity level. Patients are discharged from this unit directly to the ward.

The critical care unit balances patient needs with flexible staffing and monitoring resources. This approach may decrease cost and avoid unnecessary critical care admissions. It also allows a focused, cardiac-specific education of medical trainees, nurses and paramedical staff.

In an institution that had used a conventional critical care unit model for many years (London Health Sciences Centre, London, Ontario, Canada), adopting a specialized critical care unit model staffed by consultants in critical care, cardiac surgery and cardiac anaesthesiology was beneficial. Specifically, there was no change in mortality rates, but the rate of major complications and the duration of postoperative mechanical ventilation decreased.

Postoperative pain management of cardiac surgical patients has traditionally been opioid-based and nurse controlled. As patient-controlled analgesia (PCA) has been shown to be as effective in controlling pain postoperatively in the cardiac population, it may be that utilizing PCA more widely will decrease the nurse–patient ratio, thereby lowering costs.

Delays in diagnosis of postoperative complications can lead to substantial increases in morbidity and mortality. Therefore, it is important to establish a diagnosis as quickly as possible in haemodynamically unstable patients and initiate appropriate treatment as soon as possible. Transoesophageal echocardiography is an invaluable tool in these circumstances.

Strategies to reduce the cost of cardiac surgery and recovery

Off-pump coronary artery bypass surgery

Off-pump CABG may significantly decrease the incidence of postoperative atrial fibrillation, transfusion, inotrope requirements, respiratory infections, ventilation time, critical care unit LOS and hospital LOS when compared with conventional CABG. The subset of high-risk patients undergoing off-pump CABG additionally may have a lower rate of stroke, myocardial infarction, renal dysfunction and reoperation for bleeding when compared with conventional on-pump surgery. Because all of these factors are associated with more intense resource utilization, reducing them causes a corresponding decrease in the overall cost of CABG surgery by 15% to 35% when compared with conventional on-pump CABG.

Early tracheal extubation after cardiac surgery

In the 1970s, it was possible to extubate cardiac surgical patients within a few hours postoperatively because inhalational anaesthesia was mainly used. Cardiorespiratory complications were, however, not uncommon, probably because of the surgical techniques of the time. In the 1980s, opioid-based cardiac anaesthesia became popular because of the marked haemodynamic stability afforded by this technique as well as the concern about isoflurane-induced coronary steal. This led to an obligatory period of postoperative mechanical ventilation, often for longer than 12 to 24 hours. Concerns about the safety of extubation within a few hours (like in the 1970s) have always been present; but several studies have now shown that early extubation is safe and may decrease costs substantially.

The optimal time to extubate in relation to cost depends on the institution, and has a greater impact if the patient can be discharged from the critical care unit after extubation, or the level of care (nurse to patient ratio). Early extubation of the trachea is indeed important, but it is equally important to realize that the factor that provides the most cost-savings is a reduction in the critical care unit and hospital LOS. Therefore, the key step for effective resource management is having a clinical pathway in place that focuses on the protocols necessary for early recovery and extubation after cardiac surgery, rather than the physical act of removing a patient's endotracheal tube.

Rational use of pharmaceuticals

Drugs represent about 7% of the annual total operating costs of most hospitals, and their cost has increased by approximately 10% yearly since 1997. An issue related to the additional drugs available to the clinician is an increase in adverse drug reactions that consumes resources. A cost-effective method to encourage rational drug use is to have a dedicated pharmacist in the critical care unit, assisting with prescribing. Employing a pharmacist is associated with up to 60% reduction in the incidence of drug-related adverse events! Other strategies to reduce hospital costs related to drugs have been studied such as:

- prophylactic administration of antibiotics (even if there is no agreement of which agent to use!) – this reduces infection rate (including sternal wound) by a factor of 5; and
- use of antifibrinolytics to reduce postoperative transfusion rate.

Not all strategies have proven cost effective, and some are controversial, such as:

- prophylactic use of erythropoietin to reduce the rate of transfusion of allogeneic blood products – this has been shown in one study to increase cost by 50%; and
- administration of prophylactic amiodarone to reduce the incidence of postoperative atrial fibrillation.

Nursing care

Nursing care is the most expensive cost in the critical care unit, accounting for about 50% of overall direct critical care budget. Nursing resources should therefore be used in a cost-effective way. Early tracheal extubation may reduce nursing costs by about 25% because nurses can be shifted to the care of more acutely ill patients, and the nurse–patient ratio can be changed from 1:1 to 1:2 more readily. For optimum resource utilization, nursing management needs to support single-day critical care stay, transfer of selected patients and flexible nursing rotas. The use of CIS may also help decrease the workload of nursing staff.

Key points

- Cost containment is a major goal of sustainable health care.
- Many areas in the care of a cardiac surgical patient are amenable to interventions that maintain or improve the quality of the health care received while simultaneously decreasing cost.
- The main goals of resource management in critical care are early tracheal extubation, the rational use of pharmaceuticals, a flexible nursing model, and effective patient flow facilitated by clinical pathways and protocols.

FURTHER READING

Cheng DCH, and David TE. *Perioperative care in cardiac anesthesia and surgery*. Philadelphia: Lippincott Williams & Wilkins; 2005.

Chapter 68

Education and training in cardiothoracic critical care in the United Kingdom

J. CORDINGLEY AND C. GILLBE

Introduction

Cardiothoracic critical care has developed to provide a service to patients in the perioperative period of a cardiothoracic surgical episode. It is therefore natural this has been predominantly led by the surgeons and anaesthetists managing the patients in the operating room.

Traditionally, the cardiothoracic surgical patient has been cared for by an informal system in which the responsible surgeon cooperates to a greater or lesser degree with the anaesthetic team in the critical care area. This model is now changing as patients are older and sicker and as cardiothoracic critical care achieves increasing recognition as a specialist area of practice. Quite commonly, initial management is carried out by the cardiothoracic surgical team, with patients formally transferred to the critical care team after 24 to 48 hours.

Level of care

Increasingly, there is a perceived divide between relatively low-risk patients having surgery and higher risk patients with an anticipated high level of postoperative dependency. Different care pathways are appropriate for these groups of patients, always accepting that the occasional patient in the lower risk group will require prolonged intensive care.

This may mean that the critical care unit can be divided into separate areas with different staffing levels, depending on the patient population. Alternatively, the low-risk patients could be admitted to a different unit altogether, as is the custom in a number of centres.

Workforce constraints

The European Working Time Directive has led to junior doctors working fewer hours in UK hospitals, with on-call time considered as time working, whether resident in the hospital or at home. From 2009, the maximum working week will be limited to 48 hours. This means that trainees, who have traditionally worked as resident intensive care doctors, will increasingly be working shift patterns. This has implications for the training of anaesthetists and, perhaps more so, for surgeons whose time in the operating theatre will be severely limited if they also work shift patterns in critical care.

This has led hospitals to consider alternatives to surgeons and anaesthetists in cardiothoracic critical care. The role of the critical care practitioner (CCP) has developed to meet this need. Senior critical care nurses have undertaken further training at a high level to qualify as practitioners. Local protocols have been implemented allowing them to manage patients independently, including prescribing a limited number of drugs, fluids and blood products. This is especially the case in low-risk patients who recover quickly from surgery and may be weaned from ventilation and extubated without recourse to medical staff. Employment of CCPs may allow a reduction in the number of resident medical staff

Table 68.1 Level of critical care for adult patients

Level	Characteristics
0	Patients whose needs can be met through normal ward care in an acute hospital.
1	Patients at risk of their condition deteriorating, or those recently relocated from higher levels of care, whose needs can be met on an acute ward with additional advice and support from the critical care team.
2	Patients requiring more detailed observation or intervention including support for a single failing organ system or postoperative care and those 'stepping down' from higher levels of care.
3	Patients requiring advanced respiratory support alone or basic respiratory support together with support of at least two organ systems. This level includes all complex patients requiring support for multiorgan failure.

in the unit and may result in fewer calls to these staff during their working shift.

Medical staff

Currently, patients are managed by a combination of surgeons, anaesthetists and nurses, often using a management system that is largely protocol driven.

ANAESTHETISTS

The anaesthetic curriculum includes a minimum of 9 months of intensive care training, but there is no requirement that any of this need be in a cardiothoracic critical care. There is a requirement for a 3-month period of cardiothoracic anaesthetic training, and this includes some immediate postoperative management. Anaesthetists wishing to practice cardiothoracic anaesthesia in the United Kingdom usually undertake a minimum of 15 months of training in cardiothoracic anaesthesia, and often more with many choosing to spend some time training abroad. During this time, they work a substantial amount of time in critical care, but very few choose further formal critical care training or qualification in addition to their anaesthetic requirements. This means that the majority of anaesthetic consultant staff who practice in cardiothoracic critical care have no formal intensive medicine accreditation.

SURGEONS

Cardiothoracic surgical trainees spend a significant part of their training time working in critical care. This is considered vital because of their role in managing their patients in critical care when they achieve consultant status. However, time for specialist cardiothoracic surgical training is significantly shorter, with current recommendations that it should be reduced to 6 years. This, together with working time directives, means that surgeons in training will spend less and less time in the operating theatre. Therefore, many programs are limiting the time spent by surgical trainees in critical care units to maximize operating experience.

A new intercollegiate surgical curriculum is being developed. This sets out an ambitious syllabus that includes many of the technical competencies required for the management of patients in the critical care, but without specifically committed critical care training time. Trainees are expected to acquire these skills as part of the regular training program. For instance, surgical trainees are expected to achieve competence in the following areas:

- orotracheal intubation,
- rigid and fibreoptic bronchoscopy,
- arterial and central venous cannulation, and
- transoesophageal echocardiography.

There is therefore doubt as to whether the critical care components of the intercollegiate surgical curriculum can be delivered in addition to the surgical skills against the backdrop of reduced training time.

INTENSIVE CARE SPECIALISTS

The management of marginal or frank multiple organ failure during recovery from the surgical procedure is by necessity a complex and specialist area. There is increasing realization that intensive care specialists should provide this care, working in close relationship with the cardiothoracic anaesthetist and surgeon.

Recently published literature suggests that the management of cardiothoracic critical care by specialist critical care consultants leads to:

- a reduction in mortality, length of stay, complications and costs;
- more referrals to specialist teams;
- introduction of protocols with a view to improving quality and cost;
- fewer complications of invasive procedures; and
- streamlined and standardized admission and discharge policies.

Publications have estimated that switching from critical care management by the primary specialist to an intensivist-managed model is associated with a relative reduction in mortality rates between 15% and 60%. This has led to a substantial increase in the number of units staffed exclusively by critical care specialists.

Specialist training

Training in intensive care in the United Kingdom is now supervised by the Intercollegiate Board for Training in Intensive Care Medicine (IBTICM), which is regulated by the Medical Royal Colleges. Specifically, its remit is to determine the duration, content and assessment of training in intensive care medicine and to recommend minimum standards for intensive care units recognized by the Colleges for training. The IBTICM recognizes two levels of training in intensive care medicine, intermediate and advanced. The latter, along with competitive appointment and the acquisition of appropriate complementary specialties can lead to certification in intensive care medicine jointly with another specialty.

Principles of IBTICM training

The underlying principles of training in intensive care medicine are compatible with those laid down by the Postgraduate Medical Education and Training Board.

PATIENT SAFETY

The duties, working hours and supervision of trainees must be consistent with the delivery of high-quality, safe patient care.

QUALITY ASSURANCE, REVIEW AND EVALUATION

Postgraduate training must be quality controlled locally by deaneries, working with others as appropriate, for example, medical Royal Colleges/Faculties and specialty associations.

EQUALITY, DIVERSITY AND OPPORTUNITY

Postgraduate training must be fair and based on principles of equality.

RECRUITMENT, SELECTION AND APPOINTMENT

Processes for recruitment, selection and appointment must be open, fair and effective; those appointed must be inducted appropriately into training.

DELIVERY OF CURRICULUM, INCLUDING ASSESSMENT

The requirements set out in the curriculum must be delivered and the trainee assessed.

SUPPORT AND DEVELOPMENT OF TRAINEES AND TRAINERS

Trainees must be supported to acquire the necessary skills and experience through induction, effective educational supervision, an appropriate workload and time to learn.

MANAGEMENT OF EDUCATION AND TRAINING

Education and training must be planned and maintained through transparent processes that show who is responsible at each stage.

EDUCATIONAL RESOURCES AND CAPACITY

The educational facilities, infrastructure and leadership must be adequate to deliver the curriculum.

OUTCOMES

The impact of the standards must be tracked against trainee outcomes and clear linkages should be reflected in developing standards.

Entry to the program

Trainees must enter the certification program by appointment after open competition as laid down by national regulations. In the future, it may be possible to apply directly for a joint specialty-training program of intensive care medicine and one of the specialties of primary appointment at entry to Specialist Training. Similarly, it may be possible in the future to apply for a single specialty certification in intensive care medicine.

Structure of the program

The competency-based training program in intensive care medicine requires

- intensive care medicine training;
- anaesthesia training for doctors whose specialty of primary appointment is medicine, an acute surgical specialty or emergency medicine;
- general medicine training for doctors whose specialty of primary appointment is anaesthesia, an acute surgical specialty or emergency medicine; and
- certification in one of the specialties of primary appointment of Emergency Medicine, Anaesthesia, Medicine or an Acute Surgical Specialty.

Assessment

Formal assessment is now carried out using workplace observation and regular reviews. The workplace assessments focus on knowledge, skills, attitudes and behaviour. The competencies required at an early stage of training are mainly of knowledge and practical skills; at a later stage trainees are required to display broader professional attributes.

The four validated assessment tools that are likely to be included in specialty training assessments are multisource feedback, the mini clinical evaluation exercise, direct observation of procedural skills and case-based discussion.

Future changes

The IBTICM proposes to establish a run-through training program in Intensive Care Medicine and has begun work on a curriculum to this effect. The current intention is that it will begin with the 2-year Acute Care Common Stem, comprising 6 months each of Acute Medicine and Emergency Medicine, and a year of Intensive Care Medicine/Anaesthesia that may comprise up to 9 months of either component. The remaining 5 years of the program will probably have the following components:

- general internal medicine and medical specialties (cardiology, respiratory, renal and hepatic medicine);
- anaesthesia (including exposure to each of cardiac, neuro-anaesthesia, paediatric anaesthesia, major general surgery);
- intensive care medicine;
- imaging module;
- clinical laboratory sciences; and
- surgery as applied to intensive care medicine.

The course will significantly be based on the Competency Based Training for Intensive Care for Europe curriculum that has been developed by the European Society for Intensive Care Medicine.

Qualifications

The current structure of postgraduate medical education and training in the United Kingdom does not include examination in ICM as a prerequisite to practice in intensive care. Nonetheless, increasing numbers of trainees choose to sit one of the two available examinations, the European or the UK Diploma in Intensive Care Medicine, to demonstrate commitment to the specialty. These examinations are qualitatively different.

The European Diploma

The European Diploma has been available since 1989 and now attracts more than 100 candidates annually with a pass rate of approximately 80%. The examination was reviewed in 1994 and consists of two parts, a multiple choice question paper after a minimum of 12 months training, and a clinical and viva examination after 24 months.

The UK Diploma

The UK Diploma has been available since 1998 and attracts between 30 and 40 candidates each year. The prerequisites for sitting the examination are a previous success in the examination of the specialty of primary appointment and training recognized by IBTICM to at least intermediate level in ICM. Its popularity has been greatly enhanced by the institution of the CCT programme in ICM and the pass rate is usually more than 80%. It is taken towards the end of training and comprises three parts:

- Dissertation of 4,000 to 6,000 words and a viva thereon.
- Viva on expanded case summaries and clinical scenarios.
- Oral examination on structured domains.

Qualification in echocardiography

It is clear that echocardiography is an essential tool in intensive care medicine as well as the operating room. Many intensive care physicians therefore seek qualification and accreditation. There are three examinations available, each with differing criteria and expectations. These are managed by the British Society of Echocardiography, the European Association of Echocardiography and the National Board of Echocardiography,

The consultant post

Finally, for those who have left it too late in their primary specialty training, it must be remembered that it is not a requirement to be on the Specialist Register in the specialty of one's consultant appointment. It is therefore possible, for instance, for a certificate holder in cardiac surgery to apply successfully for a post in intensive care medicine. Appointment must be made on the basis of curriculum vitae, interview and references, all mapped against the personnel specification. For those who wish to follow this path, it would be appropriate to have covered the curriculum for training in intensive care medicine in an informal manner and to seek a letter of similarity of training from the IBTICM.

Key points

- Trained intensive care specialists caring for patients in cardiothoracic critical care may reduce mortality and length of stay.
- More formalized training allows ICM training jointly with other specialties.
- Examination by British or European Diploma and competency-based assessment is now a requirement of training.
- A formal run-through training program for intensive care medicine is under development.

FURTHER READING

British Society of Echocardiography [homepage on the Internet]. Available at: www.bsecho.org.

European Society of Cardiology [homepage on the Internet]. Available at: www.escardio.org.

European Society of Intensive Care Medicine [homepage on the Internet]. Available at: www.esicm.org/.

Intercollegiate Board of Training in Intensive Care Medicine, UK [homepage on the Internet]. Available at: www.ibticm.org/.

National Board of Echocardiography [homepage on the Internet]. Available at: www.echoboards.org.

SECTION 7 Ethics, Legal Issues and Research in Cardiothoracic Critical Care

Chapter 69

Patient's perspective

W.T. McBRIDE

Introduction

This chapter presents a frank and personal story of a consultant in cardiac anaesthesia and intensive care, who became a patient in his own critical care unit.

Preoperatively

While cutting an already fallen tree, a heavy branch crashed down on my left shoulder, crushing my back and leading to an unstable fracture of the 12th thoracic vertebra. The next day, I found myself in orthopaedic theatres in my own institution undergoing urgent spinal stabilization. A haemangioma identified at the fracture site meant that a further thoracoabdominal procedure was required through a left thoracotomy and laparotomy, with the eighth rib used to replace the body of fractured T12.

Preoperative concerns

Loss of dignity and control

Had I been asked before the accident, I would have preferred admission if required to any critical care unit other than the one in which I worked, due to a sense of embarrassment at loss of privacy before my colleagues. Nevertheless, faced with the harsh reality of making such a decision, I opted for my own unit where I knew the nurses and doctors so well. Knowing that I was not going to be there as a stranger was reassuring.

Concerns regarding my loved ones

I was worried about my elderly parents coming in and out of the critical care unit and arranged in advance for a family friend to accompany them. I later discovered that this is a significant concern, experienced by 71% of patients.

Fearing the worst, including death

I have often marvelled at the courage of my patients when facing high-risk surgery, and never speculated as to how I myself would react in such a situation. As an anaesthetist, I knew about the likelihood of considerable blood loss from the haemangioma with its attendant risks. I was also aware of the possibility of being paralysed during the procedure, although neither mortality nor morbidity were discussed with me in advance. I was spared that formality because my team knew that I understood the risks perfectly well! I had the highest respect and confidence for the team of surgeons and for my anaesthetist, who had incidentally taught me well during my training. Although I fully expected to make a swift and uncomplicated recovery, I was aware of the possibility of fatal complications. Accordingly, to spare my loved ones any concerns, I privately asked a good friend and Bible teacher to carry out my funeral service just in case that was needed.

The comfort of faith

As a diligent student from school days of the original Biblical languages, I found myself searching the familiar pages of my beloved Hebrew Bible for reassurance the night before surgery. I was not disappointed, although I knew that the next few days might be a test of my faith.

Postoperatively

Of course, I knew exactly where I was going to be nursed postoperatively, the ventilators that would be used and the procedures in place. My first recollection after surgery was while I was still ventilated. I recall feeling that I was in a very bright room albeit with my eyes closed. I felt uncomfortably warm. I was aware that I was being ventilated. I had no sense of discomfort from the endotracheal tube. However, I would have liked to breathe more quickly but was powerless to do this or signal my 'air hunger' to whoever was at the bedside. I rationalized that someone would realize that my $Paco_2$ was going up and would increase the ventilator rate. Remarkably, there was no sense of fear. Everything seemed to be under control and I felt completely relaxed and at ease. I recall moving my feet and feeling a sense of pleasure and relief that I was not paralysed. Later my colleagues were able to tell me that I moved my feet to command in the critical care and smiled around the endotracheal tube when I realized that I could move them. I have no recollection of anyone telling me to move my feet or indeed smiling, although I still distinctly remember the relief at knowing that I was not paralysed. Somewhere at this stage I coughed and I became aware of a sharp searing pain down my left side – the thoracotomy pain! I coughed on the tube again and felt an intense choking sensation: I still was able to rationalize that someone would do something quickly to help me out, such as increase the propofol infusion. I expect this is what happened, as very quickly I fell deeply asleep. Throughout all of this, my knowledge of critical care unit management proved important in allowing me to rationalize the circumstances I was experiencing.

At another point while being ventilated I recall feeling myself increasingly warm and with a considerably heightened awareness of wanting to breathe more but being unable to do so – quite an uncomfortable feeling. I could hear one of my surgical registrar colleagues who is a good friend saying, 'He's very septic.' That did not surprise me; I felt really ill. Interestingly, as I look back on this development, despite feeling utterly helpless I do not recall feeling any sense of fear. Moreover, I knew that whatever needed to be done would be done. Afterwards, when I related this experience to my friend, he was concerned that he had alarmed me. I was able to reassure him that his comment did not trouble me – if anything it was reassuring to know that the sepsis had been recognized.

After extubation

I have no conscious memory of being extubated the next day, although my colleagues tell me that when I was told that the endotracheal tube was coming out I smiled around the tube again and signalled with thumbs up that I approved of this. I experienced quite significant pain postoperatively, especially if I moved or was moved onto my left side. A morphine infusion was in process and the pain was less severe when not moving. In fact, I was pleasantly relieved that pain was not as I had suspected or feared. However, my main battle that day was with unremitting nausea and hallucinations.

Hallucinations and vivid dreams

On a small trolley beside the bed was a 'Neofract' jacket prepared preoperatively for me to wear during mobilization. When I closed my eyes, I had a recurrent and frighteningly realistic dream that this was a headless and limbless human body, which was being carved away for human consumption. I discovered that if my eyes were open that this did not happen so I tried in vain to keep awake. Again I had a recurrent dream of men wheeling people (dead or alive, I was not sure) very quickly in metal trolleys along long corridors. Remarkably, various teams would meet as they wheeled their human cargo and briefly engage each other in rapid conversation in foreign languages – although I have no memory of the content of these 'conversations.' In contrast with my time on the ventilator when I was entirely calm and free of fear, this period of confusion was accompanied by an unpleasant and completely irrational emotion of deep foreboding, none of which I felt free (at the time) to express to my caregivers. Nevertheless, my nursing colleagues who cared for me will probably never know that their calm and reassuring care helped me through that time.

I was under the impression that no one knew what I was thinking and at the time I was too disturbed to share my horror with anyone else. Later, the critical care sister was able to tell me that the staff knew I was not my usual self and suspected confusion. If I talked any nonsense, to this day they have not told me!

In a moment of lucidity, I wondered if it was the morphine infusion that was causing the problem so I asked for the morphine to be discontinued. Given the choice of pain or hallucinations I would warmly have embraced severe pain as a welcome friend, so frightening were these dreams. Obligingly, the morphine was stopped and the expected severe pain did not materialize, probably owing to alternative analgesics prescribed.

Discharge to the ward

Four days later I was discharged from the critical care unit to the ward. The following night, the unpleasant sense of impending doom came over me again. There was no rational reason for this emotion. I called the nurse and asked if she could keep an eye on me throughout the night. Her gentle reassurance meant everything. In the early hours of the morning I opened my eyes to find the nurse standing looking worried at the side of the bed. "Are you all right?" she asked. "You've been talking all night and I haven't understood one word you said" she went on.

Going home

One month after the injury I was home again. Every step was painful but paracetamol and diclofenac proved highly effective. For the first few weeks I was afflicted with nightmares. One recurring dream was of me disappearing into an underground car-park where the passageway seemed to get narrower and narrower until I was wedged head first in this tight dark tunnel. In my efforts to escape I would struggle in my sleep flinging myself across the bed violently until the pain in my wound woke me. On one occasion I flung myself out of the bed but escaped serious injury by being caught in the bedclothes. Thereafter, I made sure there were chairs at the side of the bed to prevent me falling.

Rehabilitation

I wonder if this bizarre tunnel dream reflected my sense of pain and claustrophobia in the tube of the MRI scanner a few days before my second operation. In those dark days, it was by no means clear if I would make a full recovery. I was concerned lest sleep disturbance and constant pain could feed into depression. I resolved to fight this. There was only one direction – that was forwards. I was determined not to sit at home in self-pity. I agreed to honour a commitment to give a talk at a congress in Belfast organized by my colleagues 2 weeks after hospital discharge. Well loaded with analgesics, and with a trembling hand, I delivered the presentation. The mental challenge of this was highly therapeutic. Three months later I was to talk on thoracic trauma at the Association of Cardiothoracic Anaesthetists meeting in Cambridge. The preparation for this was again most effective in my rehabilitation. Meeting all my old friends was very enjoyable, although at the time I did not like talking about the accident. At the time I did not find resurrecting the memories of this at all helpful. Immediately thereafter, and with the encouragement of my surgeon, I went on a holiday to Vancouver, planned well before the accident. Standing on the snows at the top of

Whistler mountain with friends holding on to each arm, I felt moved by the stupendous view and the invigorating effect of the still mountain air. My surgeon was absolutely right: it was just the experience I needed to finally consign the memory of my injury and subsequent critical care unit experience to a safe and manageable distance. From that moment onwards, I knew my physical and psychological recovery would be complete. Three months later I was back at work.

Discussion

Preoperative preparation

In my case, preoperatively acquired knowledge helped enormously to keep me serene and understand my circumstances during the times that I was aware of being mechanically ventilated. In the non-medically trained patient, it is all the more important to ensure adequate preoperative explanations of the routine procedures within critical care to help minimize anxiety.

I did not need preoperative visits from my critical care nursing colleagues as I already knew them all, but in general such visits can help to reduce anxiety.

There is increasing awareness of the need for medical and nursing staff, however secular in outlook, to at least be aware of and respectfully sensitive to the potential spiritual needs of their patient particularly at a time of emotional vulnerability.

My time on the ventilator

I do recall coughing while on the ventilator and experiencing a choking sensation at that time. I do not know if this accompanied chest physiotherapy or not. However, the literature highlights chest physiotherapy and endotracheal tube suction as being especially uncomfortable in the ventilated patient. Care with this procedure and accompanying reassurance and explanation are essential. My ability to respond to commands such as 'move your feet,' and be aware of my colleague saying, 'he's very septic,' emphasizes that ventilated and sedated patients may still be aware of their surroundings. Staff should be vigilant when talking in close proximity to patients. On the other hand, understanding of conscious auditory awareness in the sedated patient can be helpful for relatives who can be encouraged to whisper reassuring words in the ear of their sedated and unconscious loved one. It was many weeks later that I learned that during my time on the ventilator I was pyrexial with a high platelet count and early systemic inflammatory response to sepsis (SIRS) picture. This explains my sense of feeling ill and very hot, and the deeply uncomfortable feeling of air hunger while on the ventilator. It was a relief to lose consciousness at that time and retreat into the refuge of propofol sedation. My experience certainly highlights the importance of adequate sedation.

Dreaming in the critical care unit

Vivid and disturbing dreams, hallucinations or delusions are common with recollection of these as high as 44%. Objective diagnosis of this is difficult with observed delirium not associated with recollection of such dreams. Contributing factors include sedatives and analgesics, although sepsis, endocrine and electrolyte imbalance all contribute. Long after pain has been forgotten, the horrors of hallucinations and vivid dreams live on. Often the patient may feel that he or she is going mad and is thus afraid to express these 'unreal' experiences. It is especially helpful for a patient to describe these experiences to an understanding doctor or nurse and to be reassured that this experience is not uncommon and merely reflects the severity of the patient's illness. Such reassurance usually brings relief to the patient, who may even have feelings of guilt, especially about things they may recall saying during the mists of confusion. Routine follow-up of critical care patients may alleviate the effects of these potentially terrifying delusions. My personal experience has led me routinely to inquire of my patients as to whether or not they have been having troubling dreams or managing to sleep peacefully enough. Such an open-ended question often provides the trigger for the patient to unload this worry. Any patient for whom this is a particular problem could eventually be referred to a clinical psychologist.

Post-traumatic stress disorder

Recollection of unpleasant ICU experiences may compromise quality of life after critical care discharge. Support should be available to hasten a patient's neuropsychological recovery. In my own case, no formal diagnosis of post-traumatic stress disorder (PTSD) was given to me, but clearly this describes my neuropsychological status for the first few weeks after my return home. I quickly realized that active recollection of the stressful events, whether the accident itself or the hallucinations, was distinctly unhelpful. As a result of my personal experiences, I now encourage any patients who share with me their experiences of hallucinations or show signs of PTSD to press forwards and not look backwards in their recollection. I advise setting targets such as deadlines for excursions to the seaside, holidays and so on.

Key points

These personal experiences emphasize the need for

- Careful preoperative explanations of the critical care experience.
- Critical care staff where possible to meet the patient preoperatively.
- Care in speaking in close proximity to a sedated ventilated patient.
- Heightened awareness of delirium as a symptom.
- Caregivers to allow opportunity for patients to express concerns regarding nightmares and hallucinations so that the appropriate counselling and reassurance can be given.
- Long-term follow-up of the critical care patient several weeks after discharge to allow management of PTSD if still present.

Acknowledgement

The author wishes to record his grateful thanks to all the medical and nursing staff involved in his care both in the operating theatre and in the critical care unit at the Royal Victoria Hospital Belfast. Their devotion and professionalism was truly outstanding.

FURTHER READING

Clark C, Heidenreich T. Spiritual care for the critically ill. *Am J Crit Care* 1995;4:77–81.

Löf L, Berggren L, Ahlström G. Severely ill ICU patients recall of factual events and unreal experiences of hospital admission and ICU stay – 3 and 12 months after discharge. *Intensive Crit Care Nurs* 2006;22:154–166.

Pattison N. Psychological implications of admission to critical care. *Br J Nurs* 2005;14: 708–714.

Richter JC, Waydhas C, Pajonk FG. Incidence of post-traumatic stress disorder after prolonged surgical intensive care unit treatment. *Psychosomatics* 2006;47:223–230.

Roberts BL, Rickard CM, Rajbhandari D, *et al.* Patients' dreams in ICU: recall at two years post discharge and comparison to delirium status during ICU admission. A multicentre cohort study. *Intensive Crit Care Nurs* 2006;22: 264–273.

Van de Leur JP, Zwaveling JH, *et al.* Patient recollection of airway suctioning in the ICU: routine versus a minimally invasive procedure. *Intensive Care Med* 2003;29:433–436.

Chapter 70

Ethical management

W.E. SCOTT

Introduction

Most doctors, wherever they work, subscribe to the tenets of beneficence and nonmaleficence (*Primum non nocere* – first do no harm). There is the desire to help, to try to heal, without doing further harm. However, critical care staff have to be ruthlessly realistic about what is possible, as opposed to what is desirable, and resist the temptation to play God. Public expectations are on the increase, particularly as new treatments and cures are announced in the media regularly. The delay in such treatments becoming mainstream is variable and the time it takes for drugs to gain their product licence is often financially driven. There is the constant feeling of frustration that something that would make a seminal difference to a particular patient is just out of reach. Had they contracted their illness next year it could have been different.

Critical care, in a sense, embodies and concentrates many of the ethical issues and concerns that are prevalent but just more diluted, throughout the rest of the hospital. Because it is a highly charged place where life-and-death decisions are made on a daily basis, it is also the place where the need for professionalism is of particular importance. There is the risk, however, that the wall of professionalism becomes the barrier beyond which the carers cannot afford to go in preservation of their own emotions, feelings and often sanity.

WARNING: Each country has its own laws and this chapter cannot account for all variations in practices.

Admission/discharge criterion

A doctor's duty is to their patient, to the individual that is in their care at a particular time. There is a limitation on beds in critical care units so some kind of screening process for entry is essential. The patient has to be 'sick enough' to justify entry, but not too sick (so certain to die or where intensive treatment is futile) that admission to critical care is inappropriate.

Often the final decision about whether a patient is treated in critical care is the result of a combination of factors that, although not ideal, is the reality. A patient cannot be treated in critical care if there is no bed – no matter how ill they are. Decisions have to be made as to whether an existing patient can be discharged prematurely (and thus their condition may potentially be compromised), whether there is a 'less sick' patient than the person requiring admission and the 'less sick' patient could therefore be transferred to another unit, making room for the new admission, or whether it is the new patient that should be transferred even if their condition is severe and transfer is dangerous. These are not easy decisions; each patient has the right to the best possible care for them. In this scenario, someone's health is going to be compromised each time.

Futility and APACHE scoring

Futility is understood in medical terms as the concept that any ongoing treatment is not likely to benefit the patient. It is a medical decision but one that has been challenged in the courts. The clinical decision that a patient is too sick to be admitted to critical care is a very difficult one to make, and the majority of the time the patient will be admitted for further assessment and commencement of treatment. Response to initial treatment may allow more accurate decision making. A scoring system of likelihood of survival does not make the case for an individual patient. The current Applied Physiology and Chronic Health Evaluation (APACHE II) conveys the probability of survival and does not determine whether admission to critical care is indicated or not.

Treatment and its burdens – what is too great a burden?

There may come a point during a patient's treatment that even though the therapeutic road has not been fully exhausted, the cost to the individual is too great. The patient has 'had enough.' The paternalistic approach once so prevalent is no longer acceptable morally or legally. The patient's autonomy should always be paramount. It is more difficult when the patient is a child because someone other than the child has to make the decision as to whether treatment is too burdensome. The medical profession and the parents may hold differing opinions.

Consent issues – and what constitutes assault?

Consent in critical care is a difficult issue as patients are often unconscious, sedated or too ill to allow staff to gain valid consent. For consent to be valid, it means the patient should have been given the necessary information in a form that is readily understood by them (in the correct language or have an interpreter to translate), has had time to understand it and have the mental capacity to do so. Relatives often want to be involved in the decision making regarding the management of their loved one. It is certainly good medicine to keep relatives informed and involved, but two different factions of a family may request different things, one to let the relative die, one to fight on. Relatives do not have the right to sign consent forms for adult patients. In some countries, a living will may have been completed before admission and an executor may have been appointed to help the decision making process.

A properly completed living will is legally binding, and treating a patient against their will is assault. This is so whether it is taking blood from a patient or maintaining their life on a ventilator.

End-of-life issues/the right to life

A competent patient has the right to say whether treatment should be withdrawn. This is true whether or not the outcome will lead to the death of the patient. What exercises some doctors is whether refusal to treat because treatment would be futile, or stopping treatment once initiated, is morally different. Although withdrawing treatment may be emotionally harder to do, especially in a patient in whom a great deal of time and energy has been invested, ethically it is no different than not initiating treatment in the first place – providing both courses of action are in the best interests of the patient. Withholding or withdrawing treatment can be distressing not only for relatives but for those involved in caring for the patient.

The role of the clinical ethics committee

In complicated cases, it should not be left to the staff of the critical care unit to make all the difficult decisions. Some hospitals have a clinical ethics committee and although the decision whether to initiate treatment may have to be made in a hurry, the decision to withdraw treatment can be made after careful consideration by all concerned, including the clinical ethics committee. It is as well to involve the hospital solicitors at this stage as then they can decide if a ruling from the courts is indicated.

Off-licence drug usage

Because critical care is at the cutting edge of treatment and management, drugs may be considered useful that have not been granted a product licence for use for that particular indication. It is a slightly confused area. Drug companies have no responsibility if the drug is used for a nonlicenced use. The hospital may not be happy to apply their indemnity if it feels the clinicians have been cavalier or careless in their use of a drug. Drugs and therapeutics committees in a hospital, while seeing their role as overseeing the use and misuse of drugs, can be ultraconservative in their agreement to the use of drugs outside their product licence. Delicate negotiation may be necessary. The veto put on the use of drugs considered to be too expensive also can introduce disagreement between the intensivists and the committee (rationing issue). It is always more sensible to have a consensus agreement among the intensivists for the use of a particular drug used outside its product licence so one doctor does not put themselves at particular risk of litigation. It helps to discuss its intended use with the family, who, although they cannot insist on treatment, are less inclined to sue should the patient die if they have been involved in the decision-making processes.

Pressures on staff

Critical care staff are highly trained individuals, so when there are decisions to be made, difficult or otherwise, it is hardly surprising that there may be more than one opinion about a course of treatment. It is possible for two opinions to be different, but still both morally justified. Critical care can become dysfunctional when a clinician works in isolation, disregarding the previous day's management of a patient and imposing their own decisions without listening to other peoples' opinions. Much more successful is the unit where there is a consistent strategy to a particular patient's treatment. This is achieved when there is the same team singing from the same song sheet over a period of time. Chopping and changing treatment because of change of personnel is not always helpful and may not be in the patient's best interests.

A good critical care unit has facilities to debrief staff at regular intervals, especially after a particularly harrowing death or the death of a person who has spent considerable time in critical care and to whom staff have become attached.

Choice and responsibilities of staff

Critical care staff have a duty of care to all patients in their care. This is paramount and precludes a doctor or nurse from refusing to treat a particular patient unless in very exceptional circumstances. Reluctance by staff to treat a particular patient may be due to fear for their own particular safety because there is a risk of contracting the disease (e.g. Avian flu) or because of moral disapproval of the patient's life style. Hospitals, as corporate institutions, have more recently accepted that there are some patients that collectively will be refused treatment. Those are patients who are deliberately abusive and violent to staff. A patient who becomes abusive or violent in critical care may, however, be suffering from psychosis, confusion or delusion. It would be a failure of duty not to treat them in this situation; therefore, careful analysis over a period of time is necessary and specialist advice from mental health care teams may be required. Staff are exposed to many hazards, including needle-stick injuries, exposure to radiation and musculoskeletal damage from lifting. Although the hospital must do everything possible to protect staff, staff themselves have an obligation and responsibility to comply with workplace regulations, for example, wearing lead aprons if helping with radiographs and attending manual handling courses. There is the need for mutual vigilance in this area. The vulnerability of the unconscious patient means an advocate is required to ensure treatment is given, the patient's dignity is maintained and there is respect for the whole person.

Nurses consider themselves to be the patient's advocate. That being so, they have an obligation to know as much about the person's culture, religion and personal wishes as is possible. A vegan may wish not to be given any drugs made from animal products, but how rigidly the belief is held must be ascertained. Would they rather die than be given animal products? Hindus would rather not be given Gelofusin. It contains gelatin, which is made from cows' feet. Has the patient who is also a Jehovah's Witness signed a written statement saying that no blood is to be given them at any cost? If so and the patient bleeds, they must not be given blood. That would also be assault, a criminal offence. If they are Sikh, is it important that their ceremonial daggers are near them?

Choice and responsibility of patients and their families

Critical care may mean that the patient has less choice in what is being done to them. Staff are not obliged to go looking into peoples' life styles and religions, but are obliged to respect them when the information is provided. By reading and assimilating the information given before elective admission, it can be assumed that, by agreeing to the surgery, the patient agrees to what will happen in critical care providing they have not brought up an objection to something before surgery. Relatives of competent individuals really do not have any real rights except those due to them of common courtesy, respect and to be kept informed.

Key points

- Resolution of differing ethical views is essential for each individual patient and good multidisciplinary team work is required.
- Mutual respect and conflict resolution is in the best interests of not only the patients but also the staff who work in a critical care unit.
- A living will is a binding document, and should be adhered to.
- Treatment against a patient's or their properly appointed advocate's wishes may be constituted as assault. If in doubt the hospital's solicitor should be consulted.

FURTHER READING

British Medical Association. *Medical ethics today*. London: Blackwell Publishing Ltd; 2003.

Draper H, Scott W. *Ethics in anaesthesia and intensive care*. London: Butterworth Heinemann; 2003.

General Medical Council UK [homepage on the Internet]. Good medical practice. Available at: www.gmc-uk.org.

Chapter 71

Medicolegal issues

A.F. MERRY AND D.A. SIDEBOTHAM

Introduction

Medicolegal issues are increasingly relevant to practice in critical care, and might lead to various processes within a variety of organizations. The law is complex and variable, and although some familiarity with relevant aspects of legislation is important, the details are probably beyond the grasp of most health care professionals. However, an understanding of the underlying medicolegal issues is usually a good guide to doing the right thing.

But in the end, the best legal defence in medicine is the appropriate care of one's patients.

Ethics, morality and the law

The complexity and variability of the law

Legislation varies between countries. In some countries the law, or a substantial part of it, is *codified*, or written down. In others, *common law* pertains, under which the legal position on most issues is not specified, but is determined from case law, on the basis of precedence. Even with codified law, interpretation and precedence are important. Furthermore, policy may have greater practical importance than the law itself.

The law and doing the right thing

Decisions involving life and death are commonplace in critical care and it can be difficult to know exactly how the law applies in the particular circumstances of each individual case. For example, euthanasia is illegal (and amounts to murder) in many countries, and legislation mandating the provision of 'the necessities of life' is common, yet the withdrawal of life-sustaining treatment (e.g. mechanical ventilation, intravenous fluids) occurs regularly. To make matters more difficult, the fact that a practice is legal and/or commonly accepted in one's own society or by one's own colleagues is not always a reliable guide to ethical practice. This point can be illustrated by the atrocities committed by some doctors in Nazi Germany (disclosed at the 1946 Nuremberg Medical Trials), who were working within the rules of their society at the time. Doctors, not only those who work in critical care, should never cease evaluating and reevaluating the ethical basis of their practices.

Ethics and moral philosophy – some basic concepts

Ethics is a field of study concerned with understanding values, morals, responsibilities and obligations.

A *dilemma* is a choice in which all options are bad, and may be resolvable (when one of the options is clearly less bad than the others) or irresolvable. Dilemmas may be ethical or practical.

Beauchamp and Childress enunciated four principles relevant to resolving ethical dilemmas in healthcare. Balancing these principles depends on the weight placed on each, and on which school of ethics one subscribes to, and is not always straightforward.

Table 71.1 Some of the organizations and processes that may (often or occasionally) deal with 'medicolegal' issues

The criminal courts	Criminal prosecutions
The civil courts	Suits for compensatory damages Suits for exemplary damages Suits for breaches of contracts
Employment courts	Hearings to resolve employment disputes
Coroner's courts	Inquests
Medical councils	Disciplinary processes Competency inquiries
Medical colleges and associations	Inquiries into alleged breeches of conduct or standards (rare)
Hospitals	Internal inquiries or disciplinary processes External inquiries
Others (country specific)	

Table 71.2 The four principles described by Beauchamp and Childress

Respect for autonomy A norm of respecting the decision-making capacities of autonomous persons
Nonmaleficence A norm of avoiding the causation of harm
Beneficence A group of norms for providing benefits and balancing benefits against risks and costs
Justice A group of norms for distributing benefits, risks and costs fairly

The issue of blood transfusion in Jehovah's Witnesses illustrates this. Autonomy dictates against giving blood (even to save a life), and it is generally expected that this overrides considerations of beneficence in adult patients who are clear about their wish to avoid transfusion. It is also generally expected that parents will act as surrogates in exercising children's right to autonomy. However, for children, beneficence is widely held to outweigh this right to autonomy, and transfusions to save life are often given to children, whatever the wishes of the parents, or at times even of the child.

Nevertheless, these four principles provide a useful framework for the analysis of ethical and medicolegal issues. Principles are general (e.g. avoid causing harm), but can be translated into rules, which are more specific (e.g. never actively kill a patient, but withdrawal of treatment may be acceptable in specified circumstances). Rules may be collected into codes of conduct.

Some basic legal concepts relevant to medicine

Doctors are deemed to have a *duty of care* in relation to their patients, and are expected to observe a reasonable standard of knowledge, skill and care in fulfilling that duty. *Negligence* is usually defined as a failure to meet this 'reasonable standard' and is termed 'gross' if the failure is substantial. Negligence does not imply insight. *Subjective recklessness* involves knowing that there is a risk, and choosing to take that risk nevertheless.

Objective recklessness implies an action in which the risk would be obvious to any reasonable person, and is similar in practice to gross negligence.

Battery is a *tort* or civil wrong involving the deliberate touching of another person without their consent. Many things done by doctors to patients would constitute battery (or the related crime of assault) in the absence of consent. However, there are limits to what the law condones on the basis of consent. For example, consent would not necessarily justify euthanasia.

The legal and regulatory response to adverse events

About 2% of patients admitted to hospital suffer an adverse event involving harm that is serious, avoidable and caused by health care; some (surprisingly few) of these patients complain. Complaints may also follow care that conforms to reasonable standards. Vexatious complainants do exist, but they are the exception. Most people who complain do so for understandable reasons, including concern with standards of care (often expressed as a desire to prevent similar incidents in the future), the need for an explanation, a desire for compensation and a belief that staff and organizations should have to account for their actions. Depending on the extent (if any) of negligence or recklessness involved when a patient is harmed, compensation, accountability and punishment may each be appropriate, to varying degree.

Deliberate harm to patients warrants criminal or disciplinary sanctions, but is very rare. In England, there has recently been an alarming increase in manslaughter charges against doctors, arising from unintentional accidents during the course of normal practice, which have lead to death (the criminal law has not often been evoked in relation to adverse events involving only injury to patients).

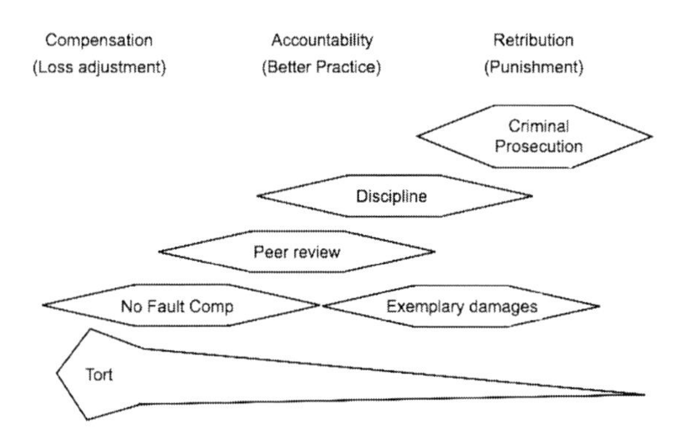

Figure 71.1 Dealing with accidental harm in health care. The elements of an appropriate response and some mechanisms by which these are usually provided (Reproduced with permission from Runciman *et al.*).

Informed consent

The *Bolam principle* held sway during much of the last century; it applied to medical practice in general and informed consent in particular. This was the standard of the reasonable doctor, established on the basis of support from some (not necessarily all or even most) responsible practitioners. It has increasingly given way to a reasonable patient standard for informed consent, and judges have assumed the right to override expert evidence, although this right is infrequently exercised. Information about the risks of the proposed treatment or procedure is important, but informed consent depends on also providing an outline of all reasonable alternatives (including the option of no treatment). Informed consent may be difficult to obtain. For instance, patients may not understand the information provided or may make it clear they do not want to receive information regarding risk. Also, patients forget what they have been told, and what patients consider reasonable disclosure of risk may change if they actually develop a complication. The courts tend to be sensitive to these difficulties, particularly if a conscientious attempt has been made to see matters from the perspective of the patient. In the context of critical care, it may often be impossible to obtain consent, because patients are frequently ventilated and sedated and because of the urgent nature of the problem. There are various approaches to this difficulty. It is usually reasonable to proceed with life-saving procedures without consent. However, appropriate explanations should be given, and the patient and family involved in decision making as soon as possible.

In critical care, it is not always obvious which procedures require explicit consent, and for which consent can be taken as implicit. For cardiac surgery, consent should be extended to cover related procedures and the possible need to treat complications such as postoperative bleeding. Practice varies considerably and local guidelines can be helpful.

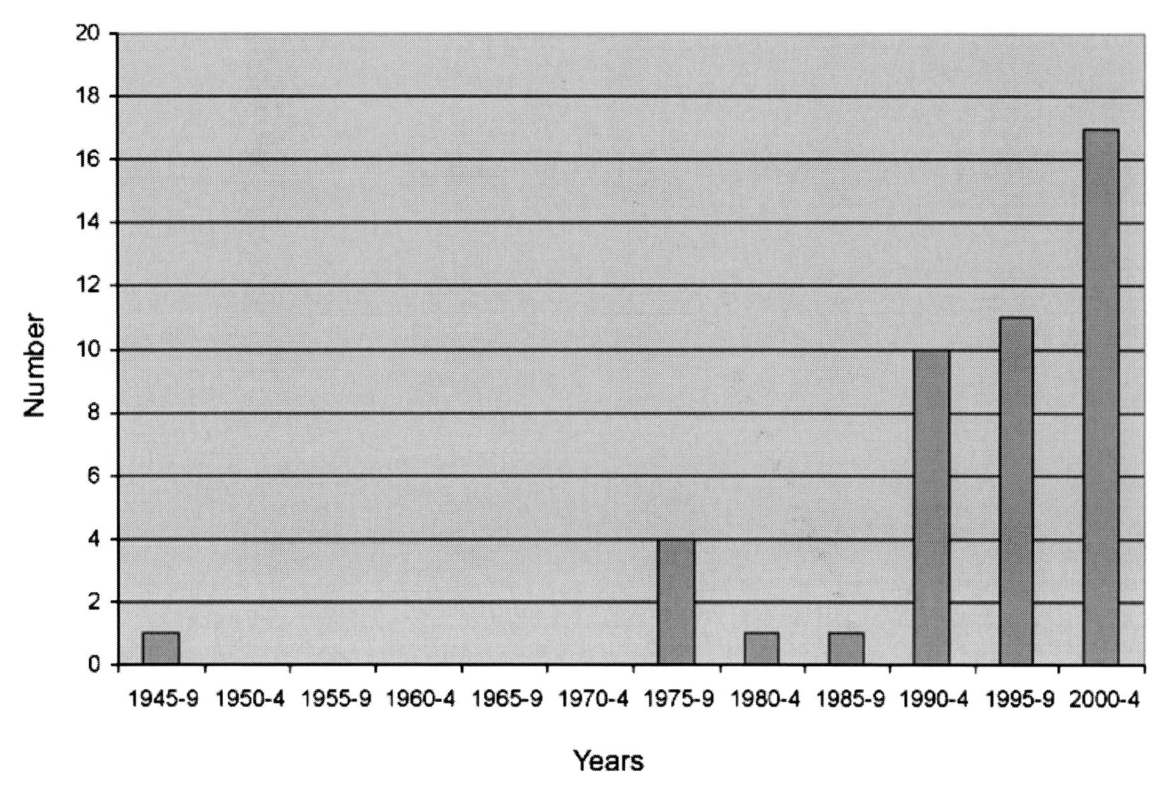

Figure 71.2 Number of doctors prosecuted for manslaughter in the United Kingdom in 5-year periods from 1945 to 2004. (Data provided by R.E. Ferner and S.E. McDowell, *J R Soc Med* 2006;99(6):309–314.) The recent increase in frequency of such prosecutions probably reflects a change in prosecution policy, because the law itself has not changed

Table 71.3 Approaches to consent in patients who do not have the capacity to provide it and for whom an enduring power of attorney has not been established

Substituted judgment Aiming to make the decision the incompetent person would make if he or she were competent; requires general evidence from previous communications (e.g. conversations, letters).
Pure autonomy As above, but requires explicit, relevant preferences expressed in advance (e.g. through a legally constituted advance directive).
Best interests Balancing the principles of beneficence and nonmaleficence; quality of life should be considered as well as the chances of survival.

End-of-life decisions

Any critically ill patient may die, and good end-of-life care should be considered at the same time as potentially life-saving therapies. Events that lead to rapid deterioration tend to create fewer dilemmas over prolonging life support than slow, progressive and inexorable deterioration. The concept of a *disease trajectory* may be helpful in determining the most appropriate balance between the objectives of 'cure' and 'comfort.' Both objectives can be pursued simultaneously, with the emphasis shifting from one to the other as the patient progresses along this trajectory. Attention to the non-medical needs of seriously ill patients should not be deferred until there is too little time for them to be met.

Table 71.4 Some components of end-of-life care important to patients and their family and close friends or other supporters
Communication
Sensitivity to language and potentially distressing terms such as 'withdrawal of care,' 'futility,' 'terminal care,' and 'passive euthanasia.'
Control of distressing symptoms
Continuity of care
Attention to emotional, psychological and spiritual needs
Access by family and close friends to the dying patient
Involvement of social workers, palliative care specialists, chaplains and other people who may assist in the nonmedical aspects of the care of the seriously ill patient
Evident compassion

Limiting and withdrawing treatment

At some point in a patient's disease trajectory, the question of withdrawing certain treatments may arise. If brain stem death is present, then, in most jurisdictions, it is reasonable to take the legal and ethical position that the patient is dead, and no dilemma arises. However, in cardiothoracic critical care, the great majority of patients who die are not brain dead. Furthermore, the lives of many desperately ill patients can be extended substantially by therapies such as ventilation, antibiotics, dialysis and mechanical cardiac support, even though this may not be in their best interests. Key principles are:

1. Care will never be withdrawn or limited, only specific therapies, and only for explicit reasons.
2. Medical knowledge is uncertain and patients may not die immediately after withdrawal of support.

Killing and letting die

The courts, and the public generally, endorse humane and sensible decisions to withdraw treatment that no longer serves the best interests of anyone, and decisions of this sort are made every day in critical care units around the world. However, the legal and ethical implications of such decisions can be subtle, and assertions made to justify them do not always withstand close scrutiny. A distinction is often made between:

- actively killing a terminally ill patient (euthanasia);
- deciding not to initiate life-supporting therapy; and
- withdrawing such therapy.

Critical care specialists (whatever their own view of the matter) should be aware that some credible moral philosophers reject the notion that there is any morally relevant difference between these three approaches to the humane management of the end of life, and any legal distinctions may also be less clear than some people imagine. The patient's wishes are clearly relevant. Patients who are competent to do so have the right to decline treatment, and doctors are generally obligated to respect such refusals (although the psychological status of the patient may need to be considered – the presence of severe depression may justify overriding patient autonomy, as in the immediate response to an attempted suicide, for example). It is not quite so clear that competent patients have the inalienable moral right to demand every possible treatment, in the face of a hopeless prognosis, and meeting such demands may be impossible for practical reasons. The necessity to balance autonomy with the requirements for (distributive) justice is widely recognized. Requests from competent patients for aid in dying are another matter again; it is generally accepted that doctors are not obligated to honour such requests. However, some moral philosophers hold that doctors may ethically elect to do so if they wish, at least in certain circumstances, and in some jurisdictions this is legal.

Organ donation

There a growing imbalance between the demand for and supply of organs for transplantation, and pressure to include donors that do not meet the criteria for brain stem death is growing.

The *dead donor rule* holds that it is unethical to cause death by procuring organs and unethical for organ procurement to precede death. Exceptions to the rule include the willing donation of organs (such as single kidneys) from living persons. Numerous ethical issues arise. The principle of autonomy suggests that it is a person's right to donate an organ, if he or she so wishes, but close family members of potential recipients may feel undue pressure to do this, at real personal risk. Poverty may also exert undue influence on a person's decision in this regard, and the purchase of organs is widespread in some parts of the world. This has been condemned by most commentators. Empirical evidence suggests that the money often does little to alleviate the poverty of paid donors. *Brain stem death* is widely taken as equating to death of the person (although that position has been disputed, primarily from certain religious perspectives). This view implies that there is therefore no question of precipitating or hastening death to obtain organs, and is supported by the fact that no one correctly diagnosed with brain stem death has ever recovered. An important corollary of this position is that criteria for brain death must be applied meticulously. All clinicians involved with organ procurement are advised to satisfy themselves that proper testing has been done and documented. The public is understandably nervous about organ donation, and an entire transplantation programme could be jeopardized by the publicity, which could follow even a single failure in this respect.

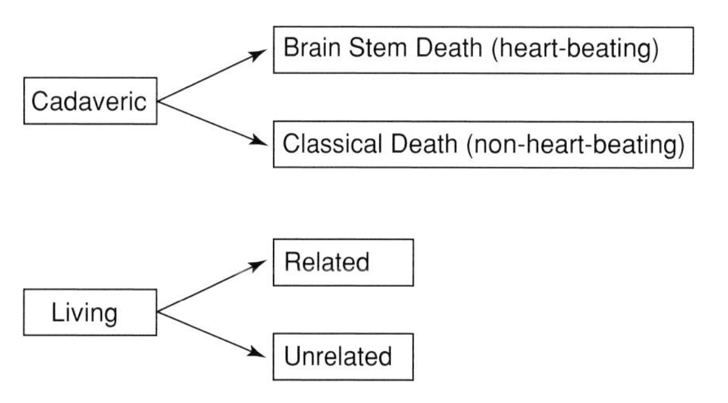

Figure 71.3 Categories of donor for transplantation of organs.

In the past, the viability of organs from patients who met brain stem death criteria was better than that of organs from non-heart-beating donors, but this is no longer necessarily the case for some organs (e.g. lungs). Non-heart-beating donation may be uncontrolled (in the context of sudden cardiac arrest), but this is generally impractical. In controlled non-heart-beating donation, permission is obtained to procure organs from patients in whom persistent treatment is no longer thought appropriate and death is considered inevitable. Support is then withdrawn, and the heart allowed to stop beating. After a certain length of time (which varies according to the criteria used) the patient is pronounced dead, and organ donation is deemed ethical and legal. This approach is fraught with difficulty.

Cardiac arrest is potentially reversible for considerable periods of time, but specifying longer periods before death can be diagnosed leads to reduced viability of the procured organs. Perfusion of the organs to be retrieved (e.g. via femoral cannulae) may circumvent this difficulty, but raises different connotations from simply allowing patients to die. In the end, society may have to choose between the benefits of organ donation and the moral disquiet associated with occasionally managing the end of life in such a way as to allow the procurement of satisfactory organs. Honesty about the issues is likely to allay some of the concerns of the public and will at least allow informed debate to occur.

Table 71.5 Issues that may raise legal and/or ethical difficulties in relation to the procurement of organs from non-heart-beating donors

Informed consent
The precise time of death, or of declaring dying as irreversible, may be unclear (note that meaningful resuscitation remains a possibility for considerable periods after cardiac arrest)
Irreversibility of death may be uncertain in the absence of brain stem death
Interventions to secure or enhance organ survival may hasten or delay the progression of dying
The possibility of sentience (which might be increased by interventions which improve cerebral perfusion, for example)
Maintenance of patients beyond the initial period of severe brain injury to allow brain stem death to declare itself could expand the permanent vegetative state population

Managing medicolegal risk

Responding to adverse events

All critical care units should have formal processes for dealing with complaints integrated into those of their hospital. Patients and their families should be informed of this process and of their rights (e.g. access to independent advocates and statutory ombudsmen). Ideally, this should occur before something goes wrong. Doctors, nurses and allied health staff should receive training in dealing with complaints. Complaints should be recorded, and when appropriate, other processes for responding to adverse events (such as root cause analysis) initiated. The aim should be to resolve complaints locally and promptly. If something goes wrong, most of the same processes can be used proactively, with the view of making a complaint unnecessary. Support is needed for all parties. Looking after the patient and his or her family is obviously the immediate priority. If serious harm has occurred, staff should not be left to continue a heavy load of other duties while stressed and preoccupied with the adverse event; they should be freed up to concentrate on the needs of the injured patient first, and then on their own emotional and medicolegal needs. They should consult their hospital's complaints officer early, and a lawyer (who should be independent of the hospital and whose interests may not align with those of staff). Medical indemnity organizations should be informed, and many will take a proactive role in providing advice on the optimal management of the situation. An early meeting with the complainant (together with family or other supporters) should be offered. The relevant staff members should attend, including someone with appropriate seniority (such as a senior critical care consultant) who was not directly involved in the incident. The presence of lawyers is not generally conducive to low-level resolution of medicolegal issues. The fact that the complainant feels aggrieved should be acknowledged empathically. A genuine apology (when appropriate) can be helpful in resolving complaints, and does not imply admission of liability (which should not occur without legal advice). Notes should be taken at the meeting, and a letter prepared in liaison with the complaints department and the consulted lawyer. It should summarise the discussion, outline a plan to resolve the complaint and include the options if the complainant wishes to take matters further.

Medical indemnity cover

All clinicians should have medical indemnity cover. Traditional insurance is based on highly specified contracts and provides a sense of certainty about the types of event covered, but the fine print is important. Not-for-profit organizations, such as the Medical Defence Union and the Medical Protection Society, provide *discretionary cover*. This concept may provoke some anxiety, but in practice allows the inclusion of events not foreseen by either party at the time the policy was bought. Cover for one's 'tail' is important to deal with complaints arising from previous events but laid in the period after one has stopped working. Experience in Australia, where several medical indemnity providers became insolvent, indicates that it is important to confirm the sound financial position of whichever organization one selects.

Key points

- The best preventative of medicolegal difficulties is the excellent care of patients; this implies proactive commitment to the quality of all aspects of critical care, with an emphasis on communication.
- Informed consent depends on providing an outline of all reasonable alternatives; this may be difficult to obtain in critical care.
- Humane and sensible decisions to withdraw treatment that no longer serves the best interests of the patient are generally supported by the legal system.
- Great care must be taken when diagnosing brain stem death, especially before organ donation; non-heart-beating donation is increasing but is fraught with difficulty.

FURTHER READING

Beauchamp TL, Childress JF. *Principles of biomedical ethics*. Oxford: Oxford University Press; 2001.

Manthous CA, DeGirolamo A, Haddad C, *et al.* Informed consent for medical procedures: local and national practices. *Chest* 2004;124: 1978–1984.

Merry AF, McCall Smith A. *Errors, medicine and the law*. Cambridge: Cambridge University Press; 2001.

Runciman W, Merry A, Walton M. *Safety and ethics in healthcare: A guide to getting it right*. Aldershot: Ashgate; 2007.

Chapter 72

Research

A.F. MERRY AND D.A. SIDEBOTHAM

Introduction

Because so many patients in critical care are very unwell, barriers to clinical research are created. Understandably, staff and patients (and their families) may feel that this is not the time for 'experiments,' and may be reluctant to deviate from practices thought optimal.

Cardiothoracic critical care is different from general critical care in that many of the admissions are planned and there is greater uniformity in the presentation of patients. On the other hand, the influences of surgery and anaesthesia have to be considered in any research design.

The need for research in critical care

Outcomes in critical care are improved by data-driven, evidence-based medicine (EBM).

Definition

One definition of EBM is that it is the conscientious, explicit and judicious use of current best evidence in making decisions about the care of individual patients. The practice of EBM means integrating individual clinical expertise with the best available external clinical evidence from systematic research. An important strategy to increase the implementation of EBM is the development and implementation of practice guidelines. This is a publishable form of research in itself that depends on understanding the principles of research in general. The steps involved include:

- defining the population and intervention of interest;
- conducting a systematic review of the literature;
- incorporating other forms of evidence;
- developing and implementing guidelines; and
- auditing compliance, and monitoring predefined outcomes before and after the introduction of the guidelines.

Types of evidence

There is a vogue for ranking evidence from different sources. This approach overlooks three points:

- the reliability of conclusions from any trial depends on its quality, and many studies are flawed; the conclusions of a well-designed and conducted observational study may be more reliable than those of a flawed randomized controlled trial;
- many important questions cannot be answered by randomized controlled trials (e.g. questions related to values, ethics, and the experiences of patients, and to the natural history of disease processes); and
- even for appropriate questions, a randomized controlled trial may be impractical and other methods may be more feasible or affordable.

In fact, the value of evidence lies more in its importance, validity and applicability to one's own patients or environment than in the type of study that generated it.

Table 72.1 Challenges particular to research in cardiothoracic critical care

The medical and humanitarian requirements of very sick patients must be balanced with those of research protocols.
Informed consent may be difficult to obtain from temporarily or permanently incapacitated patients.
Differences between samples (study patients) and populations may limit the applicability of results.
Large numbers are needed for outcome studies because of relatively low mortality rates.
Funding may be relatively difficult to obtain (from industry or other sources) because absolute numbers of patients are relatively small.
Standardized inclusion criteria may be difficult to meet in a variable patient population.
Surgery and anaesthesia, as well as management in the critical care unit, may influence results.

Generalizing research findings

To what extent can one apply the findings of a study to one's own unit? In general, conclusions apply to a population to the degree that the sample studied represents that population. Random sampling, matching of cases with controls, multivariate analysis and propensity analysis are aimed at ensuring that data from a sample applies to a population. The definition of populations is critical. If the sample comes from one unit, then the population is the patients of that unit (and perhaps only those treated over the period of the study). Results may not apply to other populations (e.g. patients at other times, in other units and particularly in units in other systems or countries). The conclusions of a large, international multicentre observational study may be more widely applicable than those of a single-centre randomized controlled trial. Research to confirm or expand the findings of others is often valuable. If similar findings emerge from several centres, then they may well apply widely.

Table 72.2 Hierarchical categories of evidence

Ia	Evidence from meta-analysis of randomized controlled trials
Ib	Evidence from at least one randomized controlled trial
IIa	Evidence from at least one controlled study without randomization
III	Evidence from nonexperimental descriptive studies, such as comparative studies, correlation studies and case-control studies
IV	Evidence from expert committee reports or opinions and/or clinical experience of respected authorities

Overview

The beginner in research is strongly advised to obtain supervision, usually from a more experienced colleague. It is helpful to use other people's published studies as models. The advice of a statistician should be obtained early, because the design of a study strongly influences the applicability for statistical analysis.

Some important concepts

Research may be theoretical or empirical. *Empirical research* involves observations and measurements of the real world; good research expands theoretical knowledge. An in-depth understanding of the theory underlying questions is critical to obtaining meaningful answers. Data can be *quantitative* (involving numbers or measurements) or *qualitative* (without numbers or measurements).

QUANTITATIVE RESEARCH

Quantitative research tends to be deductive (it starts with a question) and is hypothesis driven. It often involves the study of individuals in a sample taken from a population. Variables are typically measured (e.g. weight) and statistics estimated (e.g. the sample

Table 72.3 Examples of common deficiencies in clinical trials

Inadequate review of the literature in relation to the study
Inadequate formulation of hypothesis and/or specification of primary outcome variable
Inadequate blinding
Inadequate size and/or lack of power analysis
Incorrect statistical analyses
Inadequate discussion of limitations
Conclusions that are not sustained by the data
Claims in the abstract that differ from those in the body of the paper
Ghost or guest authorship
Publication bias (positive results are more likely to be published than negative results)
Fraud (data that has simply been fabricated or misrepresented)

mean). Parameters are inferred (e.g. the population mean) from these statistics. Commonly reported statistics are the standard deviation and the standard error. The *standard deviation* of a sample is an estimate of the standard deviation of the population, and characterizes the distribution of the parameter of interest. The *standard error* (obtained by dividing the standard deviation by the square root of *n*, the sample size) is a measure of the accuracy of the statistic as an estimate of the parameter.

QUALITATIVE RESEARCH

Qualitative research involves phenomenology (describing the world as we or our patients experience it) and the understanding of meaning. Qualitative research is often inductive (it begins with observation) and may be hypothesis generating. Qualitative research is grounded in theoretical

Table 72.4 Check list for evaluating the quality of a clinical trial (following Huwiler-Muntener and the CONSORT Statement)

Does the title identify the study as a randomized controlled trial?
Is the abstract presented in a structured format?
Are the objectives stated?
Is the hypothesis stated?
Is the study population described?
Are inclusion and exclusion criteria described?
Are the interventions described?
Are the outcome measures described?
Is the primary outcome specified?
Is a minimum important difference for the primary outcome reported?
Are power calculations described?
Is the statistical analysis described and explained?
Are stopping rules described?
Are the methods of randomization, allocation concealment and blinding described?
Are the numbers of eligible, randomized, treated and analysed patients reported?
Are withdrawals and dropouts described for each comparison group?
Are protocol deviations described for each comparison group?
Is the estimated effect of the intervention on primary and secondary outcomes stated, including a point estimate and measure of precision (confidence interval)?
Are the results stated in absolute numbers?
Are summary data and inferential statistics presented in sufficient detail to permit alternative analyses and replication?

constructs with sociological connotations. It is usually context oriented; the interest is more in understanding local situations, defined groups, or even individuals than in seeking universally applicable truths. For example, the way a patient may feel about an issue (such as a religious belief or the relevance of informed consent) may be very different when having an arthroscopy than from when he or she is in a critical care unit and desperately ill. Critical care lends itself to qualitative research because of the number of value judgments that must be made. It is often worth including qualitative questions in quantitative work, for example, by asking about the meaning of the data collected. Triangulation is the process of looking at questions from different angles, or by different methods, to gain more comprehensive answers.

Reviews of the literature

Research is about adding to the existing body of knowledge. It is a waste of resources and unethical to expose patients to the risks and inconvenience of research on a question that has already been answered. In a systematic review the method of selecting studies for inclusion is explicitly described; in a narrative review, it is not. In the former, the aim (as with any research) is to reduce bias and improve repeatability. A highly formalized methodology for systematic reviews has been defined by the Cochrane Collaboration. A systematic review usually includes:

- Defining the question to be answered.
- Defining and executing a search strategy using MedLine, PubMed or similar databases.
- Defining inclusion criteria (e.g. randomized controlled trial with >100 patients in each group published in English).
- Searching for additional references in each publication identified.
- Extending the search by consulting colleagues and identified experts, examining books of conference abstracts, and asking companies about unpublished studies.
- Optionally, specifying the weight given to different studies (and why).
- If appropriate, undertaking a meta-analysis of the data.

Meta-analysis is a statistical technique for amalgamating the results from several different studies and is not an essential part of a systematic review; it is fraught with difficulty and expert advice should be sought.

The randomized clinical trial

The randomized clinical trial is a powerful tool for answering certain types of question. Randomized allocation of subjects between groups tends to neutralize the influences of natural history, placebo and bias, but does not eliminate them. Ideally, trials should also be blinded. *Single blinding* involves subjects; *double blinding* extends to those conducting the trial; *triple blinding* includes those analysing the data as well (the potential for bias in this late stage of research is often underrecognized). A randomized clinical trial provides probabilistic answers, with an estimate of the likelihood that these are not due to chance alone. The probability (stated as a level of significance, or P value) of the answer being correct is often close to 0.05, which implies a 1:20 chance of its being wrong (known as a *type I error*, the chance of accepting an effect when there is none). Sometimes the result is negative. In this case, the chances of an error (known as a *type II error*, the chance of rejecting an effect when one is present) is typically 1:5 (or 20%). These estimates depend on the proper design and execution of the randomized clinical trial; flaws in these may totally negate the conclusions.

Writing a research protocol

Research projects begin with a protocol. Some important steps are discussed.

Reviewing the state of knowledge

Research starts with an in-depth understanding of the constructs in question. Discuss your idea with experts to facilitate progress and avoid wasting time and making obvious mistakes. Then, undertake a systematic review of relevant literature.

Formulating the research question and endpoints

Define the question you intend to answer and how you are going to answer it. An accurate, testable primary hypothesis and a primary outcome variable with which to test it are essential for deductive research. Secondary endpoints should be meaningful, and should usually add to one's understanding of the question to be studied.

Definition of the population and the sample

The value of a study is profoundly influenced by the sampling strategy. For example, including a random selection of all critical care units in the United Kingdom would provide results applicable to the entire country. It may be appropriate to impose some restrictions to the sample, such as limiting it to cardiac units.

Sample size estimation, methods of allocation and statistics

Sample size estimation defines the limits of what may be interpreted from a study. In general, the number of subjects needed depends on how much variation is likely in the primary outcome variable, on how large or small a difference one wishes to demonstrate and on the level of risk one is prepared to take that the answer will be wrong. The method of allocation of patients between interventions and control treatments must be explicit. If randomization is used, this should ideally be done formally by someone independent of the study. Statistical methods should be explicitly described.

Safety

Most clinical trials are too small to permit the conclusion that an intervention is safe, but evidence that it is not might well emerge. Safety must be addressed, and safety related endpoints defined. A Data Safety Monitoring Committee to review the results at defined intervals may be appropriate.

Ethics committee

Prior approval from the applicable ethics committee is usually mandatory for research involving patients. Few journals accept papers in the absence of ethics committee approval or an explicit waiver of the necessity for this.

Informed consent

Informed consent is required for research involving patients. Ideally, consent should be expressly given by the participants themselves, after the provision of appropriate information and explanations, time to reflect and the opportunity to ask questions or discuss the proposed project. This requires the capacity to assimilate information, understand it and make a decision. Patients in cardiac critical care units may be unable to do this for one or more of the following reasons.

- They are too sick.
- They have a neurological disability.
- They are anaesthetized.

In cardiothoracic critical care, it is often possible to recruit patients to studies before surgery, at a time when they are competent to give consent. However, patients should have the right to withdraw from research at any time, and this may be impractical. It may be possible for patients to delegate the discretion to withdraw to a third party, such as a close family member. For certain trials, particularly those involving treatment strategies for uncommon complications (e.g. dialysis dosing for acute renal failure, ventilatory strategies for treating respiratory failure) it may be not be feasible to obtain consent

Table 72.5 Types of informed consent

Types of informed consent
Express
Tacit
Deferred
Surrogates Substituted judgment standard Pure autonomy standard Best interests standard

preoperatively, because it is difficult to predict who will develop the complication. Obtaining prior consent from all patients might be one way around this, but tends to be impractical. A number of alternative approaches have been developed for obtaining consent, notably surrogate consent, in which informed consent is obtained from someone other than the patient (e.g. next of kin). In any situation of ethical compromise, it is important to minimize the extent of that compromise. For example, if surrogate consent is used, it would seem appropriate to supplement this with (so-called) deferred consent as soon as possible.

Compliance

The number of local, national and international requirements in relation to research is increasing. Failure to comply with these may have serious consequences for the study (e.g. that the data cannot be published) and for the investigator (e.g. in the form of law suits, disciplinary actions, and damage to reputation).

Contracts

Funded research often involves a contract with a company or a funding agency. It is prudent to obtain advice before signing such contracts. The principle investigator (at least) should have unrestricted access to all data. It is usually unethical to carry out clinical research under a contract that allows the sponsor to ban publication if the results turn

Table 72.6 Points to consider in relation to compliance obligations in a clinical study

Points to consider
Good clinical practice guidelines
Ethics committee approval and written, informed consent from all participants
In some countries, consultation with minority groups who might be involved with the study
Agreement with host institution
Agreement with sponsor, whether a funding agency or company
Reporting to ethics committee, funding organizations and patients at the end of the study
Retention of data (typically 10 or 15 years)
Adequate security for document storage
Privacy and confidentiality ensured for all aspects for the research
Study registration with an appropriate agency

out to be commercially unattractive. Allowing time for sponsors to file patents, and giving sponsors the opportunity to comment on any intended publication is reasonable.

Registration

The protocol must be registered in one of the international research registry before initiation of the study.

Writing the paper

Choosing a journal is important. Ideally, one would like the most impact from one's publication, but a reasonable chance of acceptance is also relevant. Follow your chosen journal's guidelines for authors.

Abstract

This is the part of the paper that will be read by most people. It must agree with the body of the paper in all respects – nothing new is permissible, and certainly nothing different. Give as much space as possible to the results, and cite actual data where possible.

Introduction

This should be short. Explain the context of the research. Then give a summary of what is known on the subject, and what is not. This should lead logically to a clear statement of the objectives of the study.

Methods

Explain precisely what has been done, in sufficient detail for another researcher to repeat the study. It is often helpful to use subsections, such as Ethics, Participants, Measures, Procedures, Statistical Analysis and so on.

Results

Give enough detail to allow the reader to verify that your data support your conclusion. Give actual values (means, standard deviations, frequencies) as well as significance levels – it is from the former, far more than from significance levels, that clinicians can interpret the clinical relevance of research.

Discussion

Focus on the study. This is not the place for an extensive literature review. State your key findings. Set these in context by reference to previous research. Make your contribution to the advancement of knowledge clear. Outline the limitations and weaknesses of the study. Indicate possible directions for future work. Draw conclusions, which should be clear, balanced, and justified by your data.

Key points

- Research is difficult, with many pitfalls and risks to patients and researchers. For the inexperienced, supervision is mandatory.
- The research question should determine the methods chosen in research.
- Theory is fundamental to research – extensive reading, discussion and thought should always precede the collection of data.
- Pay close attention to ethical issues, and to the need for compliance with regulations and contracts.
- Systematic reviews and the development of practice guidelines are useful and important forms of research, and are an ideal starting point for the tyro.

FURTHER READING

Begg C, Cho M, Eastwood S, *et al.* Improving the quality of reporting of randomized controlled trials. The CONSORT statement. *JAMA* 1996;276:637–639.

Huwiler-Muntener K, Juni P, Junker C, *et al.* Quality of reporting of randomized trials as a measure of methodologic quality. *JAMA* 2002;287:2801–2804.

Mays N, Pope C. *Qualitative research in health care.* London: BMJ Publishing Group; 2000.

Merry AF, Davies JM, Maltby JR. Qualitative research in health care. *Br J Anaesth* 2000;84: 552–555.

Myles PS, Gin T. *Statistical methods for anaesthesia and intensive care.* London: Butterworth Heinemann; 2000.

Sackett DL, Rosenberg WM, Gray JA, *et al.* Evidence based medicine: what it is and what it isn't. *BMJ* 1996;312:71–72.

Appendix

Works Cited

Carson JL, Hill S, Carless P, *et al*. Transfusion triggers: A systematic review of the literature. *Transfus Med Rev* 2002:16:187–199.

Comprehensive critical care: A review of critical care services. London: Department of Health; 2000.

Griffiths R, Jones C. *Intensive care after care*. New York: Elsevier Science.

Hogue CW, Murphy SF, Schechtmas KB, *et al*. Risk factors for early or delayed stroke after cardiac surgery. *Circulation* 1999;100:642–647.

Ivanov J, Borger MA, Rao V, *et al*. The Toronto Risk Score for adverse events following cardiac surgery. *Can J Cardiol* 2006;22: 221–227.

Lassnigg A, Hiesmeyer MJ, Bauer P, *et al*. Effect of centre-, patient- and procedure-related factors in intensive care resource utilization after cardiac surgery. *Intensive Care Med* 2002;28:1453–1461.

Runciman B, Merry A, Walton M. *Safety and ethics in healthcare: Getting it right*. Aldershot: Ashgate; 2007.

Salmeron J, Rodes J. *Oxford textbook of clinical hepatology*, 2nd ed., vol 2. Oxford: Oxford Medical Publications; 1999. pp 2023–2027.

Thistlethwaite PA, Mo M, Madani MM, *et al*. Operative classification of thromboembolic disease outcome after pulmonary endarterectomy. *J Thorac Cardiovasc Surg* 2002;124:1203–1211.

Index